Veterinary Nursing
of Exotic Pets

SECOND EDITION

Moulton College
SNVSA

Veterinary Nursing of Exotic Pets

SECOND EDITION

Simon J. Girling

DZooMed DipECZM CBiol FSB EurProBiol MRCVS, Royal College of Veterinary Surgeons Recognised Specialist in Zoo and Wildlife Medicine, European Veterinary Specialist in Zoological Medicine (Zoo Health Management)

WILEY-BLACKWELL

A John Wiley & Sons, Ltd., Publication

This edition first published 2013 © 2003 by Blackwell Publishing, Ltd, 2013 by John Wiley & Sons, Ltd

Wiley-Blackwell is an imprint of John Wiley & Sons, formed by the merger of Wiley's global Scientific, Technical and Medical business with Blackwell Publishing.

Registered office: John Wiley & Sons, Ltd, The Atrium, Southern Gate, Chichester, West Sussex, PO19 8SQ, UK

Editorial offices: 9600 Garsington Road, Oxford, OX4 2DQ, UK
The Atrium, Southern Gate, Chichester, West Sussex, PO19 8SQ, UK 2121 State Avenue, Ames, Iowa 50014-8300, USA

For details of our global editorial offices, for customer services and for information about how to apply for permission to reuse the copyright material in this book please see our website at www.wiley.com/wiley-blackwell.

Library of Congress Cataloging-in-Publication Data
ISBN: 9780470659175
Girling, Simon.
  Veterinary nursing of exotic pets / Mr Simon J Girling BVMS (Hons) DZooMed DipECZM(Zoo Health Management) CBiol MSB MRCVS. – 2nd edition.
     pages cm
  Includes bibliographical references and index.
  ISBN 978-0-470-65917-5 (pbk. : alk. paper) 1. Exotic animals–Diseases–Nursing. 2. Veterinary nursing. 3. Pets–Diseases–Nursing. I. Title.
  SF997.5.E95G57 2013
  636.089'073–dc23

2012028349

A catalogue record for this book is available from the British Library.

Wiley also publishes its books in a variety of electronic formats. Some content that appears in print may not be available in electronic books.

Cover image: © Simon J. Girling
Cover design by Meaden Creative

Set in 9/12 Minion Pro by Aptara Inc., New Delhi, India
Printed and bound in Malaysia by Vivar Printing Sdn Bhd

1 2013

Contents

Preface

Since the first edition of this textbook was published, exotic pet medicine has continued to develop at pace. More and more of the pet-owning public are turning to exotic pets whether it be due to their increased availability, physical attraction or the constraints of space making smaller pets more appealing. Veterinary nurses are now expected to understand the basics of diseases, husbandry, anatomy, and physiology of exotic pets as outlined by the RCVS examinations. Also as the veterinary nurse is often the practice–client interface, a sound knowledge base in these species is essential.

Many courses have developed over the last 12 years to support this increased need in training and this textbook acts as a companion to the City and Guilds NVQ level-4 equivalent qualification 'Veterinary Nursing of Exotic Species'. This qualification is now in its 12th year and has seen over 500 veterinary nurses qualify and is now recognised as the industry standard for veterinary nurses wishing to train in this area in the UK. This year (2012), the course has been taken back in-house by Girling and Fraser Ltd. Training and Consultancy making it available to a wider audience (see www.girlingandfraser.co.uk).

This revised and enlarged second edition of 'Veterinary Nursing of Exotic Pets' hopes to further educate and inform future generations of veterinary nurses, technicians and veterinary students in one of the most fascinating of subdisciplines of veterinary medicine.

Simon J. Girling

Part I Small Mammals

Chapter 1 Basic Small Mammal Anatomy and Physiology

Classification of small mammals

The commonly seen species of small mammals in veterinary practice are classified in Table 1.1.

RABBIT
Biological average values for the domestic rabbit

Table 1.2 gives the biological parameters for domestic rabbits.

Musculoskeletal system

The skeletal system of rabbits is light. As a percentage of body weight, the rabbit's skeleton is 7–8%, whereas the domestic cat's skeleton is 12–13%. This makes rabbits prone to fractures, especially of the spine and the hindlimbs.

Skull

The mandible is narrower than the maxilla, and the temporomandibular joint has a wide surface area, allowing lateral movement of the mandible in relation to the maxilla.

Axial skeleton

The cervical vertebrae are box-like and small and give mobility. The thoracic vertebrae possess attachments to the 12 paired ribs, which are flattened in comparison to cat's ribs. The pelvis is narrow and positioned vertically. The iliac wings meet the ischium and pubis at the acetabulum, where an accessory bone unique to rabbits, called the *os acetabuli*, lies. The pubis forms the floor of the pelvis and borders the obturator foramen which is oval in rabbits.

Appendicular skeleton

The scapula is slender and distally has a hooked suprahamate process projecting caudally from the hamate process. The scapula articulates with the humerus which in turn articulates with the radius and ulna. In rabbits, the ulna fuses to the radius in older animals and the two bones are deeply bowed. The radius and ulna articulate with the carpal bones which in turn articulate with the metacarpals and the five digits.

The femur is flatter than a cat ventrodorsally, and the tibia and fibula are fused in the rabbit. The tibia articulates distally with the tarsal bones where there is a prominent calcaneus bone. The tarsals articulate with the metatarsals which articulate with the four hindlimb digits.

The hindlimbs are well muscled and powerful.

Respiratory anatomy
Upper respiratory tract

Rabbits, like horses, are nasal breathers, with the nasopharynx permanently locked around the epiglottis; hence, upper respiratory disease or evidence of mouth breathing is problematic. The nasolacrimal ducts open onto the rostral floor of the nasal passage. The epiglottis is not visible easily from the oral cavity, making direct intubation difficult. It is narrow and elongated and leads into the larynx which has limited vocal fold development. The larynx leads into the trachea which has incomplete C-shaped cartilage rings for support.

Lower respiratory tract

The trachea bifurcates into two primary bronchi. There are two lungs, which are relatively small in proportion to the overall rabbit's body size. This means that even minor lung disease may cause serious problems. Each lung has three lobes, with the cranial ones being the smallest (see Figure 1.1).

Respiratory physiology

The impetus for inspiration derives from the muscular contraction and flattening of the diaphragm. The lung parenchyma possesses a cellular population that is well

Veterinary Nursing of Exotic Pets, Second Edition. Edited by Simon J. Girling. © 2013 John Wiley & Sons, Ltd. Published 2013 by John Wiley & Sons, Ltd.

Table 1.1 Classification of commonly seen small mammals.

Order	Lago-morpha	Rodentia						Sciuro-morpha	Carnivora	Didelphimorphia	Diprotodontia
Sub-order		Myomorpha		Hystricomorpha					Caniformia		
Family	Lepori-dae	Muridae	Cricetidae	Caviidae	Chinchilli-dae	Octodon-tidae	Sciuridae	Musteli-dae		Didelphidae	Petauridae
Species	Domestic rabbit (*Oryctolagus cuniculus*)	Rat (*Rattus norvegicus*) Mouse (*Mus musculus*)	Gerbil (*Meriones unguiculatus*) Syrian hamster (*Mesocricetus auratus*) Russian hamster (*Phodopus sungorus*) Chinese hamster (*Cricetulus griseus*)	Guinea pig (*Cavia porcellus*)	Chinchilla (*Chinchilla laniger*)	Degu (*Octodon degus*)	Siberian chipmunk (*Eutamias sibiricus*) Eastern chipmunk (*Tamias striatus*)	Domestic ferret (*Mustela putorius furo*)		Virginia opossum (*Didelphis virginiana*)	Sugar glider (*Petaurus breviceps*)

Table 1.2 Biological parameters for the domestic rabbit.

Biological parameter	Domestic rabbit
Weight (kg)	1.5 (Netherland dwarf) to 10 (New Zealand whites and Belgian hares)
Rectal body temperature (°C)	38.5–40
Respiratory rate at rest (breaths per minute)	30–60
Heart rate at rest (beats per minute)	130 (New Zealand whites) to 325 (Netherland dwarf)
Gestation length (days)	29–35 (average 31)
Litter size	4–10
Age at sexual maturity (months) Male Female	5–8 4–7
Lifespan (years)	6–10

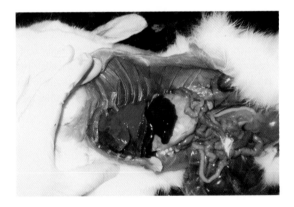

Figure 1.1 Lateral post-mortem view of a rabbit with the chest and abdominal walls removed. The structures from left to right (cranial to caudal) are the dark red heart, bright red lungs (three lobes), darker brown diaphragm and liver, pale cream stomach, yellow brown small intestines (the dark brown large intestines and caecum are reflected ventrally) and yellow-coloured urinary bladder. The left kidney may be seen dorsally as a dark brown structure in the mid-abdomen tucked under a fold of skin. (Fraser and Girling, 2009)

supplied with anaphylactic mediating chemicals. These are strong enough to cause fluid extravasation and blood pooling as well as spasms within the walls of the main pulmonary arterial supply, leading to rapid right-sided heart failure.

Digestive system

Oral cavity

The dental formula is

$$I\ 2/1\ C\ 0/0\ Pm\ 3/2\ M\ 3/3.$$

The teeth are elodont ('open rooted'), allowing continual growth throughout the rabbit's life. The molar enamel is folded providing an uneven occlusal surface with the ipsilateral jaw which allows interlocking. Wear is kept even by the lateral movement of the mandible, allowing independent left and right arcades to engage in mastication. The incisors differentiate Lagomorpha from Rodentia as rabbits and hares have two smaller incisors, or 'peg teeth', behind the upper two, whereas rodents have only two upper incisors. The larger incisors only have enamel on the labial surface, whereas the smaller maxillary peg teeth have enamel on the labial and lingual sides. This creates a wedge-shaped bite-plane where the lower incisors close immediately behind the upper large incisors and fit into a groove made by the peg teeth. The permanent incisors are present at birth, although the peg teeth are replaced by permanent peg teeth at around the second week of life. The deciduous premolars present at birth are replaced and joined by permanent molars by the fourth week of life. There are no canines; instead, there is a gap, or diastema, between the incisors and premolars (Figure 1.2).

Stomach

The stomach is a large, simple structure, with a strong cardiac sphincter (see Figure 1.1). This makes vomiting in the rabbit virtually impossible. There is a main body, or fundus, and a pyloric section with a well-formed pyloric sphincter. The lining of the stomach wall contains acid-secreting and separate pepsinogen-secreting cells. The pH of the rabbit's stomach contents is surprisingly lower than a cat's or dog's at 1.5–1.8. In addition, a healthy rabbit's stomach never truly empties.

Small intestine

The total length of the small intestine in the average rabbit may be some 2–3 feet! It is difficult to determine the divisions between duodenum, jejunum and ileum as they all have a similar diameter.

Caecum and large intestinal anatomy

At the junction of the ileum and caecum lies the *sacculus rotundus*. This is a swelling of the gut, infiltrated with lymphoid tissue and a common site for foreign body impactions. The caecum is large, sacculated and spiral-shaped, finishing in a blind-ended, thickened, finger-like projection known as the vermiform appendix, which also contains lymphoid tissue. The bulk of the caecum is thin walled and possesses a semi-fluid digestive content.

The start of the large intestine is the *ampulla coli* which sits near to the *sacculus rotundus* and caecum. It is a smooth-walled portion of the gut with some lymphoid infiltration of its walls, unlike the rest of the large intestine. It is also distinguished by having bands of fibrous tissue (known as *taeniae*) which create sacculations (also known as *haustra*). At the end of the proximal colon, the taeniae and haustra cease, and the gut is then known as the *fusus coli*, its walls becoming thickened and smooth because of the presence of large members of nerve ganglia which act as pacemakers for contraction waves in the large bowel. The distal descending colon continues through the pelvis to empty through the rectum and anus. There are a couple of anal glands just inside the anus, one on either side, emptying their secretions onto the faecal pellets.

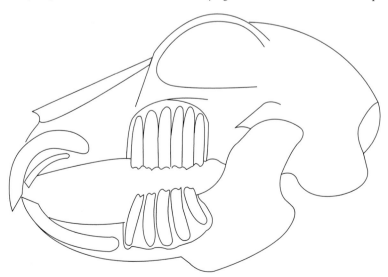

Figure 1.2 Lateral diagram of a normal rabbit skull showing the relation of tooth roots to the orbit and jawbones. Note peg-teeth incisors behind main incisors in maxilla.

Large intestinal physiology

Two types of faecal pellets are produced by the rabbit. One is a true faecal pellet, comprising waste material in a dry, light brown spherical form. The other is a much darker, mucus-covered pellet known as a caecotroph. The caecotroph is eaten directly from the anus, as soon as it is produced, which in the wild is during the middle of the day when the rabbit is underground. In captivity, they are often produced overnight, but may be produced at any time. The caecotroph contains plant material from which all of the nutrients have yet to be extracted.

The large bowel can produce two types of pellets due to the contraction waves in the large intestine and caecum. The proximal colon can separate out food as the haustra or sacculations of the colon hold on to the smaller particles. The larger particles become pushed towards the colon lumen. The haustra then push the small particles towards the caecum by contracting, and the segmental contractions of the colon itself propel the larger particles towards the rectum producing a waste pellet. When caecotrophs are produced, the haustra dramatically reduce their contractions, and instead the segmental activity drives material from the caecum through the distal colon where they are covered in mucus and then eaten directly from the anus. The caecum is thus the powerhouse filled with microbes which turn the ingesta into volatile fatty acids (VFAs) which can either nourish the caecal epithelium (butyrates) or be absorbed and converted to glucose by the liver (acetates). A high-fibre diet is important to maintain the balance of VFAs which should be made of predominantly acetates followed by butyrates and then propionates. Decreases in fibre levels increase butyrates and propionates at the expense of acetates, which results in reduction in the normal peristalsis of the gut and leads to hypomotility disorders and ileus or gut stasis.

Liver

The rabbit liver has four lobes. There is a gall bladder, which has an opening separate from the pancreatic duct into the proximal duodenum. The main bile pigment is biliverdin, rather than bilirubin seen in cats and dogs.

Pancreas

The pancreas is a diffuse organ, suspended in the loop of the duodenum. There is one single pancreatic duct, separate from the bile duct, emptying into the proximal duodenum.

Urinary anatomy

Kidney

The kidneys are bean shaped. The right kidney is more cranial than the left, and they are often separated from the ventral lumbar spine by large fat deposits. A single ureter arises from each kidney and traverses across the abdominal cavity to empty into the urinary bladder.

Bladder

The bladder lining is composed of transitional cell epithelium. The urethra in the male rabbit exits through the pelvis and out through the penis. In females, the urethra opens onto the floor of the vagina.

Renal physiology

Rabbit's urine is alkaline with a pH varying between 6.5 and 8, but it will become acidic if the rabbit has been anorectic for 24 hours or more. The urine contains varying amounts of calcium carbonate. This is because it has no ability to alter how much calcium is absorbed from the gut, and so any excess calcium must be excreted by the kidneys into the urine. This can be seen as a tan-coloured silt. Porphyrin pigments may also be seen in rabbit's urine. These are plant pigments and make the urine appear anywhere from a dark yellow to a deep wine-red in colour. This may mimic haematuria; therefore, to diagnose blood in the urine, it is necessary to examine it microscopically.

Cardiovascular system

Heart

The rabbit heart is small in relation to body size. The right atrioventricular valve has only two cusps instead of three. The pulmonary artery also has a large amount of smooth muscle in its wall which can contract vigorously during anaphylactic shock, causing immediate right-sided cardiac overload and failure.

Blood vessels for sampling

Vascular access in rabbits includes

Lateral ear vein

This runs along the lateral margin of either ear. It may be accessed using a 25 or 27 gauge needle or catheter and used for slow intravenous injections and blood sampling.

Cephalic vein

This runs in a similar position to that seen in cats and dogs. It may be split into two in some individuals, but may be used for intravenous fluids and sampling (Figure 1.3).

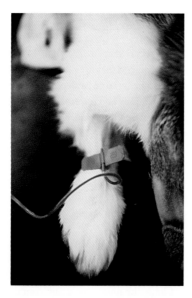

Figure 1.3 Cephalic vein access in a rabbit using a pre-heparinised butterfly catheter.

Saphenous vein

This runs across the lateral aspect of the hock, as in cats and dogs, and may also be used for venipuncture.

Jugular vein

The jugular veins are prominent in the rabbit but they form the major part of the drainage of blood from the orbit of the eye. If a haematoma or thrombus forms and blocks the lumen of a jugular vein, severe orbital oedema may occur, with possible damaging effects.

Lymphatic system

Spleen

The spleen is a flattened structure, oblong in nature and attached to the greater curvature of the stomach, and is thus found predominantly on the left side.

Thymus

The thymus is a large structure in the cranial thoracic compartment even in the adult rabbit. It provides the body with the T-cell lymphocytes.

Lymph nodes

The root of the mesentery supporting the digestive tract is well supplied with lymph nodes, as is the hilar area of the lungs where the two main bronchi diverge to supply each lung. In addition, there are superficial lymph nodes in the popliteal, prescapular and submandibular areas.

Reproductive anatomy

Male

The paired testes can move from an inguinal position within the thin-skinned scrotal sacs, to an intra-abdominal position through the open inguinal canal (see Figure 1.4). The scrotal sacs are sparsely haired and lie on either side of the anogenital area.

The accessory sex glands in the buck attached to the urethra in the caudal abdomen are: dorsal and smaller ventral prostate; bilobed vesicular gland; bilobed coagulating gland and a bilobed bulbourethral gland. The prepuce has numerous small preputial glands in the dermis, and there are a couple of inguinal glands situated on either side of the penis which secrete a brown-coloured sebum clearly seen adjacent to the anus.

Female

The ovaries are supported by the ovarian ligament and lie caudal to each respective kidney. The ovarian artery often splits into two parts after leaving the aorta, and it, along with the rest of the reproductive tract, is frequently encased in large amounts of fat.

The uterus is duplex – there is no common uterine body. Instead there are two separate uteri with separate cervices emptying into the vagina. The vagina is large and thin walled, with the urethra opening onto its floor cranial to the pelvis. The vulva therefore is a common opening for the reproductive and urinary systems unlike many rodents. It lies just cranial to the anus and is flanked on either side by the inguinal glands, as with the buck.

The doe has on average four pairs of mammary glands extending from the inguinal region to the axillary areas.

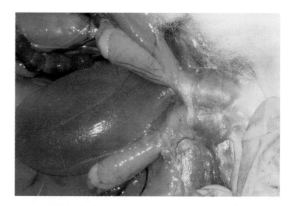

Figure 1.4 Close-up of the caudal abdomen of a male rabbit showing the retracted testes and the inguinal canals and the full urinary bladder. (Fraser and Girling, 2009)

Reproductive physiology

Male

The buck rabbit has the same sexual hormones as in cats and dogs, but they are on a seasonal time clock triggered by the lengthening daylight of spring. This is mediated through the pineal gland in the brain which has neural links from the eyes and controls the hormone melatonin. It in turn controls the pituitary release of follicle-stimulating and luteinising hormones which then act upon the testes.

Female

Does are induced ovulators. Waves of follicles swell and regress during the course of the season, starting to increase in activity in early spring. If not mated, these follicles will often dominate the cycle for 12–16 days at a time. There is no real anoestrus phase in does; instead, a slight waning in activity for 1–2 days occurs before a return to heat. During peak sexual activity, the vulva is often deeply congested and almost purple in colour and considerably enlarged.

Once mated, the male's semen may form a copulatory plug, which is a gelatinous accumulation of sperm which drops out of the doe's vagina 4–6 hours post-mating. Gestation lasts from 29 to 35 days, with the foetus forming a haemochorial placenta (where the outer chorion layer of the foetal placental membrane burrows into the lining of the uterus so that it directly attaches to the blood in the intrauterine vessels) at about day 13. This is a common time for abortions to occur. A pregnant doe will remove fur from her ventrum to line the nest in the latter few days prior to parturition.

Dystocia is uncommon. The doe only nurses the kittens once a day for 20 minutes or so, often in the early morning. It is therefore not uncommon for owners to think that the doe is neglecting her young as she will often spend the rest of the time eating and away from the litter.

Pseudopregnancy often occurs after an unsuccessful mating or mounting activity by another buck or doe. A *corpus luteum* forms and this lasts for 15–17 days during which time the doe may produce milk and build a nest. At this time, the doe is susceptible to mastitis.

Neonatology

The young kits or kittens are altricial in nature, that is they are totally dependent on the mother for nutrition and survival for the first few weeks of life. They are born blind, deaf and furless. Fur growth appears around day 5–6, the eyes open at day 8–10 and the ears at 11–12. Weaning occurs around 6 weeks of age, with the young taking solid food from 2 to 3 weeks.

Sexing

The young may be sexed from 4 to 5 weeks of age. Gentle pressure is placed on either side of the reproductive or anal area to protrude the vulva or penis. The vulva of the young doe is rounded and has a central slit in midline and projects cranially. The penis of the young buck is more conical and pointed, with no central slit and tends to project caudally when protruded. Once the buck is older, the testes descend into the scrotum.

Skin

Lop breeds, particularly does, have extra skin folds called 'dewlaps' around the ventral neck region. In addition, such extra folds of skin may be found around the anogenital area, leading to increased risk of urine and faecal soiling.

Rabbits do not have keratinised footpads. Instead they have thick fur covering the areas of the toes and metatarsals which are pressed flat to the ground.

In addition to the para-anal scent glands mentioned above, there are a series of discrete submandibular chin glands. These are used to mark territory and also, in the case of does, to mark their young to distinguish them from others.

The rabbit has no skin sweat glands except a few along the margins of the lips. This means that they are very prone to heat stress at temperatures greater than 28°C.

The presence of many vibrissae or sensitive hairs around the lips and chin are important since rabbits cannot see anything immediately below their mouths, and so rely on touch to manipulate food towards the mouth.

Eyes

Rabbits have prominent eyes, which allow a near 360° field of vision. There is a prominent third eyelid, which moves from the medial canthus of the eye and possesses a large amount of reactive lymphoid tissue within its structure and a Harderian tear gland at its base. This is often enlarged in the buck during the breeding season and possesses two lobes in both the sexes.

Haematology

The most notable feature is the staining of the rabbit neutrophil, which resembles the cat or dog eosinophil, and so is often known as the pseudoeosinophil. Many rabbits have more lymphocytes than pseudoeosinophils, resembling other mammals such as cattle, rather than cats and dogs, in which the neutrophil is the commonest white blood cell.

RAT AND MOUSE

Biological average values for the rat and mouse

The normal biological values for the rat and mouse are given in Table 1.3.

Musculoskeletal system

Skull

The skull of both species is elongated. The eyes are laterally situated, and there is a long snout and a shallow cranium. The maxilla is narrower than the mandible. The temporomandibular joint is elongated craniocaudally, allowing the mandible to move rostrally and caudally in relation to the maxilla. This allows the incisors to be engaged for gnawing, while the molars are disengaged. Alternatively, the molars may be engaged for mastication prior to swallowing, while the incisors are disengaged. The two procedures cannot occur at the same time. The rostral symphysis, joining each half of the mandible, is also articulated allowing movement of each hemimandible independently of the other.

Table 1.3 Biological parameters for the rat and mouse.

Biological parameter	Average range rat	Average range mouse
Weight (g)	400–1000	25–50
Rectal body temperature (°C)	37.6–38.6	37–38
Respiration rate at rest (breaths per minute)	60–140	100–280
Heart rate at rest (beats per minute)	250–450	500–600
Gestation length (days)	20–22	19–21
Litter size	6–16	8–12
Age sexual maturity (weeks)		
Male	8	6
Female	10	7
Oestrus interval (days)	4–5	4–5
Lifespan (years)	3–4	2–3

Axial skeleton

The pelvis of the female mouse is joined at the pubis and ischial areas midline by fibrous tissue. This allows separation of the pelvis during parturition in the mouse. There are no fibrous areas to the pelvis of the female rat and consequently no pelvic separation occurs.

Appendicular skeleton

The scapula articulates at its coracoid process with the clavicles as well as the humerus. There are four metacarpal bones in the rat, with four digits. Occasionally the vestigial remnant of digit 1 is present.

The hindlimbs have a strong laterally bowed fibula in both species. The tibia articulates with five metatarsal bones at the hock joint. Consequently there are five digits in the hindlimbs of these species. Rats and mice are plantigrade in their stance, that is they walk with the whole of the metatarsal bone area flat to the ground.

Male rats may still have open growth plates in many of their long bones well into the second year of their lives, whereas mice close their growth plates in the first 3–4 months of life.

Respiratory system

The nares of both species are prominent and surrounded by an area of hairless skin containing some sweat glands.

There is a vomeronasal organ in the floor of the nasal passages, accessed via two small stoma in the roof of the mouth just caudal to the maxillary incisors. This organ is responsible for detecting pheromones secreted by other individuals.

The right lung of the rat is divided into three distinct lobes, whereas the left lung is undivided. The chest cavity itself is smaller in proportion to the abdominal cavity than is the case in cats and dogs, meaning that rats and mice have little respiratory reserve.

Digestive system

Oral cavity

The lips of mice, and particularly rats, are deeply divided exposing the upper incisors, with large areas of loose folds of skin forming the cheeks.

Both species have pigmented yellow – orange enamel coating the labial aspect of the incisors. The maxillary incisors are one-third to one-quarter of the length of the mandibular incisors. There is a chisel shape to their occlusal surfaces due to the absence of enamel on the lingual aspect of the incisors making them wear quicker on this side. The mandibular incisors are also mobile and loosely rooted in the lower jaw. Their dental formula is

I 1/1 C 0/0 Pm 0/0 M 3/3.

There is no evidence of any deciduous or 'milk' teeth being present in either species. The molars grow extremely slowly.

Both species have a diastema. In the case of rats, this gap is particularly noticeable and large enough to allow them to draw their cheeks into the gap to effectively close off the back of the mouth. This enables them to gnaw, without consuming the material they are nibbling.

The tongue is relatively mobile and its surface is covered with small, backward-pointing papillae.

Stomach

The stomach of the mouse and rat is elongated and narrow. In the rat, in particular, the stomach is divided into two regions. The most cranial is known as the proventricular region and is covered by a thin, whitened lining of aglandular mucosa. The oesophagus enters the stomach halfway along the length of its lesser curvature. The caudal area of the stomach is covered by a redder, thicker, glandular mucosa known as the pyloric region.

Small intestine

The small intestine comprises the largest portion of the gastrointestinal tract. The bile duct enters the first part of the duodenum direct from the liver in the rat, which has no gall bladder. The mouse does have a gall bladder which empties into the first part of the duodenum.

Large intestine

The ileum enters the large intestine at the junction of the caecum and the large intestine on the left side of the abdomen. The caecum is a medium-sized organ in the mouse and rat, reflecting their omnivorous nature, and forms a blind-ended pouch which is flexed back on itself.

Liver

The liver is divided in both species into four lobes. There is a gall bladder present in the mouse but not in the rat. The liver sits cranial to the stomach. Biliverdin is the prominent bile pigment in rats and mice.

Pancreas

The pancreas lies along the proximal aspect of the duodenal loop. In both species, it empties through a series of ducts into the bile duct. Its function appears to be the same as in cats and dogs, producing both insulin and glucagon for glucose homeostasis and the digestive enzymes – amylase, lipase and trypsinogen.

Urinary system

Kidney

The kidneys are bean shaped. The right kidney sits in a depression in the right lobe of the liver, and the left kidney is slightly more caudal. Each empties through its ureter which enters the bladder at the trigone area.

Bladder

The bladder is lined with transitional epithelium and empties through the urethra. In the female mouse and rat, the urethra empties through a separate urinary papilla rather than onto the floor of the vagina as it does with higher mammals. The female mouse and rat therefore have three orifices caudoventrally: the anus most caudally, the reproductive tract entrance next cranially and the urinary papilla the most cranial of the three.

Cardiovascular system

Heart

The heart of the mouse and rat has four chambers, as in other mammals. As with rabbits, the chest compartment is relatively small in comparison to the abdomen, and the heart therefore appears relatively large in relation to the rest of the chest. The heart occupies the fourth to sixth rib spaces.

Blood vessels for sampling

Useful vessels from which to sample blood are the lateral tail veins. These are best accessed after first warming the tail, or lightly sedating the mouse or rat to allow dilation of the vessels. A 25–27 gauge needle or butterfly catheter is required. Some mild pressure at the tail base allows further dilation.

In the rat, the femoral vein may also be used for sampling. This is found on the medial aspect of the thigh, close to its junction with the inguinal area, just caudal to the femur. This vessel is best used only under anaesthetic due to the difficulty of accessing it in a conscious rat.

For small capillary samples, a microcapillary tube may be gently pushed into the medial canthus of the eye socket in the anaesthetised rat or mouse. This collects blood from the orbital sinus.

Lymphatic system

Spleen

The spleen of male mice is often twice the size of that in females. In both species, it is a strap-like organ sitting along the greater curvature of the stomach.

Thymus

The thymus is an obvious organ in the cranial chest, and may be split into several smaller islands of tissue. It is frequently present in the adult rat or mouse.

Lymph nodes

The lymph nodes follow similar patterns to those seen in the rabbit. The mesenteric lymph nodes can become very prominent in certain bacterial infections.

Reproductive anatomy

Male

The male rat and mouse reproductive systems are nearly identical in design.

The testes are large and can move between the abdomen and the scrotal sacs, although somewhat inhibited by a large fat body attached to the tail of each testicle extending through the open inguinal canal. Each testis descends into the scrotum around the fifth week of age in the rat and the third to fourth week in the mouse.

The *vasa deferentia* are joined by the opening of the small ampullary glands which open into a swelling of the vas deferens known as the ampulla just before they join the urethra. Other accessory sex glands, the vesicular glands, the coagulating glands (which are joined together) and the two parts of the prostate (the ventral and dorsal lobes), open into the urethra itself. As the urethra exits the pelvic canal, a paired bulbourethral gland empties into its lumen.

These accessory glands produce nutrients and supporting fluids for the spermatozoa. In addition, the coagulating glands are responsible for allowing a plug of sperm to form in the female's vagina immediately after mating. The penis has an os penis in both species. There is a preputial gland in the small prepuce, which is used for territorial marking. Male mice and rats have no nipples.

Female

The rat uterus has two separate uterine horns which come together at two separate cervices. From the outside these appear to merge to form a common uterine body, and so it is referred to as bicornuate in nature. The vagina itself has no lumen in the immature rat.

Instead, at puberty, the solid mass of tissue forms its own lumen, breaking through to the surface at the time of the first ovulation.

The mouse uterus is almost exactly the same except that the two separate uterine horns do fuse just before the cervix, making it truly bicornuate and so there is just the one cervical opening into the vagina. The vagina is also non-patent in the immature state.

Mammary tissue is extensive in both female rats and mice. In mice there are normally five pairs of mammary glands, three in the axillary region, with mammary tissue extending dorsally nearly to midline! The other two pairs of glands are in the inguinal region, with mammary tissue extending around the anus and tail base. In rats there are more commonly six pairs of mammary glands. Three are located in the axillary region, again with some tissue moving onto the lateral chest wall. The other three glands are inguinally located.

Reproductive physiology

The female rat is non-seasonally polyoestrus. The commonest time for heat to occur is during the night. The first cycling activity occurs around 8 weeks of age in the female rat, with the cycle lasting 4–5 days in total. Ovulation is spontaneous and occurs towards the end of the 12-hour-long heat. There is a reduction in reproductive activity in the female rat over 18 months of age.

During mating, the semen deposited in the female rat's vagina forms a copulatory plug which sits in the cranial vagina, blocking both cervices. This dries and falls out within a few hours of mating, but seems to play an important role in the success of mating. It is often eaten rapidly after being passed.

Gestation length is around 21 days. The placentation of the rat and mouse is discoidal, that is the area of attachment is disc-like with the chorion of the placenta in contact with the blood stream of the dam's uterus. There may be a bloody mucous discharge from the vagina around 14 days, which is normal. This stops within 2–3 days. Mammary development occurs at around days 12–14 and at that stage the foetuses may be palpated.

Parturition is rarely complicated. There is no separation of the pelvis in the female rat, although the female mouse's pelvis does separate at the ischial and pubic sutures. Parturition occurs in the afternoon and is followed by a post-partum oestrus.

Pseudopregnancy is seen in both rats and mice. During this time the female may build a nest; there may be some mammary development and no signs of a heat for up to 2 weeks.

There are a couple of important physiological reproductive phenomena in mice and rats. One of these is the Whitten effect. This is when a group of anoestrus females will all come into heat spontaneously some 72 hours after being exposed to the pheromones of a male. This has beneficial effects when it comes to successful rapid breeding. The other is the Bruce effect. This is when a female in the early stages of gestation will reabsorb the embryos and come back into heat when presented with a new male. By preferentially allowing successful mating with a new male, this is thought to have a beneficial effect on genetic diversity.

Neonatology

Rat and mouse pups are altricial. They are born blind, deaf and hairless. The ear canals open around days 4–5 and the eyes at around 2 weeks of age. The first few hairs are also seen in the first week of life. The pups are born without teeth, the incisors becoming visible at 1–2 weeks of age with the molars developing later.

The female rat and mouse are prone to cannibalism if disturbed with their young in the first few weeks after parturition. It is therefore important to leave the female rat and mouse alone during this period, only disturbing them to replenish food and clear the worst of any cage soiling.

Sexing

Sexing may be done from 4 to 6 weeks of age. In males the urinary papilla is slightly larger than the female and further away from the anus. It may be possible in the sexually mature female to see the small reproductive tract entrance as a transverse slit in between the anus and urinary papilla. Also, in male mice and rats, no nipples are visible. In mature males, if the rat or mouse is gently suspended in a vertical position with the head uppermost, the testes will often descend into the scrotal sacs and are then obvious.

Skin

Rats and mice possess no generalised sweat glands and so are prone to heat stress at temperatures above 26–28°C. There are some sweat glands present on the soles of the feet as well as the nares.

There is a layer of brown fat between the shoulder blades dorsally; its function is not clearly known, but it decreases with age and may play a role in thermoregulation.

The tails of rats and mice are relatively hairless. As rats age, there is an increasing number of coarse skin scales present on the tail surface making blood sampling difficult. Rats should not be grasped by the tip of the tail as the skin may slough in this region.

White fur will often yellow in rats as they age, and most rats will show evidence of a yellow hue to the skin on the back with time.

The vibrissae around the lips and nose are important for detecting vibrations and determining where food is due to their inability, as with rabbits, to see food immediately below their mouths.

Eyes

Rats and mice have a prominent set of small eyes located laterally. The albino breeds lack pigment in their irises or retinas, and so their eyes appear pink red.

Haematology

The haematological parameters are similar to those seen in cats or dogs, except that the lymphocyte, as opposed to the neutrophil, is the most common white blood cell.

GERBIL AND HAMSTER
Biological average values for the gerbil and hamster

Table 1.4 gives the average normal values for the basic biological values for gerbils and hamsters.

Musculoskeletal system
Skull

The skull of the gerbil is not dissimilar to that of the rat or mouse; in the hamster, the skull is shortened, particularly in the Russian and Chinese hamster subspecies.

Axial skeleton

The axial skeleton is much the same as for the rat and mouse, except the hamster has much fewer coccygeal vertebrae (only seven or so).

Appendicular skeleton

Gerbils have a longer femur and tibial length, giving them longer hindlimbs equipped for jumping. Their normal stance is bipedal, standing erect on their hindlimbs. Hamsters are a much shorter-legged creature, stockier in build and walk predominantly on all fours.

The forelimbs have four digits, and the hindlimbs have five in both species.

Table 1.4 Biological parameters for the gerbil and hamster.

Biological parameter	Russian hamster	Syrian hamster	Gerbil
Weight (g)	30–60	90–150 (male larger)	70–120 (male larger)
Rectal body temperature (°C)	36–38	36.2–37.5	37.5–39
Respiration rate at rest (breaths per minute)	60–80	40–70	80–150
Heart rate at rest (beats per minute)	300–460	250–400	250–400
Gestation (days)	Average 16 (Chinese hamster 21)	15–18	24–26 (up to 42 days with delayed implantation)
Litter size	4–8	4–12	2–6
Age at sexual maturity (weeks) Male Female	5–6 6–8 (Chinese hamster 14)	6–8 8–12	8–9 9–10
Oestrus interval (days)	3–4	4	4–6
Lifespan (months)	18–24	24–36	36–60

Respiratory system

As with rats and mice, the chest cavity is small in relation to the abdomen, but the situation is not so pronounced as that seen in rats.

Digestive system

Oral cavity

The incisors in both species are continuously erupting (open rooted), and both species have orange pigmentation of the enamel surfaces. The dental formula is

I 1/1 C 0/0 Pm 0/0 M 3/3.

Hamsters are born with the incisors fully erupted, and use them to grasp the nipples of the female enabling them to suck effectively.

The molars do grow continually, but at a very slow rate. In addition, there appears to be no evidence of deciduous teeth. Both species possess a diastema. The mandible is generally wider than the maxilla.

The cheek pouches of the hamster are its most distinguishing feature. These are not present at birth, but rather develop during the second week of life from a solid cord of cells which disintegrate, creating the cavities. The entrances to the cheek pouches open into the diastema. Each cheek pouch extends caudal to the respective ear. They are lined with stratified squamous epithelium, and have a reduced local immune system and lymphatic function. This can be a problem if the cheek pouch becomes infected.

Stomach

The stomach of the hamster has two separate areas. The oesophagus enters the proximal portion. This portion is non-glandular and has a bacterial population that allows limited microbial breakdown of food. It is sharply divided by a deep groove from the distal area of the stomach, which is glandular, with a redder lining composed of the acid- and pepsinogen-secreting cells that start the process of enzymatic digestion.

The gerbil has two areas to the stomach but they are less clearly demarcated, and the proximal portion does not support a significant microbial population.

Small intestine

The hamster's small intestine is extremely long, being three to four times its own body length! The gerbil has a similar layout to the mouse.

Large intestine

In the hamster the caecum is a sacculated and enlarged organ sitting in the ventral left portion of the abdomen at the ileocaecal junction. It has fine divisions within it, which may function to increase its surface area and aid fibre fermentation. The gerbil has a similar layout to the mouse.

Liver

The liver in both species is divided into four lobes. In both hamsters and gerbils, a gall bladder is present. A bile duct empties into the duodenum accompanied by the pancreatic duct.

Pancreas

The pancreas is found adjacent to the descending duodenum. It has a similar structure and function to that seen in the rat and mouse.

Urinary system

Kidney

The kidneys are similar to the rat and mouse kidney. The gerbil is very good at concentrating its urine, being a desert-dwelling species, and to do this it has very long loops of Henle which contain a countercurrent multiplier system. In the hamster, the renal papilla is particularly long and protrudes from each kidney into its ureter.

Bladder

The bladder of gerbils and hamsters is essentially the same as that seen in rats and mice.

Cardiovascular system

Heart

The heart is similar in form to the rat and mouse heart.

Blood vessels for sampling

The hamster has very few accessible external vessels for blood sampling. This is principally due to its much reduced tail length, which provides the main vascular access in the rat and mouse. The gerbil's tail breaks off easily, making its use for blood sampling very restricted. Vessels used therefore include the jugular veins and the femoral veins, both of which require the hamster or gerbil to be sedated or anaesthetised. Capillary samples may be taken from the orbital sinus as described in the rat and mouse.

Lymphatic system

Spleen

The structure and position of the spleen is much the same for both species as that seen in the rat.

Thymus

The thymus is again a prominent organ in the cranial chest and often persists in the adult. It provides the T-cell lymphocytes.

Lymph nodes

The presence of lymphatic tissue is the same as that seen in the mouse and rat.

Reproductive anatomy

Male

The male hamster has a smaller fat body attached to the testicle than has the rat. The testes are freely moveable between the abdominal cavity and the scrotal sacs. A small os penis is present in the penile structure.

The male gerbil is similar to the male rat and mouse. The main difference is the slightly smaller size of the testes in relation to the overall body size and the presence of a pigmented scrotum.

Female

The hamster uterus is bicornuate. It has two separate cervices opening into a common vagina, although the uterine horns appear to join externally to produce a common uterine body. The vagina is, as with the rat, not patent at birth. It opens after the tenth day of life, rather than at puberty as in the rat.

The gerbil reproductive tract is similar to that of the mouse. The main difference is that, while there is only one cervical opening into the vagina, the division between the left and right uterine lumens persists to within a few millimetres of this single cervical orifice.

The female hamster has six to seven pairs of mammary glands stretching in a continuous band from the axillary region to the inguinal and perianal region.

The female gerbil has four pairs of mammary glands. Two pairs are found in the axillary region and two pairs in the inguinal region.

Reproductive physiology

The female hamster is seasonally polyoestrus with cycling and fertility dropping off during the winter period. The reproductive cycle is short, lasting 4 days. The female hamster develops a creamy white vaginal discharge around the first day following oestrus. This may be mistaken for a pathological discharge as it has an odour. Ovulation is spontaneous and generally occurs overnight. Phantom pregnancy does occur in the hamster, postponing oestrus for 7–13 days. Gestation itself lasts for 15–18 days in the Syrian hamster, an average of 21 days in the Chinese hamster and an average of 16 days in the Russian hamster. Successful mating is followed by the presence of a copulatory plug of coagulated semen 24 hours later. Pregnancy can be confirmed by failure to produce the copious white discharge 5 days after mating, and an increase in weight at around day 10. There is no evidence of pelvic separation at parturition. There is reduced fertility in the female hamster after 1 year of life.

Gerbils form a monogamous pair, that is they pair for life. The female gerbil is seasonally polyoestrus and a spontaneous ovulator. The oestrus cycle lasts for 4–6 days. Oestrus lasts for 24 hours, and may occur within 14–20 hours of parturition. Gestation lasts an average of 26 days, but may take up to 42 days if mating has occurred at the post-partum heat as when the female is still feeding the young, the fertilised ova will not implant, so prolonging the interval from mating to parturition.

Neonatology

The young hamster is altricial. The pale pink colour of the skin is replaced by some darker pigmentation after the first 2–3 days, with the eyes opening at 2 weeks of age. Weaning occurs around 3–4 weeks of age, with the female hamster becoming sexually mature at 6–8 weeks (up to 14 weeks for the Chinese hamster) and the male at 8–9 weeks.

The young gerbil is also altricial. The skin is a pale pink at birth but darkens by the end of the first week with the appearance of the first few hairs. The teeth erupt in the first few days of life. The eyes open at 2 weeks of age and the ears around days 4–5. Weaning occurs at 3–4 weeks of age. The female gerbil becomes sexually mature at 9–10 weeks of age when the vaginal opening becomes patent. The male gerbil becomes sexually mature at 8–9 weeks of age, with the testes descending into the scrotal sac at 5 weeks.

It is inadvisable to disturb the female hamster with her young as cannibalism can occur. However, a common protective action of the female is to place the young into her cheek pouches to move them, and this may make it look as if she is 'eating' the young. Gerbils are less prone to abandoning or abusing their young if disturbed.

Sexing

This may be performed from 4 weeks of age. In the immature gerbil and hamster, the differences are determined by anogenital distances as with the rat and mouse. In the sexually mature hamster, the male has a pointed outline to its rear, owing to the descended testes, whereas the female has a more rounded appearance. In both, it is relatively easy to determine the sex once mature if the individual is supported in a vertical position with the head uppermost. In this position, the testes will descend into the scrotal sacs where they are clearly visible!

Skin

Hamster and gerbil skin has no sweat glands. Gerbils, however, can tolerate wider temperature ranges, up to 29–30°C, although if the humidity levels increase above 50% they will rapidly suffer from heat exhaustion.

In hamsters, there is a pair of oval, raised, flank scent glands situated on each flank cranial to the thigh region. In the mature adult, particularly the male, they may become darkly pigmented. The secretions of these glands may matt the sparsely covered fur, increasing their prominence.

In gerbils, there is a large ventral sebaceous scent gland in the region of the umbilical scar. This is devoid of fur, secretes a yellow sebaceous fluid and is more prominent in males. This is a predilection site for the development of adenocarcinoma in adults. The tail of gerbils is fully furred, but has a series of fracture planes allowing a degloving injury if a gerbil is grasped by the tail. The soft tissue structure never regrows, and the denuded vertebrae will die off leaving a stump.

Haematology

The lifespan of the gerbil erythrocyte is short, lasting only 10 days. This is why so many gerbil red cells show degenerative basophilic speckling when stained with Romanowsky stains. Gerbil blood is often lipaemic, and this has been blamed on their high-fat (sunflower seed) diet. In addition, the blood parameters vary depending on the sex. The male gerbil has a higher packed cell volume, white blood cell and lymphocyte count than the female. Hamster haematology is similar to that seen in mice.

GUINEA PIG AND CHINCHILLA
Biological average values for the guinea pig and chinchilla

The average normal values for guinea pigs and chinchillas are given in Table 1.5.

Musculoskeletal system
Guinea pig
Skull

The skull is rodent shaped, with an elongated nose, low forehead and widely spaced eyes. There are moderately large tympanic bullae which house the middle ear and are clearly visible on radiographs.

Axial skeleton

The vertebral structure is the same as that seen in the rat and mouse, except the number of coccygeal vertebrae is much reduced at 4–6 and they are less mobile. There are 13 ribs; the last two are more cartilaginous than mineralised. Guinea pigs also possess clavicles.

Table 1.5 Biological parameters for the guinea pig and chinchilla.

Biological parameter	Guinea pig	Chinchilla
Weight (g)	600–1200	400–550
Rectal body temperature (°C)	37.2–39.5	37.8–39.2
Respiration rate at rest (breaths per minute)	60–140	50–60
Heart rate at rest (beats per minute)	100–180	120–160
Gestation length (days)	59–72 (average 63)	111
Litter size	1–6 (average 3)	1–5 (average 2)
Age at sexual maturity (months) Male Female	2–3 1.5–2	6–7 8–9
Oestrus interval (days)	16	30–50
Lifespan (years)	3–8	6–10

The pelvis of the female is joined at the pubis and ischium by a fibrocartilaginous suture line, allowing separation of the pelvis prior to and during parturition. If the female guinea pig has not had a litter by the time she has reached 1 year of age, this suture line mineralises and prevents future separation. Female guinea pigs not mated before 1 year should therefore not be mated for the rest of their life as dystocia problems are common.

Appendicular skeleton
The forelimbs and hindlimbs are relatively long in comparison to the rat and mouse, but the same bone formulas exist. The main difference is that the guinea pig has four digits on each forelimb and only three digits on each hindlimb.

Chinchilla
Skull
The bones of the skull are more domed than the guinea pig, although still distinctly rodent-like (Figure 1.5). Like the guinea pig, the chinchilla has very large tympanic bullae which are clearly visible as coiled, snail-shell-like features on radiographs.

Axial skeleton
The vertebral structure is similar to that seen in the rat and mouse. Chinchillas are fine-boned and prone to fractures.

Appendicular skeleton
The hindlimbs in particular have very long femurs and tibias. The chinchilla has the usual four digits on each forelimb, but, unlike the guinea pig, has four digits on each hindlimb as well.

Respiratory system
The lung structure of the guinea pig is similar to that seen in the rat and mouse. The left lung is divided into three lobes, and the right into four. Chinchillas follow a similar pattern.

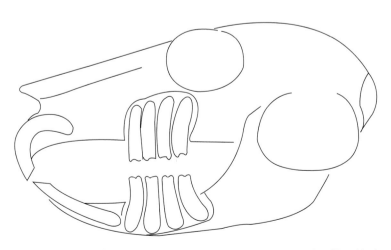

Figure 1.5 Lateral diagram of the skull of a normal chinchilla showing the relation of tooth roots to the orbit and jawbones. Note how close the roots of the third and fourth cheek teeth are to the inner aspect of the eye; hence, root elongation often causes watering of the eyes.

Digestive system
Oral cavity

The dental formula for both chinchillas and guinea pigs is

$$I\ 1/1\ C\ 0/0\ Pm\ 1/1\ M\ 3/3.$$

In both species, all of the teeth, incisors, premolars and molars, are elodont ('open rooted') and therefore continuously growing. This can lead to malocclusion, particularly in chinchillas, if an inappropriately non-fibrous diet is fed. The incisors of the chinchilla are orange yellow pigmented on their enamel surfaces, but those of the guinea pig are often white. In both cases, a diastema is present.

Both species also have a palatal ostium creating an entrance through the soft palate, allowing communication of the oropharynx with the pharynx. It exists because the soft palate is actually connected with the base of the muscular tongue.

Stomach

The whole stomach of the guinea pig is covered with a glandular epithelium containing acid- and pepsinogen-secreting cells and is usually full of food material. It has a strong cardiac sphincter, making vomiting a rare and grave occurrence. The stomach of the chinchilla is much the same.

Small intestine

The small intestine of both species is relatively long and pink in colour, measuring anywhere up to 50–60 cm in the chinchilla and more than 120 cm in the adult guinea pig!

Large intestine

The large intestine starts at the ileocaecal junction on the left side of the abdomen where the ileum enters the caecum. The caecum is a large, sacculated organ, measuring 20 cm in length, and in the guinea pig it contains 60–70% of all the gut contents. It is attached to the dorsal abdomen and has a series of three smooth muscle bands running along its length known as *taeniae coli*. These produce the sacculations of the caecum known as *haustra*. In the chinchilla, the caecum is smaller, containing only 20–25% of gut contents, but it is more folded. The caecum itself forms a blind-ending sac at one end and empties into the colon near to the ileocaecal junction.

The colon is twice as long as the small intestine in both species and is dark brown. In the chinchilla, the proximal section of the colon possesses taeniae and haustra, whereas in the guinea pig the whole of the colon is smooth surfaced. The latter half of the colon in both species can be distinguished by the presence of faecal pellets in its lumen. The large intestine of the guinea pig has a complicated series of coils, which form a spiral of bowel on the right cranial ventral aspect of the abdomen. The chinchilla's colon is much more simply arranged, and not as long.

Liver

The liver of the guinea pig has six lobes. There is also an obvious gall bladder, unlike the rat. The gall bladder empties through one bile duct into the small intestine. The chinchilla's liver has a similar format.

Pancreas

The pancreas has two limbs in the guinea pig and lies alongside the stomach and proximal duodenum. It empties via one duct into the mid-descending duodenum and performs the same functions as in other mammals.

Urinary system
Kidney

As with the hamster, the guinea pig has a relatively long renal papilla. Both kidneys in the guinea pig are surrounded by large amounts of fat, making them difficult to see at laparotomy. The chinchilla's kidneys are not so covered in fat deposits.

Lower urinary tract

The urine of the guinea pig is often yellow and cloudy in nature. Like all herbivore urine, it is alkaline under normal conditions and may contain calcium carbonate or calcium oxalate crystals. In the female guinea pig, the urethra empties just caudal to the vagina, but without a urinary papilla, giving the false impression of a common urogenital opening.

In the female chinchilla, cloudy alkaline urine is common. The urethra of the bladder, however, opens through a separate orifice from the vagina. The urinary papilla is a large structure in the female chinchilla and may easily be confused with the male penis.

Cardiovascular system
Heart

In both species, the thoracic cavity appears relatively small in comparison with the abdominal cavity; therefore, the heart appears relatively large in comparison with the lung field.

Blood vessels for sampling

The jugular veins are the vessels commonly used for blood sampling. Small doses of intravenous medications may be administered through the ear veins which are clearly visible on the non-furred ears or via the cephalic or saphenous veins which occupy the same positions as in other species.

Lymphatic system
Spleen
The spleen of the guinea pig is a wide structure attached to the greater curvature of the stomach on the left side of the cranial abdomen.

The spleen of the chinchilla is a smaller strap-like organ attached again to the greater curvature of the stomach on the left side.

Thymus
In guinea pigs, the thymus is prominent in the cranial thorax in the immature stage, but there are often only remnants left in the adult. A similar situation exists in the chinchilla.

Lymph nodes
The guinea pig is prone to *Streptococcus zooepidemicus* infections of the cervical lymph nodes, which run in a chain along the ventral aspect of the neck. Both species have prominent mesenteric lymphoid deposits.

Reproductive anatomy
Male
Guinea pig
The male guinea pig is often referred to as a boar. Its testes are prominent and occupy the scrotal sacs on either side of the anus. Each testis has a large fat body projecting through the open inguinal canal into the abdomen. The vas deferens opens, with the accessory sex glands (the vesicular glands, the coagulating glands and the ventral and dorsal prostate lobes), into the proximal urethra. The vesicular glands are the most prominent, curving cranially into the abdomen for 10 cm or more. The paired bulbourethral glands lie dorsal to the urethra just before it passes into the penis, which is Z-shaped, moving cranioventrally from the caudal brim of the pelvis and then caudoventrally so to point caudally at rest. The penis is a large structure by rodent standards and possesses a glans structure distally. There is an *os penis* which sits dorsal to the urethra when the penis is erect and pointing cranially. Ventral to the distal urethra are two invaginated spurs, which, when the penis is erect, project from the end of the glans as two slender spurs 4–5 mm in length. Their function is not fully known but they may aid in locking into similar grooves in the female reproductive system. The whole penis is contained in a prepuce, which possesses sebaceous glands, and is partly formed from a fold of perineal skin.

Chinchilla
There is no true scrotum. The tail of the epididymis sits lateral to the anus, while the testis occupies an inguinal position. A fat body projects from each testis into the abdominal cavity. The vas deferens opens into the urethra caudal to the bladder neck along with the accessory sex glands. These include the ventral and dorsal paired lobes of the prostate as well as the paired, frond-like vesicular glands. The urethra then passes caudally through the pelvis, becoming ensheathed in the ischiocavernosus muscles that control the movement of the penis and pelvic floor. The bulbourethral glands lie dorsal to the urethra in this area. The urethra then passes out of the pelvis and into the penis, which is tubular and blunt ended and points caudally when relaxed. The penis forms a Z-like flexure, similar to the guinea pig, and contains an *os penis* in its most caudal portion.

Male chinchillas are often prone to fur rings. This is when a band of fine fur becomes wound around the penis inside the prepuce. This may constrict and so may cause ischaemic damage to the penis.

Female
Guinea pig
The female guinea pig is often referred to as a sow. Its uterus is bicornuate. It has two uterine horns, a short uterine body and a single cervix. The ovaries are closely associated with the respective kidneys. The periuterine tissues and cornuate ligaments are sites for the same fat deposition that is seen in the female rabbit. The vagina opens just cranial to the urethral opening. A small clitoris sits just ventral to the urethral opening, and the two are enclosed in skin folds to create a Y-shaped slit. The entrance to the vagina is sealed by epithelial tissues at all times other than at oestrus and immediately prior to parturition.

The female guinea pig has two mammary glands in the inguinal region (the male has two vestigial glands as well).

Chinchilla
The female chinchilla has a uterus like the rabbit. There are two uterine horns but no common uterine body. Instead two separate cervices open into the vagina. The entrance to the vagina is sealed at all times except

during oestrus and just prior to parturition. The urethra opens through a separate urinary papilla.

Reproductive physiology

Guinea pig

The female guinea pig is non-seasonally polyoestrus. The cycle lasts for around 16 days, oestrus lasting for 6–12 hours, and ovulation is spontaneous. Immediately after mating (1–2 hours), a copulatory plug may be found in the cage. It is possible that this is necessary to prevent leakage of sperm back out of the reproductive tract, but it could also prevent another male from successfully mating the female. Gestation lasts on average 63 days, although it may take up to 67 days for small litters and 59 days for large ones. The average litter contains three young. Pregnancy may be detected by gentle palpation from 3 weeks. The entrance to the vagina is closed at all times other than immediately before parturition, and for 2–3 days around oestrus. There is a post-partum heat within 10 hours of parturition at which the female may be successfully re-mated.

In the last 2 days of gestation, hormones, such as relaxin and progesterone, allow the pelvic ligaments to separate the pubis and ischium by up to 2 cm, allowing the passage of the relatively large young. This occurs only if the female is less than 1 year of age or has had her first litter before 1 year. Nulliparous females more than 1 year of age have a fused pelvis, and dystocias are therefore common. Many female guinea pigs will breed through to 2 years of age.

The guinea pig placenta is haemochorial. That is the membranes of the placenta (chorion) are in contact with the blood of the mother. This allows for large amounts of immune system exchange between mother and foetus during gestation.

Chinchilla

The chinchilla is seasonally polyoestrus. The reproductive season stretches from November to May, and the cycle lasts on average 40 days. The entrance to the vagina opens at oestrus, which lasts for 12–24 hours, and stays patent for 3–4 days. At this stage, the perineum may darken in colour, and clear mucus may be seen from the vaginal opening. It also opens 2–3 days prior to parturition and remains open for the commonly seen post-partum oestrus.

Chinchillas are spontaneous ovulators. A copulatory plug is frequently found the day after a successful mating. Gestation lasts on average 111 days, with typically two kits being born. Pregnancy may be diagnosed by palpation from day 60. Female chinchillas may continue to breed up to 10 years of age.

The chinchilla placenta is haemochorial.

Neonatology

Both guinea pigs and chinchillas are precocial, that is they are born fully furred, with eyes and ears open, and often start to eat small amounts of solid food from day 1. Weaning generally occurs at 6 weeks in guinea pigs and 6–8 weeks in chinchillas. Sexual maturity occurs from 2–3 months in the guinea pig to 6–8 months in the chinchilla.

Sexing

Guinea pig

Sexing of male and female guinea pigs is relatively simple and may be performed from the first few weeks of life. The female anogenital area is oval in nature. The anus is closest to the tail base, and cranial to this is a Y-shaped slit housing the small clitoris and the entrance to the urinary and genital tracts. In the male, the distance between the anus and urogenital system is larger, and gentle pressure on either side of the prepuce will allow protrusion of an obvious penis.

Chinchilla

The female chinchilla has a large urinary papilla making identification difficult. The identification is made on the distance between the anus and the urinary papilla. The female's urinary papilla is close to the anus, and if examined closely, it may be possible to observe the transverse slit which marks the sealed (when not in heat) entrance to the reproductive tract lying between the anus and urinary papilla. The male's prepuce, which resembles the female's urinary papilla, is much larger and more cranial, and the penis may be protruded in compliant individuals.

In chinchillas, females are larger than males – the reverse of many other rodents.

Skin

The guinea pig has a prominent sebaceous gland on its back, cranial to the tail base. This secretes a yellow waxy material which frequently matts the fur in this area. There are additional glands emptying into the anal sacs in the folds of skin which enclose the anus and genitalia. These can produce a creamy white, strong-smelling discharge in the boar. Guinea pig fur is often relatively coarse in nature.

Conversely, the coat of the chinchilla is renowned for its soft silky nature. It responds badly to moisture, requiring dust baths for cleaning. In addition, the chinchilla may experience a feature known as 'fur slip'. This is when a section of fur will drop out due to fright or stress. The alopecic area left may take several weeks to regrow its fur.

In both species, the ears are prominently furless, with the chinchilla in particular having the largest pinnae.

The guinea pig has a prominent subcutaneous fat pad over the scruff region of the neck, which makes large injections at this site painful.

The chinchilla has very small claws on each digit. In comparison, the guinea pig has prominent claws on every digit. Both have defined leathery pads at the ends of each digit.

Eyes

The eyes of the guinea pig are small in comparison to the size of their heads. There is a prominent third eyelid tear gland which may prolapse. The chinchilla on the other hand has large prominent eyes, and a vertical, slit-like pupil which allows the chinchilla to virtually close off all light reaching the retina. This is to protect it from bright sunshine in its wild habitat high in the Andes of South America.

Haematology

In both species, the morphology of the red and white cells is similar to that seen in other rodents. There are predominantly more lymphocytes than neutrophils in the white cell count. In the guinea pig, an intracellular inclusion known as the Kurloff body may be seen in circulating monocytes, which are known as 'Kurloff cells'. These are rare in juvenile and male guinea pigs, but common in adult females particularly during gestation, and they may play a role in the physiological immunity relationship between mother and foetus. Their origin is not clear but they are thought to come from the thymus or spleen.

CHIPMUNK
Biological average values for the chipmunk

The normal values for the basic biological parameters for the chipmunk are given in Table 1.6.

Musculoskeletal system

The musculoskeletal system has many similarities to the rat as outlined above.

Skull

The skull is typically rodent in its long and flattened form.

Table 1.6 Biological parameters for the chipmunk.

Biological parameter	Chipmunk
Weight (g)	55–150
Rectal body temperature (°C)	37.8–39.6 (when not hibernating)
Respiration rate at rest (breaths per minute)	60–90
Heart rate at rest (beats per minute)	150–280
Gestation (days)	28–35
Litter size	2–10 (average 4)
Age at sexual maturity (months) Male Female	8–9 9–12
Oestrus interval (days)	Average 14
Lifespan (years)	8–12 (may be shorter in captivity)

Axial skeleton

The spinal vertebral layout is the same as the rat.

Appendicular skeleton

Each forelimb has four and each hindlimb five digits. Their gait is a jumping sinuous movement, which makes them excellent climbers, with forelimbs and hindlimbs a similar length. Their bodies are more elongated than those of rats or mice, and their long, prehensile tail is used for balance and support. Their bone structure is lightweight and more bird-like than the heavier structure of the rat.

Respiratory system

The lungs are divided into three lobes on the left side and four on the right. Their thoracic cavity is larger in relation to the abdomen than is the case in many other rodents.

Digestive system
Oral cavity

The incisors are open rooted, or continuously growing, and malocclusions are not uncommon. The dental formula is

I 1/1 C 0/0 Pm 0/0 M 3/3.

They have a diastema. The mouth is narrow, the tongue fleshy and fixed firmly at the base, although the rostral tip is mobile. There are small cheek pouches, communicating with the diastema of the oral cavity and extending back to the ear base. These are frequently sites for abscess formation if sharp seeds, such as unhusked oats, are fed.

Stomach

The stomach is of a simple glandular design. There is a strong cardiac sphincter which normally prevents regurgitation.

Small intestine

The small intestine is relatively long. The duodenum receives a duct from the gall bladder just after the pyloric sphincter, and one further on from the pancreas.

Large intestine

The initial part of the large intestine at the ileocaecal junction has a small, blind-ending caecum with some sacculations, or *haustra*.

Liver

The liver has four main lobes and possesses a gall bladder and bile duct which join the descending duodenum.

Pancreas

The pancreas is found along the descending duodenum and the edge of the stomach. It empties through one duct which empties into the proximal descending duodenum.

Urinary system

Kidney

The kidneys are a typical bean shape. Fat deposits are often found in this area during the late summer and early autumn. Each kidney has the usual ureter passing caudally to the urinary bladder.

Bladder

Chipmunk urine is usually alkaline in nature and may contain calcium crystals. However, due to their more omnivorous nature (they eat insects, eggs, etc.), they may also produce acidic urine.

Cardiovascular system

Heart

The heart is similar to that seen in the rat and mouse.

Blood vessels for sampling

The jugular veins make the best vessels for blood sampling. The ventral tail vein may be used but care should be exercised and the chipmunk should be sedated as the tail skin can deglove and slough relatively easily.

Lymphatic system

Spleen

The spleen is a small, strap-like organ on the greater curvature of the stomach to the left side of the cranial abdomen.

Thymus

The thymus is a prominent organ in the juvenile, and persists in the cranial thorax of the adult.

Reproductive anatomy

Male

The testes sit in a caudally placed scrotum, but only during the reproductive season. During the quiescent period, the testes are retracted into the abdomen. The scrotum and testes thus enlarge during the breeding season from January to September.

Female

The female chipmunk has four pairs of mammary glands, two inguinal and two thoracic. Otherwise, the reproductive tract follows a pattern similar to that of the rat.

Reproductive physiology

The chipmunk is seasonally polyoestrus, cycling between March and September. Chipmunks are spontaneous ovulators, with an oestrus cycle length of around 14 days. There is no evidence of a post-partum oestrus, and gestation length averages 31–32 days. Mammary development becomes prominent 24–48 hours prior to parturition.

Reproductive success drops dramatically after 6–7 years of age in the female.

Neonatology

Chipmunk young are altricial and so are born blind, deaf and hairless. Fur starts to appear around 7–10 days of age, and the eyes open at 4 weeks. The age at weaning is 5–7 weeks. Sexual maturity is reached at 8 months in the male and 10 months in the female.

Sexing

The male chipmunk has a clearly visible penis which points caudally. During the breeding season, the scrotum is noticeably enlarged. The female has a urogenital papilla, but the distance from anus to papilla is less than the distance from anus to prepuce in the male.

Skin

Chipmunks have soft fur covering the whole of their bodies. Sebaceous glands exist around the anus in both sexes. They have five digits on their forepaws and four on the hind, which possess small pads and claws. The ears are small and furred.

PET MARSUPIALS

Biological average values for some pet marsupials

Table 1.7 gives the basic normal biological values for sugar gliders (*Petaurus breviceps*) and Virginia opossums (*Didelphis virginiana*) – two of the more commonly kept marsupial pets.

Sugar gliders may enter a stage of torpor when faced with starvation in an attempt to lower energy demands. Virginia opossums may sham death when attacked (the derivation of playing possum).

Musculoskeletal system

The sugar glider has five digits on front and rear limbs, but the second and third digits of the rear limbs are part fused together into a grooming comb. The first digit of the hindlimb is opposable.

The Virginia opossum has five digits, including opposable thumbs on both front and rear limbs. The majority of marsupials have no claw on the first digit of the hindlimbs.

Most marsupials have extra pubic bones that project cranially from the floor of the pelvis and are thought to help to support the pouch in females and abdominal muscles in both sexes. They are, however, absent in sugar gliders.

Both the sugar glider and the Virginia opossum have prehensile tails.

Respiratory system

The respiratory tract is similar to that of Eutherian mammals. Respiratory rates for the sugar glider are around 16–40 breaths per minute and for the Virginia opossum around 25–40 breaths per minute.

Digestive system

The sugar glider's dental formula is

$$I\ 3/1\ C\ 1/0\ Pm\ 3/4\ M\ 4/4.$$

The incisors are specialised to gouge the bark of acacia trees to release their sap.

The Virginia opossum's dental formula is

$$I\ 5/4\ C\ 1/1\ Pm\ 3/3\ M\ 4/4.$$

The sugar glider has an enlarged caecum which may help to digest its natural diet of acacia gum. Otherwise the digestive system of omnivorous marsupials is similar to that of many omnivorous rodents with the exception that marsupials have a cloaca, similar to that in a bird or reptile as a

Table 1.7 Biological parameters for the sugar glider and Virginia opossum.

Biological parameter	Sugar glider	Virginia opossum
Weight (g)		
Male	115–160	4000–5000
Female	95–135	2000–2500
Cloacal body temperature (°C)	34–35	32.2–35
Respiratory rate at rest (breaths per minute)	16–40	25–40
Heart rate at rest (breaths per minute)	200–300	70–100
Gestation length (days)	16	12–13
Litter size	1–2	8–20 embryonic young (average 13)
Age at sexual maturity (months)		
Male	12–14	6–8
Female	8–12	6–8
Oestrus cycle length (days)	29	28
Oestrus length (days)	1–2	1–2
Lifespan (years)	12–14	3–5

common opening for the urinary, reproductive and digestive systems. Most male marsupials have anal glands just inside this (females have pouch glands), but the Virginia opossum has cloacal glands in the female as well. In the Virginia opossum, the secretions of this gland are green.

Urinary system

The urinary tract is similar to that of Eutherian mammals, except the ureters pass medial to the reproductive tract instead of lateral.

Cardiovascular system

Heart

As marsupials have a heart rate around half that of a comparative sized Eutherian mammal, their heart size is around 30% heavier than a comparative sized Eutherian mammal's heart.

Blood vessels

In the sugar glider, the cephalic, lateral saphenous, femoral, ventral or lateral tail veins may be used to collect blood samples.

In the Virginia opossum, the cephalic, saphenous, ventral or lateral tail veins may be used to collect blood samples. In addition, the female has pouch veins which may be accessed under anaesthetic.

Endocrine system

Most marsupials are unable to thermoregulate when born. This ability develops around halfway through their time in the pouch and coincides with the development of the thyroid gland.

The adrenal glands of the female marsupial are around twice the size of the male's in milligrams per kilogram body weight. This difference increases during lactation due to development of the cortex of the adrenal gland (the 'X' zone), which is due to the production of a testosterone-like hormone.

Reproductive anatomy

Male

The reproductive system of the male is much more similar to that of Eutherian mammals than that of the female. The main differences in the male are external rather than internal and comprise a bifurcate penis which is posterior to the scrotum. When flaccid, the penis is held in an S-shaped curve withdrawn into the body and lies on the ventral cloacal floor. The scrotum is obvious and pendulous.

The testes have epididymides, and the vas deferens when it leaves the scrotum enters the body and joins the large disseminated prostatic gland and one or more pairs of bulbourethral glands (Cowper's glands). The duct of the bulbourethral gland enters the urethra on the ventral surface. Marsupial males lack seminal vesicles and coagulating glands.

Female

Female marsupials have a double reproductive system. Each side has from cranial to caudal: an ovary, an oviduct and a uterine body. The caudal half of the reproductive tract is composed of paired lateral and one median vaginal canals. All marsupials give birth through the central (median) vaginal canal. In some species, for example the brushtail possum, there is a septum that blocks the median canal and that is breached during birth, and which subsequently reforms; in others, for example the grey kangaroo, this median canal remains open permanently. Caudal to the three vaginal canals is the urogenital sinus that also contains the urethral opening on its ventral floor. This then empties into the cloaca.

The female sugar glider has a well-developed pouch during the breeding season and has an average of four nipples inside, although some may only have two.

The female Virginia opossum has a well-developed pouch in which 13 nipples are arranged in an open circle with one in the centre, although there may be some variation in this layout between individuals.

Reproductive physiology

Female sugar gliders are polyoestrus with a cycle averaging around 29 days. Females may produce two litters a year. In captivity there appears to be no specific breeding season. Gestation is on average 16 days.

Female Virginia opossums are polyoestrus with a cycle of around 28 days and are in full oestrus for 1–2 days. Generally the breeding season starts in December to January in the northern hemisphere with a second peak of breeding in the early spring with an average of 110 days separating the two litters. Gestation is on average 12–13 days

Females tend to have a post-partum oestrus during which breeding and fertilisation can occur, although if there are joeys in the pouch, the fertilised egg stops development and implantation until the young have been weaned or die. This is known as foetal diapause (similar to delayed implantation in some mammals – although the placenta of marsupials never actually implants during foetal development).

Neonatology

Marsupial milk changes in consistency during the period of development of the young. However, maternal immunoglobulins are absorbed across the neonate's gut right up until weaning. This makes up for the lack of placental transfer of immunity.

In all neonates, a strong shoulder girdle of cartilage (metacoracoid) exists at birth to aid their struggle to the pouch. This regresses once the journey is made and becomes the coracoid process of the scapula. The teat once in the neonate's mouth swells up, and the neonate becomes firmly attached.

The sugar glider in the wild lives in nests containing up to seven males and females and their young as an extended family. The young weigh around 0.19 grams at birth and usually two are born. They first detach from the nipple at around day 40 or life and first leave the pouch around day 70. They are reported to become weaned from day 111.

The Virginia opossum's young are very underdeveloped but have impressive claws which they use to climb from the mother's birth canal to the pouch. They are only 10 mm long when born and weigh on average 0.13 grams. Generally around 13 young are born but as many as 56 have been reported! As there are only around 13 mammary glands, more than 13 rarely survive. The young release their grip on the mammary glands around 50 days of age and will leave the pouch for short periods from day 70 onwards. They are completely weaned and independent of the mother around 3–4 months of age with sexual maturity occurring around 6–8 months.

Sexing

The female sugar glider has a well-developed pouch with usually four mammary glands. The male has an obvious pendulous scrotum.

The female Virginia opossum has an obvious pouch with around 13 mammary glands within. The male has a pendulous scrotum.

Skin

One of the most striking features of the sugar glider is the patagium which stretches from the fifth digit of the forelimb to the tarsus of the ipsilateral hindlimb. The sugar glider has multiple scent glands on the head (often creating a bald patch in males), the chest and in the paracloacal area. Smaller scent glands are found around the corners of the mouth, the paws and the inside of the ears. The female has scent glands inside her pouch which is located ventrally over the cranial abdomen and cranially facing. The fur is soft with no guard hairs and the tail is well furred.

In the Virginia opossum, the fur consists of a soft underfur with white-tipped guard hairs which are unique to the family Didelphidae. The first tenth of the tail is covered with fur and the rest is naked skin.

Haematology

Red and white cell morphologies are similar to that of Eutherian mammals.

FERRET

Biological average values for the domestic ferret

Table 1.8 gives the basic normal biological values for the domestic ferret.

Musculoskeletal system

Skull

The skull is more rodent-like, in that it is pointed and flattened dorsoventrally. The eyes are forward-facing, giving binocular vision for prey detection.

Axial skeleton

The vertebral formula for the ferret is similar to that of most mammals and comprises the usual 7 cervical vertebrae, with the extended 15 thoracic (occasionally 14), 5–7 lumbar, 3 sacral and, on average, 18 coccygeal vertebrae.

Table 1.8 Biological parameters for the domestic ferret.

Biological parameter	Domestic ferret
Weight (kg)	
Male	1–2
Female	0.5–1
Rectal body temperature (°C)	37.8–40
Respiration rate at rest (breaths per minute)	40–80
Heart rate at rest (beats per minute)	180–250
Gestation length (days)	41–42
Litter size	2–14 (average 8)
Age at sexual maturity (months)	
Male	4–6
Female	4–8 (spring following birth)
Lifespan (years)	5–10

Appendicular skeleton

The form is basically similar to that seen in the cat. The forelimbs and hindlimbs each have five digits.

Respiratory system

Ferret lungs are split into two lobes on the left side and four on the right. The entrance to the thoracic cavity is very small and is bounded by the first ribs.

Digestive system

Oral cavity

The ferret has a set of deciduous teeth, which appear at 3–4 weeks of age. These are replaced by permanent teeth at 7–11 weeks of age. The dental formula for the adult is

$$I\ 3/3\ C\ 1/1\ Pm\ 3/3\ M\ 1/2.$$

The deciduous formula for the ferret is

$$I\ 1/0\ C\ 1/1\ Pm\ 3/3.$$

The most prominent teeth are the canines, which are responsible for holding onto the prey. The molars and premolars are shearing teeth. The tongue is fleshy and mobile.

Stomach

The stomach is of a simple form, lined with glandular epithelium containing both acid- and pepsinogen-secreting cells. It has a weak cardiac sphincter, allowing easy vomition, and a pronounced pyloric sphincter. The stomach can dilate markedly when full.

Small intestine

The descending duodenum begins at the pylorus of the stomach and passes across to the right side of the abdomen. It is entered into, after the first 5 cm or so, by the common bile and pancreatic duct.

Large intestine

The large intestine is not easily differentiated from the small intestine since it is the same width and colour, although the mesenteric lymph node marks the junction between the two. There is no caecum in the ferret. The terminal portion of the rectum has two anal glands attached which, when emptied, can give off the very unpleasant odour associated with a frightened ferret! The removal of these glands is considered an unnecessary mutilation by the Royal College of Veterinary Surgeons in the UK and so should not be done unless there is a medical reason.

Liver

The liver is divided into six lobes. The right lobe has the usual renal fossa to accommodate the right kidney. A gall bladder is present and empties via a common duct with the pancreas.

Pancreas

The pancreas is a prominent organ, with two main lobes, one along the descending duodenum and the other along the pyloric axis. A single duct merges with the bile duct to provide a common entrance to the duodenum.

Urinary system

Kidney

The kidneys are the traditional kidney-bean shape. The right kidney sits more cranially, in a fossa in the right lobe of the liver. The left kidney is more caudal and freely suspended.

Bladder

The bladder is similar to that seen in cats or dogs. The urethra passes through the penis in the male ferret, which contains a J-shaped os penis. This makes urinary catheterisation of the male difficult.

Ferret urine is naturally acidic in nature due to its carnivorous diet.

Cardiovascular system

Heart

The heart occupies rib spaces 6–8. Its tip is connected to the sternum by a ligament which frequently contains fat, making the heart appear elevated off the sternal floor on radiographs.

Blood vessels for sampling

Blood vessels for sampling include the jugular, cephalic and saphenous veins. These are found in the same places as for the cat. The ferret also has an unusual series of arteries branching from the main aortic trunk. In cats and dogs, two separate carotid arteries arise from the aortic trunk. In the ferret, a single vessel (the brachiocephalic or innominate artery 1) leaves the aortic arch. This then divides into the left and right carotid arteries, as well as into the right subclavian artery at the thoracic inlet. This prevents restriction of blood flow to the head which could occur due to the narrow chest inlet.

Lymphatic system

Spleen

The spleen varies greatly in size between individuals, and it is attached to the greater curvature of the stomach on the left side. Its ventral tip may extend across the floor of the abdomen and back up to meet the right kidney.

Thymus

The thymus is a prominent organ in the cranial thorax of the young ferret. It dwindles to a few islands of tissue in the adult.

Lymph nodes

The lymph nodes are of a similar arrangement as seen in the cat. The most notable lymph node is the mesenteric node, which can be used to differentiate between small and large intestine.

Reproductive anatomy

Male

The male ferret is known as a hob. The testes are situated in a perineally located scrotum. They enlarge in the breeding season (March to September). There is no movement of the testes from scrotal sac to abdomen.

The prostate lies at the neck of the bladder and opens into the lumen of the urethra. The urethra passes caudally through the pelvis before bending ventrally and cranially to exit at the ventrally located prepuce. The *os penis* is J-shaped.

Female

The female ferret is known as a jill. The ovaries are found close to the caudal poles of the respective kidneys. The uterus is bicornuate and similar to that seen in the cat, with two long uterine horns and a short uterine body. There is a single cervix opening into the vagina. The urethra opens into the floor of the vagina, so there is a common urogenital opening at the vulva, cranial to the anus.

Reproductive physiology

The female ferret is seasonally polyoestrus and an induced ovulator. Ovulation occurs 1–2 days after mating. The breeding season runs from March to September. Oestrus is demonstrated by the obviously swollen vulva, which returns to normal 2–3 weeks after a successful mating.

Gestation lasts on average 42 days. The placenta is zonary, similar to that seen in cats and dogs.

The most important point about the female ferret's reproductive cycle is that if she is not mated, or brought out of heat in some way, the persistent exposure to oestrogen can cause a fatal bone marrow suppression in one season. Female ferrets should therefore be mated by entire or vasectomised males, treated with progesterone hormone therapy or GnRH agonists to suppress oestrus.

Neonatology

The young ferret is known as a kit. They are born altricial, blind, furless and deaf. The average litter size is eight kits. The fur starts to appear around the second day post-partum and is pronounced by 2 weeks. The eyes open around 3 weeks and the ears around 10 days. The kit is born with a prominent fat pad on the dorsum of the neck, providing some energy reserves during the early stages of life. The female ferret is sexually mature from 4 to 8 months and the male from 4 to 6 months, usually in the spring following birth.

Sexing

The male ferret has an obvious prepuce on the ventral abdomen similar to that seen in the domestic dog. In addition, the male has a caudally located scrotum with obvious testes. The female has a vulval orifice just ventral to the anus.

Skin

The claws are not retractable. The odour of a ferret is primarily from the normal sebaceous glands present within the skin, giving it the characteristic musky smell. These glands are particularly well concentrated around the mouth, chin and perineum. The odour of the male ferret is particularly strong due to the action of testosterone on these glands and the tendency to spray and empty the anal glands to mark territory. Neutering reduces this latter problem.

Haematology

One noticeable aspect of the ferret blood count is the consistently high packed cell volume, often in the 58–63% range in healthy adults. The white cell count on the other hand tends routinely to be lower than that seen in cats and dogs. The neutrophil is generally the predominant white cell seen.

Further reading

Fraser, M.A. and Girling, S.J. (2009) *Rabbit Medicine and Surgery for Veterinary Nurses*. Blackwell-Wiley, Oxford.

Harkness, J.E. and Wagner, J.E. (2000) *Biology and Medicine of Rabbits and Rodents*, 5th edn. Lea & Febiger, Philadelphia, PA.

Keeble, E. and Meredith, A. (2009) *Manual of Rodents and Ferrets*. BSAVA, Quedgeley, UK.

Meredith, A. and Flecknall, P. (2006) *Manual of Rabbits*, 2nd edn. BSAVA, Quedgeley, UK.

Meredith, A. and Johnson-Delaney, C. (2010) *Manual of Exotic Pets*, 5th edn. BSAVA, Quedgeley, UK.

Okerman, L. (1998) *Diseases of Domestic Rabbits*, 2nd edn. Blackwell Science, Oxford.

Quesenberry, K.E. and Carpenter, J. (2003) *Ferrets, Rabbits and Rodents*, 2nd edn. W.B. Saunders, Philadelphia, PA.

Chapter 2   Small Mammal Housing, Husbandry and Rearing

DOMESTIC RABBIT

Breeds

There are many different breeds of rabbit, varying from the miniature breeds such as the Netherland dwarf, weighing in at 0.5–0.75 kg, through to the New Zealand whites and the Belgian hares at 8–10 kg. Other commonly seen breeds include the lop-eared crosses, the angora breeds, the Rex and the traditional Dutch rabbits.

Cage requirements

Size and construction

The traditional hutch is a common feature of rabbit husbandry (see Figure 2.1). The provision of a wooden enclosure that is sufficiently large to provide sleeping quarters, a feeding area and a toilet area is common. In general, a rough guide to a minimum width of a rabbit hutch is three times the length of the rabbit to be housed when it is stretched out at rest. The depth should be one rabbit length, and the height equal to that of the rabbit standing on hind legs. Anything smaller and the rabbit must be provided with an outside run, or allowed out of the hutch for regular exercise periods every day. Indeed current recommendations suggest that all rabbits should have an exercise area, fully protected from predator attack to ensure adequate environmental enrichment and exercise. Cooping a rabbit up in too small a hutch is cruel; it will also lead to muscular and skeletal atrophy and increase the risk of spontaneous spine and limb fractures when the rabbit overexerts itself. However, many commercially available hutches are in fact too small for the adult rabbit, being the correct size only for the small juvenile or dwarf.

Wooden hutches are the standard and are satisfactory in many cases. Their disadvantage is that they will tend to rot with the absorption of urine and rain unless properly protected. Care should be taken with wood preservatives to ensure an animal-friendly preservative is chosen (do not use creosote!). The roof may be further protected with the felt material used to roof garden sheds and should

slope to the rear of the hutch to avoid rain dripping into the front, or pooling on the roof. The hutches should also be raised off the floor on legs to avoid the bottom rotting from the damp ground surface. A ramp should therefore be supplied if the rabbits are to be allowed in and out of the hutch of their own accord. Wooden hutches are also much more easily destroyed by gnawing.

In commercial fur- and meat-producing situations, rabbits are kept in wire mesh hutches suspended above a solid floor. The wire mesh 'hutch' has one major advantage in that it prevents soiling of the fur by urine and faeces. However, it can cause abrasions of the hocks in older overweight rabbits and is not advised for housing pet rabbits.

Substrates

Substrates used for cage floor covering include straw, hay, shavings and newspaper. Many rabbits will preferentially select hay and straw for bedding over shavings and paper. One of the advantages of the former is that they allow urine to drop through the fibre framework and away from the rabbit, so reducing the likelihood of urine scalding in older and arthritic rabbits.

Positioning

Care should be taken to avoid overheating of the hutch, as rabbits cannot sweat and temperatures above 26–28°C will rapidly cause hyperthermia and death. Hutches should therefore be positioned out of direct sunlight, particularly in the summer months. Rabbits will shiver when cold, although they can tolerate cold better than heat. Care should still be taken to ensure that the hutch is not overly draughty or exposed during the winter months. Bringing it into a shed or garage is often advisable in the worst weather.

Food and water bowls

Feeding bowls should be a ceramic or metal. The former are preferable, as they are heavier and harder to knock

Veterinary Nursing of Exotic Pets, Second Edition. Edited by Simon J. Girling. © 2013 John Wiley & Sons, Ltd. Published 2013 by John Wiley & Sons, Ltd.

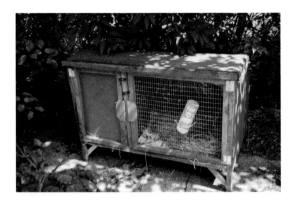

Figure 2.1 Traditional wooden rabbit hutch. Care should be taken to ensure that access is given to a run to ensure adequate exercise and enrichment.

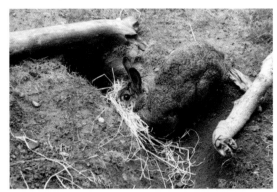

Figure 2.2 In an extensive open housing system outside, be prepared for considerable digging and creation of natural warrens!

over. Plastic feed bowls should be avoided as they are easily chewed. Water feeders are better offered with ball valve drip dispensers. They allow less contamination of the water with food, urine and faeces than an open bowl. Care should be taken with these feeders, though, as some rabbits reared with water bowls will not drink from them. In addition, the ball valve often leaks and this will lead to excessively damp substrate and mould growth. Drip feeders will also suffer from bacterial build-up and need careful cleaning once or twice a week, or even daily if a large number of rabbits are housed.

Outdoor runs

It is advisable to provide outside runs attached to the hutch in the summer months. This allows the rabbit access to unfiltered sunshine, which is important for vitamin D_3 synthesis as well as for stimulating normal annual rhythms of behaviour. Fresh grass is also the food item rabbits are supremely adapted to eat. The fibre content, in particular, is vital for wear of the teeth and stimulation of normal gut motility. Grass should not be cut first and then offered however, as this rapidly ferments and can produce colic.

Care should be taken when securing outside runs to make them both rabbit proof and predator proof. For this reason, it may be necessary to bury the wire sides to any run a foot or so beneath the ground surface as does in particular will burrow regularly (see Figure 2.2). To prevent foxes and cats gaining access to the run, a meshed roof should be provided. Finally, all outdoor rabbits should be vaccinated against myxomatosis, the viral condition spread by fleas and mosquitoes from wild rabbits, and preferably against viral haemorrhagic disease as well.

House rabbit

Many rabbits are now kept as house rabbits, with sleeping quarters and a litter tray. Rabbits can be toilet-trained relatively easily. The first steps in this are to keep the rabbit in a small area with a sleeping area, the litter tray and a feeding area. Once the litter tray has been associated with urination in particular, the rabbit may then be allowed more freedom to roam.

Hazards in the home include electrical cabling, which should be hidden beneath carpets or protected inside heavy-duty cable trunking, which is available from hardware stores. Houseplants are another problem. Many of the exotic tropical houseplants are poisonous. Examples include African violet, Dieffenbachia, cheese plant and spider plant.

Social grouping

Rabbits are in general a social species, preferring to live in a group rather than singly. Problems arise though with keeping a number of entire males together, as bullying and sexual harassment will occur. Neutering is therefore advised where more than one male is to be kept and may be performed in bucks from 4 to 5 months of age. Mixed sex groups will work well if the does are spayed. This may be safely done from 5 to 6 months of age and is advisable even in solitary does due to the high risk of developing a malignant uterine cancer, known as a uterine adenocarcinoma, in middle age.

Some owners advocate the grouping of guinea pigs with rabbits. This is to be discouraged for two important reasons. One is that the rabbit has very powerful hind legs, and the guinea pig, a long and fragile spine. Consequently, one well-placed kick from the rabbit can do a great deal of damage. The other reason is that rabbits are frequently asymptomatic carriers of the bacteria *Bordetella bronchiseptica* in their airways. These bacteria can cause a severe pneumonia in guinea pigs. Other domestic pets are not advised to be mixed with rabbits, as both cats and dogs are potential predators!

Behaviour

Rabbits are a prey species and therefore communicate in a very different manner from the more commonly understood cats and dogs. Indeed, it may seem that rabbits are very poor at communicating their feelings to their owners, when in fact they may be communicating, but in a much more subtle manner.

Affection is shown by mutual grooming of a companion, or owner, with licking of the hands in the latter case common. Other signs of relaxation include coming to the owner to be fed treats, following an owner around the house and, in many rabbits, making a buzzing noise from the larynx. This may be mistaken for a disease problem by inexperienced owners as it can be quite loud!

Aggression is shown by scratching, boxing with the front legs and biting. Aggression may be initiated because of a hormonal state, such as those caused by coming into season or bucks fighting for territory in the early spring, or it may be fear or pain driven. Aggression may also become a learnt behaviour if an act of aggression results in a desired effect, such as immediate backing off by the victim or replacing of a rabbit that has just been picked up by an owner.

Fear is shown initially by the regular thumping of the hind legs. This is a warning signal. As the object of fear approaches, the rabbit will either then freeze and remain motionless or suddenly bolt towards an exit.

Chewing of almost everything in the rabbit's environment is a perfectly normal behaviour and no amount of training will alter this fact. Owners of house rabbits should be warned of this and take appropriate action to prevent chewing of electric cables and other hazardous items of household furnishing.

Fostering

Rabbit kittens are difficult to hand-rear. Many females will not foster a strange doe's kittens, but does kept together and lactating at the same time will often allow others' young to suckle. This is the best scenario if another known lactating doe is available. If not, as is often the case, hand-rearing may be attempted.

A rearing formula has been derived (Okerman, 1998): 25 mL of whole cow's milk to 75 mL of condensed milk and 6 g of lyophilised skimmed milk powder. To this a vitamin supplement may be added. The kitten is fed only twice a day, from 2 to 10 mL depending on its age. This should continue until the kitten is 2 weeks old when more and more good quality hay and pellets should be introduced, aiming to wean the kitten at 3 weeks. The anogenital area should be stimulated with a piece of damp cotton wool after every feed to stimulate urination and defecation for the first 2 weeks.

RAT AND MOUSE
Varieties
Rat

The common albino laboratory rat is widely domesticated. Other common varieties include the hooded rat and Rex groups. These are all variations on the *Rattus norvegicus* species, and the fancy rat numbers are ever increasing.

Mouse

As with rats, there are many different varieties of domesticated mouse. These vary from albinos through to the Rex, whole body colour types, etc.

Cage requirements
Construction and temperature

These are similar for both rats and mice. The traditional solid, plastic-bottomed and wire mesh upper cages are advisable. These allow good air circulation at the level of the rat or mouse. The fish-tank style of housing is much less ventilated and allows the build-up of ammonia from urine-soaked bedding. Ammonia is a heavy gas and sits just above substrate level, that is at the rat's or mouse's nose level, and is thus inhaled often in high concentrations in this style of housing. Ammonia is highly irritant to the sensitive mucous membranes of the airways and will inflame and damage them, allowing secondary bacterial infection. This leads to the all-too-common problem of pneumonia seen in these species.

Environmental temperatures should range from 18°C to 26°C. Because they lack skin sweat glands, temperatures above 28–29°C will rapidly induce hyperthermia and death in rats and mice. Rats can tolerate cooler temperatures better than mice, because of their lower surface area to body mass ratio and deposits of brown fat beneath the skin. However, temperatures consistently below 10°C will lead to poor health and hypothermia.

Substrate

Wood shavings are well tolerated by rats and mice, but be aware that many pine and coniferous woods contain resins which may cause skin and airway irritation. Alternatively, newspaper or paper towelling may be used. Straw and hay may be used, but again beware that parasites may be introduced from wild rodents inadvertently with these bedding materials.

Cage furniture

As with hamsters, wheels are enjoyed by mice in particular. But these should be solid in construction rather than open wired to avoid damage to limbs. Rats are less keen to use wheels, although they do enjoy climbing and hiding inside cardboard tubes and other enclosed items.

Food and water bowls

As with rabbits, sip feeders are ideal, as they lead to minimal wastage and contamination. Ceramic or stainless steel bowls are preferable to plastic.

Social grouping

Rat

Male rats may be kept with other males, particularly if reared together from an early age, without fighting. Females may also be paired with other females and seem to benefit from the company. Intersex groups also work well, although care should be taken to neuter the males (which may be performed from 3 to 4 months of age) if unwanted pregnancies are to be avoided. This may be done from 3 to 4 months of age. If breeding is intended, male rats may be 'paired' with 1–6 females. The pregnant female should be removed to a separate cage from the male rat 4–5 days prior to parturition to avoid disturbing the female at this sensitive time.

Mouse

Females may be kept in groups, particularly if reared together from a young age. Males should always be housed singly, as severe fights and even death may result from aggression between sexually mature males. If breeding is intended, male mice may be 'paired' with 1–6 females. It is then advised to remove the pregnant female from the male some 4–5 days prior to parturition.

Behaviour

Rat

Rats are generally docile and rarely do they bite. Female rats are prone to cannibalism of the young if disturbed in the first few days following parturition. Food and water should therefore be provided prior to whelping, to last for the following 7–10 days, and the female then left. The female rat builds a relatively poor nest in comparison to other members of the rodent family.

Mouse

Mice are generally relatively docile, although male mice may be more aggressive than females. The latter though will be aggressive in the defence of her young. In addition, although cannibalism towards her young is rare, a female mouse should be left undisturbed for a minimum of 2–3 days post-partum. It is advisable to remove the female to a separate tank once she has mated to allow her to give birth and rear her young undisturbed.

Fostering

It is extremely difficult to rear young rats and mice successfully. Attempts may be made using a 1:1 dilution of evaporated milk to previously boiled water fed every 2 hours for the first 1–2 weeks. Weaning may be performed at 3 weeks. Stimulation of the anogenital area should be performed to encourage urination and defecation.

GERBIL AND HAMSTER
Varieties
Gerbil

There seems to be one main breed common in captivity, although a separate species known as the fat-tailed gerbil (*Pachyuromys duprasi*) has become more popular recently. There are however several different fur colour types, with albinos, black variants and greys as well as the normal tan colouration now available.

Hamster

There are four main species: Syrian, European, Chinese and Russian. Within these species there are many colour variations, from albino to red to black, with differing fur types such as the fluffy 'teddy bear' version of the Syrian hamster in addition to the more common short-coated varieties.

Cage requirements
Cages and substrates
Gerbil

These enjoy tunnelling through deep litter substrates. It is important that the environment is kept dry, as humid conditions lead to poor fur quality and increased skin and respiratory infections. Shavings are an ideal substrate and should be at least 10–15 cm deep (see Figure 2.3). Placing ceramic or cardboard tubes through the substrate can help tunnel formation and provide environmental enrichment. Peat and other soil substrates should however be avoided due because they are more likely to encourage damp. Environmental temperatures are usually kept around 20–25°C if possible.

Hamster

Cages for hamsters are best constructed of solid walls. The Rotastak®-style cage is ideal, with multiple tunnels for the hamster to manoeuvre from enclosed space to enclosed space. Wire cages are not so good, as hamsters have a habit of climbing up the sides, and then hand-over-hand across the roofs of these cages. They will often lose their grip suffer back injuries or compound fractures of the tibia as they land on the cage floor. It is advised to keep housing temperatures between 18°C and 26°C. Temperatures less than 5–6°C will result in the hamster hibernating. In this state, respiration and heart rates slow considerably, making it difficult in many instances to detect if the hamster is still alive. Temperatures above 29–30°C will result in hyperthermia and death.

Cage furniture

Hamsters enjoy wheels much, but these should be of a solid type, rather than the open wire format. This is to prevent the inadvertent damaging or even fracturing of a hind leg if it gets pushed between the wire slats. Tubes are ideal to entertain gerbils as mentioned above.

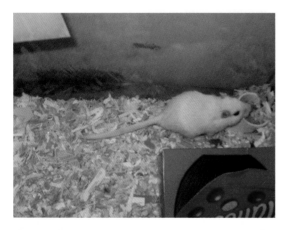

Figure 2.3 Deep substrate using shavings or paper is important for gerbils to allow burrowing.

Food and water bowls

Food bowls for both species are best made of a ceramic material, as these resist gnawing, are easily cleaned and difficult to tip over. Water is usually supplied in the traditional drip feeders, although care should be taken especially with gerbils that the valve is not leaky, as this leads to excessively wet substrate conditions and resultant dermatitis.

Social grouping

Gerbil

Gerbils are best housed singly, as a female pair or a neutered male and female pair. In the wild they will often bond, male to female, for life. Males housed together though will fight, inflicting severe wounds. Female gerbils will rarely cannibalise their young, unlike hamsters, although care should still be taken not to disturb the female and young too much in the first week post-partum.

Hamster

Males of the European, Chinese and Syrian species will fight. To a certain extent males of the Russian species will also fight, although this is lessened somewhat if they are reared from a young age together. Females may also be aggressive and so it is advised that hamsters in general be housed individually. For breeding purposes it is better to introduce a male hamster to a female's cage, rather than the other way around, to minimise fighting. A female hamster that has recently given birth should not be disturbed for a minimum of 10 days as the incidence of cannibalism of the young is high. To avoid this, enough food, water and bedding material (too little bedding is another reason for a female hamster killing the young) should be placed in the female's cage a few days prior to parturition and the female left undisturbed for the next 10–14 days.

Behaviour

Gerbil

Gerbils can be difficult to handle if not acclimatised to it from an early age. They will often bite if frightened or handled roughly. They are rarely vocal, but they will communicate their alarm through regular drumming of the floor of the cage with one hind leg, in much the same way as a rabbit will do. Gerbils spend the day dozing and they are most active at night; that is, they are nocturnal.

Hamster

Hamsters are frequently accused of being aggressive. They will certainly bite readily if handled roughly, disturbed or

frightened. Chinese and Russian hamsters are more aggressive than Syrian and European ones. Hamsters are
also nocturnal and much of the aggression is due to being
disturbed from their nest during the day. Therefore, they
really do not make good pets for children. Females may
be aggressive towards their young if disturbed.

Fostering
Gerbil
See rats and mice. Young gerbils are extremely difficult to
rear artificially.

Hamster
See rats and mice. Young hamsters are extremely difficult
to rear artificially. They do not foster well onto another
female in any of the species, except perhaps the Russian
hamster where a lactating female may accept another's
young.

GUINEA PIG AND CHINCHILLA
Breeds
Guinea pig
There are several different varieties of domesticated
guinea pig: the Abyssinian, which possesses whorls of fur
over the body and head; the Peruvian, which is particularly long-furred; the English or short-furred variety; and
the Rex varieties, with short fuzzy fur. Colour variations
are many and varied from whole body colours of tan,
white and black, through mixtures of two or three colours
and albinos.

Chinchilla
There are just two subspecies of chinchilla recognised.
Chinchilla lanigera is the standard domestic long-tailed
chinchilla, which comes in a variety of colours from
silver, to white, to champagne, to black. Some authori-
ties also recognise a subspecies known as *Chinchilla
brevicauda*, which is a short-tailed, larger version of the
above.

Cage requirements
Guinea pig
A hutch system similar to that outlined above for rabbits
is advised, although the whole structure should be on one
level. The same substrate and bedding materials are offered. In addition, it is often advised that lengths of tubing, such as drainpipe, should be offered as bolt holes for
the guinea pigs to use when frightened. Access to grazing is useful, and guinea pigs cannot climb or dig so pen

requirements are easier to provide than for rabbits. Care
should be taken to ensure that any steps or ramps are not
so steep that a guinea pig could fall, as their long and fragile backbone is easily damaged. Guinea pigs are expert
chewers so, if allowed access to the home, precautions
should be observed as with rabbits. Bowls and drinkers
for food and water are as for rabbits.

Chinchilla
Space requirements for chinchillas are greater than for
guinea pigs as they are extremely active. Recommendations
include enclosures in excess of 2 m^3. They appreciate vertical space, unlike the ground-dwelling guinea pig. Cage
construction should be of wire mesh, with a solid or mesh
floor. This is because chinchillas are particularly good at
chewing wood, and rapidly destroy wooden hutches.
Chinchillas prefer an actual nest box rather than plentiful
substrate. This should ideally be 20 cm^3 or more in size
and can be lined with hay or straw, although the rest of
the cage is often left bare. The floor is often a wire grid
structure, to prevent any fluid accumulating, as this may
lead to damage of the fur. The provision of lengths of
drainpipe tubing is also advised, as for guinea pigs, to allow the shy chinchilla to hide from public gaze.

Water can be provided in the traditional drip feeders. Chinchilla fur mats very quickly when wet, so care
should be taken to prevent the cage from becoming damp
from any leakage. Because of this tendency to mat easily, chinchillas should not be allowed to bathe in water,
but instead provided with daily access to a fine, pumice
sand and fuller's earth mixture as a dust bath. This can be
provided in a metal box which may be clipped onto the
inside of the cage or in a cat litter tray. The latter is less
satisfactory as the chinchilla may chew the plastic. The
sand bath should only be provided for short periods each
day as otherwise the chinchilla tends to spend all day in
the bath! Environmental temperatures should not exceed
20–22°C as heat stress may occur with that thick fur coat.

Social grouping
Guinea pig
Guinea pigs are a social species, and they live a much
more contented life in the presence of other guinea pigs.
Entire males can fight, although this is less likely if they
are reared together from an early age. Even so, males will
form a hierarchical system, and subordinate males may
be bullied and bitten on a regular basis. Females live
happily together, and the sexes may be mixed, although
castration of the males (which may be done from 4 to 5

months of age) is advised to prevent unwanted pregnancies. In addition, females are unusual among the species so far discussed in that they will allow the nursing of other young than their own.

Chinchilla

Chinchillas will often form bonded pairs, although they will equally live happily in multi-sex and multi-chinchilla groups. If breeding is to be prevented, one or both of the sexes should be neutered. Males may be castrated from 5 to 6 months and females from 6 to 7 months.

Behaviour
Guinea pig

Guinea pigs make good pets for the older child. They are docile and easily handled and rarely bite. Unlike many of the other species discussed here, they are very vocal. Their normal, contented vocal sounds include a series of chirrups and chattering noises which are low pitched. When alarmed, though, they will emit higher pitched squeaks of warning. They will also run around the perimeter of their enclosure at high speed when stressed, and may flatten any younger guinea pigs in the process!

Chinchilla

Chinchillas are shy and retiring creatures. They are very affectionate and will make chirruping noises when contented. When frightened they will bite, bark and often exhibit fur-slip, where fur will drop out leaving alopecic areas which last for many weeks. When distressed, many chinchillas will urinate at the handler. This includes females who, having a large urinary papilla, can direct their urination as accurately as males!

Fostering
Guinea pig

Use of a foster mother for any orphaned guinea pigs is advisable, even though they are precocious and may start to eat solids from day 3 post-partum. Even so, rearing milk formulas are still advised to be fed. Recipes for these include commercial feline weaner formulas, or using a 1:2 mixture of evaporated milk to previously boiled and then cooled water, thickened with a proprietary vegetable baby food powder (Richardson, 1992). This may be given through a kitten-rearing feeder every 2 hours for the first week, but the young should be encouraged to take solids as early as possible as a high incidence of cataracts is noticed in young guinea pigs fed for too long on cat, dog or cow's milk replacers. For the first 7–10 days the anogenital area of the young guinea pig should be stimulated with damp cotton wool to encourage urination and defecation.

Chinchilla

Even though young chinchillas are precocious at birth, they can be difficult to rear successfully. A rough guide to a rearing formula is to feed a 50:50 mix of a commercial cat- or dog-rearing formula added to evaporated milk. Alternatively, a 1:2 mix of evaporated milk with cooled, previously boiled water, thickened with a little fruit or vegetable baby food (Milupa or Farex) may be used. This should be fed through a kitten feeder every 2 hours for the first week, dropping to every 3–4 hours once the young chinchilla starts nibbling small volumes of solid. Chinchillas may be weaned early at 4 weeks if eating sufficient dry foods. Their weight should be measured daily to ensure regular gains. After each meal, the anogenital area should be stimulated with a piece of damp cotton wool to stimulate urination and defecation, although this is really only necessary for the first 7–10 days.

CHIPMUNK
Species

The two main species seen in captivity are the Siberian chipmunk and, to a lesser extent, the North American chipmunk. The coat variations are limited, but the basic pattern is with a light brown base coat with darker longitudinal stripes. Albinos do exist.

Cage requirements
Cages and substrates

Chipmunks appreciate a combination of cage environments. The enclosure itself resembles more closely an aviary system designed for cage birds, with a wire mesh wall. The most successful examples combine a deep litter floor with bark chippings to allow foraging for food for environmental enrichment and roost boxes attached a few feet off the ground. These are constructed along similar lines to bird boxes. The cage may be further enhanced by stringing ropes from side to side to create aerial walkways.

Positioning

It is important not to house chipmunks near any source of electrical radiation in the 50–60 Hz range. This includes television sets and many strip lights and computer terminals. The radiation waves given off by these electrical items cause high degrees of stress to the chipmunks, which will exhibit manic behaviour. This occurs even when they are turned off but still plugged in to the mains socket.

Social grouping

Chipmunks prefer to be grouped together. Males are territorial and will fight during the breeding season, but females will tolerate each other well. In general, family groups are preferred, but the parents will chase away the young when weaned.

Behaviour

Chipmunks are extremely nervous and highly strung creatures. They will bite if handled, and are difficult to tame, even when hand-reared. They will chatter excitedly to each other when stressed and often emit high-pitched squeaks. Some will also drum their hind legs as a warning signal. Tail flicking occurs almost continually, but becomes even more excited when stressed.

Fostering

Young abandoned chipmunks are difficult to rear. A rearing formula has been proposed using a mixture of one part evaporated milk to two parts water, adding vegetable baby foods to this as the chipmunk ages. Minerals and vitamins may then be added, and the whole fed through a kitten-rearing feeder every 4 hours for the first 2 weeks of life, dropping down to every 8 hours from 3 weeks until they are weaned at 5–6 weeks. The young chipmunk should be stimulated to urinate and defecate with a piece of damp cotton wool rubbed over the anogenital area immediately after feeding.

MARSUPIALS
Cage requirements
Sugar glider

Minimum cage dimensions for an adult pair would be 2 m × 2 m floor space with a height of 1.8 m. Mesh size should be 1 cm². A nest box should be provided such as a wooden cylinder with a narrow opening. Branches should also be provided within the enclosure as sugar gliders are arboreal in nature. Additional heating is usually required to maintain environmental temperatures above 25°C with humidity of 60–80%. Substrate can be shredded paper or shavings.

Virginia opossum

Minimum cage dimensions should be 2 m × 2 m unless they are regularly allowed out of their cages.

Rabbit hutches and runs may be adapted for use but some facility for climbing should be provided. Substrate can be shredded paper, shavings or bark. Environmental temperature ranges of 12–25°C should be achieved with relative humidity levels above 60%.

Social grouping
Sugar glider

They are social animals and should not be kept singly as self-mutilation may occur. The most suitable group structure is to keep an adult male and an adult female together plus young. The young in a breeding pair of adults will usually comprise last year's joeys plus the current year's joeys in the pouch. When the former are sexually mature and need to be removed from the group then the latter will have been weaned.

Virginia opossum

These are usually kept as pairs or individuals. Young should be removed 4–6 weeks after weaning. Neutered adults can be kept together in larger groups assuming sufficient space is allowed.

Behaviour
Sugar glider

These are very vocal when frightened and will make small barking noises as well as screeches. They will vigorously scent-mark and are very territorial, particularly the males.

Virginia opossum

These are very vocal and will hiss, click and growl as well as making a screeching sound when frightened. They can also 'play possum' that is feign death when threatened.

Fostering

Orphaned joeys must first be brought up to the correct body temperature (35–37°C) before being fed. Any milk replacer should be warmed to 35°C before being offered. Frequency depends on maturity with non-furred joeys being fed every 2–3 hours and furred ones being fed every 4–6 hours. Volumes fed should be between 10% and 20% of the joey's body weight over a 24-hour period. Teats on feeding bottles should have small needle holes and be long and thin in shape.

MacPherson (1997) derived a formula for sugar gliders using 1 scoop of Puppy Esbilac® powder to 3 scoops of Pedialyte® (or equivalent small animal electrolyte replacer). A similar replacer can be used using 1 part Puppy Esbilac® to 3–5 parts water.

FERRET
Cage requirements
Cages and substrates
Many ferrets are kept in outside hutches in a fashion similar to rabbits in the United Kingdom, particularly during the summer months (see Figure 2.4). Increasingly though, ferrets are being kept as house pets in the United Kingdom, and of course have been kept as such in the United States of America for many years now. The problem with wooden hutches is that the often strong-smelling urine of the ferret will penetrate the wood. This is not so bad in ferrets that are kept outdoors, but for indoor ones this may be a considerable downside! Therefore the use of steel-bottomed and wire upper cages is preferred for indoor ferret keeping, as this type of cage can be easily disinfected. The size of the ferret cage should be a minimum of two ferret lengths in each direction. Ferrets like to make use of vertical space, so the provisions of a shelf and raised sleeping quarters are useful. Care should be taken to ensure that the wire mesh is no larger than 2.5 cm^2 to avoid smaller ferrets escaping. Substrate in the cage may be newspaper, hay, shavings or straw. The nest box is best lined with towelling or a similar material. Ferrets enjoy hiding in plastic tubing and investigating every nook and cranny of a house. It is therefore essential not to allow a ferret access to rooms where there are holes in the walls for pipes, such as the kitchen, as they usually end up disappearing down them!

Hacking boxes
These are used for working ferrets to transport them to and from the area of rabbiting (see Figure 2.5). They tend to be capable of carrying two ferrets separately and are of a simple design in wood with ventilation holes and a shoulder strap for carrying. They are not designed for keeping a ferret in for any length of time.

Social grouping
Female ferrets get on well together, and ferrets in general like company, so it is often advisable to house them together. Male ferrets (hobs) though may fight and so care should be taken when housing multiples. Chemical neutering using deslorelin implants of male ferrets is advised on grounds of reducing odour in any case and this makes them more malleable and less likely to fight as well. The female ferret (jill) is not susceptible to cannibalism of the young if disturbed, although care should be exercised when interfering with the young as the jill will defend them vigorously if she feels threatened.

Behaviour
Ferrets are extremely inquisitive creatures and will explore everything and anything! They are generally docile when reared in the company of humans, but they can give a ferocious bite when frightened, from which it may be difficult to disengage.

Management
Ferrets are currently kept in the United Kingdom mainly as working pets, for hunting, chiefly, of rabbits. Ferrets may be 'trained' to flush out rabbits from their warrens, although this is merely taking advantage of their natural hunting tendency.

Ferrets may be walked on a harness, and they can be litter trained with perseverance.

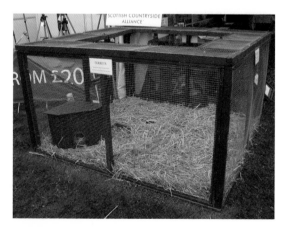

Figure 2.4 A typical temporary outside ferret run and housing for the summer months.

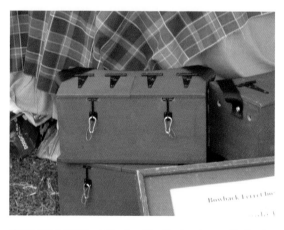

Figure 2.5 A typical working ferret hacking box to carry the ferret to and from the area of rabbiting.

The odour of ferrets is reduced in the case of the hobby castration. However this has now been shown to be associated with adrenal gland neoplasia, therefore the use of gonadotropin releasing hormone agonist such as desolrelin has been advocated instead. The removal of the anal glands is prohibited as an unnecessary mutilation in the United Kingdom.

Fostering

Care should be taken to ensure correct nursing of the kit after failure of the jill to nurse, produce milk or when mastitis occurs. This is best done by fostering the kits onto another lactating jill, but this is often difficult. If the affected jill is still well enough the kits should be left with her to gain what little milk they may. Supplemental feeding may then be given using a proprietary feline milk replacer enriched with whipping cream to increase the fat content. A rough guide is 2–3 parts feline milk replacer to one part whipping cream. This needs to be fed every 2 hours or so via a nipple feeder, preferably warmed prior to feeding. Weaning may be brought forward to 3 weeks, and the kits trained to drink milk replacer from a saucer. Generally kits cannot manage to survive on solid foods alone until they are over 5 weeks of age. As with neonatal cats and dogs, kits require stimulation of their anogenital areas with damp cotton wool after each feed to encourage urination and defecation.

References

MacPherson, C. (1997) *Sugar Gliders. A Complete Owner's Manual.* Barron's Educational Series, Hauppage, NY.

Okerman, L. (1998) *Diseases of Domestic Rabbits*, 2nd edn. Blackwell Science, Oxford.

Richardson, V. (1992) *Diseases of Domestic Guinea Pigs*. Blackwell Publishing, Oxford.

Further reading

Booth, R. (2003) Sugar gliders. *Seminars in Avian and Exotic Pet Medicine*, **12**(4), 228–231.

Fraser, M.A. and Girling, S.J. (2009) *Rabbit Medicine and Surgery for Veterinary Nurses*. Wiley-Blackwell, Oxford.

Harkness, J.E. and Wagner, J.E. (2000) *Biology and Medicine of Rabbits and Rodents*, 5th edn. Lea & Febiger, Philadelphia, PA.

Keeble, E. and Meredith, A. (2009) *Manual of Rodents and Ferrets*. BSAVA, Quedgeley, UK.

Meredith, A. and Flecknall, P. (2006) *Manual of Rabbits*, 2nd edn. BSAVA, Quedgeley, UK.

Meredith, A. and Johnson-Delaney, C. (2010) *Manual of Exotic Pets*, 5th edn. BSAVA, Quedgeley, UK.

Quesenberry, K.E. and Carpenter, J. (2003) *Ferrets, Rabbits and Rodents*, 2nd edn. W.B. Saunders, Philadelphia, PA.

Chapter 3 Small Mammal Handling and Chemical Restraint

Before attempting to restrain a small mammal patient, we must first be sure that it is necessary. Points to be considered include

- Is the patient severely debilitated and in respiratory distress? Examples include the pneumonic rabbit with obvious oculonasal discharge and dyspnoea, or the chronic lung disease so often seen in older rats. Excessive or rough handling of these patients is contraindicated.
- Is the species a tame one? Examples of the more unusual small mammals that may be kept include chipmunks, sugar gliders, marmosets and raccoons. All of these are potentially hazardous to handlers and themselves as they will often bolt for freedom when frightened, or turn and fight!
- Is the small mammal suffering from a metabolic bone disease? This is often seen in small primates, young rabbits and, to a lesser extent, guinea pigs. The diet may have been deficient in calcium and vitamin D_3 and exposure to natural sunlight may be absent. Therefore, long-bone mineralisation during growth will be poor leading to easily fractured bones.
- Does the small mammal patient require medication or physical examination, in which case restraint may be essential?

Handling techniques

Because of the wide range of species grouped under the heading small mammal, this section is easier if considered under specific groups and orders. Always approach small mammals from the sides and low levels to avoid mimicking the swooping action of a bird of prey.

Domestic rabbit

The majority of domestic rabbits are docile. In the occasional aggressive rabbit, the main dangers are from the claws, which can inflict deep scratches, and the incisors, which can produce deep bites. Aggression is worse at the start of the breeding season in March and April, or when

the rabbit is frightened. In addition, a struggling rabbit may lash out with its powerful hindlimbs and fracture or dislocate its spine. Severe stress can even induce cardiac arrest in some rabbits. Rapid and safe restraint is therefore essential.

If aggressive, the lagomorph may be grasped by the scruff with one hand while the other supports the hind legs. If the rabbit is not aggressive, then one hand may be placed under the thorax, with the thumb and first two fingers encircling the front limbs, while the other is placed under the hind legs to support the back (see Figure 3.1).

When transferred from one room to another the rabbit must be held close to the handler's chest. Nonfractious individuals may also be supported with their heads pushed into the crook of one arm, with that forearm supporting the length of the rabbit's body. The other hand is then used to place pressure on or grasp the scruff region (see Figure 3.2).

Once caught the rabbit may be calmed further by wrapping it in a towel, so that just the head and ears protrude. There are also specific rabbit papooses that encircle the rabbit, but leave the head and ears free. This allows ear blood sampling and oral examinations, but controls their powerful hindlimbs. It is important not to allow them to overheat in this position, as rabbits do not have significant sweat glands and do not actively pant. They can therefore overheat quickly with fatal results if their environmental temperature exceeds 23–25°C.

Rat and mouse

Mice will frequently bite an unfamiliar handler, especially in strange surroundings. First, grasp the tail near to the base and then position the mouse on a non-slip surface. While still grasping the tail, the scruff may now be grasped firmly between thumb and forefinger of the other hand.

Rats will rarely bite unless roughly handled. They are best picked up by encircling the pectoral girdle immediately behind the front limbs with the thumb and fingers

Veterinary Nursing of Exotic Pets, Second Edition. Edited by Simon J. Girling. © 2013 John Wiley & Sons, Ltd. Published 2013 by John Wiley & Sons, Ltd.

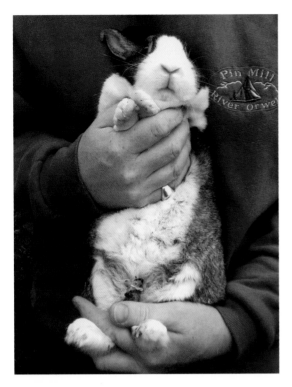

Figure 3.1 Method of restraining a tame rabbit for examination.

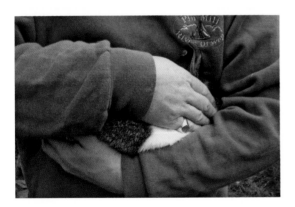

Figure 3.2 Method of transporting a rabbit from one place to another.

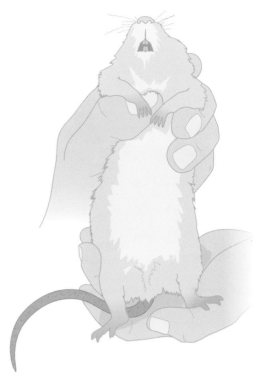

Figure 3.3 Method of restraining a hand tame rat. Note support of hind quarters with free hand.

Gerbil and hamster

Hamsters can be difficult to handle. If the hamster is relatively tame, cupping the hands underneath the animal is sufficient to transfer it from one cage to another.

Some breeds of hamster are more aggressive than others, with the Russian hamster (also known as the Djungarian or hairy-footed hamster) being notorious for its short temper. In these cases, the hamster should be placed onto a firm flat surface, and gentle but firm pressure placed onto the scruff region with finger and thumb of one hand. As much of the scruff should then be grasped as possible, with the pull in a cranial direction, to ensure that the skin is not drawn tight around the eyes (hamsters have a tendency to proptose their eyes if roughly scruffed) (Figure 3.4). If a very aggressive animal is encountered, the use of a small glass or perspex container with a lid for examination and transport purposes is useful.

Gerbils are relatively docile, but can jump extremely well when frightened and may bite. For simple transport they may be moved from one place to another by cupping the hands underneath them. For more rigorous restraint, the gerbil may be grasped by the scruff between thumb

of one hand, while bringing the other hand underneath the rear limbs to support the rat's weight (Figure 3.3). The more fractious rat may be temporarily restrained by grasping the base of the tail before scruffing it with thumb and forefinger.

Under no circumstances should mice or rats be restrained by the tips of their tails as de-gloving injuries to the skin covering them will occur.

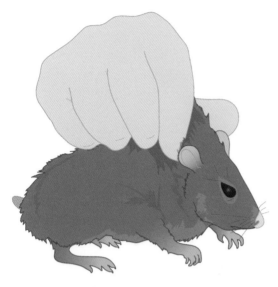

Figure 3.4 Method for restraining a hamster. Note the large amount of loose skin which must be grasped and the high position at which it is grasped immediately behind the ears to avoid eye proptosis.

and forefinger of one hand after placing it onto a flat level surface. It is vitally important not to grasp a gerbil by the tail. The skin will strip off, leaving denuded coccygeal vertebrae, and the skin will never regrow. Jerds and jerboas are related species and handling techniques are the same.

Guinea pig and chinchilla

Guinea pigs are rarely aggressive, but they are highly stressed when separated from their companions and normal surroundings. Dimming the lighting, and reducing noise and other stress can aid in control.

The guinea pig should be grasped behind the forelimbs from the dorsal aspect with one hand, while the other is placed beneath the hindlimbs to support its weight. This is particularly important as the guinea pig has a large abdomen but slender bones and spine. Without supporting the rear end, spinal damage is risked.

Chinchillas are equally timorous and rarely if ever bite. They too can be easily stressed and reducing noise and dimming room lighting can be useful. When restrained they must not be scruffed under any circumstances as this will result in the loss of fur at the site held. This fur-slip will leave a bare patch which will take many weeks to regrow. Chinchillas may actually lose some fur due to stress of restraint, even if no physical gripping of the skin occurs. Some chinchillas, when particularly stressed, will rear up on their hind legs and urinate at the handler with surprising accuracy! It is therefore essential to pick

up the chinchilla calmly and quickly with minimal restraint, placing one hand around the pectoral girdle from the dorsal aspect just behind the front legs, and the other hand cupping the hind legs and supporting the chinchilla's weight. Degus may be handled in a similar fashion, although they are less prone to fur-slip.

Chipmunk

Chipmunks are highly strung, and the avoidance of stress and fear aggression is essential to avoid fatalities. They are difficult to handle without being bitten, unless hand-reared, when they may be scruffed quickly, or cupped in both hands. To catch them in their aviary-style enclosures the easiest method is to use a fine-meshed aviary or butterfly net, preferably made of a dark material. The chipmunk may then be safely netted and quickly transferred to a towel for manual restraint, examination, or injection or induction of chemical restraint.

Marsupials

Sugar gliders are very docile and may be restrained with minimal force. If they need to be held firmly for any reason, one hand can hold the base of the tail and the other the dorsal aspect of the neck. For Virginia opossums that are tame, one had may be used to grasp around the pectoral girdle and the other to support the rear end in a similar fashion to that described for domestic rats. For more aggressive animals leather gardening gloves/gauntlets should be used. They may also be wrapped in towels in a fashion similar to rabbits.

Ferret

Ferrets can make excellent house pets and many are friendly and hand-tame. However, in the United Kingdom, ferrets are most frequently kept for rabbit hunting; hence, many ferrets are not regularly handled and so may be aggressive.

For excitable or aggressive animals, a firm grasp of the scruff, high up at the back of the neck is advised. The ferret may then be suspended while stabilising the lower body with the other hand around the pelvis. In tamer animals, they may be suspended with one hand behind the front legs, cupped between thumb and fingers from the dorsal aspect, with the other hand supporting the hindlimbs. This hold may be varied somewhat in the more lively individuals by placing the thumb of one hand underneath the chin, so pushing the jaw upwards, and the rest of the fingers grasping the other side of the neck. The other hand is then brought under the hindlimbs as support.

Aspects of chemical restraint

Chemical restraint may be necessary for a number of reasons in small mammals:

- Sample collection, such as blood testing or urine collection
- For procedures such as radiography
- Oral examinations

Is the patient fit enough for chemical restraint?

It is important to assess whether the patient is fit enough for a chemical restraint before it is attempted. Factors that should be considered prior to the anaesthesia of small mammals are outlined below.

Low-grade respiratory infections

Many rodents and lagomorphs suffer from low-grade respiratory infection all of their lives. Most will cope with this, but when anaesthetised the respiratory rate slows and respiratory secretions, already thickened or increased due to chronic infection, become more tenacious. This can cause physical blockage of the airways.

Respiratory system anatomy

The majority of the species considered are nose breathers, with their soft palates permanently locked around the epiglottis. Therefore, if the patient has a blocked nose, whether it be due to pus, blood, tumours or abscesses, then respiratory arrest is made much more likely under anaesthetic.

Hypothermia

Because of their small size and resultant high body surface area to volume ratios, these small mammals are prone to hypothermia during anaesthesia. This is due to the cooling effect of the inhaled gases and reduced muscular activity. It is dangerous, therefore, to anaesthetise a patient that is already hypothermic without first treating this condition.

Dehydration

Respiratory fluid losses during drying gaseous anaesthetic procedures are much greater than in cats, dogs or larger species. Hence, putting a severely dehydrated small mammalian patient through an anaesthetic without prior fluid therapy is not advisable.

Pre-anaesthetic management
Weight measurement

It is vitally important to weigh the patient accurately. A mistake of just 10 g in a hamster, say, will lead to an under- or overdosage of 10%! The use of scales that will read accurately down to 1 g in weight is therefore essential.

Blood testing

Blood testing is starting to become much more common in small mammals and should be considered in every clinically unwell or senior patient where a sufficiently large sample may be obtained. Sites for venipuncture are detailed below.

Rabbit: A 25–27 gauge needle may be used in the lateral ear vein. Prior to sampling, apply a local anaesthetic cream to the site and warm the ear. Alternatively, the cephalic or the jugular veins may be used. The latter should be used with caution as it is the only source of blood drainage from the eyes, and so, if a thrombus forms in this vessel, ocular oedema and permanent damage or even loss of the eye may occur.

Rat and mouse: The lateral tail veins may be used. These run on either side of the coccygeal vertebrae and are best seen when the tail is warmed as for the lateral ear vein in lagomorphs. A 25–27 gauge needle is required.

Ferret: The jugular vein is the easiest to access, but may be difficult in a fractious animal. One handler holds onto both front limbs with one hand, clamping the body with forearm and elbow, the other hand placed under the chin and raising the head. Towel restraint may also be utilised to papoose the ferret. Cephalic veins may also be used. Needles of 23–25 gauge suffice.

Guinea pig and chinchilla: The jugular veins are the most accessible. One handler holds both front limbs with one hand and brings the patient to the edge of the table, raising the head with the other hand. The other operator may then take a jugular sample with a 23–25 gauge needle. Lateral saphenous veins may be used in guinea pigs, but chinchillas rarely have any other peripheral vessel large enough to sample.

Gerbil and hamster: These are difficult. With care (particularly in gerbils) the lateral tail veins may be used. Frequently cardiac puncture under anaesthetic is often necessary to obtain a sufficient sample.

Chipmunk: Jugular blood samples may be taken, but in nearly every case anaesthesia is required first.

Marsupials: The lateral or ventral tail vein, cephalic or lateral saphenous may be used. Anaesthesia may be required first though due to the small size of some and potential aggression of others.

Fasting

Rabbit: These do not need to be fasted prior to anaesthesia, as they have a very tight cardiac sphincter preventing vomiting. Starving may actually be deleterious to the patient's health as it causes a cessation in gut contractility and subsequent ileus. It is important, though, to ensure that no food is present in the mouth at the time of induction, hence a period of 30–60 minutes starvation should be ensured.

Rat and mouse: Because of their high metabolic rate and likelihood of hypoglycaemia, rats and mice need only be starved a matter of 40–60 minutes (mice) to 45–90 minutes (rats) prior to anaesthetic induction.

Guinea pig and chinchilla: These may be starved for 3–6 hours prior to surgery to ensure a relatively empty stomach and reduce pressure on the diaphragm. Again, prolonged starvation (>4 hours) will lead to hypoglycaemia and gut stasis.

Gerbil and hamster: As for Muridae, a period of 45–90 minutes is usually sufficient. Any longer than 2 hours and post-operative hypoglycaemia is a real problem.

Chipmunk: Periods of fasting of 2 hours have been reported as safe.

Marsupial: Smaller marsupials may be starved for 1 hour with larger ones requiring 3–6 hours.

Ferret: These may be starved for 2–4 hours. Many have insulinomas and will develop hypoglycaemia. Also mustelids have a high metabolic rate and short gut transit times.

Pre-anaesthetic medications

Pre-anaesthetic drugs are used because they provide a smooth induction and recovery from anaesthesia, or because they ensure a reduction in airway secretions, act as a respiratory stimulant or prevent serious bradycardia.

Antimuscarinics

Atropine is used in some species such as guinea pigs and chinchillas where oral secretions are high and intubation is difficult. Doses of 0.05 mg/kg have been used subcutaneously 30 minutes before induction. Atropine also acts to prevent excessive bradycardia, which often occurs during the induction phase.

It is not useful in lagomorphs, as around 60% of rabbits have a serum atropinesterase that breaks down atropine before it has a chance to work. Glycopyrrolate, which functions in a similar manner, may be used instead at doses of 0.01 mg/kg subcutaneously.

Tranquilisers

Tranquilisers are used to reduce the stress of induction. Many species will breath-hold during gaseous induction, to the point where they may become cyanotic. In rabbits, the 'shock' organ is the lungs, and during intense stress the pulmonary circulation can go into spasm, making the hypoxia due to breath-holding even worse, even to the point of collapse and cardiac arrest!

Acepromazine: Acepromazine (ACP) can be used at doses of 0.2 mg/kg in ferrets, 0.5 mg/kg in rabbits and 0.5–1 mg/kg in rats, mice, hamsters, chinchillas and guinea pigs. In general, it is a very safe premedicant even in debilitated animals. However, it is advised that it not be used in gerbils, as ACP reduces the seizure threshold, and many gerbils suffer from hereditary epilepsy. This author uses a dose of 0.2 mg/kg ACP in combination with 0.05 mg/kg atropine as a premedication for chinchillas.

Diazepam: Diazepam is useful as a premedicant in some species. In rodents, doses of 3 mg/kg can be used, even in gerbils. In rabbits, the benefits are somewhat outweighed by the larger volumes required. In addition, as the drug is oil based, the intramuscular route is employed and this may be painful.

Neuroleptanalgesics

The fentanyl/fluanisone combination (Hypnorm®) may be used at varying doses as a premedicant, a sedative or as part of an injectable full anaesthesia. As a premedicant, doses of 0.1 mL/kg for rabbits, 0.08 mL/kg for rats, 0.2 mL/kg for guinea pigs (one-fifth the recommended sedation doses) can produce sufficient sedation to prevent breath holding and allow gaseous induction. These doses are given intramuscularly 15–20 minutes before induction. However, Hypnorm® is an irritant and large doses in one site may cause post-operative lameness. It can be reversed after the operation with butorphanol at 0.2 mg/kg or buprenorphine at 0.05 mg/kg intravenously. Should a vein not be available, both may also be given intramuscularly.

Fluid therapy

Fluid therapy is a vitally important pre-anaesthetic consideration and will be mentioned below and elsewhere in the book.

Induction of anaesthesia
Injectable agents
Table 3.1 outlines some of the advantages and disadvantages of injectable anaesthetics in small mammals.

Propofol
It may be used in ferrets at 10 mg/kg after the use of a premedicant such as ACP. However, in rabbits and hystricomorphs, apnoea can be a problem, and because it must be given intravenously it is difficult to use in the smaller rodents. Doses of 5–10 mg/kg have been used intravenously in rabbits.

Alfaxalone
Alfaxalone has also been used at 5 mg/kg intravenously in rabbits, but it must be given slowly as apnoea can result.

Ketamine
Ketamine is a dissociative anaesthetic commonly used in small mammals.

Ferret: Ketamine may be used alone for chemical restraint in the ferret at doses of 10–20 mg/kg but, as with cats and dogs, the muscle relaxation is poor and salivation can be a problem. More often, ketamine is combined with other drugs such as the alpha-2 agonists xylazine and medetomidine. In ferrets, 10–30 mg/kg ketamine may be used with 1–2 mg/kg xylazine (Flecknell, 1998), preferably giving the xylazine 5–10 minutes before the ketamine.

Rabbit: Ketamine is used at a dose of 5–10 mg/kg in conjunction with medetomidine at 0.1–0.25 mg/kg and butorphanol at 0.5 mg/kg or with xylazine at 5 mg/kg (Flecknell, 2000). The advantages are a quick and stress-free anaesthetic, but the combination will cause blueing of the mucous membranes due to peripheral shut-down, making detection of hypoxia difficult. Respiratory depression may become a problem and intubation is often advised. Medetomidine may be reversed using atipamezole at 1 mg/kg.

Table 3.1 Advantages and disadvantages of injectable anaesthetics.

Advantages	Disadvantages
Easily administered	Delay in reversal
Minimal stress	Hypoxia and hypotension common
Prevent breath-holding	Tissue necrosis
Inexpensive	Organ metabolism required

Rat, mouse, gerbil and hamster: Ketamine can be used at 90 mg/kg in combination with xylazine at 5 mg/kg intramuscularly or intraperitoneally in rats and 100 mg/kg ketamine with 5 mg/kg xylazine in hamsters (Harkness & Wagner, 1989). Mice require 100 mg/kg of ketamine and 10 mg/kg xylazine (Orr, 2001). These combinations provide 30 minutes or so of anaesthesia.

In gerbils, the dose of xylazine may be reduced to 2–3 mg/kg as they appear more sensitive to the hypovolaemic effects of the alpha-2 drugs, with ketamine doses at 50 mg/kg (Flecknell, 1998).

Ketamine may also be used at 75 mg/kg in combination with medetomidine at 0.5 mg/kg in gerbils (Keeble, 2001) and rats (Orr, 2001). Mice may require as much as 1 mg/kg medetomidine (Orr, 2001). The advantages of the alpha-2 agonists are that they produce good analgesia (which ketamine does not) and that they may be quickly reversed with atipamezole at 1 mg/kg. Their disadvantages include severe hypotensive effects, and that once administered they are more difficult to control than a gaseous anaesthetic. Alpha-2 agonists also increase diuresis and may exacerbate renal dysfunction.

Guinea pig and chinchilla: Ketamine at 40 mg/kg in conjunction with xylazine at 5 mg/kg can be used in guinea pigs to produce a light plane of anaesthesia (Mason, 1997). Ketamine at 40 mg/kg may also be used with medetomidine at 0.5 mg/kg for guinea pigs (Flecknell, 2001), or ketamine at 30 mg/kg with medetomidine at 0.3 mg/kg for chinchillas (Mason, 1997). These doses may be reversed with 1 mg/kg atipamezole. The response to both of these combinations may be improved after an ACP premedication of 0.25 mg/kg. Alternatively, for chinchillas, a ketamine (40 mg/kg) and ACP (0.5 mg/kg) combination can be used (Morgan *et al.*, 1981). Induction takes 5–10 minutes and typically lasts for 45–60 minutes, but recovery may take 2–5 hours for the non-reversible ACP combination, hence reducing the dose of this drug and using the reversible alpha-2 antagonists may be beneficial. This author uses a combination of 0.2 mg/kg ACP plus 0.05 mg/kg atropine as a premedication followed by 2–4 mg/kg ketamine and 0.02–0.04 mg/kg medetomidine as induction in chinchillas which is suitable for radiography, dental examinations/molar burring and minor invasive procedures.

Fentanyl/fluanisone (Hypnorm® Vetapharma Ltd)
This drug combination is a neuroleptanalgesic licensed for use in rats, mice, rabbits and guinea pigs. Fentanyl is a morphine-/opioid derivative, and fluanisone is the

neuroleptic. It is mentioned here particularly because it is specifically licensed for use in rabbits, rats and mice and guinea pigs in the United Kingdom.

Rabbit: Sedation at doses of 0.5 mL/kg intramuscularly (see data sheets) produces sedation and immobilisation for 30–60 minutes, but the analgesic effect from the opioid derivative fentanyl will persist for some time longer. It may however be reversed with 0.5 mg/kg butorphanol intravenously, or 0.05 mg/kg buprenorphine, both of which will counteract the fentanyl and its analgesia and substitute their own pain relief.

Alternatively, to provide anaesthetic depth fentanyl/fluanisone may be combined with diazepam at a dose of 0.3 mL Hypnorm® to 2 mg/kg diazepam given intraperitoneally or intravenously (but in separate syringes as they do not mix). It may also be combined with midazolam (0.3 mL Hypnorm® to 2 mg/kg midazolam) and given intramuscularly or intraperitoneally in the same syringe. Hypnorm® may also be given intramuscularly first and then followed 15 minutes later by midazolam given intravenously into the lateral ear vein. These two combinations provide good analgesia and muscle relaxation with duration of anaesthesia of 20–40 minutes.

The fentanyl part may be reversed with buprenorphine or butorphanol given intravenously. In emergencies, naloxone at 0.1 mg/kg intramuscularly or intravenously may be given, but this provides no substitute analgesia.

Fentanyl/fluanisone combinations are well tolerated in most rabbits, but they can produce respiratory depression and hypoxia.

Rat and mouse: Hypnorm® may be used as sedation only on its own at a dose of 0.01 mL/30 g body weight in mice and 0.4 mL/kg in rats. This produces sedation and immobilisation for 30–60 minutes and may be reversed with buprenorphine or butorphanol as above.

Alternatively, it may be combined with diazepam (mice 0.01 mL/30 g Hypnorm® with 5 mg/kg diazepam intraperitoneally; rats 0.3 mL/kg Hypnorm® with 2.5 mg/kg diazepam intraperitoneally). In this case the diazepam and Hypnorm® are given in separate syringes as they do not mix. Midazolam is miscible with Hypnorm® and for rodents the recommendation is that each drug is individually mixed with an equal volume of sterile water first. These solutions are then mixed together in equal volumes. Of this stock solution, mice receive 10 mL/kg and rats receive 2.7 mL/kg as a single intraperitoneal injection. These two combinations provide anaesthesia for a period of 20–40 minutes.

Guinea pig and chinchilla: Hypnorm® may be used for sedation only on its own at a dose of 1 mL/kg intramuscularly. This may be problematic in guinea pigs as large volumes are required. Hypnorm® is an irritant and may cause lameness when the whole dose is placed in one spot – multiple sites are therefore preferred. It should be noted that it is not licensed for use in the chinchilla in the United Kingdom.

Alternatively, it may be combined with diazepam (1 mL/kg Hypnorm® and 2.5 mg/kg diazepam) in separate syringes and given intraperitoneally, or with midazolam by making the stock solution as described above for rats and mice, and then administering 8 mL/kg of this solution intraperitoneally. Hypnorm® may be reversed with the partial opioid agonists buprenorphine and butorphanol, or with the full antagonist naloxone.

Gaseous agents

Table 3.2 gives some advantages and disadvantages of gaseous anaesthetics in small mammals.

Isoflurane

Usually a premedication is used as due to its mildly irritant effects on mucus membranes, breath-holding is common, particularly in rabbits. Its advantage over previous gases such as halothane is in its safety for the debilitated patient. Only <0.3% of the gas is metabolised hepatically, the rest merely being exhaled for recovery to occur. Recovery is therefore rapid.

Induction levels vary at 2.5–4% and maintenance usually is 1.5–2.5% assuming adequate analgesia. Breath-holding can still be a problem, even with premedication, but the practice of supplying 100% oxygen to the patient for 2 minutes prior to anaesthetic administration helps

Table 3.2 Advantages and disadvantages of gaseous anaesthetics.

Advantages	Disadvantages
Faster alteration of depth of anaesthesia possible	Increased drying effect on respiratory membranes
Recovery times shorter	Hypothermic effect from drying
Less organ metabolism	Difficulty in some species which breath-hold
Delivered in 100% oxygen so better oxygenation than injectables on their own	May be considerably more expensive

minimise hypoxia. Isoflurane is then gradually introduced, first 0.5% for 2 minutes, then, assuming regular breathing, increased to 1% for 2 minutes and so on until anaesthetic levels are reached. This allows a smooth induction.

Sevoflurane

This gas anaesthetic is used commonly in small mammals now, and has an advantage over isoflurane in that breath-holding, when it is used as an induction agent is much reduced, particularly in rabbits. At levels exceeding 4% on induction it can still induce breath-holding, so it is preferable to use it at 4% for induction and 2–3% for maintenance. In guinea pigs, profuse lacrimation as well as salivation occurs with both isoflurane and sevoflurane and therefore it is advisable to use atropine or glycopyrrolate as a premedicant.

Maintenance of anaesthesia

Intubation

As with all gaseous anaesthetics, the placement of an endotracheal tube for maintenance after induction is to be recommended whenever possible. This is relatively straightforward in ferrets, being much the same procedure as for cats.

In rabbits, the use of a number 1 Wisconsin flat-bladed paediatric laryngoscope and a 2–3 mm tube is advised. The rabbit is first induced either with an injectable anaesthetic or with an inhalational one. It is then placed in dorsal recumbency, allowing the larynx to fall dorsally and into view. The tongue should be pulled out to one side and the laryngoscope and endotracheal tube are inserted (see Figure 3.5). A guide wire may first be passed through the laryngeal opening, and, once in, the endotracheal tube is threaded over the top and the wire withdrawn.

Alternatively the rabbit may be intubated blindly. This is performed in sternal recumbency, after initial induction. The head is lifted vertically off the table and the endotracheal tube is inserted orally in the midline until slight resistance and a cough is elicited. It is then advanced slowly, and air passage through the tube checked to ensure correct placement.

Intubation is a specialised procedure for rodents such as rats and mice where rigid guide tubes and wires and smaller scopes are used to guide the tube into the larynx. If intubation is not possible, then oxygen on its own or with an anaesthetic gas may be supplied via an intranasal catheter as rodents are obligate nose breathers.

Intubation of omnivorous marsupials is more straightforward as they have a large oral opening. However, the small overall body-size of the sugar glider may still make it a challenge.

Intubation of ferrets is similar to that for cats. They should be first induced by face mask (see Figure 3.6) or by using injectable anaesthetics before intubation is attempted.

In rabbits and ferrets it is helpful to use xylocaine spray on the larynx to reduce laryngospasm and aid intubation (see Figure 3.7).

Intermittent positive pressure ventilation

Intermittent positive pressure ventilation (IPPV) may be necessary in some individuals who breath-hold during induction. The patient should receive ventilation at their

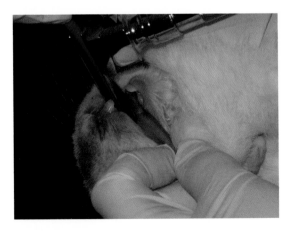

Figure 3.5 Insertion of a laryngoscope and ET tube in an already anaesthetised rabbit in dorsal recumbency. Note the careful lateral displacement of the tongue to avoid laceration on the incisors.

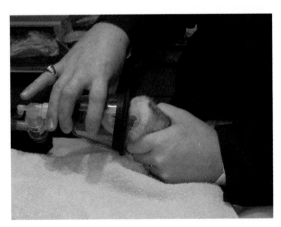

Figure 3.6 Induction of a ferret is easily achieved using a face mask and isoflurane or sevoflurane in 100% oxygen.

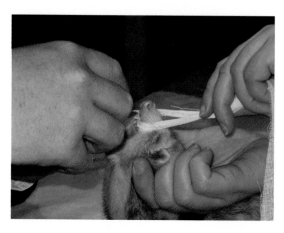

Figure 3.7 Spraying the larynx, which is easily visualised, is advised prior to inserting an ET tube in the ferret.

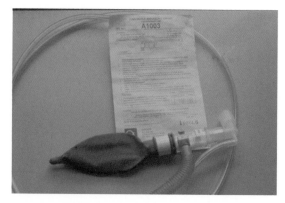

Figure 3.8 A Mapleson C circuit with a 0.25 L rebreathing bag is deal for smaller species.

resting respiratory rate. If intubation is not possible then three options are available:

1. Ensure a tight-fitting face mask and use an Ayres T-piece, Mapleson C or modified Bain circuit with 0.5 L bag attached to attempt ventilation.
2. Place a nasopharygeal tube, via the medial meatus of the nose, into the pharyngeal area. Then supply 4 L or so of oxygen (to combat the resistance of the small diameter tubing of 1–2 mm) via this route. This cannot be done in mammals smaller than a young guinea pig.
3. Perform an emergency tracheostomy with a 25–27 gauge needle attached to the oxygen outlet, placing the needle between the supporting C-shaped laryngeal cartilages ventrally.

Anaesthetic circuits

Most of the small mammals described here are less than 2 kg in weight. For this reason an Ayres T-piece, modified (mini) Bain or Mapleson C circuit are the best ones to use, as they provide the minimum of dead space (Figure 3.8). For larger rabbits, an Ayres T-piece is usually sufficient.

Supportive therapy during and after anaesthesia

Recumbency

For most surgical procedures, the positioning for restraint or recumbency will be dependent upon the area being operated on. This may necessitate being placed in dorsal recumbency. Because small herbivores rely on their gut flora to aid digestion, most of them have developed an enlarged hindgut. When in dorsal recumbency there is a lot

of weight on the diaphragm, and as the majority of small mammals considered here are diaphragm breathers, the hindrance to inspiration is significant. During lengthy surgical procedures, this may lead to apnoea and hypoxia. Therefore, place the patient with its cranial end elevated above the caudal when in dorsal recumbency. This allows gravity to draw the intestine away from the diaphragm.

Maintenance of body temperature

Maintenance of core body temperature is vitally important in all patients to ensure successful recovery from anaesthesia, but is particularly important in small mammals. This is primarily due to their increased surface area to volume ratio, allowing more heat to escape per gram of animal. To help minimise this, the following actions may be taken:

- Perform minimal surgical scrubbing of the site, and minimal clipping of fur from the area. Do not use surgical spirit as this rapidly cools the skin.
- Ensure the environmental room temperature is at the warm end of comfortable.
- Place the patient onto either a water-circulating heat pad or a hot air blankets, or use latex gloves/hot water bottles grouped around the patient (making sure that the containers are not in direct contact with the patient as skin burns may ensue).
- Administer warmed isotonic fluids subcutaneously, intravenously or intraperitoneally prior to and during surgery.

Anaesthetic gases have a rapidly cooling effect on the oral and respiratory membranes, and so patients maintained on gaseous anaesthetics will cool down quicker than those on injectable ones. This effect will worsen as the length of the anaesthesia increases.

It is worth noting, however, that hyperthermia may be as bad as hypothermia. Small mammals generally have few or no sweat glands, so heat cannot be lost via this route. In addition, very few actually pant to lose heat, so if over-warmed the core body temperature rises and irreversible hyperthermia will occur. A rectal thermometer is useful to monitor body temperature. Normal body temperature ranges are given in Table 3.3.

Fluid therapy

Intra-, pre- and post-operative fluid therapy is important in small mammals, even for routine surgery. The small size and relatively large body surface area in relation to volume of these patients means that they will dehydrate much faster, gram for gram, than a larger cat or dog. Studies have shown that the provision of maintenance levels of fluids to small mammals during and immediately after routine surgery improved anaesthetic safety levels by as much as 15% in some cases, with higher levels if the surgery was being performed on severely debilitated animals.

It is therefore recommended that all small mammal patients receive fluids during and after an anaesthetic be it routine or not. For further information see chapter 6.

Monitoring anaesthesia

No one factor will allow you to assess anaesthetic depth. Indeed, in small mammals many of the useful techniques used in cats and dogs are irrelevant. Eye position, for

Table 3.3 Normal body temperatures for selected small mammals.

Species	Normal body temperature range (°C)
Rabbit	37–39.4
Guinea pig	37.2–39.5
Chinchilla	37.8–40
Rat	38 (average)
Mouse	37.5 (average)
Gerbil	37.4–39
Hamster	36.2–37.5
Chipmunk	38 (average)
Ferret	37.8–40
Marsupial	32 (sugar glider) 32.2–35 (Virginia opossum)

example, should not be used to assess depth of anaesthesia in small mammals. Instead, a useful method is to assess the response to noxious stimuli such as pain.

The first reflex lost is usually the righting reflex – the animal is unable to return to ventral recumbency.

The next reflex to be lost, for example in rabbits and guinea pigs, is the swallow reflex. However, this may be difficult to assess. Palpebral reflexes (the response of blinking when the peri-ocular area is lightly touched) are generally lost early on in the course of anaesthetic, but rabbits may retain this reflex until well into the deeper planes of surgical anaesthesia. The palpebral reflex is also affected by the anaesthetic agent used. Most inhalant gaseous anaesthetics cause loss of the reflex early on, but it is maintained with ketamine.

The pedal withdrawal reflex is useful in small mammals, with the leg being extended and the toe firmly pinched. Loss of this reflex suggests surgical planes of anaesthesia, but again rabbits will retain the pedal reflex in the forelimbs until much deeper (and often dangerously deep!) planes of anaesthesia are reached. Other pain stimuli such as the ear pinch in the guinea pig and rabbit are useful. Loss of this indicates a surgical plane, as does the loss of the tail pinch reflex in rats and mice.

Monitoring of the heart and circulation may be done in a conventional manner, with stethoscope and femoral pulse evaluation, or, in the larger species, an oesophageal stethoscope may be used. Increases in the respiratory and heart rates can indicate lightening of the plane of anaesthesia.

Pulse oximetry may be used in rabbits, but many oximeters will not read heart rates above 250 beats per minute, so care should be taken in selection of these. The ear artery may be used, as may the ventral tail artery or a toe artery in larger rabbits.

As with cats and dogs, the aim is to achieve 100% saturation, and levels below 93% would indicate significant hypoxaemia and the initiation of assisted ventilation. The ear artery is useful for this in rabbits, using the clip-on probe, while the linear probes may be used successfully on the ventral aspect of the tail in most other species. Other forms of cardiac monitoring include ECGs, which are adapted to minimise trauma by substituting fine needle probes for alligator forceps, or by blunting the alligator teeth. Oesophageal ECG probes are generally too large to be of use in small mammals.

Doppler probes that can detect blood flow in the smallest of vessels up to the heart itself are also useful. The Doppler probe converts blood flow into an audible signal, which is transmitted through a speaker device. This can then be assessed by the anaesthetist during surgery for changes in strength of output and heart rate.

Respiratory monitors may be used if the patient is intubated and many pulse oximeters have outlets for these. Their use allows for assessment of respiratory rates, which for rodents are typically 50–100 breaths per minute and for rabbits and ferrets, around 40–50 breaths per minute. A reduction by 50% or more in this rate would give cause for concern. Capnographs can also be used but obviously neither of these is useful for patients maintained on face masks or on injectable anaesthetics alone. In addition, because of the small lung capacity and the need to minimise dead space, only side-stream capnographs can be used and these may not give accurate readings. However, changes in the trend can still be more useful than relying on absolute figures.

Recovery and analgesia

Recovery

Recovery from anaesthesia is improved with the use of suitable reversal agents, if available. Examples include atipamezole after medetomidine anaesthesia or sedation, and naloxone, butorphanol or buprenorphine after opioid or Hypnorm® anaesthesia or sedation. Gaseous anaesthesia, particularly with isoflurane, tends to result in more rapid recovery than injectable anaesthetics, but recovery from all forms of anaesthesia is improved by ensuring adequate maintenance of body temperature and fluid balance during and after anaesthesia.

Most small mammals will benefit from a quiet, darkened and warm recovery area. Subsequent fluid administration the same day is frequently beneficial, as many of these creatures will not be eating as normal for the first 12–24 hours.

Recovery temperatures of 28–30°C are recommended for most small mammals. This should be reduced to their normal thermal range (see chapter on husbandry) as soon as they are recovered to prevent hyperthermia.

Analgesia

Recognising pain

This can be one of the most challenging aspects of small mammal medicine. The species that we are dealing with here are all prey species and as such there is a survival benefit in not showing signs of illness or pain. When in pain, many small mammals will become

anorexic and due to their high metabolic rates will rapidly lose weight. Heart and respiratory rates will often increase – but remember that small mammals in strange surroundings with a fear response will also have elevated respiratory and heart rates. Additionally, as most rodents will have a heart rate in excess of 300 beats per minute, this can be a difficult parameter to measure with accuracy.

The following clinical signs may indicate pain in rodents (Miller & Richardson, 2011):

- Abnormal appearance, including lack of grooming, piloerection, hunched position and porphyrin staining, in rats; facial changes in mice: for example orbital tightening, nose bulges and cheek bulges
- Changes to normal behaviour: for example a decrease in normal exploratory behaviours – such as walking, sniffing – and an increase in sleeping; also, a decrease in food and water consumption
- Guarding behaviour with alteration in body posture, preventing contact with the affected area
- Self-mutilation with excessive grooming, licking, biting, scratching of the painful area
- Vocalisation when the painful area is palpated. In guinea pigs, there may be a reduction in vocalisation with pain
- Specific behaviour changes: for example belly pressing (particularly rats and mice with abdominal pain), abdominal contractions, twitching, back arching, raised tail (particularly mice) and increased aggression

Analgesia is vitally important to a quick and smooth recovery process. The time taken to return to normal activity such as grooming, eating, drinking has been shown to be considerably shortened following adequate analgesia. Dosages for analgesics frequently used in small mammals are given in Table 3.4. The administration of analgesia prior to the onset of pain makes for the most effective control. In NSAIDs COX-2 inhibitors are preferable, for example meloxicam or carprofen. Meloxicam has been used at 1.5 mg/kg once daily orally for 5 days with no significant changes in biochemistry or detectable deterioration in the health of the rabbit (Turner *et al.*, 2006). Indeed, there is evidence that the routinely published doses of meloxicam are not sufficient for post-surgical analgesia in rabbits. Meloxicam at 1 mg/kg *per os* post-surgery followed by 0.5 mg/kg once daily on the following 2 days produced a significant reduction in some pain-associated behaviours associated with ovariohysterectomy (Leach *et al.*, 2009). As always,

Table 3.4 Analgesics used in small mammals.

Drug	Ferret	Rabbit	Myomorph rodent	Chinchilla and degu	Guinea pig	Chipmunk	Marsupial
Butorphanol	0.3 q4h	0.3 q4h	1–5 q4h	0.5–2 q4–8h	0.5–1 q4–8h	1–5 q4h	0.2–0.5 q4h
Buprenorphine	0.01–0.03 q8–12h	0.01–0.05 q8–12h	0.01–0.05 q8–12h	0.01–0.05 q8–12h	0.01–0.05 q8–12h	0.01–0.05 q8–12h	0.01–0.03 q8–12h
Tramadol	3–5 q8–12h	10 q12–24h	5 q8–12h	5 q8–12h	5 q8–12h	5 q8–12h	–
Morphine	2–5 q3–4h	2–5 q3–4h	2–5 q3–4h	2–5 q3–4h	2–5 q3–4h	2–5 q3–4h	–
Carprofen	2–4 q24h	2–4 q24h	5 q24h	5 q24h	5 q24h	2–4 q24h	–
Meloxicam	0.2 q24h	0.3–0.6 q24h	0.5–1 q24h	0.3–0.6 q24h	0.3–0.6 q24h	0.3–0.6 q24h	0.2–0.4 q24h

Source: Data from Johnson-Delaney (2010), Flecknell (1998) and Mason (1997).
Values are in mg/kg body weight.
q4h, every 4 hours; q8h, every 8 hours; and so on.

care should be exercised in the use of NSAIDs in renally compromised animals.

Full opioid agonists may slow intestinal motility and therefore their use in hindgut fermenters such as rabbits, chinchillas and guinea pigs should be accompanied by gut motility enhancing medications. They can of course also produce respiratory suppression. Buprenorphine does have some of these effects but as a partial agonist they are significantly less than morphine. Tramadol has been used successfully at 10 mg/kg in the rabbit. However, pharmacokinetic data suggested that 11 mg/kg orally did not achieve the necessary levels in the blood stream to provide analgesia in humans (Souza *et al.*, 2008).

Multimodal analgesia is also important as with other mammals, as the combination of NSAIDs and opioids are of greater benefit than the separate sum of their individual parts.

Local anaesthesia may be used in rabbits and rodents at a maximum of 2 mg/kg lidocaine. This is useful for head surgery where infraorbital nerve, mental nerve, mandibular nerve, maxillary nerve and palatine nerve blocks may be performed as with cats and dogs.

Choice of analgesic depends on the level of pain and other factors, such as concurrent disease processes. Flunixin, for example, is not a good analgesic to use in dehydrated animals or those with renal disease. Opioids depress respiration and so may be contraindicated in cases of severe respiratory disease. Buprenorphine requires 2 to 3 times daily administration, while carprofen and meloxicam have been shown to be useful when given only once daily.

References

Flecknell, P.A. (1998) Analgesia in small mammals. *Seminars in Avian and Exotic Pet Medicine*, **7**(1), 41–47.

Flecknell, P.A. (2000) Anaesthesia. *Manual of Rabbit Medicine and Surgery* (ed. P. Flecknell), 1st edn. BSAVA, Cheltenham, UK.

Flecknell, P. (2001) Guinea pigs. In: *Manual of Exotic Pets* (eds A. Meredith & S. Redrobe), 4th edn. BSAVA, Quedgeley, UK.

Harkness, J.E. and Wagner, J.E. (1989) *The Biology and Medicine of Rabbits and Rodents*, 3rd edn, pp. 61–67. Lea & Febiger, Philadelphia, PA.

Johnson-Delaney, C. (2010) Marsupials. In: *Manual of Exotic Pets* (eds A. Meredith & C. Johnson-Delaney), 5th edn, pp. 103–126. BSAVA, Quedgeley, UK.

Keeble, E. (2001) Gerbils. In: *Manual of Exotic Pets* (eds A. Meredith & S. Redrobe), 4th edn, pp. 34–46. BSAVA, Cheltenham, UK.

Leach, M.C., Allweiler, S., Richardson, C., *et al.* (2009) Behavioural effects of ovariohysterectomy and oral administration of meloxicam in laboratory housed rabbits. *Research in Veterinary Science*, **87**(2), 336–347.

Mason, D.E. (1997) Anaesthesia, analgesia and sedation for small mammals. In: *Ferrets, Rabbits and Rodents* (eds E.V. Hillyer & K.E. Quesenberry), pp. 378–391. W.B. Saunders, Philadelphia, PA.

Miller, A.L. and Richardson, C.A. (2011) Rodent analgesia. *Veterinary Clinics of North America: Exotic Animal Practice*, **14**, 81–92.

Morgan, R.J., Eddy, L.B., Solie, T.N. and Turbe, C.C. (1981) Ketamine–acepromazine as anaesthetic agent for chinchillas (*Chinchilla laniger*). *Laboratory Animals*, **15**, 281–283.

Orr, H. (2001) Rats and mice. In: *Manual of Exotic Pets* (eds A. Meredith & S. Redrobe), 4th edn, pp. 13–25. BSAVA, Cheltenham, UK.

Souza, M.J., Greenacre, C.B. and Cox, S.K. (2008) Pharmacokinetics of orally administered tramadol in the domestic rabbit (*Oryctolagus cuniculus*). *American Journal of Veterinary Research*, **69**(8), 979–982.

Turner, P.V., Chen, H.C. and Taylor W.M. (2006) Pharmacokinetics of meloxicam in rabbits after single and repeat oral dosing. *Compendium of Medicine*, **56**(1), 63–67.

Further reading

Booth, R. (2003) Sugar gliders. *Seminars in Avian and Exotic Pet Medicine*, **12**(4), 228–231.

Fraser, M.A. and Girling, S.J. (2009) *Rabbit Medicine and Surgery for Veterinary Nurses*. Blackwell-Wiley, Oxford.

Harkness, J.E. and Wagner, J.E. (2000) *Biology and Medicine of Rabbits and Rodents*, 5th edn. Lea & Febiger, Philadelphia, PA.

Keeble, E. and Meredith, A. (2009) *Manual of Rodents and Ferrets*. BSAVA, Quedgeley, UK.

Meredith, A. and Flecknell, P. (2006) *Manual of Rabbits*, 2nd edn. BSAVA, Quedgeley, UK.

Meredith, A. and Johnson-Delaney, C. (2010) *Manual of Exotic Pets*, 5th edn. BSAVA, Quedgeley, UK.

Okerman, L. (1998) *Diseases of Domestic Rabbits*, 2nd edn. Blackwell Science, Oxford.

Quesenberry, K.E. and Carpenter, J. (2003) *Ferrets, Rabbits and Rodents*, 2nd edn. W.B. Saunders, Philadelphia, PA.

Classification

One way of classifying small mammals is according to their diet. There are three main categories of the commonly seen small mammals as defined by their diet.

Carnivores

The main carnivore seen in small mammal practice is the ferret, which, like the cat, is totally carnivorous. To cope with this diet, the ferret has developed sharp shearing teeth and powerful crushing jaws. In addition, because its diet consists of highly digestible fats and proteins, it has a very short gastrointestinal tract.

Herbivores

A variety of species, from lagomorphs to hystricomorphs, are herbivores. Their teeth are grinding in nature. Some species have continually growing molars and incisors, and their gastrointestinal tracts are long and often sacculated. This increases their volume and allows the bacterial fermentation that assists digestion of the relatively indigestible cellulose, which forms a large part of their diet in the wild.

Omnivores

Some rodents will eat a mixed diet. Rats and chipmunks will consume meat and eggs if offered, but both species are primarily herbivorous by preference, and true omnivores, such as humans, are uncommon among the small mammals seen routinely. The two species of marsupials we have looked at so far – the sugar glider and the Virginia opossum are both omnivores.

Individual species have become highly evolved to cope with certain types of food. In addition to the above generalisations, we also know that in the wild, many of these creatures have a changing food supply throughout the year.

General nutritional requirements

Water

Maintaining good water quality is important. Many small mammals will dunk food in their water supply or, if the water feeders are poorly situated (in bowls rather than in sip-feeders), some animals may actually defecate in their water bowls. This can cause massive bacterial population explosions which may lead to gastroenteritis. Enriching the water with mineral and vitamin supplements will also allow rapid bacterial growth.

The amount of water an individual small mammal consumes will obviously depend on the diet being offered and the species considered. On dry biscuit or seed-based diets, water consumption will be much higher than for small mammals such as rabbits and guinea pigs, which consume large amounts of fruit and vegetables. A gerbil, for example, is a desert, seed-eating rodent and may only drink 5–10 mL of water in a 24-hour period whereas an average 2 kg rabbit may drink 200 mL or more. Sugar gliders have been reported to require 103 mL water per kilogram bodyweight on a daily basis either as free water or more usually as part of the wet food they consume (Hume, 1999).

Maintenance energy requirements

Every species has a level of energy consumption per day that is needed to satisfy basic maintenance requirements. It is the energy used purely to maintain current status under minimal activity and hence is frequently the lowest energy requirement during that mammal's life. As with other species a formula has been derived as maintenance energy requirements (MER) is dependent on the basal metabolic rate (BMR = the energy requirement when at complete rest) and metabolic body weight as follows:

$$\text{MER} = \text{constant } (k) \times (\text{body weight}) \, 0.75$$

The constant, k, varies with family groups and has been estimated at 100 for adult rabbits, going up to 200 for growth and 300 for lactation (Carpenter & Kolmstetter, 2000). Other small mammals are similar, having much higher metabolic rates than their larger dog and cat counterparts. Marsupials have much lower energy requirements and their k factor is around 40–60 which means that obesity is common as owners often feed them the equivalent amount of food that would be fed to a same-sized Eutherian mammal. Studies by Dierenfield *et al.* (2006) suggest that young male sugar gliders require energy levels of between 105 and 147 kJ/day.

Energy requirements give a guide to what a small mammal must consume per day in order to continue to maintain good health and body weight. Hence, if the foods offered are so low in energy content that the small mammal has to eat more of it than will fit into its digestive system in 24 hours, the animal will rapidly lose condition.

An example is that of meat-based foods such as rodent prey which have an energy content of 19–21 kJ/g dry matter (6.3–7.5 kJ/g real or wet weight), whereas high water-content vegetable foods such as lettuce have a lower energy density of 12.5 kJ/g dry matter (0.75 kJ/g real or wet weight). The latter is therefore unlikely to meet the requirements of a high-energy-demanding ferret (irrespective of the fact it is a carnivore!) which has a requirement of 837–1255 kJME/kg per day (Carpenter & Kolmstetter, 2000).

Conversely, many pet small mammals will continue to eat until their digestive tracts are full. If all they are offered are the energy-dense seed types (the all-sunflower seed diet) then they will rapidly achieve their MER and then exceed it, leading to obesity.

Protein and amino acids

The 10 essential amino acids required by birds and reptiles are also needed by the small mammals considered here, and the concept of biological value of a protein is just as applicable. In addition, it is known that an extra supplement of the amino acid glycine is required for diets low in the amino acids methionine or arginine.

For small mammals, levels of dietary protein required have been shown to vary from maintenance to reproductive needs (Hillyer *et al.*, 1997; Dierenfield *et al.*, 2006), and from species to species:

- 35% for ferrets
- 14–20% in rodents
- 18–20% in guinea pigs
- 15–18% in rabbits as dry matter
- 16–20% for chinchillas and guinea pigs
- Reported as low as 7% but advised to be 19–25% for sugar gliders

The majority of this protein in granivorous rodent diets seems to come from seeds. Some seeds are very high providers of certain amino acids. Sunflower seeds, white millet and rapeseed, for example, provide high levels of the sulphur-containing amino acids methionine and cystine,

useful when moulting. In rabbits and other grazing herbivores, the majority of the proteins are from plant sources such as clover, alfalfa hay and good quality grass hays.

Deficiencies in amino acids have been shown to cause certain diseases. An example of this is urolithiasis seen in ferrets that are fed on plant protein sources, which are deficient in several essential amino acids. In addition, the lack of arginine in plant proteins will cause the young growing ferret to develop hyperammonaemia and neurological signs such as fitting (Bell, 1993).

Fats and essential fatty acids

Fats provide high concentrations of energy, but also supply the small mammal with essential fatty acids. These are required for cellular integrity and as the building blocks of internal chemicals such as prostaglandins, which play a part in reproduction and inflammation.

Fats also provide a carrier mechanism for the absorption of fat-soluble vitamins such as vitamin A, D, E and K.

The primary fats and essential fatty acid (EFA) for small mammals is linoleic acid, as it is for larger mammals, with the absolute dietary requirement being 1% of the diet. If the diet becomes deficient, a rapid decline in cellular integrity occurs. This is manifested clinically by the skin becoming flaky and dry and prone to recurrent infections. Fluid loss through the skin is also increased, even to the extent of causing polydipsia. It is, however, unlikely that any seed-eating small mammal will be deficient in linoleic acid as it is widely found in sunflower seeds and safflower seeds among others. It is also present in the animal protein fed to ferrets.

The latter species has a requirement for arachidonic acid as well, similar to cats, without which they will develop a number of problems such as skin diseases, including intense pruritus. Ferrets have an overall fat requirement of 20–30% of dry matter fed. Rabbits require no additional dietary fat other than the 2–5% provided in their vegetable-based diet, similar to the rodent, chinchilla and guinea pig families. Sugar gliders have been reported typically fed fats at 6–14% dry matter (Dierenfield *et al.*, 2006).

Another essential fatty acid which is thought to be important for rodents is alpha-linolenic acid which is necessary for some prostaglandin and eicosanoid synthesis.

The problem of overconsumption of fats in small mammals which are not exercising regularly is well-known, and high-fat oil seeds are the prime culprits in this case. Obesity can also be a problem for overfed, underworked ferrets fed overweight laboratory rats, for example.

Saturated animal fats provide cholesterol, often in excessive amounts, to ferrets, and hepatic lipidosis can be the result. Because rodents and rabbits have a much lower requirement for fat, excess plant fats can also cause severe hepatic lipidosis and, in rabbits, atherosclerosis in the aorta. Sources of sunflower and other high-fat oil-based seeds are often the culprits.

Carbohydrate

Carbohydrates are primarily used for rapid energy production. This is particularly important for herbivorous small mammals that constantly demand rapid supplies of energy for their often hyperactive and high-metabolic-rate lives. Small mammals that are debilitated in some way will particularly benefit from the supply of high carbohydrate foods. Ferrets have no requirement for carbohydrates (similarly to cats) with blood glucose being provided by hepatic gluconeogenesis from amino acid sources.

Fibre

Dietary fibre does not seem to be important for ferrets. Indeed, their extremely short gastrointestinal tract and minimal bacterial microflora show an inability to cope with any fibre at all. Herbivorous small mammals, particularly the guinea pig, the chinchilla and the rabbit, rely more heavily on fibre. Fibre in these species is important for a number of reasons.

First, it provides a source of abrasive food, as most of the fibre-providing foods, such as grasses, contain silicates, which wear down the teeth. This is important as these species have open-rooted or continually growing teeth, which need to be kept in check (Figures 4.1–4.3).

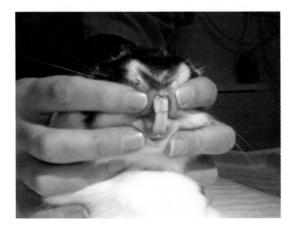

Figure 4.1 Incisor malocclusion in a rabbit may be due to inappropriately low levels of fibre in the diet, leading to molar overgrowth. This forces the mouth open so that the incisors do not wear against each other and so overgrow.

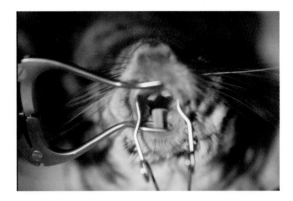

Figure 4.2 A chinchilla showing cheek tooth elongation leading to mouth ulcers and anorexia.

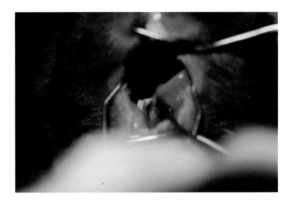

Figure 4.3 A guinea pig showing cheek tooth elongation and buccal spurs leading to ulceration of the tongue and anorexia.

Second, the fibre is essential to stimulate gut motility. These species are hind gut fermenters and rely on the microflora of the hind gut to digest food by breaking down the cellulose. Fibre is converted by the intestinal microflora into volatile fatty acids, which decrease the pH of the caecum and large bowel, so preventing bacterial overgrowth and minimising enteritis problems. Without sufficient fibre, the hind gut fermenting species develop a mucoid enteropathy, with intermittent constipation, diarrhoea and colic.

Rabbits may also be inclined to overgroom themselves, consume large volumes of fur as a 'fibre source' and so develop fur balls (trichobezoars) which may completely block the stomach. Rabbits have a requirement for 12–16% crude fibre, which is similar to guinea pigs, but chinchilla dietary fibre levels have been quoted as varying from 15% to 35% (Hoefer, 1994). The high levels for chinchillas are explained by their natural diet, which is chiefly composed of poor-quality, highly abrasive and fibrous grasses in the arid and high altitude Andes Mountains of South America. The lack of such fibre in pet diets may well account for the chinchilla's appalling susceptibility to molar malocclusion problems. It is recommended that chinchillas and rabbits are fed good quality hay, dried grass or dried grass pellets as 30–50% of their diet as a minimum. The sole feeding of pelleted and dry mix foods currently available leads to a major fibre shortage which leads to lack of dental wear, gastrointestinal upsets and obesity.

Unlike rabbits and other species, guinea pigs do not eat until their calorific requirements are satisfied and then stop, but instead eat until their digestive system is full, irrespective of how diluted the energy of the diet is by increased fibre. Recommended minimum crude fibre levels for guinea pigs are 10%, with an average of 13% being routinely offered (Hillyer *et al.*, 1997).

Vitamins

Fat-soluble vitamins

Vitamin A: In small herbivores the diet frequently contains only the vitamin A precursors, as carotenoid plant pigments, whereas in ferrets, vitamin A itself is obtained from animal proteins and does not need to be synthesised. In small herbivores, the most important form of these precursors in terms of how much vitamin A can be produced from it is beta-carotene. Because it is fat-soluble, vitamin A can be stored in the body, primarily in the liver.

Hypovitaminosis A is an uncommonly seen problem in small mammals. This is because green vegetables are good providers of the beta-carotenes. A problem can arise with rodents that develop an addiction to seeds such as sunflower seeds and peanuts. Hypovitaminosis A in rabbits can cause infertility, foetal resorption, abortion, stillbirth and neurological defects such as hydrocephalus. In ferrets it can cause infertility, poor coat and fluid retention (anasarca). Recommendations for dietary levels include 7000 IU/kg for rabbits (Carpenter & Kolmstetter, 2000). The low levels may be met by as little as 200 g of carrot per day for a 2 kg rabbit, but would require 70 kg of oats to provide the same levels!

Hypervitaminosis A rarely occurs naturally, but may be induced by overdosing with vitamin A injections at 1000 times or more the daily recommended doses. If this occurs, acute toxicity develops with mucus membrane and skin sloughing, liver damage and frequently, death within 24–48 hours. It may also be seen in ferrets fed predominantly the livers of prey items. In these cases excess bony production may occur similar to the syndrome seen in cats.

Vitamin D: This vitamin is primarily concerned with calcium metabolism. Cholecalciferol is manufactured in the small mammal's skin, a process enhanced by ultraviolet light. Small mammals kept indoors therefore produce much less of this compound, and this can lead to deficiency. Cholecalciferol must then be activated in the liver and kidneys before it can function in calcium metabolism. Once formed into its active metabolite it acts in concert with parathyroid hormone to increase reabsorption of calcium at the expense of phosphorus from the kidneys, to increase absorption of calcium from the intestines and to mobilise calcium from the bones, all of these functions increasing the blood's calcium levels.

Hypovitaminosis D_3 causes problems with calcium metabolism and leads to rickets. This is exacerbated by low-calcium-containing diets, a typical sufferer being an indoor kept small mammal, fed an all seed diet in the case of a rodent or an all meat and no calcium supplement diet for a ferret. This leads to well-muscled, heavy rodents or ferrets, with poorly mineralised bones, flaring of the epiphyseal plates at the ends of the long bones and concomitant bowing of the limbs, especially the tibiotarsal bones. Recommended minimum levels are 3.5–9 IU/g of feed for rodents and lagomorphs (Wallach & Hoff, 1982) and 0.5–1.5 IU/g dry matter for sugar gliders.

Hypervitaminosis D_3 occurs due to over supplementation with D_3 and calcium and leads to calcification of soft tissues, such as the medial arterial walls, and the kidneys, creating hypertension and causing organ failure. Recommended maximum levels are 2000 IU/kg dry matter of food fed for most small mammals (Wallach & Hoff, 1982).

Vitamin E: This compound is found in several active forms in plants, the most active being alpha-tocopherol. It is used as an antioxidant and in immune system function.

Hypovitaminosis E in ferrets results in a yellow discolouration in body fat deposits, haemolytic anaemia and a progressive paresis of the limbs. In addition, a series of firm swellings underneath the skin in the inguinal area may be seen. In rabbits a similar disease is seen with hindlimb paresis and white muscle degeneration. In hamsters, deficiencies have been reported as causing muscular weakness, ocular secretions and death, often due to cardiac muscle damage. Hypovitaminosis E may occur due to a reduction in fat metabolism or absorption as can occur in small intestinal, pancreatic or biliary diseases, or due to a lack of green plant material, the chief source of the compound, in the diet. Recommended levels for rabbits are 40 mg/kg dry matter of food offered (National Research Council, 1978).

In addition, feeding diets high in unsaturated fats (such as oily fish) may use up the body's reserves of vitamin E and so induce signs of hypovitaminosis E. This has occurred in ferrets and mink fed such a diet.

Hypervitaminosis E is extremely rare.

Vitamin K: Because of its production by bacteria, it is very difficult to get a true deficiency of vitamin K, although absorption will again be reduced when fat digestion or absorption is reduced, as in, for example, biliary or pancreatic disease.

Ferrets eating prey which has been killed by warfarin will show signs of deficiency. Rabbits and guinea pigs eating large amounts of sweet clovers can also experience a relative deficiency. The signs of disease that are seen are due to increased internal and external haemorrhage, but vitamin K also has some function in calcium/phosphorous metabolism in the bones and this may also be affected.

Water-soluble vitamins

Vitamin B_1 (thiamine): Hypovitaminosis B_1 is uncommon, but may be seen in ferrets fed raw saltwater fish which contain thiaminases. When a relative deficiency occurs, neurological signs such as opisthotonus, weakness and head tremors are seen. Ferrets can suffer from a condition known as Chastek syndrome. The symptoms may include salivation, paralysis, incoordination, pupillary dilation and easily induced convulsions, which are characterised by strong ventral flexion of the neck. Evidence of dilated cardiomyopathies is seen at postmortem. The recommended minimum level for most small mammals is around 6–7 mg/kg of diet dry matter (Wallach & Hoff, 1982). Sugar gliders fed primarily on pollen/nectar replacers may develop thiamine deficiencies owing to the low levels of thiamine in these food sources. Clinically this can present with seizures. Ensuring adequate mineral vitamin pre-loading of insects in the sugar glider diet will prevent this.

Vitamin B_2 (riboflavin): Hypovitaminosis B_2 is very rare and produces growth retardation, roughened coat, alopecia, excess scurf and cataract formation.

Niacin: Rodents fed a high proportion of one type of seed such as sweetcorn can become deficient in niacin. They exhibit blackening of the tongue (known as pellagra) and oral mucosa, retarded growth, poor coat quality and scaly dermatitis. Rats may also have anaemia and porphyrin-encrusted noses.

Biotin: Deficiency may occur in animals fed large amounts of unfertilised, raw eggs, the whites of which contain the antibiotin vitamin, avidin. This can be seen in ferrets and chipmunks when greater than 10% of the diet is composed of raw egg. Deficiency produces exfoliative dermatitis, toes may become gangrenous and slough off and ataxia may be observed. The recommended minimum requirement is 0.12–0.34 ppm food as dry matter for small mammals (Wallach & Hoff, 1982).

Folic acid: Deficiency occurs mainly because of the folic acid inhibitors that are present in some foods such as cabbage and other brassicas, oranges, beans and peas. The use of trimethoprim sulphonamide drugs also reduces gut bacterial folic acid production. Deficiency causes a number of problems, such as failure in reproductive tract maturation, macrocytic anaemia due to failure of red blood cell maturation and immune system cellular dysfunction.

Choline: Because of their interactions, the need for choline is dependent on levels of folic acid and vitamin B_{12}. That is, a deficiency may be caused if the latter are deficient, as may occur in an animal fed a diet high in fats. Deficiency causes retarded growth, disrupted fat metabolism and fatty liver damage. Recommended minimum requirements for small mammals are 880–1540 mg/kg food as dry matter.

Vitamin C: There is no direct need for this vitamin in small mammals other than the guinea pig, as vitamin C may be synthesised from glucose in the liver. In some marsupials it can be synthesised in the kidney. In the sugar glider it is not currently known whether it can synthesise vitamin C, but the Virginia opossum can do so in its liver. The guinea pig lacks the enzyme L-gluconolactone oxidase and therefore cannot convert glucose to ascorbic acid, so has a dietary requirement for vitamin C. However, during disease processes, particularly those conditions that affect liver function, it may be beneficial to the recovery process in all species to provide a dietary source of vitamin C.

Vitamin C is required for the formation of elastic fibres and connective tissues and is an excellent antioxidant, similar to vitamin E. Deficiency leads to 'scurvy'. Signs of scurvy include poor wound healing, increased bleeding due to capillary-wall fragility, gingivitis and bone alterations. These include the swelling of long bones close to joints (the epiphyseal plates), which become very painful. In addition, crusting occurs at mucocutaneous junctions such as the eyes, mouth and nose, as well as loosening of the teeth due to periodontal ligament weakening.

Vitamin C also helps in the absorption of some minerals, such as iron, from the gut.

The daily recommended requirement for guinea pigs is 10 mg/kg body weight for maintenance, increasing to 30 mg/kg body weight during gestation, although treatment of scurvy recommends levels of 50–100 mg/kg until resolution of clinical signs (Harkness & Wagner, 1995). This may be given by injection, or soluble human vitamin C tablets may be placed in the drinking water each day if the guinea pig is still drinking adequately. In addition, fresh fruit and vegetables as well as a specific supplemented guinea pig diet, should always be fed. Many deficiencies occur due to guinea pigs being housed with rabbits and therefore fed only dry rabbit food which has no supplemental vitamin C.

Minerals
Macro-minerals

Calcium: Calcium has a wide range of functions, the two most obvious being its role in the formation of the skeleton and mineralisation of bone matrix, and its use in muscular contraction. The active form of calcium in the body is the ionic double-charged molecule Ca^{2+}. Low levels of this form, even though the overall body reserves of calcium may be normal, lead to hyperexcitability, fitting and death.

Calcium levels in the body are controlled by vitamin D_3, parathyroid hormone and calcitonin.

The ratio of calcium to phosphorus is very important. As one increases the other decreases and vice versa. A ratio therefore of 2:1 calcium to phosphorus is desirable in juvenile and lactating small mammals and 1.5:1 for adults. Excessive dietary calcium (>1%) though reduces the use of proteins, fats, phosphorus, manganese, zinc, iron and iodine. In rabbits, this is exacerbated by their unique method of calcium control, in that they have no ability to reduce calcium absorption from the gut, as do other species. Instead, all available calcium is absorbed from the diet, and any excess must then be excreted through the kidneys. This leads to excess calcium excretion into the urine, the formation of calcium carbonate crystals and urolithiasis. In addition, as rabbits are herbivorous, their urine pH is alkaline, and as calcium carbonate (limestone) is less soluble in alkaline environments it precipitates more readily in the urine, forming crystals.

Levels of calcium >4% dry matter for rabbits will lead to soft tissue mineralisation in sites such as the aorta and kidneys. Calcium deficiency and metabolic bone disease problems are common in omnivorous marsupials such as the sugar glider which consume sap and insects in large quantities – both of which are deficient in calcium. Hypocalcaemic tetany has also been reported in sugar gliders.

Phosphorus: Like calcium, phosphorus is used in bone formation, but it is also used in cell structure and energy storage. It is widespread in plant and animal tissues, but in the former it may be bound up in unavailable form as phytates. Levels of phosphorus are controlled in the body as for calcium, the two being in equal and opposite equilibrium with each other. Therefore, if dietary phosphorus levels exceed calcium levels appreciably (a maximum of twice the calcium levels on average) the parathyroid glands become stimulated to produce more parathyroid hormone in an effort to restore the balance. This causes nutritional secondary hyperparathyroidism which leads to progressive bone demineralisation and then renal damage due to the high circulating levels of parathyroid hormone. High dietary phosphorus also reduces the amount of calcium which can be absorbed from the gut, as it complexes with the calcium present there. This can be a big problem for ferrets that are fed pure meat diets with no calcium or bone supplement, and in rodents that are predominantly seed eaters, as cereals are high phosphorus/low calcium foods. Feeding green vegetables or supplementation with calcium powders may therefore be necessary. In the case of ferrets a standard ferret complete diet, or whole rodent prey, should be fed to avoid this.

Potassium: As with larger mammals, this is the major intracellular positive ion. Rarely is there a dietary deficiency. Severe stress can cause hypokalaemia due to increased kidney excretion of potassium due to elevated plasma proteins, as can persistent diarrhoea. Hypokalaemia can lead to cardiac dysrhythmias, muscle spasticity and neurological dysfunction. Other symptoms are stunted growth, ascites, abnormally short hair and reduced appetite. Potassium is present in high amounts in certain fruits, such as bananas. It is controlled in equilibrium with sodium by the adrenal hormone aldosterone which promotes sodium retention and potassium excretion.

Sodium: This is the main extracellular positive ion and regulates the body's acid–base balance and osmotic potential. In conjunction with potassium, it is responsible for nerve signals and impulses. Rarely does a true dietary deficiency occur, but hyponatraemia may occur due to chronic diarrhoea or renal disease. This disrupts the osmotic potential gradient in the kidneys and water is lost leading to further dehydration. Excessive levels of sodium in the diet (>10 times recommended) lead to poor coat, polyuria, hypertension, oedema and death.

Chlorine: This is the major extracellular negative ion and responsible for maintaining acid–base balances in conjunction with sodium and potassium. Deficiencies are rare, but if they do occur, retarded growth and kidney disease are commonly seen.

Micro-minerals (trace elements)

Copper: Copper is used in haemoglobin synthesis, collagen synthesis and in the maintenance of the nervous system. Copper toxicosis has been reported in ferrets in the United States as a possible hereditary storage disease. The symptoms are of liver disease, as seen in Bedlington Terriers (Brown, 1997). Deficiency has been reported in hamsters as a cause of poor coat quality and generalised alopecia. Minimum recommended levels are 13–20 ppm (Wallach & Hoff, 1982).

Iodine: Iodine's sole function is in thyroid hormone synthesis, which affects metabolic rate. Deficiency causes goitre, and has knock-on effects on growth causing stunting, stillbirths and neurological problems. It is a relatively uncommon finding in small mammals but may occur in species such as rabbits that are fed large volumes of goitrogenic (iodine inhibiting) plants such as cabbage, kale and Brussels sprouts.

Iron: This is essential, as with larger mammals, for the formation of the oxygen-carrying part of the haemoglobin molecule. Absorption from the gut is normally relatively poor, as the body is very good at recycling its own iron levels. Vitamin C enhances iron uptake from the gut. In sugar gliders Dierenfield *et al.* (2006) recommend less than 50 μg/g of dry diet of iron to avoid iron storage disease, which can damage the liver.

Manganese: Deficiency has been reported as causing poor bone growth, with limb shortening as a consequence. Recommended daily requirements are from 40 to 120.7 ppm with the higher dosages for guinea pigs (Wallach & Hoff, 1982).

Selenium: The main role of selenium is as part of the antioxidant enzyme glutathione peroxidase, with which vitamin E is also involved. Its functions are therefore similar to those of vitamin E in that it helps keep peroxidases from attacking polyunsaturated fats in cell membranes. A general deficiency in both selenium and vitamin E will lead to liver necrosis, steatitis and muscular dystrophy. The selenium content of plants is dependent on where they were grown and the levels of selenium in the soil. Recommended minimum requirements are still not clearly defined for small mammals in general.

Zinc: This is a vital trace element for wound healing and tissue formation, forming part of a number of enzymes. Deficiencies can occur in young, rapidly growing guinea pigs and chinchillas fed on plant material high in phytates such as cabbage, wheat bran and beans. In addition, high dietary calcium decreases zinc uptake. Deficiency produces retarded growth and poor skin quality with increased scurf and hyperirritability. Zinc deficiency alopecia is particularly seen at about day 50 of gestation in chinchillas with hair regrowth occurring 2–3 weeks after parturition (Smith *et al.*, 1977). Minimum recommended requirements are 20–122 ppm for small mammals (Wallach & Hoff, 1982). Zinc toxicosis has been reported in ferrets, with anaemia, lethargy and hindlimb paresis, and was associated with feeding from zinc galvanised buckets (Donnelly, 1997).

Requirements for young and lactating small mammals

Rabbit

Neonatal rabbits nurse for only 3–5 minutes at a time once or twice in a 24-hour period and are totally dependent on their mother's milk up to day 21 postpartum (Okerman, 1994). At this time they should be weighed, as solid foods offered will be increasingly consumed, and weight losses may be seen if they do not eat enough of this. The doe may be offered increasingly more pelleted dry foods before weaning, as her energy demands increase to 3.5 times maintenance by peak lactation. *Ad-lib* dry food is therefore often advocated for the doe at this stage. It should be noted though that levels of food for the doe should not start to be dramatically increased until 5–7 days after parturition. Early overfeeding can cause excessive milk production, and mastitis will result if the kits do not have enough appetite to empty the mammary glands at each sitting. For hand-rearing formulas, see page 28.

Growing kits require higher levels of vitamin D_3 and calcium than their adult counterparts. To ensure that this is received, a balanced diet should be offered, combining pelleted food, good quality grass hay and some greens.

Dry foods should be carefully chosen. Many are balanced nutritionally, but only if the rabbit consumes all parts equally. Rabbits are concentrate selectors (that is they will preferentially pick out those foods containing the highest calories in their environment and eat them first). Therefore, if offered one of the 'muesli'-type diets, it will eat all of the fatty, carbohydrate foods first, and, if provided *ad-lib*, they will not get around to eating the high fibre, calcium-containing grass pellets. Hence, it is advised either to use a homogenous pelleted diet where all of the pellets are exactly the same, or to feed enough in 24 hours so that the bowl is completely emptied before offering more. Access to unfiltered natural sunlight is also advised, even if for only 15–20 min/day, to ensure sufficient vitamin D_3 synthesis. Lactating does will also have higher calcium requirements, and so their consumption of pelleted diet and grass products (both high in calcium) will increase. Care should be taken, though, not to overdo pelleted diets at the expense of good quality hay/grass, as excessive amounts of calcium and vitamin D_3 can come to be present, leading to reno- and urolithiasis as well as soft tissue mineralisation.

Ferret

Young ferrets have a higher calorific requirement than adults, as do lactating jills, needing 1.5–2 times maintenance adult calorie levels. The protein requirement is a minimum of 35% in young growing ferrets and lactating jills with a fat level of a minimum of 25% as dry matter (Kupersmith, 1998). For rearing formulas see page 35.

Rodents, chinchilla and guinea pig

The guinea pig sow, when lactating, has a requirement for vitamin C which increases from 10 to 30 mg/kg per day. She also has the usual increases in calcium, energy and protein demands. The demands for increased calories are particularly important, as the long gestation of the guinea pig (average 63 days) and the frequent litter size of 3–4 piglets, place huge stresses on the sow. If these increased requirements are not met, then a condition known as pregnancy toxaemia, or ketosis ensues. This is when a lack of available calories leads to increased fat mobilisation. If this is combined with a glucose deficit the fats are converted into chemicals known as ketones. These produce metabolic acidosis in addition to the hypoglycaemic state. Death can follow within 24 hours. Prevention is geared towards avoiding obesity and sudden dietary change, both of which set up the condition.

Young guinea pigs are frequently not hungry for the first 12–24 hours after birth because they have brown fat reserves. They should not be force-fed during this time. Young chinchillas and guinea pigs eat solid foods practically from day 1 after parturition. It is important therefore to ensure high-fibre foods are offered preferentially at this stage so as to avoid them developing into fussy eaters in later life.

Rodents such as rats and gerbils have been quoted as needing a dietary protein level of 20–26% during and prior to pregnancy and lactation, as opposed to their more usual 16–18%.

For rearing formulas see page 29.

Omnivorous marsupials

Energy requirements increase significantly in sugar gliders from around 46 kJ/day as basal requirements to 229 kJ/day for growth and activity. Lactation has much higher demands on the female marsupial than gestation, due to the altricial nature of the joeys when born. Many insectivorous marsupials can enter a state of torpor when food sources (mainly the insect source which provides most of the protein, fats and calories) are scarce to conserve energy. Their body temperature will drop and they will appear to be unrousable. It is not uncommon for these periods to last up to 11 hours.

For rearing formulas for sugar gliders and Virginia opossums see page 33.

Requirements for debilitated small mammals

In general, requirements for debilitated animals will vary from 1.5 to 3 times maintenance levels, with the lower levels being for mildly injured or infected animals and the upper levels for burns victims and cases of serious organ damage or septicaemia.

Fluid therapy as additional support is essential, particularly for the herbivorous mammals, which have very high maintenance requirements when compared with cats and dogs (on average 80–100 mL/kg per day). Also, herbivore gut contents are voluminous and need to be kept fluid. For further details see chapters 6 and 8.

Rabbit

The debilitated rabbit may be supported with nasogastric or oral syringe feeding of vegetable-based baby foods (lactose free varieties), or, for preference, with a gruel composed of ground dry rabbit pellets and water as this will supply a better fibre level for gut stimulation.

Amounts suggested to feed at any one sitting vary from 3 to 15 mL four to six times daily.

A nasogastric tube (more correctly a naso-oesophageal tube as the tubing must not allow reflux of acid stomach contents into the oesophagus) is placed after first spraying the nose with lignocaine spray. A 3–4 French tube is pre-measured from the extended nose to the seventh rib or caudal end of the sternum and then inserted. Sterile water should be flushed through the tube before and after feeding to ensure it is correctly placed and does not become blocked. The tube may then be glued, taped or sutured to the dorsal aspect of the head and a bung inserted when not in use. It may be necessary to put an Elizabethan collar on the rabbit to prevent removal.

The use of cisapride at a dose of 0.5 mg/kg orally every 8–24 hours (Smith & Bergmann, 1997) is to be advocated in rabbits to stimulate large bowel activity, and encourage the return of normal appetite.

Older rabbits often do better on lower protein (14%) and higher fibre (18%) diets as these reduce the risk of obesity, kidney and liver damage.

Ferret

The debilitated ferret may be supported with nasogastric or oral syringe feeding of meat-based baby foods, or commercially prepared liquid meat-based formulas designed for cats and dogs such as Reanimyl® and Hill's a/d. Amounts suggested for feeding at any one sitting vary from 2 to 10 mL three to six times daily. It is vitally important that no debilitated ferret goes longer than 4 hours without nutritional support, as they will become rapidly hypoglycaemic.

A feline 3 French nasogastric tube can easily be placed via the nostril after first spraying the area with lignocaine spray. The tube should be premeasured to extend from the nose tip to the level of the seventh rib (i.e. it is really a naso-oesophageal tube, to avoid the acid contents of the stomach refluxing and causing an oesophagitis) and cut to this length. It may then be secured with tissue glue, or taped or sutured to the skin over the forehead. It is advised to fit an Elizabethan collar to prevent the ferret removing the tube. The tube should be flushed with sterile water before and after feeding to ensure the tubing is in the correct position and does not block.

Rodents, chinchilla and guinea pig

Syringe feeding orally or using a straight avian crop tube to administer liquid food directly into the oesophagus are advised. The latter may be stressful, as the rodent must be scruffed prior to administration. Volumes suggested vary from 0.5 mL for a mouse, up to 2.5 mL for a rat at any one sitting, the dose to be repeated 6–8 times daily to ensure correct calorie administration. Diets such as dry rodent pellets ground in a coffee grinder and then added to water to form gruel, or the use of vegetable-based, lactose-free baby foods may be used. Guinea pigs and chinchillas benefit from the use of oral cisapride to stimulate gut motility, as well as the use of gruels made from higher-fibre chinchilla or rabbit pellets. Naso-oesophageal tubes can be attempted for the larger individuals of these two species.

Marsupials

For sugar gliders a typical diet would include the following (Johnson-Delaney, 2010): 15 mL of Leadbeater's mix (which is in itself made of 150 mL warm water plus 150 mL honey plus one shelled, hard-boiled egg plus 15 g of baby cereal (rice-based) plus 5 g of powdered avian vitamin and mineral supplement); 15 g of an insectivore/carnivore diet; and then various additions as treats such as chopped fruit and live gut fed insects, which should not exceed 10% of the diet. The practice of gut-loading insects with vitamin/mineral supplements is useful and should be familiar to anyone keeping reptiles.

Probiotics

The use of oral probiotics is recommended for small herbivores, to encourage normal digestive function by providing enzymes and to encourage normal pH conditions. Probiotics are best added to the drinking water but may be added to the syringed food to ensure consumption.

References

Bell, J. (1993) Ferret nutrition and diseases associated with inadequate nutrition. *Proceedings of the North American Veterinary Conference*, Orlando, FL, pp. 719–720.

Brown, S.A. (1997) Basic anatomy, physiology and husbandry. *Ferrets, Rabbits and Rodents: Clinical Medicine and Surgery* (eds E.V. Hillyer & K.E. Quesenberry), pp. 3–13. W.B. Saunders, Philadelphia, PA.

Carpenter, J.W. and Kolmstetter, C.M. (2000) Feeding small exotic mammals. *Hill's Nutrition*, pp. 943–960. Mark Mervis Institute, Marceline, MO.

Dierenfield, E.S., Thomas, D. and Ives, R. (2006) Comparison of commonly used diets on intake, digestion, growth and health in captive sugar gliders (*Petaurus breviceps*). *Journal of Exotic Pet Medicine*, **15**(3), 218–224.

Donnelly, T.M. (1997) Basic anatomy, physiology and husbandry. *Ferrets, Rabbits and Rodents: Clinical Medicine and Surgery* (eds E.V. Hillyer & K.E. Quesenberry), pp. 147–159. W.B. Saunders, Philadelphia, PA.

Harkness, J.E. and Wagner, J.E. (1995) *The Biology and Medicine of Rabbits and Rodents*, 4th edn, p. 230. Lea & Febiger, Philadelphia, PA.

Hillyer, E.V., Quesenberry, K.E. and Donnelly, T.M. (1997) Biology, husbandry and clinical techniques. *Ferrets, Rabbits and Rodents: Clinical Medicine and Surgery* (eds E.V. Hillyer & K.E. Quesenberry), pp. 243–259. W.B. Saunders, Philadelphia, PA.

Hoefer, H.L. (1994) Chinchillas. *Veterinary Clinics North American Small Animal Practice*, **24**, 103–111.

Hume, I. (1999) Metabolic rates and nutrient requirements. *Marsupial Nutrition* (ed. I. Hume), pp. 1–34. Cambridge University Press, Cambridge.

Johnson-Delaney, C. (2010) Marsupials. *Manual of Exotic Pets* (eds A. Meredith & C. Johnson-Delaney), 5th edn, pp. 103–126. BSAVA, Quedgeley, UK.

Kupersmith, D.S. (1998) A practical overview of small mammal nutrition. *Seminars in Avian and Exotic Pet Medicine*, **7**(3), 141–147.

National Research Council (1978) *Nutrient Requirements of Laboratory Animals*. National Academy Press, Washington, DC.

Okerman, L. (1994) *Diseases of Domestic Rabbits*, 1st edn. Blackwell Science, Oxford.

Smith, D.A. and Bergmann, P.M. (1997) Formulary. *Ferrets, Rabbits and Rodents: Clinical Medicine and Surgery* (eds E.V. Hillyer & K.E. Quesenberry), pp. 392–403. W.B. Saunders, Philadelphia, PA.

Smith, J.C., Brown, E.D. and Cassidy, W.A. (1977) Zinc and vitamin A: interrelationships of zinc metabolism. *Current Aspects in Health and Disease*. Alan R. Liss, Inc., New York.

Wallach, J.D. and Hoff, G.L. (1982) Nutritional diseases of mammals. *Noninfectious Diseases of Wildlife* (eds G.L. Hoff & J.W. Davis), pp. 133–135 and 143–144. Iowa State University Press, Iowa.

Further reading

Booth, R. (2003) Sugar gliders. *Seminars in Avian and Exotic Pet Medicine*, **12**(4), 228–231.

Fraser, M.A. and Girling, S.J. (2009) *Rabbit Medicine and Surgery for Veterinary Nurses*. Blackwell-Wiley, Oxford.

Harkness, J.E. and Wagner, J.E. (2000) *Biology and Medicine of Rabbits and Rodents*, 5th edn. Lea & Febiger, Philadelphia, PA.

Keeble, E. and Meredith, A. (2009) *Manual of Rodents and Ferrets*. BSAVA, Quedgeley, UK.

MacPherson, C. (1997) *Sugar Gliders. A Complete Owner's Manual*. Barron's Educational Series, Hauppage, NY.

Meredith, A. and Flecknall, P. (2006) *Manual of Rabbits*, 2nd edn. BSAVA, Quedgeley, UK.

Meredith, A. and Johnson-Delaney, C. (2010) *Manual of Exotic Pets*, 5th edn. BSAVA, Quedgeley, UK.

Okerman, L. (1998) *Diseases of Domestic Rabbits*, 2nd edn. Blackwell Science, Oxford.

Quesenberry, K.E. and Carpenter, J. (2003) *Ferrets, Rabbits and Rodents*, 2nd edn. W.B. Saunders, Philadelphia, PA.

Chapter 5   Common Diseases of Small Mammals

DISEASES OF THE DOMESTIC RABBIT

Skin disease

Ectoparasitic

Mites

Cheyletiella parasitivorax produces dense, white scurf along the dorsum, starting around the nape of the neck and spreading outwards and caudally. The fur drops out and new fur regrows rapidly. The condition may not appear pruritic, although in severe cases rabbits will self-traumatise. Microscopically it appears as a large mite, with an obvious waist. The mouthparts have claws, and the ends of the legs possess combs rather than suckers. Owners may be bitten by this mite in the classical pattern of three bites.

Psoroptes cuniculi lives in the external ear canal of rabbit, where it irritates the lining making it weep serum. The serum dries in brown crusts which in severe cases may obliterate the lumen completely (see Figure 5.1). Infestation can lead to serious secondary bacterial ear infections which can cause vestibular disease. The mites are large enough to be seen with the naked eye. Microscopically they have pointed mouthparts and conical suckers to the ends of the legs.

Leporacarus (Listrophorus) gibbus is a non-pathogenic fur mite of rabbits. It is an oval mite with short legs, and so may be distinguished from the above two mites on clinical signs and the absence of a 'waist' and having conical suckers and combs on the end of its legs.

Neotrombicula autumnalis is the harvest mite. It is not a true parasite, but the juvenile (six-legged) bright orange-red mite may irritate the skin of rabbits which have access to hay, grass or straw. It causes irritation of the skin surface chiefly over the palmar/plantar aspect of the feet, the face and ears. Its typical orange-red colour is visible to the naked eye, and its six-legged form distinguishes it from other mites.

All of the above mites are surface-dwelling, and may therefore be harvested for identification using a flea comb, or Sellotape® strip applied to the affected area and then stuck to a microscope slide for examination.

Burrowing mites are rare in rabbits, the two main ones being *Sarcoptes scabiei* and *Notoedres* spp. They produce intensely pruritic skin lesions, and are diagnosed after skin scrapings and microscopic examination.

Lice

Haemodipsus ventricosis is an uncommon louse in domestic rabbits, and belongs to the sucking (Anoplura) family. It is slender and often blood filled, and may cause significant anaemia in young kits.

Fleas

The rabbit flea is *Spillopsyllus cuniculi* and is the chief vector for myxomatosis. It tends to concentrate around the ears of the rabbit and may be distinguished from the cat and dog flea by the presence of obliquely arranged genal ctenidium. These are the fronds which line the mouthparts of the flea, and which are horizontal in the cat and dog fleas.

Blow-fly

Blow-flies cause a condition called myiasis ('fly strike').

This horrible condition is common in outdoor rabbits that have perineal soiling due to urine scalding or diarrhoea. It is caused by flies including the blue, black and green bottle families. These lay their eggs on the skin of the rabbit. In warm conditions these eggs hatch into larvae within 2 hours. The larvae then mature and burrow into the rabbit.

Other parasites

Coenurus serialis, which is the intermediate host for the adult tapeworm of dogs *Taenia serialis*, may form large, fluid-filled cysts in subcutaneous sites containing the scolices of the tapeworm.

Veterinary Nursing of Exotic Pets, Second Edition. Edited by Simon J. Girling. © 2013 John Wiley & Sons, Ltd. Published 2013 by John Wiley & Sons, Ltd.

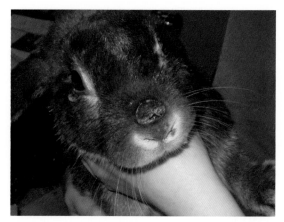

Figure 5.2 Myxoma lesions on the nose of a rabbit with partial immunity to myxomatosis.

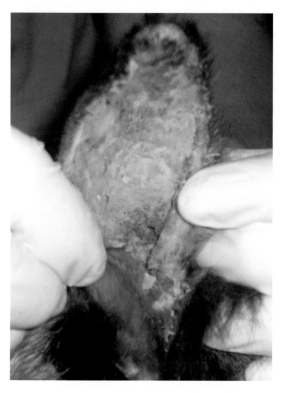

Figure 5.1 *Psoroptes cuniculi* infection in a rabbit. Note the extensive tan-coloured crusting and ulceration inside the pinna.

Viral

Myxomatosis

In rabbits with partial immunity, myxomatosis produces crusting nodules on the skin of the nose, lips, feet and base of the ears (see Figure 5.2). In these rabbits, death can still occur up to 40 days after the initial signs, but many will recover. The acute form of myxomatosis causes oedema of the periocular region, the base of the ears and the anal and genital openings. The virus attacks internal organs as well, and in the unvaccinated domestic rabbit is almost invariably fatal, running a course of 5–15 days.

The myxomatosis virus is a member of the pox virus family, and is transmitted by biting insects, chiefly fleas, but mosquitoes and lice may also provide a source of infection.

Bacterial

Rabbit pus is thick and inspissated. Abscesses are common in the head where they are invariably associated with dental disease. Bacteria involved include *Pasteurella multocida* and *Staphylococcus aureus* although, after prolonged antibiotic treatment, many anaerobic bacteria will flourish.

'Blue fur disease' is caused by *Pseudomonas aeruginosa*, which produces a blue pigment, staining the fur, and is common in outdoor rabbits, or those kept in damp conditions. It will infect damaged skin, such as occurs in the dewlap area of many lop breeds, where wet skin chafes.

Rabbit syphilis, due to *Treponema paraluiscuniculi*, affects the anogenital area, the nose and lips, producing brown crusting lesions. These may progress over the face. This bacterium is thought to be passed from doe to young during parturition, and may be sexually transmitted from buck to doe and vice versa. It is not infectious for humans.

Fungal

The two commonly seen are *Microsporum canis*, which will fluoresce under ultraviolet Wood's lamp, and the environmental *Trichophyton mentagrophytes*, which does will not. The lesions are dry, scaly, often grey plaques appearing over the head initially, but then spreading to the feet and the rest of the body. Culturing brushings of the lesions on dermatophyte medium is advised for definitive diagnosis.

Managemental

The fur of fine- and long-haired breeds, such as the Angoras mats easily, particularly when the animal is bedded on straw, hay or shavings. Owners are advised to keep them on paper or wire mesh, and to groom their rabbit once or twice daily.

Overgrown claws are common, particularly in hutch-kept rabbits with little access to the outside. Claws should be regularly assessed and, if necessary, trimmed on a 4–6-week basis. Overgrown claws can lead to lateral twisting of digit joints and deformity of the foot.

Perineal soiling may be due to faecal soiling from diarrhoea, or inability to consume the caecotrophs which are softer than the faecal pellet. Urine scalding is also common. Older rabbits may have spinal arthritis, which prevents them from positioning correctly to urinate, and lop breeds have excessive folds of skin around the urogenital area. For mild cases, provision of absorbent bedding underneath a deep layer of straw is advised. Attention to cage and rabbit hygiene on a daily basis is essential to prevent blow-fly strike and secondary bacterial skin infections.

Digestive disease
Oral

Dental disease may present from salivation and anorexia, through jaw bone swellings, to full-blown abscesses. Overgrown teeth may be obvious, as with incisor malocclusions, or may be hidden from external view, as with cheek teeth malocclusions. Dental problems may affect other parts of the head, creating abscesses behind the globe of the eye, or the tear duct as it runs over the cheek teeth and maxillary incisor roots, causing pus to appear at the eye or nares.

Causes of dental disease include hereditary defects (Netherland dwarf and lops), due to a shortened rostrocaudal length of skull and abnormal bite (Figure 5.3), or dietary deficiencies. The two most commonly cited dietary deficiencies include a lack of suitable abrasive foodstuffs for dental wear, and a lack of calcium and vitamin D$_3$ for proper jawbone mineralisation.

Rabbits have adapted to survive on a diet consisting of 85% grass, and 15% leafy herbage. Meadow grass is very high in silicates. These are abrasive and are naturally very wearing. Rabbits' normal dental growth has therefore evolved to cope with this. With a reduced abrasive diet, teeth won't wear as rapidly and overgrowth will occur. As the rabbit's mandible is narrower than its maxilla, even wear occurs by lateral movement of the mandible across the maxilla. In less abrasive, easier-chewed diets, this happens less effectively, and so the outer or buccal edges of the mandibular cheek teeth wear, and the inner or lingual edges of the maxillary cheek teeth wear, causing sharp points to form on the tongue side of the mandibular teeth and the cheek side of the maxillary. These points grow, the teeth tilt, and the mandibular teeth then cut into the tongue, and the maxillary teeth into the cheeks leading to deep ulcers, pain and anorexia.

The roots of the cheek teeth may grow back into the jaws as they elongate, due to a lack of space inside the mouth. The roots then push through the ventral aspect of the mandible, and may be felt as a series of lumps underneath the angle of the lower jaw. In the maxilla, the roots of the last two cheek teeth can push into the orbit of the eye, causing ocular pain and epiphora.

Incisors may overgrow due to elongation of the molars pushing the mouth open wider. The maxillary incisors are tightly curved whereas the mandibular incisors are more gently curving. If the mouth is forced slightly open, the maxillary incisors no longer close rostral to the mandibular ones, and overgrowth ensues. The maxillary incisors curl back and into the mouth like ram's-horns, the mandibular incisors grow up in front of the nose. Maxillary root elongation may also occur when incisors meet end on end, causing constriction of the tear duct which bends around them. This leads to dacryocystitis (inflammation of the tear duct). The duct then dams back and a milky white discharge appears at the eye. This is often misdiagnosed as a primary conjunctivitis (see Figure 5.4).

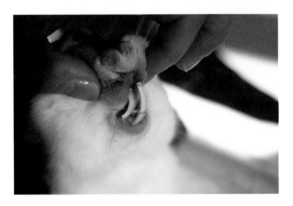

Figure 5.3 Brachygnathism is hereditary and may be a cause of malocclusion in rabbits.

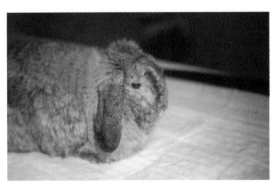

Figure 5.4 Ocular disease may be associated with rabbit snuffles but often starts in the tear duct (dacryocystitis) due to pinching of the duct by overgrown (usually incisor) teeth roots.

Other causes of dental disease include physical trauma to the head and inappropriate 'clipping' of the teeth with nail clippers. This twists and cracks the tooth root causing further deformity and predisposing to infection.

Radiography of the rabbit head plus close oral examination under sedation or anaesthesia is essential to examine the full extent of the dental problem. Positive contrast techniques may be used in the tear ducts to highlight areas of narrowing or blockage (see Chapter 7).

Gastrointestinal

Dietary

Dietary causes, for example, a sudden change in diet, will lead to temporary diarrhoea. Other dietary factors include the type of food fed. Spoiled foods and part-fermented grass cuttings will inevitably lead to diarrhoea.

Iatrogenic

Iatrogenic causes include the oral administration of certain antibiotics, for example penicillin and clindamycin. These destroy the normal flora of the gut, leaving bacteria such as *Clostridium spiriformae* or *Clostridium perfringens* to flourish. These are found in small quantities in the normal gastrointestinal flora of the rabbit, but once they achieve a critical threshold level, they can release toxins which are absorbed into the bloodstream and cause toxaemia and death.

Bacterial

Bacteria, for example *Escherichia coli*, common in young weaner rabbits, are a cause of sudden death, due to the release of enterotoxins. Death may occur before any signs of diarrhoea. An unknown agent, suspected to be bacterial, is the cause of Epizootic Rabbit Enteropathy (ERE) which is the single biggest cause of mortality in rabbits fattened for the meat industry in Europe. Clinical signs include loss of appetite, over-full stomachs and watery diarrhoea with a high mortality rate. Disease can be stopped by rapid treatment with antibiotics such as tiamulin and bacitracin (Huybens *et al.*, 2008).

Parasitic

Coccidia, for example *Eimeria* spp., are single-celled protozoal parasites which destroy the lining of the small intestine, causing diarrhoea and death in heavy infestations. In mild cases it may simply cause poor growth and stunting in young rabbits. *Eimeria stiedae* is of particular importance in rabbits as it will also damage the liver. Coccidial oocysts may be detected in the faeces.

The stomach worm *Graphidium strigosum* and the small intestinal worm *Trichostrongylus retortaeformis* are usually only found in rabbits with access to the outside, where they may pick up the eggs of these worms directly from wild rabbits' faeces or indirectly via passive spread from wild birds, etc. A large intestinal pinworm, *Passalurus ambiguus*, is commonly seen, but rarely causes disease. All of these worms' eggs may be detected in the faeces by flotation methods.

Hypomotility disorders

Aetiology and clinical signs: One of the most important factors is the level of indigestible fibre in the diet. A lack of fibre results in reduced motility both by a lack of physical stimulation of the colon due to the absence of large fibre particles and a decreased production of volatile fatty acids in the caecum. Other causes include: increased adrenergic stimulation due to stress or pain resulting in reduced motility (e.g. dental disease, osteoarthritis, etc.); and intestinal infectious diseases, all of which can cause varying effects on gut motility. Most cases in domestic rabbits are due to stress and a long-term dietary deficiency in indigestible fibre.

Stomach impaction seen in cases of hypomotility usually comprises a matt of fur and food material. These trichobezoars in rabbits have been blamed for occlusion of the pylorus so causing gastrointestinal motility disorders. The stomach of the rabbit, however, has been shown to always contain food material and groomed fur (Okerman, 1994). Gastric foreign bodies were artificially created using latex, but rabbits affected showed no reduction in appetite or in weight (Leary *et al.*, 1984). It is now widely assumed that trichobezoar formations are due to reduced gastrointestinal motility rather than the cause of it. Intestinal obstructions though can occur and will also lead to stomach distension (see Figure 5.5).

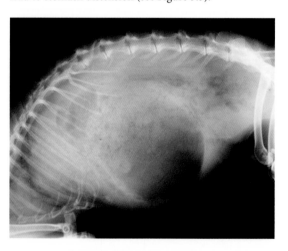

Figure 5.5 Lateral radiograph of a rabbit with a suspected small intestinal obstruction and a massively dilated stomach.

Onset can be rapid or more insidious. The rabbit is often dull, anorexic and lethargic, may show signs of dehydration and is often suffering from hepatic lipidosis and ketoacidosis. Death, when it occurs, is usually due to liver and kidney failure.

Leporine dysautonomia is another cause of hypomotility. Clinical signs include dry mucus membranes, reduced tear production, dilated pupils, bradycardia, urinary retention (with overflow incontinence), caecal and large intestine impaction, loss of anal tone and proprioceptive deficits. Aspiration pneumonia may also be seen due to megaoesophagus.

Diagnosis: Radiographs of the abdomen may show a distended stomach with food material and an accumulation of gas in stomach and caecum. Blood results show hepatic dysfunction, elevation of hepatic associated leakage enzymes (AST) lipaemia, metabolic acidosis and hyperglycaemia although early cases may show hypoglycaemia, and dehydration as witnessed by an elevated packed cell volume (usually over 45%). Cases where hepatic lipidosis and ketoacidosis are advanced may see damage to the kidneys and resultant elevation in urea, creatinine, phosphate and potassium.

Diagnosis of dysautonomia include absence/reduction of tears on a Schirmer tear test (<3 mm in a minute), dramatic miosis when 0.1% pilocarpine is applied to the eyes, radiography demonstrating aspiration pneumonia, megaoesophagus, impacted/distended caecum and large intestine and distended urinary bladder. Histopathology reveals chromolytic degeneration of the autonomic neurons similar to that seen in equine grass-sickness cases.

Prevention: Ensure all rabbits are fed on a high-fibre diet, for example freshly grazed grass, good quality hay or dried grass. Any stressful procedure where significant catecholamine release is likely to occur, for example postoperatively – it is beneficial to use prokinetic drugs such as metoclopramide and ranitidine and to provide adequate analgesia.

Hepatic lipidosis
Aetiology: Hepatic lipidosis is seen most commonly in overweight indoor rabbits that go through a period of anorexia or food withdrawal.

In rabbits we generally assume that increased mobilisation of fat deposits from a period of anorexia/food deprivation/pregnancy is the main cause. However, stress can increase fat mobilisation in overweight rabbits and minor invasive procedures such as saline injections induced an increase in plasma free fatty acid and glycerol levels in obese rabbits (Lafontan & Agid, 1979). A high-fat diet increases the risks of ketonaemia and so ketoacidosis during anorexia (Jean-Blain & Durix, 1985). Pregnant does between days 24 and 30 are insulin resistant adding to the likelihood they will develop pregnancy ketosis (McLaughlin & Fish, 1994).

The longer the anorexia, the worse the lipid mobilisation and the more the liver is swamped with lipids and free fatty acids. The lipids affect hepatocyte function and make them less able to successfully perform the TCA cycle which is further exacerbated by an absence of glucose in the bloodstream.

Once the liver has become lipidotic, the kidneys frequently follow.

Clinical signs: The early stages may be imperceptible. Most cases are triggered by a period of anorexia, the main clinical signs being reduction in food intake and faecal output. As the condition progresses, the rabbit becomes comatose, hypoglycaemic and acidotic, and dies of liver and kidney failure. Any rabbit anorexic for 12 hours or more (6–8 hours in pregnant does) should be given assisted feeding.

Diagnosis: There is no liver specific leakage enzyme in the rabbit; therefore, aspartate aminotransferase (AST), lactate dehydrogenase (LDH) and creatine kinase (CK) are measured together as AST is found in the liver and skeletal muscle, LDH in liver, cardiac and skeletal muscle and CK only in skeletal muscle. GGT elevations are associated with hepatobiliary disease rather than hepatocellular damage, and therefore have been associated with conditions such as hepatic coccidiosis by *E. stiedae*.

Elevations in triglycerides and cholesterol levels will also occur. There may be hypoglycaemia in severe cases, and levels of β-hydroxybutyrate will be elevated where ketosis is present.

Serum proteins may also be elevated, particularly alpha-2- and beta-2-lipoprotein increases. Finally, ultrasound and endoscopic biopsy of the liver gives a reliable indication of hepatic lipidosis but obviously gives no indication of the degree of ketoacidosis present.

Respiratory disease
Pasteurellosis
Pasteurella multocida causes 'rabbit snuffles'. It is commonly found in the airways of unaffected rabbits, but it can lead to purulent oculonasal discharge, and wet, matted fur of the forepaws. This can develop into pneumonia. *P. multocida* contains a dermonecrotic toxin similar to that causing atrophic rhinitis in pigs. Hence many rabbits with these

infections are left with permanent upper and lower respiratory tract damage. Poor housing, with damp, ammonia-laden bedding can irritate the airways and allow rapid infection to occur. Dental disease and myxomatosis are other factors. Similarly, overcrowded hutches and concurrent disease elsewhere in the body may lower immunity.

Pasteurella infections may also be found in tooth abscesses and middle ear disease. Infections may result in chronic abscessation of the lungs, mediastinum, pleurae and pericardium.

Other bacterial infections

Bordetella bronchiseptica may be found as a commensal of the upper airways of the rabbit but it can also produce disease. Some strains are cytotoxic and so enhance infections of *Pasteurella multocida*.

Staphylococcus aureus and *S. albus* are commonly isolated from the upper respiratory tract of healthy and diseased rabbits. *S. aureus* can produce toxins which destroy neutrophils as well as protein A which can bind to immunoglobulins. It has been associated with abscessation of the head, lungs, mediastinum and middle ears.

Viral haemorrhagic disease

This is a calicivirus and has been in the United Kingdom since 1992. It does not cause respiratory disease exclusively, as it will attack all organs within the body, particularly the lungs, digestive system and liver. It is spread via contact, and in naïve rabbits it is 100% fatal, often with no obvious clinical disease. Post-mortem examination reveals widespread internal haemorrhage. The disease does not affect rabbits under the age of approximately 10 weeks, as the virus requires the presence of a liver enzyme which is not produced until after this age. Therefore very young kits are protected from the disease.

Cardiovascular disease
Arterial wall calcification

With an excess of calcium/vitamin D_3, calcium becomes deposited in the walls of the major blood vessels, reducing their elasticity and leading to increased blood pressure. This is common in the aorta, and may also occur within the kidney parenchyma itself. Some rabbits may be genetically predisposed to this problem. There is no cure. Prevention is aimed at avoiding over-supplementation with calcium and vitamin D_3.

Cardiomyopathy and valvular disease

Cardiomyopathy, atherosclerosis and valvular insufficiency with resultant congestive heart failure are also seen in rabbits. The cause of cardiomyopathy is not always clear and rabbits may be asymptomatic. Endocardiosis is seen in older rabbits with the mitral valve being most commonly affected. Alpha-2 drugs such as medetomidine have been associated with myocardial ischaemia and cardiomyopathy development, as has stress. Stress induces catecholamine release resulting in coronary arterial constriction in the rabbit and myocardial ischaemia. End-stage dilated cardiomyopathy may present with congestive heart failure with ascites, dyspnoea and tachypnoea.

Arrhythmias

The most commonly seen arrhythmia in rabbits is bradycardia associated with a heart block. It may also be a cause of syncope and collapsing bunny syndrome.

Lead poisoning

This may lead to anaemia with basophilic stippling of the erythrocytes with Romanowsky stains. Clinically, profound chronic non-regenerative anaemia and neurological signs have been reported. Lead levels above 1.1 µmol/L on heparinised blood are diagnostic.

Urinary tract disease
Urolithiasis and cystitis

Cystitis and urolithiasis are common, as rabbits absorb all of the calcium they can from their diet, and then excrete any excess into the urine via the kidneys. The commonest urolith is calcium carbonate, which forms readily in the rabbit's alkaline urine, and is radio-dense, often filling the bladder outline on radiographs. Secondary bladder infections are common as the crystals irritate the lining of the bladder. See Table 5.1 for details of urinanalysis.

Table 5.1 Urinanalysis results for healthy domestic rabbits.

Urine volume	10–35 mL/kg/day average (depending on diet)
Urine specific gravity	1.003–1.036
Urine erythrocyte numbers	<5 erythrocytes per high power field
Urine protein levels	Trace to absent (may be more in juveniles)
Urine colour	Varies from pale yellow to deep red depending on presence/absence of porphyrins
Urine average pH	8.2
Urine crystals	Small volumes of ammonium magnesium phosphate or calcium carbonate are normal.

Haematuria

The presence of red-coloured urine in the rabbit does not necessarily indicate haematuria. Many red porphyrin pigments from the diet (particularly some leafy greens such as beetroot) will be excreted in the urine. Causes of haematuria include cystitis, uterine tumours, aneurysms and kidney infections.

Renal disease

Aetiology

In general, chronic renal failure cases are associated with: *E. cuniculi*; pyelonephritis; chronic progressive nephrosis; amyloidosis; renal calcinosis; congenital polycystic kidneys (which tend to produce CRF by 2–3 years of age); neoplasia (lymphoma) and renoliths/ureteroliths.

Acute renal failure may be seen associated with: *E. cuniculi*; pyelonephritis; drug toxicity and renoliths/ureteroliths causing hydronephrosis.

Clinical signs

Chronic renal failure: This is associated with weight loss, dehydration, loss of appetite, polydipsia and polyuria. In addition, a reduction in gastro-intestinal motility, with caecal impaction may be observed. Clinical anaemia may be present and other signs associated with specific conditions (e.g. neurological signs with *E. cuniculi* infection) may also be demonstrable.

Acute renal failure: The rabbit is usually in good bodily condition, with a history of recent medication administration (e.g. nephrotoxic drugs such as the aminoglycosides, or NSAIDS) or in does in late pregnancy with toxaemia or in obese animals which undergo a period of anorexia where fatty infiltration may occur.

Encephalitozoon cuniculi: This can be a cause of chronic and acute renal failure, and of course, may be associated with neurological signs, for example torticollis, fitting, cataracts and uveitis (often unilateral), muscle tremors, paresis and paralysis of hindlimbs and urinary overflow with urine scalding. Death may occur due to heart failure, renal failure or meningoencephalitis. The organism is a microsporidian parasite found in a wide range of mammals, including rabbits and is a potential zoonotic disease in immunocompromised humans (e.g. AIDS affected individuals). There are different strains of *E. cuniculi* – strain I (found in rabbits and humans), strain II (found in rodents) and strain III (found in dogs and humans). Infection is by ingestion of food contaminated by infected urine, although vertical transmission is possible in utero.

Replication occurs in the kidneys and spreads to the CNS as well as the cardiac muscles. The most common renal presentation is chronic renal disease due to a granulomatous interstitial nephritis and tubular degeneration.

Pyelonephritis/renoliths: Rabbits affected may be in severe pain, sometimes vocalising when passing urine. Urine may be obviously turbid with pus, or blood. Individuals may also have GI associated signs such as increased borborygmi or GI stasis. The patient is often hunched and anorectic. However, some individuals with early renoliths may be clinically unaffected.

Diagnosis

Chronic renal failure: The major acute phase protein in rabbits is C-reactive protein travelling in the beta-globulin fraction. With acute renal failure due to nephritis an increase in alpha-2 globulins is also seen (alpha-2 macroglobulin), as is the case with the nephrotic syndrome. In the nephrotic syndrome (chronic renal disease), there is also an increase in beta-1 globulins (due to transferrin and beta-2 lipoprotein). In chronic renal failure, there is often a significant drop in albumin whereas in acute renal failure there is often elevation (due to dehydration) or normal levels.

In chronic renal failure, urea, creatinine and phosphate levels will be raised, and the patient is often anaemic. Only when <25% of renal functional mass has been destroyed will these blood parameters become elevated, so these are not sensitive. A better assessment of glomerular filtration rate may be made using endogenous clearance rates for creatine. Weisbroth *et al.* (1974) calculated the normal rate at 2.2–4.2 mL/kg/minute. This requires bladder catheterisation and accurate urine output. Urine protein levels should be minimal or absent, therefore, presence of protein and casts in the urine is significant and may indicate chronic renal failure and/or infection. An assessment of urine protein:creatinine levels can be made using in-house kits for cats (e.g. Idexx), although no definitive normal values exist for rabbits – this author and others use the cut-off range for cats as a reference point.

Ionised and total calcium levels may be elevated and soft tissue mineralisation seen radiographically – most commonly the aorta and kidneys. Hypermineralisation of the bones may also be seen which is not seen in cats and dogs. Hypermineralisation is exacerbated by diets supplemented with vitamin D as rabbits are sensitive to toxicosis.

Ultrasonographically, the renal outline may be smaller than normal (<3 cm craniocaudally and <2 cm ventrodorsally).

Acute renal failure: Blood parameters will be elevated as for chronic renal failure, but there is often renal shutdown and anuria. The main difference between acute and chronic failure is the loss of body condition and generally slower onset of debilitation and polydipsia/polyuria in chronic failure.

Ultrasonographically, the renal outline may be larger than normal (>4 cm craniocaudally and <2.5 cm ventrodorsally).

Pre-renal azotaemia: These can be differentiated from acute renal failure by the presence of other clinical signs, usually cardiovascular/hypovolaemic shock in conjunction with a urine SG of >1.030. Confirmation occurs with reduction of renal parameters with rehydration and treatment of hypovolaemia.

Encephalitozoon cuniculi: Antibodies are produced 2–3 weeks after infection. There is no correlation between antibody levels and degree of spore shedding, or with the severity of lesions at post-mortem. A rising titre over 3–4 weeks is suggestive of recent infection. An IgG and IgM antibody test and a PCR test to detect spores in urine are available.

Hydronephrosis: This may be diagnosed using intravenous pyelography using an iodine-based radiopaque medium (0.5–1 mL/kg) injected through a peripheral vein. Ultrasonography may be used to determine if there is hydropic degeneration. Doppler flow ultrasound may also help to ascertain renal arterial blood flow.

Renoliths/ureteroliths: These may be easily diagnosed via radiography or ultrasonography. Renoliths are usually bilateral. The prognosis is generally guarded as renal damage is common and may be either acute or more commonly chronic. Pyelonephritis may also be present.

Reproductive tract disease
Uterine
Uterine adenocarcinoma

This is a common condition seen in does over the age of four years with reported incidence at nearly 80%. The condition is fatal if not detected early as the tumour readily metastasizes, primarily to the lungs. Radiography of the chest is therefore advised if the condition is suspected, to determine if spread has occurred.

Venereal spirochaetosis

Rabbit syphilis is caused by the bacteria *Treponema paraluiscuniculi*. The condition is self-limiting, but produces crusting of the anogenital area, the nose and lips.

Pyometra

Pyometras occur in older does, and are often due to *E. coli* infections of hyperplastic endometrial tissues.

Mammary gland

Mastitis occurs following pregnancy when the kittens are lost or in phantom pregnancy. Many of the coliform type of bacteria involved will release endotoxins into the bloodstream causing rapid toxaemia, fever and death of the doe. Others may just cause severe mastitis with abscess formation.

Mammary gland neoplasia can be seen in older rabbits and is usually benign.

Musculoskeletal disease
Splayleg

Splayleg is an inherited congenital disease wherein the kit cannot position one or more hindlimbs underneath itself. Instead the affected limb sticks out awkwardly. There is no treatment for this condition.

Fractured or dislocated spine

This is common in indoor-reared, poorly fed rabbits. The close confinement leads to weakening of bones and muscles due to disuse atrophy, and the absence of sunlight can exacerbate vitamin D_3 and calcium deficiency in a poor diet. Osteoporosis occurs, with spontaneous fractures, often in the lumbosacral area. Compression fractures of vertebral bodies are more commonly seen in the thoracolumbar area.

Other bone fractures

The rabbit skeleton forms a smaller proportion of total body weight than mammals such as dogs, cats or humans. Rabbit long bones also have a thinner, more brittle cortex, and are prone to fissure propagation, shattering with rough handling. Displacement of the superficial flexor tendons in the hindleg may mimic a spinal problem with a shuffling gait and arched back.

In contrast to cats and dogs, in rabbits, distal tibial fractures are the most commonly present fracture, followed by metatarsal fractures and then radius/ulna fractures.

Common causes of hindlimb lameness that may be missed are metatarsal and hindfeet phalangeal fractures.

Osteoarthritis

This is common in large breeds, even in young animals and can affect any joint. Most commonly though the stifles, (due to caudal cruciate damage rather than cranial), hips (often associated with dysplasia) and spine are affected. This may lead to limb disuse, pain, urine staining of the perineum and faecal soiling due to an inability to flex the spine to allow urination and caecotrophy and muscle wasting.

Neurological disease

Encephalitozoonosis

Encephalitozoon cuniculi affects the kidneys and the CNS, and may remain latent for years, producing no clinical signs. Alternatively, paresis/paralysis of the fore- and/or hindlimbs, fitting, head tilt or other vestibular symptoms and blindness may be seen (see Figure 5.6). Diagnosis is as previously described.

Vestibular disease

One cause of vestibular disease is encephalitozoonosis. Others include tumours or infarcts of the hindbrain, and more commonly *Pasteurella multocida* or other bacterial infection of the middle and inner ear. Bacteria gain access to the middle ear via the Eustachian canal, or less commonly via a perforated ear drum (e.g. in ear mite infestations). Many are unable to stand. Prognosis in advanced cases may be poor. Dorsoventral radiography of the middle ear bullae can demonstrate sclerosis of the bullae and loss of trabecular detail indicating infection. Pus is observed in the external ear canal as the disease originating from the middle ear tends to result in tympanic membrane rupture. For this reason ear drops should not be used in rabbits.

Lead poisoning

Lead poisoning may cause anaemia, and also neurological signs such as fitting, depression and sudden death.

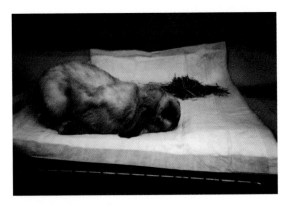

Figure 5.6 An extreme example of encephalitozoonosis neurological disease with forelimb paralysis.

Ophthalmic disease

Uveitis

This is commonly seen in rabbits with *Encephalitozoon cuniculi* infections where leakage of the lens contents stimulates a phacoclastic uveitis. This is frequently unilateral. Uveitis can also be seen with bacterial infections, for example *Pasteurella multocida* and, of course, glaucoma.

Glaucoma

New Zealand white rabbits have a recessive *bu* gene where intraocular pressures may reach 26–48 mmHg. N.B.: most tonometers underestimate intraocular pressure in rabbits. Corneal oedema occurs, but the condition does not appear painful and the eye pressure returns to normal as increased pressure results in damage to the ciliary body which produces the intraocular fluid.

Cataracts

These are commonly associated with *E. cuniculi* infection, and unilateral. However, congenital and spontaneous idiopathic cataracts have been reported.

Conjunctivitis

The milky discharge seen in rabbit eyes is often mistaken for primary conjunctivitis when dacryocystitis due to dental disease pinching the tear duct occurs. Narrowing of the tear duct can be shown by injecting iodine-based dye into the tear duct through the ventral punctum and radiographing the head (see Figure 5.7). True conjunctivitis may also be seen, and is one of the clinical signs in myxomatosis.

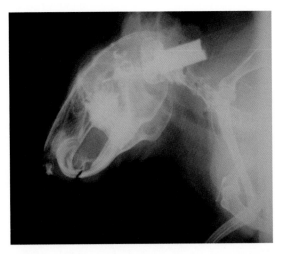

Figure 5.7 An iodine-based positive contrast study of the tear duct of a rabbit with dacryocystitis. Note the syringe with the iodine and catheter to the right and follow the contrast media down to the root of the maxillary incisor where it becomes narrowed.

PART I: SMALL MAMMALS

Aberrant conjunctival overgrowth

This is unique to the rabbit where a fold of conjunctival tissue develops from the limbus of the eye and looks like limbal keratitis. The tissue is not attached to the cornea, but overlies it and may be easily removed. The condition is a congenital abnormality with an unknown aetiology.

Exophthalmos

This is seen due to a cranial mediastinal mass surrounding the anterior vena cava which restricts venous drainage from the eyes. The exophthalmos is not permanent but occurs with stress, often disappearing when the stressful incident goes away. Examples include cranial mediastinal abscesses, lymphoma, thymoma and carcinomas.

Retrobulbar abscesses may result in (usually) unilateral exophthalmos and are associated with cheek tooth abscesses.

DISEASES OF THE RAT AND MOUSE
Skin disease
Ectoparasitic
Mites

Myobia musculi tends to affect the head of mice causing intense pruritus inducing self-mutilation. Some mice may be asymptomatic carriers, but equally some may be so severely affected as to die of secondary bacterial infection (see Figure 5.8).

Myocoptes musculinus causes disease over the body of the mouse. It may produce intense pruritus, but does not tend to induce the large areas of ulceration which are associated with *Myobia musculi*.

In the rat, the fur mite is *Radfordia ensifera*. In the tropics, the blood sucking mite *Liponyssus bacoti* can cause anaemia and general debilitation.

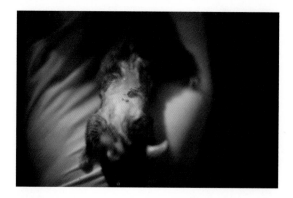

Figure 5.8 A mouse with *Myobia musculi* infestation and ulceration.

Notoedres muris is a burrowing mite of rats and causes crusting lesions on the ear tips and tail which may then spread to the rest of the body. It is extremely pruritic in the rat and secondary bacterial infections are common.

Diagnosis of these mites is based on the clinical signs and discovering them on skin scrapings.

Lice

The common sucking louse seen in both rats and mice is *Polyplax spinulosa*. This seems to be mildly pruritic, but if present in sufficient numbers (the louse may be seen with the naked eye), it can cause anaemia.

Fleas

In most pet households, infestation of pet rats and mice with either *Ctenocephalides felis* or *Ctenocephalides canis* is possible. These may cause significant anaemia. *Xenopsylla cheopis* is the main vector for the bacterium *Yersinia pestis,* the cause of bubonic plague. It is not found in the United Kingdom, but is in parts of Africa, China, South America and the western states of the United States.

Viral

Both species may be affected by their own form of pox virus. These are rare, although the mouse pox virus (ectromelia) can cause problems in laboratories.

Sialodacryoadenitis virus (rat coronavirus) infection is a disease affecting the tear glands and periorbita of rats and mice. It causes local swelling and epiphora. The tears contain porphyrin pigments making them red (chromodacryorrhoea) and mimicking dried blood. The disease is not treatable, but is generally self-limiting, although red tears may reappear in rats at times of stress.

Bacterial

Generalised bacterial skin problems are common as a sequel to any self-induced trauma. Bacteria such as *Staphylococcus aureus* and *Streptococcus* spp. and *Pseudomonas* spp. are seen commonly.

Pododermatitis

Sores commonly develop on the hocks of older, overweight rats. They start as pressure sores, allowing secondary infections to occur. Causes include osteoarthritis, excessive weight carriage and poor bedding.

Fungal

In rats and mice dermatophytes such as *Trichophyton mentagrophytes* produce lesions on the head and neck, with a typical scaling and dry crust. The tail may also be affected, and the lesions do not appear to be pruritic. This ringworm does not fluoresce under Wood's lamp.

Miscellaneous
Barbering
Barbering of the whiskers and fur is common particularly in male mice kept together. The whiskers and fur is chewed short and may proceed to more serious injuries. For this reason male mice should not be kept together.

Ringtail
Ringtail is seen in rats where circular constrictions of the skin covering the tail occur, stopping the blood supply and causing skin sloughing. It is thought to be due to a reduction in the relative humidity of the environment of the rat. Levels of humidity below 40–50% have been associated with this problem.

Atopy
Atopy is hypothesised to exist in rats. This is an allergic skin condition similar to that seen in dogs, and can occur due to contact with any potential allergen in their environment. Classically, the rat is pruritic and is covered in scabs. There is no evidence of mites on skin scrapings, and no response to ivermectin medication.

Digestive disease
Oral
Dental disease is uncommon in rats and mice. If seen it is usually incisor malocclusion.

Gastrointestinal
Endoparasitic
Pinworms such as *Syphacia obvelata* (chiefly in mice), *Syphacia muris* (chiefly in rats) and *Aspiculuris tetraptera* (chiefly in mice) are common. They may cause no disease at all, but the characteristic asymmetrical eggs may be found in the faeces, or around the anus, where *Syphacia* spp. may cause irritation. Diarrhoea, if present, is generally mild, but severe infestations may cause rectal prolapses.

Protozoal
These include *Entamoeba muris, Trichomonas muris* and *Giardia muris*. All protozoans can cause mild diarrhoea, but many may cause no disease signs at all when present in low numbers.

Bacterial
Salmonellosis: Mice and rats may remain subclinical carriers of the bacteria for years. Diarrhoea is not always seen, treatment is difficult, as clearing a rat or mouse of *Salmonella* spp. is almost impossible. Euthanasia may be advised due to the human health risk.

Transmissible murine colonic hyperplasia: Transmissible murine colonic hyperplasia (TMCH) is an infection of mice caused by the environmental bacteria *Citrobacter freundii*. It causes progressive thickening of the mucosa of the large intestine, diarrhoea, abdominal pain, anorexia and sometimes rectal prolapse, particularly in young mice, 2–4 weeks of age. Death occurs in a small number of cases. The more common outcome is stunting of the mouse. It is highly infectious, and poor cage hygiene allows rapid spread through a colony.

Tyzzer's disease: This is an infection by *Clostridium (Bacillus) piliformis*. It is common in rats, where it can cause sudden death, or watery diarrhoea, perineal staining, heart and liver disease. It is highly infectious and spread in the faeces.

Viral
Rotavirus: Rotavirus infection is seen before weaning. Chronic infections, yellow diarrhoea and stunted growth are common.

Mouse hepatitis virus: Mouse hepatitis virus (MHV) is a highly pathogenic coronavirus affecting suckling mice. It causes rapid deterioration, a yellow diarrhoea, muscle tremors, fitting and death in infected individuals, and is spread via the respiratory and faecal–oral routes.

Respiratory disease
Mycoplasma pulmonis
The bacteria *Mycoplasma pulmonis* is widespread in rats and mice. It is carried in the upper airways and the reproductive tract. Transmission is by close contact between male and female at mating, mother and young during nursing and by aerosol spread from individual to individual over greater distances. It is highly infectious.

Signs of disease include snuffles, head tilts (inner and middle ear infections), dyspnoea, hyperpnoea and death from advanced bronchopulmonary disease. The course of the infection can be chronic, with repeated bouts of bronchitis and pneumonia. They will exhibit poor body condition, a dull staring coat, chromodacryorrhea, anorexia and lethargy. Another presentation includes infertility, reduced fertility and early abortions.

Some factors will encourage onset of the infection and these include other respiratory tract infections, (e.g. Sendai virus) and unsanitary conditions. Urine soiling which leads to a build-up of ammonia gas which then leads to respiratory tract irritation and infection has also been implicated.

Other bacterial respiratory infections

Streptococcus pneumoniae (a cause of pneumonia and meningitis in humans and therefore a zoonosis), *Pasteurella pneumotropica*, *Bordetella bronchiseptica*, *Corynebacterium kutscheri* and the cilia-associated respiratory bacillus (CAR) may all occur in rats and mice. Clinical signs are respiratory and reproductive disease. *Chlamydophila muridarum* is the mouse pneumonitis (MoPn) agent, but experimentally mice are also susceptible to *C. psittaci* and *C. trachomatis*. In all cases infection is via the respiratory route. Severe acute infections produce ruffled fur, hunched stance, laboured breathing and an interstitial pneumonia. Many will die quickly, but more chronic cases will produce cyanosis of the ear and tail tips.

Sendai virus

This is a paramyxovirus type 1, transmitted by sneezing, direct contact, via food bowls or fomites. It is commonest in recently weaned mice as younger mice are protected by maternal antibodies. Signs of disease include dullness, dyspnoea, chattering of the teeth, weight loss, anorexia and a dull coat. In young mice the mortality rate may be high.

Other viral respiratory diseases

Mouse cytomegalovirus infection

Also known as murid herpesvirus 1 (MuHV-1). Pathology is found in the salivary glands but it can also affect the lungs. Neonates of all mice strains can be affected. Transmission can be via saliva, tears, urine and semen. Clinically apparent disease is rare.

Mouse hepatitis virus

Also known as murine hepatitis virus (MHV) it is a coronavirus. Natural infections are generally subclinical. The virus can infect nasal mucosa, pulmonary vascular endothelium and the draining lymph nodes. It is highly contagious and spread by aerosol and faeces. It is a problem in laboratories. Elimination of the virus may be achieved by stopping breeding of seropositive animals for 8 weeks plus environmental decontamination.

Pneumonia virus of mice

This can infect mice, rats, hamsters, guinea pigs and gerbils. It is a Paramyxoviridae *Pneumovirus*. In non-immunocompromised rodents it generally produces subclinical infections. In immunodeficient mice it can produce rhinitis, cyanosis, dyspnoea and chronic wasting.

Poxvirus

Cowpox virus can be carried by rodents and may result in disease in other domestic and wild animals (Girling *et al.*, 2011). It is subclinical in rodents. Turkmenian rodent poxvirus has been recorded in laboratory rats in Europe and Russia. Dermal and respiratory lesions with severe respiratory interstitial pneumonia and oedema have been reported.

Diagnosis of viral respiratory disease in rodents

Many laboratories can offer serological testing for rodent viruses. Virus isolation may also be attempted if fresh tissue or lung washes can be submitted.

Fungal respiratory disease

Pneumocystosis

Pneumocystis carinii is an opportunistic pathogen of the respiratory tract of mice, rats and probably all domestic mammals and humans. Transmission occurs by the inhalation of infective cysts. Mice or rats that are immunosuppressed may develop a fatal pneumonia. Affected mice are hunched, tachypneic, with weight loss. Decreased reproductive efficiency is commonly observed in colonies of immunodeficient mice. Histology of the lungs and PCR are used for diagnosis.

Aspergillus spp.

This fungus has been reported as a cause of fatal pneumonia and rhinitis in rats. Corncob bedding was implicated in the source of the fungus.

Other respiratory tract disease

Acidophilic macrophage pneumonia

This can occur in older mice, particularly where there are pulmonary tumours, pneumocystosis or chronic pneumonia. Grossly the lungs appear tan to red in discolouration and do not collapse.

Amyloidosis

This is seen in older mice and hamsters. It can affect any organ and is common in cases of chronic infection and neoplasia. Clinically, the signs depend on the organ affected. It can be more commonly found in male mice, particularly those under stress in overcrowded housing.

Eosinophilic granulomatous pneumonia and asthma

This tends to be a problem in Brown Norwegian rats. It has been associated with asthma, which is common in this breed. However, it has been reported in rats not exposed to allergens, and may be associated with an unknown infectious agent. Incidence can be up to 100% at 3–4 months of age.

Neoplasia

This has regularly been reported in older rats and is often due to primary lung tumours. Metastasis from mammary adenocarcinomas is possible in female mice.

Cardiovascular disease

Atrial thrombosis is common in aged mice, usually in the left atrium; it may be accompanied by amyloidosis. Amyloid is deposited in the walls of the great vessels. Cardiac disease is seen clinically as dyspnoea, tachypnoea and abdominal distension.

Cardiomyopathy and myocardial fibrosis are the two most commonly seen cardiac abnormalities. Cardiomyopathy (usually dilated) is particularly common in male rats that are over-fed, and can be seen as early as 3 months of age. The incidence of myocardial disease can be reduced by 25–30% by dietary restriction.

Endocardiosis and atrial thrombus formation are common in older rats. Myocardial mineralisation may be seen secondary to chronic renal disease. Congestive heart failure will result.

Myocardial abscesses can be seen with Tyzzer's disease.

Urinary tract disease
Chronic progressive nephrosis

Chronic progressive nephrosis is common in ageing rats and mice. The kidneys become progressively more damaged by protein deposits in the tubular lumens. In certain strains of mice an autoimmune factor is seen. In rats, a high-protein, low-potassium diet has been implicated, with males more susceptible than females. Recurrent disease equally may have a role to play. An increase in thirst and urination may be seen, with weight loss and dehydration. Blood samples demonstrate increased urea and creatinine with low blood albumin.

Urolithiasis

This is common in older rats and mice, especially males, where uroliths may block the narrower urethra proximal to the *os penis*. The composition varies, but is frequently calcium carbonate, ammonium phosphate or calcium oxalate. There is often a secondary cystitis.

Nephritis/pyelonephritis

Often seen in older rats and involving bacteria such as *Pseudomonas* spp., *E. coli*, *Proteus mirabilis* and *Klebsiella* spp. Culture and sensitivity testing of cystocentesis collected samples is advisable.

Interstitial nephritis can occur with *Leptospira* spp. (such as *L. ballum*) in most rodents and this can be a zoonotic disease. Lymphocytic choriomeningitis virus (LMCV) can cause interstitial nephritis and is also zoonotic. Clinically, the rodent presents with anorexia, lethargy, dehydration and abdominal pain.

Renal coccidiosis and bladder worms

Renal coccidian *Klossiella hydromyos* has been reported in rats, sporocysts being found in the urine. Sulphonamides are effective in most cases.

Trichosomoides crassicauda (bladder threadworms) have also been reported in rats (8–12 weeks of age) (see Figure 5.9). Clinical signs include poor growth, staring coats and difficulty urinating/cystitis. Worm eggs may be seen in the urine.

Nephrocalcinosis

This can be seen in older rats and is thought to be associated with a high-calcium, low phosphorus diet, combined with high levels of vitamin D_3. It is believed that oestrogens have a role in causing the disease as it is found more frequently in older females. Radiography is diagnostic.

Hydronephrosis and polycystic disease

Hydronephrosis can occur due to urolithiasis of the ureters. More commonly it is seen as an inherited condition in rats (e.g. Brown Norway, Sprague Dawley and Gunn breeds).

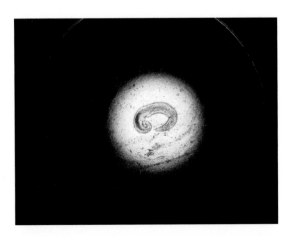

Figure 5.9 An example of the bladder nematode *Trichosomoides crassicauda* found in the urine of a 12-week-old rat.

Reproductive tract disease
Uterine
Dystocias are uncommon in rats and mice. Uterine infections do occur infrequently, with pyometras being seen in rats.

Mammary gland
The mammary glands are commonly affected by cancer in both rats and mice.

In rats, the most frequent is the fibroadenoma. This is a benign, but rapidly growing tumour, and can occur in any of the mammary tissue which extends from cranially at the forelimbs to the inguinal region (see Figure 5.10). The masses are well defined and easily removed surgically, although the predisposition appears to be hereditary, and the likelihood of further tumours occurring is high. Many are prolactin sensitive. Fibroadenomas can occur in male rats as well as females. Adenocarcinomas do occur in 10% of cases and may metastasise.

In mice, the mammary cancer most commonly seen is malignant and caused by an RNA virus, the Bittner agent, which, in a susceptible strain of mouse, causes mammary adenocarcinoma. Surgery is often unsuccessful.

Testicular
A form of testicular cancer, a Leydig cell adenoma, is seen in old male rats. It is benign and causes a soft swelling, and may be accompanied by some hair loss.

Musculoskeletal disease
Spondylosis is common in older rats, and may cause incontinence and reduction of function of the hindlimbs. Typically, the lumbosacral area is affected by the osteoarthritis, reducing mobility, causing pain and irritating spinal nerve function.

Neurological disease
Vestibular disease
Head tilts are common in rats. Causes include infections by *Mycoplasma pulmonis* and *Streptococcus pneumoniae*, which can affect the inner ear or hindbrain, affecting the vestibular centres. Other causes are tumours, with pituitary tumours reported commonly in older female rats on high-calorie/protein diets.

Lymphocytic choriomeningitis virus
This is mainly seen in wild mice. It is shed in the urine and saliva, and affected mice may show no symptoms, or they may show neurological signs such as head tilts, fitting and death. It is a zoonotic disease and can cause meningitis in humans and other primates.

Degenerative radiculoneuropathy
This is a condition in aged rats similar to that seen in German Shepherd dogs where a progressive, primary segmental demyelination is seen in rats over 18 months old (Gilmore, 2005).

Ocular disease
Sialodacryoadenitis virus causing red tears has been mentioned above, and will infect rats, mice, hamsters and gerbils. Chronic infections may cause permanent reduction in tears, leading to *keratitis sicca*. Conjunctivitis may occur secondary to this, or to the presence of finely chopped or dusty bedding, creating a foreign body reaction.

Cataracts are often associated with a hereditary deformed eye seen as microphthalmia.

Many young rats and mice have a persistent hyaloid artery which may bleed into the vitreous humour and appear as haemorrhages at the front of the eye.

Albino rats and mice must be given shelter from light, as their retinas are prone to damage. Even normal-coloured rats and mice require a shelter that is light proof.

DISEASES OF THE GERBIL
Skin disease
Ectoparasitic
Demodex merioni rarely causes disease. It has a typical cigar shape under microscopy of skin scrapings. Other mite infestations are rare, although cases of *Notoedres muris* and *Sarcoptes scabiei* have been reported.

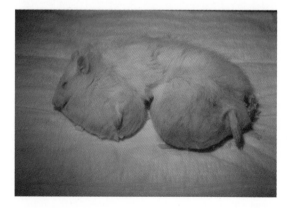

Figure 5.10 Fibroadenomas in a female rat.

Storage mites have been reported as causing irritation to the nose and facial area which is in contact with food.

Bacterial

Staphylococcus aureus infections of the nose and face occur secondary to wet substrate conditions. Sialodacryoadenitis virus infection of the tear glands, can also lead to wet dermatitis in the perinasal area, allowing *Staphylococcus aureus* to create a pyoderma.

Fungal

The dermatophyte, *Trichophyton mentagrophytes* is the commonest seen, causing areas of hyperkeratosis with grey scaling of the skin, particularly in the head region. Diagnosis is made on microscopy and culture.

Skin tumours

Ventral scent gland adenomas/adenocarcinomas, which develop from 2 years of age onwards predominantly in the male gerbil, are significant (see Figure 5.11).

Other skin tumours, such as melanomas, are seen, particularly on the extremities. Squamous cell carcinomas of the ears and nose have been reported.

Endocrine

Cystic ovarian disease (see below) has been associated with symmetrical hair loss over the flanks of female gerbils, along with a swollen abdomen.

Miscellaneous

Tail skin degloving injuries are common in gerbils that have been roughly handled or restrained by the end of the tail. The denuded vertebrae will die off later on, and the tail never regrows.

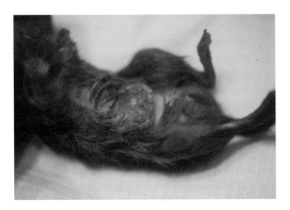

Figure 5.11 Ventral scent gland adenocarcinoma in a male gerbil.

Digestive disease

Oral

Dental disease is relatively uncommon in the gerbil, although traumatic damage to the incisors leading to fractures and overgrowth may occur.

Gastrointestinal

Bacterial

Tyzzer's disease – Clostridium (Bacillus) piliformis: Tyzzer's disease causes enteritis, but rarely diarrhoea, and often spreads to the liver and heart. The disease lasts for 1–4 days and may produce sudden death or a more lingering disease with dullness, lethargy, a hunched posture, scant or soft faeces and a dull staring coat.

Proliferative ileitis: Due to the intracellular bacteria *Lawsonia intracellularis* also causes wet-tail in hamsters. It is passed from gerbil to gerbil via the faecal–oral route, and causes thickening of the ileum resulting in maldigestion and malabsorption, producing the classical 'wet tail' of matted damp fur around the rear. The condition is much less common in gerbils than hamsters, but can nonetheless be a serious and fatal condition.

Endoparasitic

The mouse pinworm *Syphacia obvelata* and the rat pinworm *Syphacia muris* rarely cause clinical disease.

The potentially zoonotic cestode *Rodentolepis (Hymenolepis) nana* can be found and is discussed in hamsters. The gerbil is the definitive host for the pinworm *Dentostomella translucida*, which is considered non-pathogenic.

Respiratory disease

The gerbil is affected by more or less the same respiratory conditions as the rat and mouse, although it is less susceptible.

Cardiovascular disease

Tyzzer's disease may cause myocarditis, otherwise cardiovascular disease is uncommon.

Urinary tract disease

Gerbils are prone to ageing changes involving gradual scarring of renal tissue and the nephrotic syndrome, but the incidence of this is much less than in the rat or mouse.

Reproductive tract disease

Uterine infection

Uterine infections are uncommon in gerbils.

Ovarian cysts

Ovarian cysts are common. The cysts may be quite large and cause distension of the abdomen. The condition is hereditary and bilateral and causes disruption of the oestrus cycle. The cyst secretes low levels of oestrogens which have an effect on fur growth, causing mild alopecia over the flanks.

Uterine and ovarian neoplasia

After cancer of the adrenal gland, cancer of the ovaries and the female reproductive tract are the most common tumours in the gerbil. Uterine cancers may cause bleeding from the reproductive tract, or abdominal swelling. Diagnosis may be made on clinical signs, or ultrasound and radiographical examination.

Musculoskeletal disease

Fractures are uncommon in gerbils, as are other musculoskeletal problems, other than the degloving tail injuries mentioned above.

Neurological disease

Vestibular disease

Vestibular disease is common and is usually due to bacterial inner ear disease, often *Mycoplasma pulmonis, Pasteurella pneumotropica* or *Streptococcus pneumoniae*, which gain access from the oropharynx via the Eustachian canals and the middle ear. Pus may be observed at the external ear canal in some cases.

Aural cholesteatoma, papilloma and polyp formation with secondary bacterial infection are also common.

Epilepsy

Epilepsy in gerbils appears to be hereditary, and it is advisable not to keep susceptible individuals in rooms with strip lighting, television sets or computer terminals, as these all emit electromagnetic radiation of around 50–60 Hz, which may induce a fit. In addition, handling gerbils from a young age to familiarize them with human contact can reduce the likelihood of seizures in later life.

DISEASES OF THE HAMSTER
Skin disease

Ectoparasitic

Demodex criceti and *Demodex aurati* both infest hamsters and can cause clinical disease. *D. criceti* is shorter and rounder, whereas *D. aurati* is longer and more like *D. canis*. The clinical disease is manifested by alopecia over the dorsum caudally and intense white scurf (see Figure 5.12). The lesions are mildly pruritic.

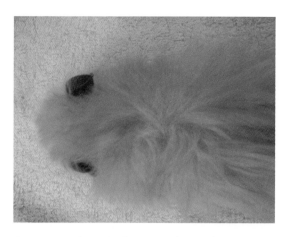

Figure 5.12 Fur loss and scaling over the dorsum of a hamster with early demidocosis.

Crusting lesions of the ears, face and other extremities have been reported in Syrian hamsters affected by the sarcoptiform mite *Notoedres notoedres*. Diagnosis in all cases is made based on positive skin scrapings.

Fungal

The dermatophyte *Trichophyton mentagrophytes* can be found as a secondary cause of skin disease in hamsters as a sequel to mange or mycosis fungoides.

Bacterial

Primary bacterial skin disease is uncommonly seen in hamsters. The main bacteria isolated from wounds include *Pasteurella pneumotropica* and *Staphylococcus aureus*. Secondary infections of skin ulcers associated with T cell lymphoma are common.

Skin tumours

The commonest is a form of T-cell lymphoma known as mycosis fungoides. This infiltrates the epidermis, producing chronic thickening of the skin and is pruritic. Alopecia is seen due to the obliteration of the hair follicles. The cancer eventually metastasises.

Melanomas affecting the head, ears and flank scent glands are also seen. These are usually pigmented, fast growing and occur more frequently in males than females.

Cutaneous epitheliomas are associated with a Hamster papovavirus (see Figure 5.13). The virus is host specific and lesions are found in hamsters from three months to a year old. The lesions are wart-like and occur most often around the face or perianal area. The virus is highly contagious and is passed through urine. It has a long incubation

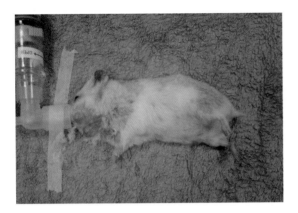

Figure 5.13 Papovavirus- induced neoplasia in a hamster.

period and is very resistant. It will also induce lymphoma in other organs. There is no spontaneous resolution.

Endocrine

Hyperadrenocorticism is due to a chromophobe adenoma in the pituitary gland. This secretes excessive levels of ACTH which causes bilateral adrenal gland hyperplasia, increased levels of cortisol producing polydipsia, polyuria, symmetrical alopecia, increased appetite and thinning of the skin and coat over the flanks. Plasma cortisol levels should be between 13.8 and 27.6 nmol/L in healthy hamsters. Serum alkaline phosphatase may also be raised in hamsters with hyperadrenocorticism (>40 U/L), normal values being 8–18 U/L. It has been suggested that hamsters may secrete both cortisol and corticosterone; therefore, diagnosis based on blood cortisol levels alone may not be accurate. Ultrasonography of the adrenal gland may show enlargement or abnormalities.

Irritant

Skin irritation has been reported in hamsters kept on cedar pine chips. These are highly resinous and can cause intense skin irritation, particularly over the ventrum and nasal areas. Removal of the hamster from these shavings produces improvement within days.

Digestive disease
Oral
Cheek pouch impaction

Impaction of the cheek pouch may occur because the hamster may have overfilled the pouch or have become ill before emptying it. Because the hamster uses his hindlimb to empty the pouch, losing a hindleg may also lead to impaction on that side.

Cheek pouch prolapse

Prolapse may occur after the hamster has emptied the cheek pouch. The sac, now everted, may not return to normal and protrudes as a pink mass from the mouth. It may also occur due to infection or neoplasia.

Gastrointestinal
Proliferative ileitis ('wet-tail')

The bacterium *Lawsonia intracellularis* produces hypertrophy of the ileum, reducing digestion and absorption which leads to diarrhoea. It can lead to rectal prolapse and intussusceptions. Some hamsters die within 24 hours of contracting the disease without showing any obvious signs.

Salmonellosis

Salmonellosis is uncommon. The bacterium *Salmonella enteritidis* is the most frequently reported and this is a zoonotic disease. Signs include sudden death, frequently before any diarrhoea is produced. Younger animals seem more susceptible.

Parasitic

Rodentolepis (Hymenolepis) nana is a dwarf tapeworm which is zoonotic. It appears to cause little or no disease in hamsters. A diagnosis may be made by finding cestode egg sachets in the faeces, or by seeing the cream coloured, 1–2-mm long egg packet wriggling on the perianal fur!

Miscellaneous

Examples of other causes of diarrhoea include rapid diet changes. Certain foods should be avoided altogether, for example, those containing lactose and over-sugary fruit such as grapes, kiwi fruit and bananas.

Respiratory disease
Sendai virus

This is an RNA paramyxovirus (parainfluenza 1) virus and affects rats, mice, guinea pigs and hamsters. Hamsters are rarely severely affected by infection.

Pasteurella pneumotropica

In hamsters it can cause acute or chronic respiratory disease – see section on rats and mice for clinical signs.

Corynebacterium kutscheri

Hamsters may act as carriers but seem not to develop disease from this bacterium.

Other causes of respiratory disease

Hamsters suffer from pulmonary thromboembolisms due to atrial thrombotic lesions which may prove fatal, and are a cause of sudden death.

Cardiovascular disease

Cardiomyopathy and atrial thromboses

Pathophysiology suggests that cardiomyopathy occurs first followed by left atrial thrombosis and death as a result of coagulopathy. Hypertrophic cardiomyopathy has also been reported as a cause for thrombus formation. In one study the incidence of cardiac disease was assumed to be around 6% (Schmidt & Reavill, 2007). Interestingly, androgens protect the heart from heart disease in hamsters. The age of onset of heart disease in females is therefore younger (around 13.5 months) than males (21.5 months). Neutering male hamsters therefore removes this effect and so means that they are more likely to develop heart disease at a younger age.

Diagnosis is based on the signs and the demonstration of an enlarged heart on radiography and ultrasound examination. The latter are often able to show the thrombi in the atria.

Other causes of cardiovascular disease

Bacterial disease such as Tyzzer's and salmonellosis can lead to myocarditis and heart failure. Amyloidosis is common in all rodents with age and chronic disease and may lead to thickening of arterial walls and organ failure.

Urinary tract disease

Kidney disease

Chronic progressive nephropathy is seen as in mice and rats. They are also prone to amyloidosis. Clinical signs vary, but may include weight loss, lethargy, polydipsia and polyuria with or without proteinuria.

Polycystic disease is seen in older male hamsters and may also involve the liver. It is congenital in nature and presents as a rapidly enlarging abdomen. Diagnosis is most easily made using ultrasound. Drainage of the cysts can help, but they tend to reform within 2–4 weeks.

Bladder

Like mice and rats, hamsters can suffer from cystitis and urolithiasis. Calcium oxalate and calcium carbonate are the two commonly seen uroliths.

Endocrine disease

Hyperadrenocorticism

See above under the discussion of skin diseases.

Diabetes mellitus

In the Chinese hamster, diabetes mellitus is a hereditary condition. Clinical signs include polydipsia (drinking often in >50 mL of water per day) and polyuria, cystitis, lethargy and weight loss. Glucosuria of 2% is common and blood glucose is often in excess of 25–30 mmol/L.

Reproductive tract disease

Uterus

Pyometra is seen, but may be mistaken for the normal reproductive tract discharge found during the oestrus cycle. Pyometras, however, persist, and smell much worse! Closed pyometras are more difficult to diagnose due to the absence of a discharge, but the hamster is often lethargic, anorectic, polydipsic, dehydrated and has a tender, swollen abdomen.

Ovaries

Cystic ovaries are common in female hamsters over the age of 8 months. The condition is bilateral, and may be accompanied by some mild symmetrical alopecia of the flanks.

Ocular disease

Chinese hamsters are prone to cataract development as a result of diabetes mellitus.

Musculoskeletal disease

Compound fractures of the tibia are the commonest, especially from hamsters falling from the roof or the sides of wire cages up which they have climbed, and leg amputation may be required. Other fractures commonly seen are fractures of spinal vertebrae, or more commonly vertebral subluxations, usually in the lumbar area, again due to falls. These will present as bilateral hindlimb paresis or paralysis.

Neurological disease

Lymphocytic choriomeningitis virus generally produces little or no clinical signs in the hamster. It is excreted in the urine and saliva. It is relatively rare in captive hamsters, being found more commonly in wild mice, but it is a serious zoonotic disease causing meningitis in man.

DISEASES OF THE GUINEA PIG

Skin disease

Ectoparasitic

Mites

The scabies mite *Trixicara caviae* causes intense pruritus and distress. The affected individual may scratch itself deeply and may be so severe as to cause abortion in heavily pregnant females. Diagnosis is made on clinical signs and skin scrapings under the microscope.

The fur mite, *Chirodiscoides caviae*, seems to cause little trouble.

Cheyletiella parasitovorax occasionally produces pruritus and scaling along the dorsum.

Demodex caviae is commonly found but rarely causes clinical disease. Diagnosis is made by collecting skin scrapings and examining them microscopically.

Lice

Gliricola porcelli and *Gyropus ovalis* are Mallophagan lice and so live off cellular debris, but rarely cause disease.

Bacterial

Cervical lymphadenitis

Cervical lymphadenitis is a disease of the cervical lymph nodes caused by the *Streptococcus zooepidemicus*. It is also found in the airways and mouth of the healthy guinea pig, and causes problems when the mucosa of the oropharynx becomes abraded by rough food particles. This leads to local lymphadenitis, with subcutaneous abscessation. The disease may gain access to the bloodstream causing septicaemia which is rapidly fatal.

Pododermatitis

Pododermatitis is commonest in overweight, older guinea pigs, which will spend more time resting, and which will walk on the flat of the hock. It can also be seen in older guinea pigs with osteoarthritis. Bacteria involved include *E. coli*, *Corynebacterium pyogenes*, *Staphylococcus aureus* and *Streptococcus* spp.

Fungal

Dermatophytosis due to *Microsporum canis* and *Trichophyton mentagrophytes* produces lesions over the head, paws and rear with brittle hairs, grey crusts and some scabs. Diagnosis is as for rats and mice.

Viral

A pox virus has been detected in association with cheilitis in two guinea pigs with crusting ulcerated lesions around the lips and philtrum.

Skin tumours

Lymphosarcoma affecting the superficial lymph nodes caused by a retrovirus can also produce a blood-borne leukaemia affecting the spleen and liver. The course of the disease is 3–4 weeks, with rapid deterioration, weight loss, secondary infections and organ failure. Treatment with chemotherapeutic agents is frequently unsuccessful.

Benign trichofolliculomas appear as solid, cyst-like structures, over the lumbosacral area dorsally. Sebaceous adenoma, fibroma, fibrosarcoma, lipoma, liposarcoma and schwannomas have also been reported.

Hormonal

Cystic ovarian disease is extremely common in aged female guinea pigs (a 76% incidence in animals between 1.5 and 5 years old has been reported). The aetiology is unknown, although oestrogenic substances in hay have been implicated. Some are embryological in origin (cystic rete ovarii). Abdominal enlargement and infertility can occur and bilateral non-pruritic alopecia is common. Diagnosis is as for gerbils and hamsters.

Miscellaneous

Guinea pigs may barber each other in the same way as rats and mice. Increasing fibre in the cage and providing more space and tubing or other hides, may help to prevent this. Cheilitis is common, and may be due to a lack of vitamin C, although a pox virus and *Candida* spp. yeasts have also been implicated.

Digestive disease

Oral

Molar overgrowth most commonly in the mandibular cheek teeth which results in entrapment of the tongue is common. The normal occlusal plane of the cheek teeth in the guinea pig is actually oblique and slopes from a dorsal position buccally to a ventral position lingually. Causes are similar to those in rabbits.

Gastrointestinal

Salmonellosis

Salmonella enteritidis and *Salmonella typhimurium* can both cause enteritis in guinea pigs. The young and debilitated are most at risk. Diarrhoea is uncommon; instead, a dull staring coat, weight loss and abortion are seen.

Other bacterial disease

Yersinia pseudotuberculosis can produce intestinal abscesses, chronic wasting and diarrhoea or acute death. *Mycobacterium tuberculosis*, *Listeria monocytogenes* and *Clostridium perfringens* can also cause intestinal disease. Guinea pigs are also prone to Tyzzer's disease, due to *Clostridium piliformis*.

Endoparasitic

Balantidium coli is a zoonosis and causes large intestinal inflammation and profuse diarrhoea in an immuno-compromised guinea pig. A coccidial organism, *Eimeria caviae*, may also cause diarrhoea in piglets.

Cryptosporidium wrairi has been reported as a major cause of small intestinal disease in young guinea pigs resulting in stunting, bloating, diarrhoea and weight loss. Most immunocompetent animals will recover within 4 weeks. Diagnosis is by PCR of faeces or by modified acid fast stains demonstrating the oocysts.

Faecal impaction

This is seen in older guinea pigs, particularly males. It occurs when excessive folds loose skin around the ano-genital opening trap faecal pellets. This can create serious constipation problems, and localised infection.

Respiratory disease

Bacterial disease

Lung infections are common in guinea pigs housed with rabbits, as the latter often carry the bacteria *Bordetella bronchiseptica* asymptomatically. This bacterium causes a severe bronchopneumonia in guinea pigs. It can also cause otitis media and interna, abscesses and metritis. Other pathogenic bacteria include *Streptococcus pneumoniae*, which is zoonotic, *Klebsiella pneumonia*, *Moraxella* spp., *Pasteurella pneumotropica* and *Pseudomonas* spp. *S. zooepidemicus* may also result in bronchopneumonia. *Chlamydophila caviae* has been reported in guinea pig breeding colonies and affects guinea pigs between 2 and 8 weeks of age. It is usually asymptomatic although conjunctivitis and rhinitis may be seen, as may abortions and urogenital tract infections.

Diagnosis can be made on history, clinical signs, auscultation of the harsh-sounding chest and, if necessary, radiography showing consolidation of the lungs and bronchioalveolar patterns.

Viral disease

Sendai virus has been reported in guinea pigs and may exacerbate bacterial disease. An adenovirus has also been reported in debilitated animals but is generally subclinical.

Lung neoplasia

Pulmonary adenoma has been recorded in guinea pigs. The tumour is slow growing and does not metastasise but causes a reduction in functional lung volume. It may be discovered on radiography or may cause clinical dyspnoea in conjunction with a respiratory pathogen. Lymphoma due to type C cavian leukaemia virus has also been reported.

Avocado toxicity

This has been reported, causing respiratory distress, hydropericardium, generalised congestion, anasarca and death. It appears that the leaves, fruit, bark and seed of avocados are toxic for a number of rodent and avian species.

Cardiovascular disease

Pericarditis has been recorded in conjunction with respiratory tract infection involving *Streptococcus pneumoniae* and may cause heart failure and death. Hypertrophic and dilated cardiomyopathies have been reported. In addition, metastatic and dystrophic mineralisation and pericardial effusions may also be seen. Calcification may be asymptomatic in guinea pigs older than 1 year of age but may equally have been associated with poor growth, muscle stiffness, bone deformities and death. Causes include magnesium deficiency, renal failure and diets high in calcium.

Urinary tract disease

Kidney disease

Chronic progressive interstitial nephritis may be a sequel to diabetes mellitus and staphylococcal pododermatitis. Clinically, the guinea pig is polyuric and polydipsic and loses weight. Blood parameters may indicate elevated urea and creatinine levels, often with low blood albumin due to urinary protein losses. Urinalysis may detect cystitis, and commonly reveals proteinuria.

Bladder

Calcium oxalate or calcium carbonate crystals are found in the bladder. Older boars may experience urethral obstruction due to dried accessory sex gland secretions, as well as being more susceptible to urolith blockage of the urethra at the *os penis*.

Secondary, or primary bacterial cystitis is often seen, the former due to irritation of the bladder by the uroliths, the latter leading to clumps of bacteria around which uroliths form. Clinically the affected guinea pig is dull, lethargic, vocalises and may periodically strain, passing small volumes of blood-stained urine. Diagnosis can be confirmed with examination of the sediment of a centrifuged urine sample. Radiography is also helpful, although calcium oxalate crystals are less radio-dense than struvite.

Endocrine disease

Cystic ovarian disease

See reproductive tract disease.

Diabetes mellitus

Spontaneous diabetes mellitus has been reported in guinea pigs. They may present with concurrent scurvy and poor hair coat, as well as polydipsia, polyuria and cataracts. Possible aetiologies include an unclassified infectious agent in Abyssinians (possibly viral in origin), hereditary factors, congenital manganese deficiency in juveniles and high sugar, high carbohydrate diets, such as apples and carrots, which exacerbate the problem.

Diagnosis is based on elevated blood glucose levels, often greater than 20 mmol/L (normal values are 3.3–6.9 mmol/L), hyperlipidaemia and results of glucose tolerance tests. For this the guinea pig is fasted for 18 hours. Blood glucose levels are measured, and then a dose of oral glucose is given at 1.75 g/kg body weight. Blood glucose levels 4 hours later are over twice the pre-dose value in diabetic animals and only 1–1.5 times the pre-dose value in normal animals.

Treatment of diabetes in both guinea pigs and hamsters consists of a high-fibre diet. Insulin therapy is rarely indicated and spontaneous recoveries are common. Where insulin is required, NPH insulin at 1 IU q12 hours has been used.

Reproductive tract disease

Cystic ovarian disease

Cystic ovarian disease is common in female guinea pigs over 15 months. It is often bilateral causing a swollen abdomen (see Figure 5.14). There is often bilateral symmetrical alopecia over the flanks.

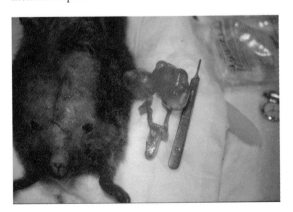

Figure 5.14 Surgically removed cystic ovaries and uterus from a guinea pig.

Reproductive tract tumours

Ovarian granulosa cell tumours often follow cystic ovaries. Other forms of reproductive tract cancer include: benign leiomyomas; and uterine adenocarcinomas, which are malignant. Diagnosis is made on palpation of an enlarged womb, radiographical or ultrasonographic evidence of enlargement of the tract, or reproductive tract discharge, which may be haemorrhagic.

Dystocia

If a sow has not given birth before 12 months, the fibrocartilaginous ligament which holds the two sides of the pubis and ischium together will become mineralised and fuse. This ligament normally stretches just before parturition under the influence of the hormone relaxin. If it does not, it significantly narrows the birth canal, and this will lead to dystocias. Any maiden sow older than 7–8 months of age should not be mated.

Pregnancy toxaemia

This is common in late pregnancy and early lactation in overweight first-time mothers. It is most likely to happen in the presence of concurrent disease, (e.g. *Trixicara caviae* mange), which may reduce the sow's appetite. A rapid mobilisation of body fats occurs, producing ketones. These cause a ketoacidosis that is rapidly fatal. Blood glucose levels are very low (<3 mmol/L) and there is an increase in the acidity of the blood. The urine becomes acidic. The sow becomes dull, lethargic and hyperpnoeic and then collapses and becomes comatose. Death can occur within two days, the sow fitting and convulsing *in extremis*.

Mammary gland tumours

Mammary gland adenomas are common in older sows. They are slow growing but may reach appreciable sizes. In 20–30% of cases the tumour may be a malignant adenocarcinoma.

Mastitis

Poor hygiene predisposes the guinea pig to this condition. The bacteria involved (such as *E. coli*) may release endotoxins into the bloodstream which can rapidly cause endotoxic shock.

Musculoskeletal disease

Scurvy

The daily requirement for vitamin C is 10 mg/kg. If this is not met then it will develop scurvy within 4–5 days. Guinea pigs lack the gene that controls the production of

L-gulonolactone oxidase which converts l-gulonolactone to ascorbic acid (vitamin C). Clinical signs include a dull staring coat, dental malocclusions, anorexia, slobbers, diarrhoea and immobility due to painful, swollen joints. The guinea pig is in constant pain and clinical signs and history are enough to make a diagnosis. Radiographically though, it can be seen that the epiphyses of the long bones and the costochondral junctions of the ribs are flared laterally, hence younger, still-growing guinea pigs are more susceptible.

Fractures

Fractures of the spine are common in guinea pigs that are housed with rabbits due to trauma. Clinically there is paresis or paralysis of the rear limbs, urinary incontinence etc. depending on the severity of the lesion. This may be confirmed as a fracture or subluxation on radiography. The prognosis is poor.

Ocular disease

Hypovitaminosis C can cause flaking of the skin of the eyelids and periocular area, as can dermatophytosis.

Conjunctivitis is often seen in guinea pigs kept on deep shavings or fine-chopped straw due to foreign bodies.

A primary cause of conjunctivitis is *Chlamydophila psittaci*, which causes crusting of the lids, reddening of the conjunctiva, increased tear production and a white-green tinged mucus discharge.

Other ocular problems include: hereditary and diabetic cataracts, and 'pea eye' – where subconjunctival fat accumulates in the ventral fornix area, making the tissue protrude.

Neurological disease

Drug toxicity

Aminoglycosides can induce renal failure; an ascending flaccid paralysis and death in guinea pigs has been reported.

Ulcerative pododermatitis

This is a particularly common condition in guinea pigs that have a more plantigrade stance with non-furred metatarsal areas. See the section on dermatological diseases. This may lead to osteomyelitis.

Pregnancy toxaemia

See page 79 for details.

Spinal trauma

See above heading 'Fractures' for details.

DISEASES OF THE CHINCHILLA
Skin disease

Fur slip

Stress and rough handling will cause clumps of fur to fall out spontaneously. This will regrow, but often not for some time.

Fur ring

In male chinchillas, a ring of fur can become wrapped around the penis inside the prepuce. This must be removed before it causes ischaemia. Males should be checked monthly, but more frequently during the breeding season – every 2–3 days – as it can be caused by mounting behaviour.

Fur matting

This is common if the fur is allowed to become damp. Chinchillas should never be washed, shampooed or allowed to live in damp environmental conditions. Fine pumice sand and Fuller's earth should be provided once or twice daily as a dust bath for fur hygiene and grooming.

Barbering

This is a common problem in chinchillas housed in pairs or groups. The fur of the tail and the whiskers are the most commonly chewed parts, and this increases when environmental stresses such as overcrowding are high, and when the diet is lacking in fibre or when dental disease is present.

Fungal disease

The dermatophyte *Trichophyton mentagrophytes* can cause alopecia in chinchillas, particularly over the nose and pinnae where non-pruritic grey crusts form.

Digestive disease

Oral

Dental disease is very common in chinchillas. Dental (cheek teeth) malocclusion occurs, as with rabbits, usually due to a lack of abrasive foods in the diet, and possibly combined with a lack of calcium and vitamin D_3 during growth. There is probably a hereditary component to the disease. Elongation of the crowns of the maxillary cheek teeth occurs laterally, so that they penetrate the cheek mucosa, with the crowns of the mandibular cheek teeth flaring medially, impinging on the tongue.

Elongation of the roots of the third and fourth maxillary cheek-teeth can cause pain and discomfort, as they penetrate the ocular orbit causing epiphora. The first and second maxillary cheek teeth enter the floor of the nasal passages/sinuses causing sneezing and nasal discharge. The mandibular cheek teeth roots penetrate the ventral aspect of the jaw and can be felt as a series of bumps along its lower border.

When the molars overgrow, gaps form between individual molars. These allow food particles to become wedged between the molars. The food particles then decay, creating periodontal disease and eventually abscesses.

Diagnosis of these problems can be made on clinical signs and radiography. Clinically, the chinchilla is often seen to be drooling saliva (the so-called 'slobbers'). It may also be anorectic, have lost weight and started consuming softer fresh foods rather than the harder dry pellets.

Gastrointestinal
Colic
Gas-colic is often due to feeding sugary food items such as banana. Clinically there may be teeth grinding, inappetence and a hunched appearance.

Caecocolic disease
Caecocolic disease occurs rarely in chinchillas, but is more likely if the chinchilla is suffering from severe diarrhoea. The caecum or proximal colon may become involved in an intussusception or a torsion. The chinchilla is in severe pain, hunched in posture, often grinding its teeth and drooling saliva, and occasionally rolling around the cage. Loops of bowel in the caudal and ventral portions of the abdomen, grossly swollen with gas, are seen on radiograph.

Constipation
Constipation due to ileus is seen most commonly as a sequel to: dental disease; obesity; late stage pregnancy; intestinal or abdominal surgery; sudden change in diet to a less fibrous, higher protein (such as an all-seed diet) diet. The chinchilla may produce scant, small faecal pellets for a number of days, and then none at all. Chinchillas so affected are often uncomfortable, and may sit hunched with tucked in abdomens.

Diarrhoea
Bacterial: Any of the bacteria mentioned in the section on guinea pigs may cause diarrhoea, with the *E. coli* and *Salmonella* spp. families appearing frequently. *Clostridium* spp. enterotoxaemia will occur if inappropriate antibiotics are used (e.g. oral penicillin).

Endoparasitic: Giardia is a single-celled protozoal parasite found in healthy and sick chinchillas alike, and therefore its role in disease is not fully understood. It is, however, a potential zoonosis. It is currently thought that poor diet, stress or concurrent disease allows the normally present *Giardia* spp. parasite to multiply up to sufficient numbers in the large bowel to cause diarrhoea. There is often the presence of soiled fur around the rear, and a general dullness. Diagnosis is by finding the motile, single-celled organisms on microscope examination of fresh faeces samples suspended in isotonic saline.

Hepatic lipidosis
Many chinchillas are overweight. They may then go on to develop dental problems or other conditions which may cause anorexia. Fat reserves are mobilised and the liver becomes swamped in fat compounds to the point at which failure may occur, with dullness and anorexia being the two most commonly seen non-specific signs. Diagnosis is made on finding elevated bile acid levels in conjunction with elevated AST and often GGT (gamma-glutamyl transferase) levels in the blood, and an enlarged liver shadow on radiography.

Respiratory disease
Pneumonia is common in chinchillas housed in damp and drafty conditions, but it may occur in any individual. The pathogens chiefly involved are bacteria such as *Bordetella bronchiseptica, Streptococcus pneumoniae, Pasteurella pneumotropica,* and *Pseudomonas* spp. Diagnosis is as for guinea pigs.

Cardiovascular disease
Chinchillas are prone to both hypertrophic and dilated cardiomyopathies. In addition, metastatic and dystrophic mineralisation and pericardial effusions may also be seen. Calcification may be asymptomatic and causes are thought to be similar to guinea pigs. In chinchillas, ventricular septal defects and tricuspid regurgitation have been reported.

Urinary tract disease
Urinary crystalline deposits have been seen in chinchillas and resemble those found in guinea pigs. Diagnosis is as for guinea pigs.

Reproductive tract disease
Dystocia occurs infrequently. There appears to be no associated significant separation of the pelvis as is seen in

the guinea pig, and therefore age at first breeding is not so critical.

Musculoskeletal disease

Fractures are common in chinchillas, and tend to occur in the longer, more slender bones such as the tibia and femur. Chinchilla bones are more brittle than other rodents'.

Ocular disease

Conjunctivitis presents epiphora. It may be due to excessive dust bathing with resultant foreign body irritation, or to the bacteria *Chlamydophila psittaci*. Alternatively, dental disease may be present, so the problem may not be a true conjunctivitis.

Neurological disease

Several causes of fitting have been described in chinchillas. These include the virus which causes lymphocytic choriomeningitis, as well as the bacteria *Listeria monocytogenes*, which may be spread by wild rodents.

DISEASES OF THE CHIPMUNK
Skin disease
Ectoparasitic

Burrowing mites such as *Notoedres muris* as well as *Sarcoptes* spp. have been reported. In addition, they are susceptible to the harvest mite *Neotrombicula autumnalis*, as well as the avian red mite *Dermanyssus gallinae*. The latter can cause anaemia and is commonly found where birds nest and roost.

Bacterial

Bacteria such as those described for rats and mice are commonly isolated from the skin of chipmunks and their associated abscesses. Abscesses are common in chipmunks housed in groups as they frequently fight.

Digestive disease
Oral

Overgrown incisors are common due to trauma. Overgrowth or damage of the incisors may cause them to impinge on the floor of the nasal passage. The chipmunk often shows signs of a runny nose with a copious discharge.

Gastrointestinal

Chipmunks suffer diarrhoea from bacteria seen in rats and mice, with *Yersinia pseudotuberculosis* and *Salmonella* spp. being reported. Tyzzer's disease (*Clostridium (Bacillus) piliformis*), which may cause liver damage, is also seen.

Respiratory disease

Pneumonia is frequently bacterial, and often occurs after periods of stress such as re-homing and handling. In addition, it is thought that the human influenza virus may be transmissible to chipmunks.

Cardiovascular disease

Chipmunks are very nervous and care should be taken to handle them carefully and in dimmed lighting. Rough handling and high levels of stress can lead to fitting and cardiac arrest.

Urinary tract disease

Struvite crystals and calcium oxalate are seen. *E. coli* bacterial cystitis is often associated. Since they have a longer urethra and an *os penis*, urolithiasis causes more problems for males than for females. Haematuria may be seen, and a swollen penis found on close physical examination. The calculi may be demonstrated radiographically and in urine samples.

Reproductive tract disease
Hypocalcaemic paralysis

This can occur soon after parturition, particularly if the chipmunk is on a poor-quality all-seed diet. The female appears lethargic, often is not suckling the young and may become unconscious.

Uterine disease

Uterine infections such as pyometras may be seen. There may be a vulval discharge, sometimes tinged with blood, and the female chipmunk is often anorectic, lethargic and polydipsic. Metritis may be seen shortly after parturition, with the female presenting as collapsed and weakened with a swollen abdomen and signs of peritonitis.

Mammary gland disease

Mastitis is uncommon, but bacteria such as *E. coli*, *Klebsiella* spp. and *Staphylococcus* spp. have been isolated. Mammary gland fibroadenomas and adenocarcinomas have been recorded.

Musculoskeletal disease

Chipmunks are acrobatic and fractures are common and often involve the spine. If a spinal fracture is suspected, radiography may be performed. The prognosis is poor and euthanasia is advised in these cases.

Neurological disease

Fitting is a problem in chipmunks housed in rooms with 50–60 Hertz wavelength equipment (TVs etc.). In addition, some chipmunks may be prone to hereditary epilepsy. Finally, bacteria such as *Listeria monocytogenes* and *Streptococcus pneumoniae*, protozoa such as *Toxoplasma gondii*, as well as viruses such as LCMV may also cause central nervous system disease.

DISEASES OF SUGAR GLIDERS AND VIRGINIA OPOSSUMS

Skin disease

Bacterial skin disease

Similar pyoderma problems as those seen in Eutherian mammals have been reported in marsupials. Fight wounds may be common where stocking densities are high or where sexually mature entire males are housed together.

Fungal skin disease

Dermatophyte *Trichophyton mentagrophytes* has been associated with scaling lesions in Virginia opossums.

Ectoparasites

Specific mites such as *Petauralges rackae* in sugar gliders and *Haemogamasus* spp. in Virginia opossums have been associated with mange. Marsupials also appear susceptible to *Sarcoptes scabei* mites. Harvest mites (*Neotrombicula autumnalis* and *Guntheria kowanyam*) have also been seen to cause pruritus and self-mutilation.

Common cat and dog fleas are not host specific and so could also infest both species of marsupial.

Neoplasia

Cutaneous lymphoma has been reported in sugar gliders and lymphoma in appears common in this species.

Self-trauma

Sugar gliders may self-traumatise digits, genitalia and their tails when stressed, initially, just removing the hair and then causing tissue injuries.

Miscellaneous

Virginia opossums have been reported with scaling of the non-haired portion of the tail. Some cases have been determined as ectoparasite associated disease and some have resolved when the environmental humidity has been increased.

Digestive disease

Dental disease

Tartar build-up with periodontal disease and abscesses are common in sugar gliders and Virginia opossums and are worsened by sugar rich soft food diets.

Bacterial disease

Gastrointestinal infections with bacteria such as *Yersinia pseudotuberculosis, Salmonella* spp. and *Clostridium* spp. have been reported in sugar gliders and Virginia opossums. Yersiniosis may result in acute death or a more chronic wasting condition, with granulomata formation in the intestines. Clostridiosis has been associated with acute death, but it and *E. coli* enteritis may also result in diarrhoea, tenesmus and rectal prolapses in sugar gliders. Mycobacterial infections of marsupials have been reported in the wild but are relatively uncommon in captivity.

Parasitic disease

Giardia spp. have been reported in both species and resulted in small intestinal disease with diarrhoea and dehydration.

Cryptosporidium spp. has been reported in neonate sugar gliders and in immunocompromised individuals has resulted in diarrhoea and a malabsorption maldigestion problem.

Various nematodes have been reported in the gut of the sugar glider including *Parastrongyloides* spp., *Paraustrostrongylus* spp. and *Paraustroxyuris* spp. In the Virginia opossum nematodes such as *Capillaria* spp., *Physaloptera* spp., and *Cruzia* spp., have been reported. Intestinal flukes (trematodes) have also been reported in Virginia opossums and may be associated with diarrhoea.

Liver flukes (*Athesmia* spp.) have been reported asymptomatically in sugar gliders but theoretically heavy infestations could result in liver damage.

Respiratory disease

Bacterial disease

Infections with *Pasteurella multocida, Streptococcus pneumoniae* and *Klebsiella* spp. have all been reported resulting in pneumonia in sugar gliders and Virginia opossums.

Fungal disease

Cryptococcus neoformans, a yeast, has been reported as the cause of pneumonia in sugar gliders. It produces a granulomatous reaction which may be seen radiographically and is difficult to treat. Sources of infection are contaminated feed/environmental plants.

Cardiovascular disease

Cardiomyopathy (dilated) has been reported in both sugar gliders and Virginia opossums and can produce congestive heart failure. Hypertrophic cardiomyopathy may also be seen in Virginia opossums, particularly those over 2 years of age and may present with tachycardia and also renal failure.

Microabscessation of the myocardium and associated heart failure may also be seen in various bacterial infections, particularly those associated with *Clostridium* spp. bacteria.

Heartworm – *Dirofilaria immitis* has also been reported as a cause of heart failure in Virginia opossums. It is transmitted principally by mosquitoes and is not currently found in the United Kingdom although it is present in parts of continental Europe and the USA.

Mineralisation of the aorta and main arteries has also been reported in Virginia opossums due to oversupplementation with calcium and vitamin D_3.

Urinary tract disease

Leptospira spp. infections of the urinary tract have been associated with interstitial nephritis, hepatitis and death of marsupials.

Urolithiasis and cystitis have been reported in sugar gliders and may be associated with urinary retention due to a lack of territory (overcrowding).

Prostatic hypertrophy and prostatitis resulting in dysuria have been reported in Virginia opossums.

Reproductive tract disease

Infections of the pouch can be seen in both species. Bacteria involved include *Pseudomonas* spp., *E. coli* and *Staphylococcus aureus.*

Infections of the reproductive tract have also been reported as a cause of ill-health and infertility and may result in uterine prolapse in Virginia opossums. Neoplasia of the reproductive tract is also relatively common in older females.

Male sugar gliders are known to self-mutilate the penis and scrotum when kept on their own.

Infertility may also be seen in individuals that are obese and in situations where there is overcrowding.

Musculoskeletal disease

Nutritional osteodystrophy

Also known as metabolic bone disease, it is common in captive marsupials, particularly in sugar gliders. As with other animals, it is associated with a lack of calcium and vitamin D_3. Clinically, it can present with bowing of long bones, spontaneous fractures and collapse of the spinal column, with resultant paresis/paralysis. Radiographs reveal poor bone mineralisation/density and hypocalcaemia and hypoproteinaemia may be seen on blood biochemistry. Diets that contain large amounts of unsupplemented fruit or meat are common culprits.

Neurological disease

Paresis or paralysis, usually of the hindlimbs, associated with nutritional osteodystrophic collapse of the spinal column resulting in spinal cord damage is common.

In sugar gliders, seizures associated with hypovitaminosis B_1 have been reported where diets have not been supplemented with this vitamin (home-made sugar/nectar formulas are often deficient in this).

All marsupials are very susceptible to *Toxoplasma* spp. infection which can result in fever, seizures and usually death. Sources are typically contamination of food/environment by the faeces of domestic cats, although the Virginia opossum is known to scavenge dead rodents which can also provide a source.

Migration through the spinal cord of the nematode *Bayliascaris* spp. has also been reported as a cause of paralysis in sugar gliders.

Many aged Virginia opossums will show evidence of fine and intention tremors due to fibrosis of the vasculature within the brain leading to reduced oxygenation.

Ocular disease

Cataracts have been reported in sugar gliders associated with both hypovitaminosis A and with diabetes mellitus. Senescent cataracts have been reported in both marsupials.

DISEASES OF THE FERRET
Skin disease
Ectoparasitic

Mites

The ear mite *Otodectes cynotis* causes intense irritation, and the production of copious black wax. This may lead to facial dermatitis, otitis externa, otitis interna and vestibular syndrome. Diagnosis is by finding the typical mites on wax samples (see Figure 5.15).

Less common is *Sarcoptes scabei* which can cause intense pruritus over the head, ears, paws and tail. Diagnosis is made on skin scrapings.

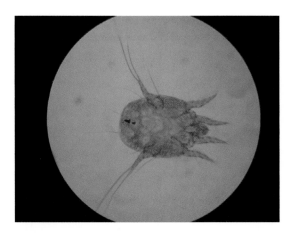

Figure 5.15 *Otodectes cynotis* ear mite from a ferret.

Fleas

The domestic cat and dog fleas *Ctenocephalides felis* and *C. canis* may infest ferrets. Many ferrets are used in the United Kingdom for hunting, and therefore rabbit fleas *Spilopsyllus cuniculi* or 'stick tight' fleas *Echidnophaga* spp. may also be seen.

Ticks

Ixodes ricinus are commonly found in ferrets used for hunting.

Bacterial

Abscesses frequently develop, particularly in the cervical area, due to intraspecific fighting. Bacteria include Streptococcus spp., *Staphylococcus* spp., *Arcanobacterium (Actinomyces) pyogenes*, *Pasteurella* spp., and *E. coli*. *A. pyogenes* infections often produce copious green-coloured pus, and may be associated with immunosuppressive conditions.

Fungal

Dermatophytosis due to *Microsporum canis* or *Trichophyton mentagrophytes* is relatively uncommon in the ferret.

Viral

Canine distemper virus (CDV), a paramyxovirus, may affect the skin with a rash over the chin and ventrum followed by brown crusts, particularly around the eyes and chin a week after infection. A nasal discharge may be present. Unless vaccinated, most ferrets will die from canine distemper between 7–21 days after contracting the virus.

Skin tumours

Squamous cell carcinomas are the most frequently reported skin neoplasm in ferrets, occurring on the head, along the nose and ear tips in particular. They are malignant tumours and rapidly spread. Sebaceous epitheliomas and basal cell tumours are seen on the head, neck and shoulders and are well-defined, benign tumours, but may ulcerate. Fibrosarcomas have been reported in response to injection site reactions, as in cats. Mast cell tumours are also common in ferrets but many will spontaneously resolve being generally less aggressive than those seen in dogs and cats (see Figure 5.16).

Hormonal

Hyperadrenocorticism is the most commonly seen cause of non-pruritic alopecia in the ferret (although around 40% may be pruritic!). Hair loss is mainly over the dorsum and flanks initially. Secondary signs of hyperadrenocortical disease including pendulous abdomen, thinning of the skin, weight gain etc. are also seen – see Endocrine diseases

In male ferrets, Leydig/interstitial cell tumours can produce excess testosterone and Sertoli cell tumours can produce excess oestrogen resulting in fur loss. In females, granulosa cell tumours of the ovaries have been associated with hair loss, as has the common hyperoestrogen condition of unmated entire females.

Digestive disease

Oral

Dental disease is common in ferrets over 18 months of age on wet diets, which cause tartar and periodontal disease.

Oesophageal

Megaoesophagus has been reported in ferrets and results in regurgitation, wasting and aspiration pneumonia. It

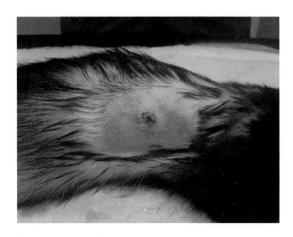

Figure 5.16 Mast cell tumour in a ferret prior to excision.

appears to be an acquired disease rather than congenital but the cause is unknown. Diagnosis is made using positive contrast radiography.

Gastric

Gastric ulceration is a common problem in ferrets and may be associated with *Helicobacter mustelae* infection. Gastric tumours and renal disease may also lead to gastric ulcer development, as will gastric foreign bodies.

The clinical signs vary from: dullness: abdominal guarding; salivation; vomiting; melaena and weight loss. Further tests involve blood tests for renal disease, radiographs, both plain and barium studies, and ultimately gastric biopsy to demonstrate/culture *Helicobacter mustelae*.

Intestinal

Proliferative ileitis

Proliferative ileitis is similar to the 'wet tail' seen in hamsters and is due to *Lawsonia intracellularis*. Clinically, a green, mucoid, bloody diarrhoea and weight loss are seen. Diagnosis is made on clinical signs primarily which are unlike almost any other condition. Biopsy can be confirmatory.

Intestinal lymphoma

This is relatively uncommon, but lymphoma of the mesenteric lymph nodes and the liver are seen in older ferrets. This may present with vague gastrointestinal signs, such as constipation, liver disease or even as apparently acute liver failure with jaundice.

Endoparasitic disease

Coccidiosis and giardiasis have both been described as causes of lethargy, diarrhoea and dehydration. Nematode and cestode parasites are rarely seen, although hunting individuals are more likely to be exposed to these parasites, with *Toxocara* spp. and *Toxascaris* spp. being the most commonly seen. Rarely do they cause clinical disease.

Viral disease

A parvovirus known as Aleutian disease is particularly lethal to mink, but in ferrets it produces unpleasant diarrhoea, although it is rarely fatal. It may produce melaenic faeces, fever, loss of weight and a number of other immune-system mediated symptoms.

Canine distemper can produce gastrointestinal signs such as diarrhoea. In addition, the influenza virus C may also be responsible for mild diarrhoea.

A member of the rotavirus family can cause diarrhoea in young, unweaned and recently weaned ferrets.

Other bacterial causes of diarrhoea

Salmonellosis due to *Salmonella typhimurium* has been reported and is a potential zoonosis.

Liver disease

The liver is commonly affected by lymphoma, although primary cancer of the liver is uncommon. Hepatic lipidosis has been recorded in persistently anorectic ferrets. In all of these cases the ferret may simply appear to be vaguely unwell, jaundice being an uncommon feature. Blood results may suggest a rise in ALT above 275 IU/L (Hillyer *et al.* 1997), but it often requires ultrasonographic and biopsy tests to make a diagnosis.

Liver disease associated with copper poisoning has also been reported in ferrets.

Respiratory disease

Viral

Canine distemper virus (CDV) is a paramyxovirus. The virus is spread by aerosol from one infected ferret or canid to another, when they sneeze or breathe. It may also be transmitted on a handler's hands and clothing. The virus gains access through the upper airways and incubates inside the ferret for 7–10 days, spreading throughout the body via the bloodstream.

The first signs of the disease occur on the skin (see skin diseases). The ferret is pyrexic and may have a serous oculonasal discharge. Secondary bacterial infections of the lungs on top of widespread immunosuppression often results in the death of an infected ferret. Towards the end of the disease fitting, nystagmus and generalised incoordination are all seen. The condition is fatal in nearly all cases of unvaccinated ferrets. Diagnosis is made on clinical signs, demonstration of viral antigens/antibodies in the bloodstream and/or mucus secretions of the ferret.

Human influenza C virus, an orthomyxovirus, is transmissible from human to ferret and back again. It causes a mainly upper airway disease with a systemic phase, producing pyrexia for 3–4 days.

Bacterial

Bacteria such as *Pasteurella* spp., *Bordetella bronchiseptica*, *Klebsiella pneumonia*, *Streptococcus pneumonia*, *Nocardia* spp. have all been associated with pneumonia in the domestic ferret. Diagnosis is made on lung radiographs, lung washes and isolation of the bacteria.

Parasitic

The lungworm *Aelurostrongylus abstrusus* can cause chronic coughing in ferrets. The adult worm sits in the pulmonary vasculature and sheds its eggs into the bloodstream which burst into the alveoli and are coughed up, swallowed and passed in the faeces. This parasite uses molluscs (e.g. slugs and snails) as intermediate hosts. The lungworm *Capillaria aerophila* has also been reported in ferrets and will cause coughing. It sits in the actual airways as an adult worm. Again eggs are coughed up and passed in the faeces, where they may be ingested by earthworms or rodents which may act as a paratenic host.

Cardiovascular disease

Cardiomyopathy

Dilated cardiomyopathy is the most commonly seen, and may lead to congestive cardiac failure with lethargy, fluid respiratory noises, weight loss, polydipsia, ascites and audible systolic murmurs on auscultation of the chest. Diagnosis is made on radiographic signs of lung congestion, occasionally pleural effusion and an enlarged cardiac shadow, ECG changes and ultrasonographic demonstration of heart-wall thinning and valvular incompetence. Hypertrophic cardiomyopathy is rarely seen. Vertebral heart scores have been derived for ferrets to assess the radiographic size of the heart relative to the thoracic vertebrae – see Chapter 7 for further information.

Endocardiosis

Endocardiosis is common in ageing ferrets. The presenting signs are similar to those seen in dogs with productive coughs, lethargy and, in more serious cases, heart failure with ascites and cyanosed membranes. Diagnosis is by auscultation, clinical signs and ultrasonographic demonstration of valvular incompetence and thickening.

Heartworm

Again, although it is not endemic in the United Kingdom, heartworm due to *Dirofilaria immitis* can be seen in ferrets from overseas. The parasite is transmitted by mosquitoes and the adult develops in the right ventricle of the heart. Ferrets affected may present with right-sided heart failure, that is, pleural effusion and ascites. An ELISA test is available but ferrets often produce false-negative results. Right-sided enlargement of the heart may be seen on radiographs and abnormalities may be seen on echocardiographic examination of the heart. In the United Kingdom, it is also possible to see the heartworm *Angiostrongylus vasorum*. This nematode uses slugs and snails as the intermediate host. The adult worms live in the right side of the heart and pulmonary vasculature with eggs being shed into the blood stream, entering the airways and being coughed and swallowed and passed in the faeces. Severe cases may show signs of right-sided heart failure.

Lymphoma

Blood-borne leukaemia is uncommon; however, the tissue-associated lymphoma is very common – being the third most frequently seen neoplasia in the ferret after adrenal gland neoplasia and insulinomas. Some authors believe that there are two types of lymphoma: one is a juvenile, aggressive (lymphoblastic) form of lymphoma seen in ferrets under 14 months of age, often found in one site (e.g thymus or spleen), develops rapidly and responds well to chemotherapy; the other is a more chronic (lymphocytic) lymphoma typically seen in ferrets over 14 months, which affects more than one site and responds poorly to chemotherapy. Other authors agree that this is what is seen clinically but believe that a staging protocol similar to that used in dogs is more useful (Schoemaker, 2009):

- Stage 1: a single site is involved (typically but not restricted to the spleen or thymus)
- Stage 2: Multiple non-contiguous sites on the same side of the diaphragm
- Stage 3: Multiple lymphatic sites on both sides of the diaphragm
- Stage 4: Multiple sites on both sides of the diaphragm including non-lymphatic tissue or bone marrow

Obviously stage 1 has the best prognosis for chemotherapy or surgery and the prognosis steadily worsens to stage 4.

Urinary tract disease

Kidney

Polycystic kidney disease is inherited in ferrets and is rare. Discrete renal cysts are asymptomatic but can be as common as 10–15%.

Pyelonephritis (e.g. *E. coli*) is seen in ferrets. In addition, interstitial nephritis due to *Leptospira* spp. is common in working ferrets coming into contact with wild rodents, which are the reservoir for this disease. Chronic interstitial nephritis is also common in all ferrets and is progressive from 2 years of age resulting in renal failure from 4 to 5 years of age.

Aleutian disease can produce a strong antibody response and result in circulating antibody–antigen complexes. These can damage the glomerular membranes of the kidneys, and produce membranous glomerulone-phritis and tubular interstitial nephritis which may result in renal failure.

Renal function can be assessed using blood urea and creatinine levels – the latter of which are lower normally than in other mammals (17–46 µmol/L).

Bladder

Urolithiasis is seen in ferrets that are fed protein from a plant source, such as is found in dog food. This creates an alkaline urine pH and allows these salts to precipitate. The provision of solely animal proteins in the diet leads to acidic urine and dissolution of the calculi. Pregnant jills are susceptible, as they are mobilising large volumes of minerals from their bones for foetal development and milk production. Uroliths are struvite or magnesium ammonium phosphate.

Male ferrets may experience obstruction at the *os penis* if it is of large enough calculi form. Clinically they are dull, straining to urinate and sometimes prolapsing the rectum. Often, the prepuce is swollen and the abdomen tense; occasionally crystals may be seen on the hairs around the prepuce. Radiography will confirm the diagnosis.

Stranguria and dysuria may be seen in male ferrets with prostatic hypertrophy and prostatic/paraprostatic cysts which are associated with hyperadrenocorticism.

Endocrine disease

Adrenal

The cause of adrenal disease in ferrets is still not fully understood, but a correlation between neutering and development of the disease has been deduced. The pathophysiology is thought to be due to ferrets (like mice and humans) having luteinising hormone (LH) receptors in their adrenal tissue, which increase in number with elevated circulating LH which occurs after gonadectomy. This triggers the production of sex steroid hormones by the adrenal glands, so clinical disease (as well as hypertrophy and neoplastic change of the gland). Some suggest that certain genetic lines of ferrets are more predisposed. In ferrets, adrenal gland hyperplasia accounts for 56% of adrenal disease, adrenocortical adenoma accounts for 16% and adenocarcinoma for 26%, both producing sex steroid hormones, particularly oestradiol. In addition, the left adrenal gland seems more likely to develop disease than the right.

Diagnosis of adrenal disease is based on clinical signs, for example, polyuria/polydipsia; bilateral hair loss,

starting over the tail rump and dorsum and spreading over the flanks and rest of the body; pruritus in 40% of cases; and swelling of the vulva or prepuce in a ferret that has been previously surgically neutered. In male ferrets, prostatic cysts and hyperplasia are seen which may present with dysuria or stranguria. Ultrasound may show enlargement of the adrenal gland, but this can be difficult in early cases. Urinary corticoid: creatinine ratio (UCCR) is often increased and resistant to dexamethasone suppression. The adrenocorticotrophin hormone (ACTH) level is often depressed and an increase in plasma cortisol levels has been observed after an injection of human chorionic gonadotrophin (hCG) (Schoemaker *et al.*, 2008). In general a panel of oestradiol, androstenedione, 17-hydroxyprogesterone and dehydroepiandrosterone sulphate (DHEAS) +/− cortisol has been recommended by many as effective in detecting adrenocortical disease in ferrets.

Diabetes mellitus

Diabetes mellitus is uncommon in ferrets, but presents as a disease similar to that seen in cats.

Insulinoma

Hypoglycaemia may occur due to prolonged fasting (ferrets should not be fasted for more than 4–6 hours due to their high metabolic rates), overdosage with insulin in a diabetic case or due to an insulinoma (an insulin secreting pancreatic tumour). Insulinomas have been reported as the most commonly seen neoplasm in older ferrets (>4 years) with an incidence varying from 21.7% (Williams & Weis, 2003) to 25% (Li *et al.*, 1998). Tumours secrete insulin continuously and are not altered by the production of hypoglycaemia. Rebound hypoglycaemia can also occur though, if a brief period of hyperglycaemia has occurred, as the tumours can increase their production of insulin. Metastatic spread is low in ferrets with insulinomas.

Diagnosis of insulinoma is based on clinical signs, which include weakness of hindlimbs, ataxia, collapse, opisthotonus and drooling saliva with pawing at the mouth. Rarely do ferrets exhibit full seizures as is seen in dogs with insulinomas. Blood levels of glucose lower than 3.3 mmol/L are suggestive of insulinoma but not diagnostic. Elevated insulin levels (normal range reported as 35–250 pmol/L (Jenkins, 2000) in the presence of hypoglycaemia are confirmatory. Some ferrets, however, may present with normal glucose levels with elevated insulin due to recent food consumption. These can be very carefully fasted for 3–4 hours to watch for the development of hypoglycaemia in the presence of persistent hyperinsulinaemia.

Hyperoestrogenism
For details, see below.

Reproductive tract disease
Pregnancy toxaemia
Pregnancy toxaemia is similar to that seen in the guinea pig. It occurs in late gestation, often in a first-time mother, during a period of anorexia. Ketoacidosis develops, leading to dullness, lethargy, vomiting, dehydration, alopecia, neurological signs, abortion and death of the jill.

Dystocia
Dystocia is relatively uncommon in the ferret. It is more common in jills carrying a small litter due to low levels of foetal corticosteroid produced. If the jill exceeds day 43 of gestation, labour may need to be induced.

Mastitis
Mastitis may occur as an acute illness immediately after parturition. Bacteria commonly present in these cases are *Streptococcus* spp. and *E. coli*. Toxaemia may develop.

A more chronic condition is seen due to the bacteria *Staphylococcus intermedius*. This form of mastitis is highly infectious between jills and destroys much of the mammary tissue, leaving scar tissue and pockets of infection.

Pyometra and metritis
Metritis occurs immediately after parturition and may cause an acute toxic reaction in the jill. The jill may be very dull and pyrexic at this stage, and have no milk production.

Pyometra occurs at any stage, and is manifested by a dark, foul-smelling vulval discharge, polydipsia and sometimes toxaemia. Occasionally, a closed pyometra with no external discharge may occur. Palpation of the abdomen reveals a swollen uterus in the caudal dorsal abdomen. The diagnosis may be confirmed with radiography or ultrasonography.

Hyperoestrogenism
An entire female will remain in oestrus for the whole of the breeding season (March–October), unless she is mated or chemically brought out of oestrus as ferrets are induced ovulators. This chronic, long-term exposure to oestrogen results in fatal anaemia from bone marrow suppression. The jill presents as tachypnoeic, with pale, petechiated mucous membranes, lethargic and collapsed. Early signs are a prominently swollen vulva, symmetrical alopecia of the flanks, and often a vulval discharge. Current recommendations are for the jill to be brought out of heat by (1) being mated by an entire or vasectomised male; (2) being injected with proligestone (Delvosteron® MSD Animal Health) a synthetic progesterone; or (3) Implanted with a gonadotrophin releasing hormone (GnRH) agonist such as deslorelin (Suprelorin® Virbac Animal Health). Surgical neutering is not recommended due to adrenal neoplasia.

Prostatic disease
Prostate cysts are particularly common in ferrets with an actively secreting adrenal gland tumour. If enlarged, the prostate will obstruct the urethra, and therefore prevent urination. Large prostatic and paraprostatic cysts are commonly seen with this condition.

Musculoskeletal disease
Fractures in ferrets are uncommon, although the spine is the most commonly affected. Posterior paresis or paralysis is often associated with vertebral fractures, but may also be a sign of cardiovascular disease, hypoglycaemia or anaemia. Diagnosis is by radiography and tests already discussed.

Neurological disease
Fitting may be seen towards the end stages of CDV infection; hypoglycaemic syndrome; as well as in severe anaemia. Posterior paresis may be associated with spinal trauma, cardiovascular disease, hypoglycaemia, anaemia and CDV.

Mild incoordination, posterior ataxia and paresis can be associated with spinal disease due to trauma, abscessation or neoplasia. Aleutian disease can result in antigen–antibody complex-mediated vasculitis which can also produce these clinical signs. Diagnosis of Aleutian disease is often made using serum protein electrophoresis with a gamma globulin level in excess of 20% of the total serum protein level.

Ocular disease
Ophthalmia neonatorum, a failure of the kits' eyes to open, is often due to bacteria from the *Staphylococcus* and *Streptococcus* spp.

Other ocular problems include crusting and weeping associated with CDV, photophobia associated with the influenza virus, conjunctivitis, night blindness and cataracts associated with hypovitaminosis A. Corneal ulcers due to trauma and local infections are common in ferrets.

References

Gilmore, S.A. (2005) Spinal nerve root degeneration in aging laboratory rats: a light microscopic study. *Anatomical Record*, **174**(2), 251–257.

Girling, S.J., Pizzi, R., Cox, A. and Beard, P. (2011) Fatal cowpox infection in two squirrel monkeys (*Saimiri sciureus*). *Veterinary Record*, **169**(6), 156.

Hillyer, E.V., Quesenberry, K.E. and Donnelly, T.M. (1997) Biology, husbandry and clinical techniques. *Ferrets, Rabbits and Rodents: Clinical Medicine and Surgery*, pp. 243–259. WB Saunders, Philadelphia, PA.

Huybens, N., Houeix, J., Szalo, M., Licois, D., Mainil, J. and Marlier, D. (2008) Is epizootic rabbit enteropathy (ERE) a bacterial disease? *Proceedings of the 9th World Rabbit Congress*, pp. 971–975. Verona, Italy.

Jean-Blain, C. and Durix, A. (1985) Effects of dietary lipid level on ketonemia and other plasma parameters related to glucose and fatty acid metabolism in the rabbit during fasting. *Reproductive Nutritional Development*, **25**, 345–354.

Jenkins, J.R. (2000) Ferret metabolic testing. *Laboratory Medicine: Avian and Exotic Pets* (ed. A.M. Fudge), pp. 305–309. WB Saunders, Philadelphia, PA.

Lafontan, M. and Agid, R. (1979) An extra-adrenal action of adrenocorticotrophin: physiological induction of lipolysis by secretion of adrenocorticotrophin in obese rabbits. *Journal of Endocrinology*, **81**, 281–290.

Leary, S.L., Manning, P.J. and Anderson, L.C. (1984) Experimental and naturally occurring gastric foreign bodies in laboratory rabbits. *Laboratory Animal Science*, **34**(1), 58–61.

Li, X., Fox, J.G. and Padril, P.A. (1998) Neoplastic diseases in ferrets: 574 cases (1968–1997). *Journal of American Veterinary Medical Association*, **212**(9), 1402–1406.

McLaughlin, R.M. and Fish, R.E. (1994) Clinical biochemistry and haematology. *The Biology of the Laboratory Rabbit* (eds P.J. Manning, D.H. Ringler & C.E. Newcomer), 2nd edn, pp. 111–124. Academic Press, London.

Okerman, L. (1994) Inherited conditions and congenital deformities. *Diseases of Domestic Rabbits*, 2nd edn, pp. 109–112. Blackwell, Oxford.

Schmidt, R.E. and Reavill, D.R. (2007) Cardiovascular disease in hamsters: review and retrospective study. *Journal of Exotic Pet Medicine*, **16**, 49–51.

Schoemaker, N.J. (2009) Endocrine and Neoplastic Diseases. *Manual of Ferrets and Rodents* (eds E. Keeble & A. Meredith), pp. 320–329. BSAVA, Quedgeley, UK.

Schoemaker, N.J., Kuijten, A.M. and Galac, S. (2008) Luteinizing hormone-dependent Cushing's syndrome in a pet ferret (*Mustela putorius furo*). *Domestic Animal Endocrinology*, **34**, 278–283.

Weisbroth, S., Flatt, R.E. and Kraus, A.L. (1974) Anatomy, physiology and biochemistry of the rabbit. *The Biology of the Laboratory Rabbit* (eds Manning *et al.*), 2nd edn, p. 65. Academic Press, London.

Williams, B.H. and Weis, C.A. (2003) Ferret neoplasia. *Ferrets, Rabbits and Rodents: Clinical Medicine* (eds K.E. Quesenberry & J.W. Carpenter), 2nd edn, pp. 91–106. WB Saunders, St Louis.

Further reading

Fraser, M.A. and Girling, S.J. (2009) *Rabbit Medicine and Surgery for Veterinary Nurses*. Blackwell-Wiley, Oxford.

Heatley, J.J. (2009) Cardiovascular anatomy, physiology and disease of rodents and small exotic mammals. *Veterinary Clinics of North America: Exotic Animal Practice*, **12**, 99–113.

Hinton, M. (1981) Kidney disease in the rabbit: a histological survey. *Laboratory Animals*, **15**, 263–265.

Keeble, E. and Meredith, A. (2009) *Manual of Rodents and Ferrets*. BSAVA, Quedgeley, UK.

Lowe, J.A. (1998) Pet rabbit feeding and nutrition. *The Nutrition of the Rabbit* (eds De Blas and Wiseman), pp. 304–331. CABI Publishing, Cambridge.

Meredith, A. and Flecknall, P. (2006) *Manual of Rabbits*, 2nd edn. BSAVA, Quedgeley, UK.

Meredith, A. and Johnson-Delaney, C. (2010) *Manual of Exotic Pets*, 5th edn. BSAVA, Quedgeley, UK.

Quesenberry, K.E. and Carpenter, J. (2003) *Ferrets, Rabbits and Rodents*, 2nd edn. WB Saunders, Philadelphia, PA.

Chapter 6 An Overview of Small Mammal Therapeutics

FLUID THERAPY

Maintenance requirements

In small mammals there is little water lost as sweat, as rodents, and lagomorphs have little or no skin sweat glands, and most do not pant either. Increased metabolic rates, and their small size, lead to a large lung surface area in relation to volume and the loss of large amounts of fluids during normal respiration. In addition, glomerular filtration rates are higher. This makes their daily maintenance fluid requirement per kilogram nearly double those seen in larger mammals. Some values are given in Table 6.1.

The effect of disease on fluid requirements

Respiratory disease is common in small mammals, especially rabbits, rats and mice. In these animals often chronic levels of lung infection are present, with increased respiratory secretions being the result. Fluid loss can therefore be appreciable via this route.

Individuals suffering from diarrhoea will experience fluid loss and often metabolic acidosis due to the prolonged loss of bicarbonate.

Another route of fluid and electrolyte loss is through skin disease. Rabbits (in particular, those kept in wet or unsanitary conditions) will contract skin infections from environmental bacterial organisms such as *Pseudomonas* spp. These produce lesions, which resemble chemical or thermal burns, and leave large areas of weeping, exudative skin causing further fluid loss.

Post-surgical fluid requirements

Surgical procedures may cause intrasurgical haemorrhaging, necessitating vascular support with isotonic crystalloids or, in more serious blood losses (>10%), colloidal fluids or even blood transfusions. Even if surgery is relatively bloodless, there are inevitable losses via the respiratory route due to the drying nature of the gases used to deliver the anaesthetics.

In addition, many patients are not able to drink immediately after surgery. Some forms of surgery, such as incisor extraction in rabbits suffering from malocclusion, will lead to inappetence for a period of time. Dehydration will result, as many rabbits gain the majority of their fluid intake from their vegetable diets.

Electrolyte replacement

Electrolyte replacement can be necessary in cases of chronic diarrhoea such as in coccidiosis in rabbits or wet tail in hamsters. The main electrolyte losses are bicarbonate and potassium, leading to metabolic acidosis.

Small herbivores, particularly rabbits, rarely vomit and so electrolyte loss by that route is unlikely to occur. Ferrets can vomit, for example, stomach ulceration due to bacteria such as *Helicobacter mustelae*. In these cases, metabolic alkalosis may result.

Fluid types used in small mammal practice

Lactated Ringer's/Hartmann's

Lactated Ringer's solution is useful as a general-purpose rehydration and maintenance fluid. It is particularly useful for small mammals suffering from metabolic acidosis, such as those described above with chronic gastrointestinal problems, but can also be used for fluid therapy after routine surgical procedures.

Glucose/saline combinations

Glucose/saline is useful for small mammals, as they may have been through periods of anorexia prior to treatment, and therefore may well be borderline hypoglycaemic. Glucose/saline combinations are also useful for cases of urethral obstruction, such as ferret urolithiasis.

Hypertonic saline

This may be used in small mammals with acute hypovolaemia. It works by rapidly drawing fluid from the cellular and pericellular space into the circulation to

---

Veterinary Nursing of Exotic Pets, Second Edition. Edited by Simon J. Girling. © 2013 John Wiley & Sons, Ltd. Published 2013 by John Wiley & Sons, Ltd.

Table 6.1 Maintenance fluid values for selected small mammals.

Species	Fluid maintenance values (mL/kg per day)
Rabbit	80–100
Guinea pig	100
Chinchilla	100
Other rodent	90–100
Sugar glider	80–100
Ferret	75–100

support central venous pressure. See Chapter 8 for further details of its use. It must be administered intravenously or intraosseously.

Protein amino acid/B vitamin supplements

Protein and vitamin supplements are useful for nutritional support (e.g. Duphalyte® at 1 mL/kg per day). These supplements are particularly good in cases where the patient is malnourished or has been suffering from a protein-losing enteropathy or nephropathy. It is also a useful supplement for patients with hepatic disease or severe exudative skin diseases.

Colloidal fluids

These are of use in small mammals which may be given an intravenous bolus. They are used when a serious loss of blood occurs in order to support central blood pressure. This may be a temporary measure while a blood donor is selected, or, if none is available, the only means of attempting to support such a patient.

Blood transfusions

If the packed cell volume (PCV) starts to drop below 20%, blood transfusions may be required. They must be same species-to-species transfers (i.e. rat to rat, guinea pig to guinea pig). The donor may have 1% body weight in blood removed, assuming it is healthy. The sample is best taken directly into a pre-heparinised syringe, or using citrate acid dextrose at 1 mL of anticoagulant to 5–6 mL of blood, and immediately transfers it in bolus fashion to the donor. The use of intravenous catheters is advised, as administration should be slow, giving 1 mL over a period of 5–6 minutes. Therefore sedation, or good restraint, is required. Very little information is currently available about crossmatching blood groups of small mammals, although ferrets, it seems, do not have detectable groups.

Intraosseous donations may be made if vascular access is not possible. Calculations for volumes are based on those available for cats, that is

$$\text{Vol. of donor blood required(mL)} = 60 \times \text{BW(kg)} \times \frac{\text{Desired change in PCV}}{\text{PCV of tranfused blood}}$$

where BW is body weight of the recipient in kilograms.

Oral fluids and electrolytes

Oral fluids may be used in small mammal practice for those patients experiencing mild dehydration, and for home administration. The most useful products contain pro/prebiotics which aid the return to normal digestive function.

Calculation of fluid requirements

Fluid within food is difficult to take into consideration when calculating fluid needed, and therefore it is safer to assume that the debilitated small mammal will not be eating enough for it to matter. Once it is appreciated that maintenance for most small mammals is double that required for the average cat or dog, then deficits may be calculated in the same manner. Assume that 1% dehydration equates with needing to supply 10 mL/kg fluid replacement, in addition to maintenance requirements.

Then estimate the percentage of dehydration of the patient as follows:
- 3–5% dehydrated – increased thirst, slight lethargy, tacky mucous membranes
- 7–10% dehydrated – increased thirst, anorexia, dullness, tenting of the skin and slow return to normal, dry mucous membranes, dull corneas
- 10–15% dehydrated – dull to comatose, skin remains tented after pinching, desiccating mucous membranes.

Alternatively, if a blood sample may be obtained, a 1% increase in PCV, associated with an increase in total proteins, may be assumed to equate to 10 mL/kg fluid deficit (see Table 6.2).

These deficits may be large and difficult to replenish rapidly. Indeed, it may be dangerous to overload the patient's system with these fluid levels all in one go. Therefore, the following protocol is worth following to ensure fluid overload, renal shutdown and pulmonary oedema are avoided:
- Day 1: Maintenance fluid levels +50% of calculated dehydration factor
- Day 2: Maintenance fluid levels +50% of calculated dehydration factor
- Day 3: Maintenance fluid levels

If the dehydration levels are so severe that volumes are still too large to give at any one time, it may be necessary

Table 6.2 Comparison of normal PCV and total proteins for selected small mammals.

Species	PCV range (L/L)	Total protein (g/L)
Ferret	0.44–0.60	51–74
Rabbit	0.36–0.48	54–75
Guinea pig	0.37–0.48	46–62
Chinchilla	0.32–0.46	50–60
Rat	0.36–0.48	56–76
Mouse	0.39–0.49	35–72
Gerbil	0.43–0.49	43–85
Hamster[a]	0.36–0.55	45–75
Sugar glider	0.45–0.53	51–61
Virginia opossum	0.34–0.47	56–78

[a] The range given for hamsters is an average of Syrian and Russian hamster values.

to take 72 hours rather than 48 hours to replace the calculated deficit.

In addition, in those species such as ferrets, which can vomit, the fluid lost in vomitus expelled should be considered, assuming 2 mL/kg per vomit.

In other species such as the small herbivores, where diarrhoea only is the norm, it is much more difficult to make estimations, although fluid losses may approach 100–150 mL/kg per day.

Equipment for fluid administration

Catheters

The blood vessels available for intravenous medication are often 30–50% smaller than their cat and dog counterparts. Small paediatric butterfly catheters may be used. It is advisable to flush with heparinised saline, prior to use, to prevent clotting. Catheters of 25–27 gauge are recommended and will cope with venous access for rabbits, guinea pigs, chinchillas and ferrets. Occasionally a 28- or 29-gauge catheter may be needed to catheterise a lateral tail vein in a rat or mouse, although 27-gauge catheters often suffice.

Hypodermic or spinal needles

Hypodermic and spinal needles are useful for the administration of intraosseous, intraperitoneal and subcutaneous fluids. The intraosseous route may be the only method of giving central venous support in very small patients, or patients where vascular collapse is occurring. The proximal femur, tibia or humerus may be used. Entry can be gained by using hypodermic or spinal needles. Spinal needles are preferable because they have a central stylet to prevent

clogging of the needle lumen with bone fragments after insertion. Spinal needles of 23–25 gauge are usually sufficient.

Hypodermic needles may be used for the same purpose, although the risks of blockage are higher. Hypodermic needles may also be used for the administration of intraperitoneal and subcutaneous fluids. Generally, 23–25 gauge hypodermic needles are sufficient for the task.

Nasogastric tubes

Nasogastric tubes are often used in small mammals to provide nutritional support in as stress-free a manner as possible. They are useful as a route for fluid administration. It should be noted though that in severely dehydrated individuals, there is no way that all of the fluid deficits may be replaced via this route alone. This is due to the limited fluid capacity of the stomach of these species, as well as the real possibility that gut pathology may exist. This route is therefore restricted for use in facilitating fluid replacement and is used mainly for nutritional support and rehydrating the gut microflora.

Syringe drivers

For continuous fluid administration, such as is required for intravenous and intraosseous fluid administration, syringe drivers are recommended. Their advantage is that small volumes may be administered accurately. An error of 1–2 mL in some of the species dealt with over an hour could be equivalent to an over-perfusion of 50–100%! In addition, it is almost impossible to keep gravity-fed drip sets running at these low rates.

Intravenous drip tubing

Fine drip tubing is available for attachment to syringes and syringe-driver units. It is useful if these are luer locking, as this enhances safety and prevents disconnection when the patient moves. It may be necessary to purchase a sheath, such as is available for protecting household electrical cables, to cover drip tubing, as most of the small herbivores are experts at removing or chewing through plastic drip tubing!

Elizabethan collars

It may be necessary to place some of the small herbivores into an Elizabethan-style collar as they are the world's greatest chewers! These can be purchased as cage bird collars and adapted to fit even the smallest of rodents.

Routes of fluid administration

These routes have their advantages and disadvantages, given in Table 6.3.

Table 6.3 The advantages and disadvantages of various fluid therapy routes in small mammals.

Route	Advantages	Disadvantages
Oral	Reduced stress Well accepted Physiological route Minimal tissue trauma Rehydration of gut flora	May increase stress in guinea pigs Risk of aspiration pneumonia in some Not useful in cases of gut disease Slow rates of rehydration Maximum volume is 10 mL/kg
Subcutaneous	Large volumes may be given reducing dosing frequency Minimal risk of organ puncture	Guinea pigs react badly to scruff injections and fur slip is common in chinchillas Slow rehydration time May impede respiration due to pressure on chest wall Hypotonic or isotonic crystalloid fluids only
Intraperitoneal	Large volumes may be given at one time Uptake faster than subcutaneous if mild dehydration is present Minimal discomfort	Risk of organ puncture Stressful positioning (dorsal recumbency) Pressure on diaphragm may increase; respiratory effort needed Isotonic or hypotonic crystalloids only
Intravenous	Rapid central venous support May be used for continuous perfusion Can be used for colloidal fluids, hypertonic saline, dextrose/glucose and blood transfusions/replacers	Minimal peripheral access in some species (e.g. hamsters, gerbils) Increased vessel fragility due to small patient size Requires increased levels of operator skill
Intraosseous	Rapid support of the central venous system Useful in collapsed and very small patients where vascular access is difficult May still be used for blood transfusions/replacers Minimal risk of organ damage (puncture)	Not useful in fragile bones or metabolic bone disease Not useful in bone fractures or osteomyelitis Increased risk of infection (osteomyelitis) Painful procedure requiring sedation/analgesia Continuous perfusion required (syringe drivers) otherwise maximum boluses are small (0.25–0.5 mL for myomorph rodents and sugar gliders, 1–2 mL for hystricomorph rodents, 2–3 mL for rabbits, Virginia opossums and ferrets)

Oral

Rabbit

The oral route is not good for seriously debilitated rabbits, but it is useful for those with naso-oesophageal feeding tubes in place. It may also be useful for mild cases of dehydration where owners wish to home treat their pet. This route is restricted to small volumes, with a maximum of 10 mL/kg administered at any one time.

Rat, mouse, gerbil and hamster

Gavage (stomach) tubes or avian straight crop tubes can be used to place fluids directly into the rodent oesophagus. The rodent needs to be firmly scruffed to adequately restrain it with the head and oesophagus in a straight line. This method is often stressful but the alternative is to syringe fluids into the mouth, which often does not work as rodents can close off the back of the mouth with their cheek folds. Maximum volumes which can be given via the oral route in rodents vary from 5 to 10 mL/kg. Naso-oesophageal or gastric tubes are not a viable option in rodents due to their small size.

Guinea pig and chinchilla

Naso-oesophageal tubes may be placed and doses of 10 mL/kg may be administered at any one time. Guinea pigs and chinchillas are more likely to regurgitate than rabbits, especially when debilitated, so care is needed.

Marsupial

Gavage (stomach) tubes or avian straight crop tubes can be used to place fluids directly into the marsupial oesophagus. The marsupial needs to be firmly scruffed to adequately restrain it and to keep the head and oesophagus in a straight line. Alternatively, fluids may be drip fed from a syringe or teaspoon into the lip sulcus either side of the mouth and lapped up from there.

Ferret

Naso-oesophageal tubes are not well tolerated in ferrets, but many will accept sweet-tasting oral electrolyte solutions from a syringe. Ferrets, especially when debilitated, can regurgitate, so care is needed.

Subcutaneous

The advantages and disadvantages of this method are given in Table 6.3.

Rabbit

The scruff or lateral thorax makes ideal sites. This is a good technique to use as routine post-operative administration of fluids for minor surgical procedures such as spaying or castration. It is possible to give a maximum of 30–60 mL split into two or more sites at one time depending on the size of rabbit.

Rat, mouse, gerbil and hamster

The scruff area is easily utilised for volumes of 3–4 mL of fluids for smaller rodents and up to 10 mL at any one time for rats. The use of a 25-gauge needle is recommended.

Guinea pig and chinchilla

This is an easily used route for post-operative fluids and mild dehydration in these species. The scruff area and lateral thorax are preferred sites (Figure 6.1). The scruff may be painful for guinea pigs as it is a site of brown fat deposition and well innervated. Doses of 25–30 mL may be given at one time, preferably at two or more sites. Fur slip is a problem in chinchillas.

Marsupial

This is an easily used route for post-operative fluids and mild dehydration in these species. The scruff area and lateral thorax are preferred sites. Volumes of 3–4 mL in sugar gliders and 15–20 mL in adult Virginia opossums may be administered.

Ferret

Volumes of 15–20 mL may be given in two or more sites over the scruff.

Intraperitoneal

The advantages and disadvantages of the intraperitoneal route in small mammals are given in Table 6.3.

Rabbit

The rabbit is placed in dorsal recumbency to allow the gut contents to fall away from the injection zone. The needle is inserted in the lower right quadrant of the ventral abdomen, just through the abdominal wall and the syringe plunger drawn back to ensure that no puncture of the bladder or gut has occurred. A maximum volume of 20–30 mL may be given at one time depending on the size of the rabbit. Previous notes regarding concurrent respiratory or cardiovascular disease should be considered. If positioned correctly, there should be no resistance to injection.

Rat, mouse, gerbil and hamster

The positioning and administration site for rodents is as for rabbits (Figure 6.2). The needle should be 25 gauge or smaller and maximal volumes of 1–4 mL in smaller rodents, up to 10 mL in large rats, may be given.

Guinea pig and chinchilla

Similar principles apply for this route as for rabbits and other rodents. Doses of 15–20 mL may be given. This is a good route for more serious cases, as intravenous fluids are not so well tolerated, particularly in chinchillas and guinea pigs.

Marsupial

Similar principles apply for this route as for rabbits and rodents. Doses of 2–4 mL in sugar gliders and 15–20 mL in Virginia opossums may be given.

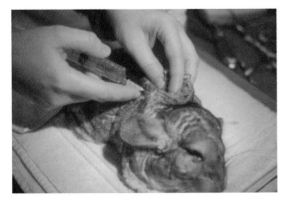

Figure 6.1 Subcutaneous fluids being administered in the scruff region in a chinchilla post-operatively.

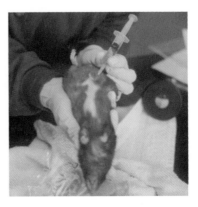

Figure 6.2 Intraperitoneal fluids administered to a rat showing positioning required for safe administration to avoid organ puncture.

Ferret

The technique is as for rabbits. Restraint may be difficult in the conscious patient, and maximum volumes are 20–25 mL.

Intravenous

The advantages and disadvantages of intravenous fluid therapy in small mammals are given in Table 6.3.

Rabbit

The blood vessel that is best tolerated is the lateral ear vein. The technique for using it is described below.

Lateral ear vein: The following technique should be used (Figure 6.3):

1. The area should be shaved and surgically prepared. Warm the ear under a lamp or hot water bottle or apply local anaesthetic cream to dilate the vessel. (NB. If the rabbit is sedated with Hypnorm®, the ear veins will dilate anyway.)
2. Use the lateral ear vein. Do not be tempted to use the apparently larger vessel that runs in the midline of the pinna as this is the central ear artery. Catheterisation of this vessel may lead to thrombosis followed by ear tip necrosis!
3. Use a 25–27 gauge butterfly catheter, pre-heparinised. Once in place, tape it in securely and reflush. Attach the intravenous drip tubing or catheter bung to the end of the butterfly catheter.
4. Fit the rabbit with an Elizabethan collar or apply an intravenous drip guard to the intravenous tubing to prevent chewing, and attach this to the syringe driver. It is possible to tape the butterfly catheter to the back of the

rabbit's head if using intermittent intravenous boluses, but it is important to ensure the catheter is regularly flushed with heparinised saline.

Cephalic vein: This may be used as for the cat and dog, although this vein may be split in some rabbits: A 25–27 gauge over-the-needle or butterfly catheter may be used for access and taped in as for cats and dogs.

Saphenous vein: For this, it is better to use a 25–27 gauge butterfly catheter as it is relatively fragile. It runs over the lateral aspect of the hock (Figure 6.4).

All of these routes can be used for intravenous boluses of up to 10 mL for larger rabbits and 5 mL for smaller dwarf breeds; but for continuous therapy, a syringe driver is required.

Rat, mouse, gerbil and hamster

The intravenous route in hamsters and gerbils is extremely difficult, as they have few peripheral veins and the tail veins in gerbils are dangerous to use due to the risk of tail separation. In mice and rats, the lateral tail veins may be used. An intravenous bolus of fluids can be given using a 25–27 gauge insulin needle or by insertion of a butterfly catheter (Figure 6.5). Warming the tail and applying local anaesthetic cream will help to dilate the vessels and make venipuncture easier. Volumes of 0.2 mL in mice and up to 0.5 mL in rats as a bolus may be given. It is also possible to perform a cut-down jugular catheterisation, but this requires anaesthesia.

Guinea pig and chinchilla

The cephalic and saphenous veins may be used – but generally these are very small and difficult to catheterise. A

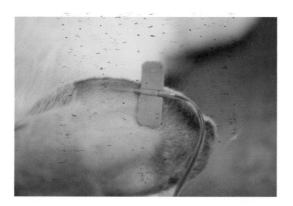

Figure 6.3 Catheterisation of the lateral ear vein in a rabbit using a butterfly catheter.

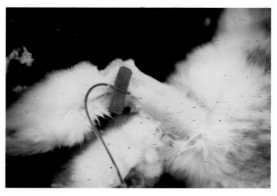

Figure 6.4 Catheterisation of the saphenous vein in a rabbit using a butterfly catheter.

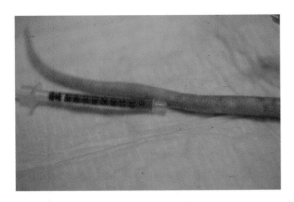

Figure 6.5 Blood transfusion in a rat. Blood is administered to an anaesthetised patient via the tail vein, here in a pre-heparinised syringe.

cut-down technique may be used to access the jugular veins in an emergency.

Jugular vein catheterisation: Sedation or anaesthesia is necessary for this procedure, which is as follows:

1. The guinea pig or chinchilla is sedated and placed in dorsal recumbency. The ventral neck is surgically prepared.
2. An incision is made lateral to the midline and parallel to the trachea, through the skin, and the underlying tissues are bluntly dissected to expose the jugular vein.
3. An over-the-needle catheter is preferred, preferably a 25 gauge with wings which can be sutured to the skin after insertion.
4. The catheter is flushed with heparinised saline, a bung is placed over the port and the catheter bandaged in place.

Marsupial

Sugar gliders are difficult to catheterise consciously because of their small size. The jugular vein is the easiest to catheterise in the sedated animal for significant fluid administration but tolerance of these catheters is poor. Other peripheral vessels such as the saphenous and cephalic are only accessible with 25–27 gauge needles. In Virginia opossums, the cephalic or saphenous veins are the most accessible. In addition, the lateral tail vein may also be used. However, tolerance of indwelling catheters in the conscious animal is poor and so maintenance is difficult.

Ferret

Ferrets are difficult to catheterise when fully conscious. The cephalic vein may be used with 24–27 gauge over-the-needle catheters; however, movement once consciousness has been regained frequently dislodges these catheters, and ferrets will often chew the dressings off. Bolus therapy, when unconscious, may be preferable with 5–10 mL given over several minutes.

Intraosseous

The advantages and disadvantages of this route in small mammals are given in Table 6.3.

Rabbit

The proximal femur is the easiest to use. The landmark to aim for is the fossa between the hip joint and the greater trochanter. A 20–23 gauge hypodermic needle or spinal needle is used, and the procedure requires sedation. The area is surgically prepared and the needle is screwed into position in the same direction as the long axis of the femur. It may be necessary to cut down through the skin with a sterile scalpel blade in some rabbits. This method will require a syringe-driver perfusion device.

It is possible to use the proximal tibia but this is less well tolerated due to interference with the stifle joint. There is frequently a need for tubing guards or Elizabethan collars for all intravenous or intraosseous techniques.

Rodents

The proximal femur may be tolerated as for rabbits in larger rats but smaller species often have a too small medullary cavity for needles to be safely inserted.

Hystricomorphs

This is the preferred route for severely dehydrated chinchillas and guinea pigs with the proximal femur being the easiest site. Access is via the natural fossa created by the hip joint and the greater trochanter. Infusion devices such as syringe drivers are advised for this route of administration (Figure 6.6).

Marsupial

The proximal femur is the easiest bone to use for intraosseous fluid administration. The landmark to aim for is the fossa between the hip joint and the greater trochanter. Insertion is as for rabbits and guinea pigs. In the sugar glider, due to their small size, a 25-gauge needle is required. In Virginia opossums, a 21–23 gauge needle may be used. These are slightly better tolerated than intravenous catheters.

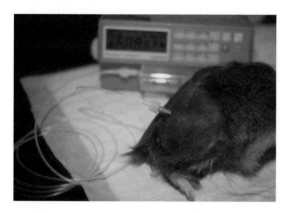

Figure 6.6 Intraosseous catheter placement in a guinea pig using the proximal femur, showing attachment to drip set and infusion device, and before bandaging in place.

Ferrets

The proximal femur is the easiest bone to use for intraosseous fluid administration. The landmark to aim for is the fossa between the hip joint and the greater trochanter. Insertion is as for rabbits.

Drug toxicities in small mammals

Lagomorpha

Drugs of the penicillin family should not be used orally due to their ability to cause an enterotoxaemia with *Clostridia* spp. gut overgrowth. The same is true of the cephalosporin and the macrolide family such as clindamycin. Other antimicrobial additives to avoid in rabbits include procaine, which is often added to penicillin preparations.

Muridae

Medications containing procaine (such as procaine penicillin) and streptomycin have been reported as causing toxicity in mice and rats.

Gerbils (Cricetidae)

Gerbils are sensitive to streptomycin and dihydrostreptomycin containing antimicrobials. They are mildly affected by potentiated penicillins orally, and these should be used with care. It is not advised to use any macrolides in gerbils (e.g. clindamycin, erythromycin).

Hamsters (Cricetidae)

The following antimicrobials should never be used in hamsters because of their ability to cause a fatal enterotoxaemic condition and in the case of the aminoglycosides because of the risks of renal damage and ototoxicity: all penicillins, all cephalosporins, all macrolides (clindamycin, erythromycin, etc.), the aminoglycosides, streptomycin, dihydrostreptomycin and oral gentamicin.

Guinea pigs (Hystricomorpha)

The following antimicrobials should not be used in guinea pigs for fear of causing a fatal enterotoxaemic condition: all penicillins, all cephalosporins and all macrolides.

Chinchillas (Hystricomorpha)

The following antimicrobials should not be used in chinchillas for fear of inducing a fatal enterotoxaemia: all penicillins, all cephalosporins and all macrolides. Metronidazole has been associated with liver failure in chinchillas, but this author has not experienced this problem.

Chipmunks (Sciuromorpha)

Avoid the macrolide family and oral penicillins as both can cause diarrhoea, particularly the former.

Marsupials

Omnivorous marsupials such as the sugar glider and the Virginia opossum seem to be generally unaffected by most antimicrobials.

Ferrets

Ferrets are generally unaffected by most antimicrobials.

TREATMENTS FOR DISEASES IN SMALL MAMMALS

The tables in this section are intended to give an overview of the therapies available and are by no means comprehensive. Readers are advised to consult one of the many excellent texts listed at the end of this chapter for further information.

Lagomorph disease therapies

Tables 6.4–6.8 discuss common treatments for selected diseases of lagomorphs on a system basis.

Muridae disease therapies

Tables 6.9–6.11 discuss common treatments for selected diseases of Muridae (rats and mice, chiefly) on a system basis.

Cricetidae disease therapies

Tables 6.12–6.15 discuss common treatments for selected diseases of Cricetidae (gerbils and hamsters, chiefly) on a system basis.

Table 6.4 Treatment of selected skin diseases in lagomorphs.

Diagnosis	Treatment
Mites, lice and fleas	Ivermectin/selamectin are the drugs of choice for mites and lice. Various preparations of ivermectin are available under the small animal exemption scheme (SAES) in the United Kingdom (e.g. Xeno450®, Dechra Veterinary Products). Imadocloprid (Advantage®, Bayer) is licensed for treating fleas in rabbits and combined with moxidectin (Advocate®, Bayer) for ferrets in the United Kingdom.
Blowfly strike	Prevention by removing urine and faecal soiling. Fine mesh to cover outdoor hutch openings. The use of topical growth inhibitor cyromazine (Rearguard®, Novartis Animal Health) preventing maggot maturation. Once infected, manually remove maggots and use ivermectin, covering antimicrobials and fluid therapy.
Bacterial diseases	Based on culture and sensitivity results. Blue fur disease requires a fluoroquinolone (e.g. enrofloxacin). Rabbit syphilis (*Treponema paraluiscuniculi* infection) requires injectable penicillin.
Dermatophytosis	Miconazole spray licensed under the SAES (Mycozole®, Dechra Veterinary Products) in rabbits in the United Kingdom. Oral itraconazole may be used at 5 mg/kg once daily. Oral griseofulvin can be used, although not in pregnant does due to its terratogenic side effects.
Myxomatosis	No treatment. Prevention is by vaccination, which recently has changed to a combined myxomatosis/VHD vaccine in the United Kingdom (NobiVac Myxo-RHD®, MSD Animal Health).

Table 6.5 Treatment of selected digestive system diseases in lagomorphs.

Diagnosis	Treatment
Dental disease	Prevention by access to good quality hay, dried grass or fresh grazing is essential. Homogenous pelleted grass-based foods are also useful. Once teeth are overgrown, regular burring to a normal shape must be performed every 6–8 weeks.
Gastrointestinal foreign body	Digestive lubricants, liquid paraffin, fluid therapy and prokinetic drugs, if there is no evidence of a complete obstruction. Surgery should be considered if tests indicate a complete obstruction.
Diarrhoea	Fluid therapy. Cause must be determined before treatment. If suspect clostridial overgrowth, then use oral cholestyramine (Questran®, Par Pharmaceutical Inc., a human product) to bind toxins and prevent absorption plus potentially metronidazole to kill the clostridia. The suspected bacterial cause of ERE has been treated by using tiamulin (licensed in feed product Denagard 2% or Denagard 10% w/w Medicated premix for pigs, chickens, turkeys and rabbits®, Novartis Animal Health Ltd.). Coccidiosis: Use oral sulfadimidine at 1 g/L of drinking water for 7 days. Repeat after 7 days. Alternatively, infeed preparations are licensed for rabbits in the United Kingdom containing diclazuril (Clinacox 0.5% Premix®, Huvepharma NV), robenidine hydrochloride (Cycostat 66G®, Pfizer Animal Health Ltd.). Nematode infections treated with an ivermectin injection at 0.2 mg/kg (various products licensed under the SAES in the United Kingdom, see Skin Diseases) or oral fenbendazole at 20 mg/kg once daily for 4 days (various products licensed under the SAES in the United Kingdom, e.g. Lapizole®, Dechra Veterinary Products; Panacur Rabbit 18.75% oral paste®, MSD Animal Health). Bacterial enteritis may be treated according to culture and sensitivity results. Loperamide may be used to symptomatically reduce diarrhoea.
Hypomotility disorder	Dietary management is important. Use of prokinetics, e.g. cisapride (0.5 mg/kg q12 hours), ranitidine (2–5 mg/kg q12 hours) and metoclopramide (0.5 mg/kg q8–12 hours), is required. Fluid therapy is essential with oral pre/probiotics or transfaunation (taking caecotrophs from a healthy rabbit and mixing them with food to administer to the patient).
Hepatic lipidosis	Prokinetics (if obstructive cause ruled out), e.g. ranitidine, metoclopramide and cisapride. Assisted feeding is important with soluble carbohydrates initially to ensure correct calorie supply. Transfaunation of caecotrophs from a healthy donor or pre/probiotics are helpful. Use of L-carnitine, extract of milk thistle and inositol are helpful in supporting hepatocyte function.

Table 6.6 Treatment of selected respiratory and cardiovascular diseases in lagomorphs.

Diagnosis	Treatment
Pasteurellosis	Fluid therapy. Treatment with fluoroquinolone (in the UK, Baytril 2.5% Injection® or Baytril 2.5% oral solution®, Bayer Animal Health, are licensed) or sulphonamide antimicrobial is advised. In commercial rabbit production, tilmicosin in feed is licensed in the United Kingdom for treating pasteurellosis (Pulmotil G100 Premix for medicated feedstuff®, Elanco Animal Health). Mucolytics (e.g. bromhexine hydrochloride orally or acetylcysteine via nebulisation) and manual cleaning of the nares.
Viral haemorrhagic disease (VHD)	No treatment. Vaccination is possible using a combined myxomatosis/VHD vaccine in the United Kingdom (NobiVac Myxo-RHD®, MSD Animal Health). This is currently at time of press dosed as one dose per rabbit from 5 weeks of age and boostered at yearly intervals. Alternatively, single VHD vaccines are available (e.g. Cylap®, Pfizer Animal Health; Lapinject VHD®, CEVA Animal Health Ltd.).
Congestive heart failure	This is the end-stage of heart disease and may have multiple initial causes. Treatment is based on reducing fluid congestion with diuretics, e.g. furosemide (1–4 mg/kg as required) and spironolactone (1–2 mg/kg q24 hours); reducing the afterload, the heart has to work against with ACE inhibitors (watch for hypotension as rabbits are more sensitive to this than cats and dogs, so usually a lower dose of drugs such as benazepril is advised at 0.1–0.2 mg/kg (Girling, 2003); positive inotropes such as pimobendan (0.25 mg/kg twice daily). If atrial fibrillation is present, then digoxin has been used at 0.005–0.01 mg/kg orally q24–48 hours. If heart blocks and bradycardia are seen, then glycopyrrolate at 0.01 mg/kg.

Table 6.7 Treatment of selected urogenital tract diseases in lagomorphs.

Diagnosis	Treatment
Urolithiasis	Catheterising, flushing bladder and aggressive fluid therapy. Surgery occasionally required. Reduce dietary calcium and restrict dry food to maximum 25–30 g/day. Antimicrobials and analgesia may be needed, if concurrent cystitis. Radiographs are helpful to look for renoliths, which will worsen the prognosis.
Chronic renal failure	Aggressive fluid therapy – initially intravenously or intraosseously, but may be supported by subcutaneous fluids once stabilised. Treatment of exacerbating conditions, e.g. pyelonephritis, urolithiasis/renolithiasis and encephalitozoonosis. ACE inhibitors, e.g. benazepril, have been shown to be helpful in increasing renal perfusion as has been seen in domestic cats, but rabbits are more prone to hypotension and so dosages should be reduced (0.1–0.2 mg/kg q24 hours) (Girling, 2003). Anabolic steroids to prevent catabolism every 3–4 weeks along with multiple B vitamins can help with appetite. Prokinetics, e.g. cisapride, ranitidine or metoclopramide, may also be required to maintain gut motility. The reduction of protein in the diet as well as phosphate salts may help preserve renal function – that is, reducing pelleted portion of the diet and increasing leafy greens.
Uterine adenocarcinoma	Treatment by surgical spaying. Prevention is by surgical spaying at 4–5 months of age.
Venereal spirochaetosis	Penicillin G, single dose, subcutaneously at 40 000 IU/kg. May need to repeat after 7 days. Care should be taken as it can be toxic if given orally.
Mastitis	Antibiosis based on culture and sensitivity (fluoroquinolones such as enrofloxacin usually effective as bacteria are frequently *E. coli* or *Pasteurella* spp.). Analgesia with carprofen 5 mg/kg, meloxicam 0.3–0.6 mg/kg daily. Fluid therapy and supportive treatment is essential.

Table 6.8 Treatment of selected musculoskeletal, nervous system and ocular diseases in lagomorphs.

Diagnosis	Treatment
Osteoarthritis	NSAIDs, e.g. meloxicam, at 0.3–0.6 mg/kg q24 hours have proved useful. More advanced cases may require multimodal analgesia with drugs such as tramadol (10 mg/kg q24 hours) or buprenorphine (0.03 mg/kg q8–12 hours).
Fractures	Spinal dislocations and fractures with hindlimb paresis carry poor prognosis, but shock doses of short-acting corticosteroids, e.g. methylprednisolone, are considered if administered within 12 hours of injury. Otherwise, use NSAIDs such as meloxicam. Limb fractures carry a better prognosis. Most require external/tie-in fixators as rabbit bones are brittle with large medullary cavities. Consider calcium and vitamin D3 supplementation in cases of metabolic bone disease.
Vestibular disease due to otitis media	Fluoroquinolone or sulphonamide antimicrobials are useful where *Pasteurella* or *Streptococcal* infections are present. Anaerobic infections may require injectable penicillins. Surgical removal of the lateral wall of the external ear canal can relieve pressure in the short narrow horizontal canal. Bulla osteotomy is difficult and failure rates are high due to the tenacious pus, deep seated nature of the bullae and their small size. Prognosis is guarded for full recovery, but generally not life-threatening if due to uncomplicated otitis media.
Encephalitozoonosis	Fenbendazole at 20 mg/kg orally once daily for 28 days (Suter *et al.*, 2001). Short-acting corticosteroids have been used in severe cases with some success in addition to fenbendazole (Harcourt-Brown & Holloway, 2003). Management of renal disease may also be required (see urogenital section). Prognosis guarded once neurological disease is apparent.
Lead poisoning	Removal of larger particles by surgery may be possible but frequently the particle size is very small. Treatment with chelating agent, e.g. sodium calcium edetate (27.5 mg/kg q6–8 hours for 5 days), combined with fluid therapy to reduce nephrotoxicity.
Anterior uveitis	Test for encephalitozoonosis and treat if positive (see above). Analgesia with systemic NSAIDs plus use of topical tropicamide drops to prevent synechiae formation. Phacoemulsification of the lens and removal may be necessary.
Dacryocystitis	Not a true ocular problem but a dental problem with constriction of the tear duct by elongating maxillary incisor root. Treatment is reliant on controlling the dental problem and cannulating and flushing the tear duct.
Conjunctivitis	This may occur secondarily to dacryocystitis or as a primary problem. Topical eye drops using fucidic acid (e.g. Fucithalmic Vet®, Dechra Veterinary Products) or gentamicin (e.g. Tiacil®, Virbac Animal Health) are licensed for use in rabbits with conjunctivitis in the United Kingdom.

Table 6.9 Treatment of skin diseases in Muridae.

Diagnosis	Treatment
Mites	Ivermectin at 0.2 mg/kg is advised (several products licensed under the SAES in the United Kingdom, see rabbit skin diseases).
Lice and fleas	Ivermectin orally/spot-on.
Bacterial disease	Based on culture and sensitivity results. Pododermatitis may require surgical debridement, analgesia (carprofen/meloxicam) and hydrating gels/dressings, as well as improving cage substrate to increase padding. Weight loss also advisable.
Dermatophytosis	Topical miconazole available under the SAES in the United Kingdom (Mycozole®, Dechra Veterinary Products). Oral griseofulvin has been used, but beware of terratogenicity in pregnant females. Oral itraconazole has also been used (5 mg/kg q24 hours) but beware of hepatotoxicity and anorexia.
Atopy	Topical soothing shampoos (e.g. Episoothe®, Virbac) and oral essential fatty acids (oil of evening primrose). Oral corticosteroids have been used in acute flare-ups but long-term use has side effects. Oral antihistamines have also been tried with varying success.

Table 6.10 Treatment of selected digestive, respiratory and cardiovascular system diseases in Muridae.

Diagnosis	Treatment
Dental disease	Burring, every 3–4 weeks with a low speed dental burr, is advised for incisor malocclusion.
Parasitic disease	Ivermectin at 0.2 mg/kg once (see Skin Disease) or fenbendazole at 20 mg/kg orally once daily for 5 days for nematodes. For coccidiosis, use sulfadimidine in water at 200 mg/L for 7 days. Metronidazole is useful for other protozoa.
Bacterial disease	Enrofloxacin (Baytril 2.5% oral solution®, Bayer Animal Health) is effective against a wide range of Gram-negative bacterial infections and is licensed for use in rodents in the United Kingdom. Oxytetracycline is used for Tyzzer's disease at 0.1 g/L drinking water. Other treatments based on culture and sensitivity.
Respiratory disease	Culture and sensitivity advised. Oxytetracycline, doxycycline, azithromycin and enrofloxacin are useful against *Mycoplasma* spp., *Streptococcus pneumonia* and *Klebsiella* spp. infections. Consider mucolytics, e.g. bromhexine hydrochloride orally or acetylcysteine by nebulisation. Nebulisation of antimicrobials may also be helpful.
Cardiovascular disease	See protocols and drugs for rabbits.

Table 6.11 Treatment of selected urogenital tract, musculoskeletal, neurological and ocular diseases in Muridae.

Diagnosis	Treatment
Chronic renal failure	Reduce dietary protein, but increase the biological value. Reduce phosphate in diet (if necessary, use aluminium hydroxide orally to bind phosphorus in the gut and prevent absorption). Fluid therapy – preferably intravenously/intraosseously initially to stabilise. Anabolic steroids and B vitamin supplementation.
Urolithiasis	Removal of blockages manually. Reduce calcium content of diet and increase bran levels. Antimicrobials for preputial gland abscess/cystitis.
Spondylosis	Meloxicam at 0.5–1 mg/kg orally once/twice daily for pain relief.
Fractures	Splinting and strict confinement plus analgesia (NSAID); allow rapid callus formation and repair (2–3 weeks).
Vestibular disease	If bacterial, use fluoroquinolone or sulphonamide antimicrobials. If caused by a pituitary tumour, surgery rarely possible.
Keratoconjunctivitis sicca	Topical cyclosporin has been used successfully.

Table 6.12 Treatment of skin diseases in gerbils.

Diagnosis	Treatment
Demodicosis	Amitraz washes (1 mL solution to 0.5 L water) once every 2 weeks until negative scrapings. Beware toxicity. Alternatively ivermectin at 0.4 mg/kg once weekly for 6 weeks has been used.
Bacterial disease	Oral or parenteral antibiosis based on culture and sensitivity results. Enrofloxacin orally or in water, oxytetracycline at 0.8 mg/L water may be useful.
Dermatophytosis	Topical miconazole available under the SAES in the United Kingdom (Mycozole®, Dechra Veterinary Products). Oral griseofulvin has been used, but beware of teratogenicity in pregnant females. Oral itraconazole (5 mg/kg q24 hours) but beware of hepatotoxicity and anorexia.
Neoplasia	Surgical excision of ventral scent gland adenocarcinomas or melanomas is advised.
Degloving injuries	Fluid therapy. Topical anticoagulants (calcium sprays) or pressure to stem bleeding. Topical/parenteral antimicrobials advised. May need surgery to remove denuded coccygeal vertebrae.

Table 6.13 Treatment of selected digestive, respiratory and urogenital system diseases in gerbils.

Diagnosis	Treatment
Proliferative ileitis (wet tail – *Lawsonia intracellularis* infection)	Difficult, but oxytetracyclines and chloramphenicol have been suggested.
Parasitic disease	Ivermectin at 0.2 mg/kg for nematode infestations. Praziquantel at 10 mg/kg orally once for *Rodentolepis nana* may need to repeat after 2 weeks.
Respiratory disease	Treatment is as for Muridae
Cystic ovarian disease	Surgical spaying is curative. Alternatively, percutaneous drainage or human chorionic gonadotrophin at 100 IU/kg may remove the cysts for a time but they will re-occur.

Table 6.14 Treatment of selected skin and digestive system diseases in hamsters.

Diagnosis	Treatment
Demodicosis	Amitraz is the treatment of choice but ivermectin may also be used (see Gerbils). However, the problem is often an underlying immunosuppressive disease that allows the mites to proliferate and so without correcting this treatments may be unsuccessful.
Sarcoptiform mange (*Notoedres notoedric*)	Ivermectin at 0.2 mg/kg once weekly on 2–4 occasions.
Dermatophytosis	See dermatophytosis in Table 6.12.
Hyperadrenocorticism	This is often untreatable. Surgery is generally too complicated with high failure rates. Metapyrone has been used at 8 mg orally once daily, but this is potentially toxic and may result in the death of the hamster.
Cheek pouch impactions	Milking the contents manually or with a dampened cotton bud is advised. Flushing the pouches with dilute chlorhexidine can remove any superficial infection.
Cheek pouch prolapse	Surgical replacement with a cotton bud under anaesthesia. A suture may be placed through the skin into the cheek pouch behind the ear to keep in place.
Proliferative ileitis (wet tail due to *Lawsonia intracellularis* infection)	Extremely difficult, see Gerbils.

Table 6.15 Treatment of selected cardiovascular, endocrine, reproductive and musculoskeletal diseases in hamsters.

Diagnosis	Treatment
Aortic thrombosis and cardiomyopathy	Use of furosemide at 0.25–0.5 mg/kg may be useful, as may the ACE inhibitor enalapril at 0.25 mg/kg orally once daily. Beware of hypotensive effects.
Hyperadrenocorticism	See Skin Diseases.
Diabetes mellitus	Protamine zinc insulin therapy at 0.5–1 unit/kg (requires dilution in saline). Aim for 0.25–0.5% glucose in urine and water consumption 10–15 mL/day. Use glucose/saline intraperitoneally and human glucose oral gels on membranes if evidence of hypoglycaemic overdose.
Pyometra	Surgical neutering after fluid therapy and antimicrobial stabilisation.
Cystic ovarian disease	Surgical spaying is curative. Alternatively, percutaneous drainage or human chorionic gonadotrophin at 100 IU/kg may remove the cysts for a time but they will re-occur.
Fractures	Compound fractures of the tibia may require leg amputation. If closed they may heal conservatively with rest and analgesia. Intramedullary pinning with 25–27 gauge needles are possible.

Hystricomorph disease therapies

Tables 6.16–6.20 discuss common treatments for selected diseases of hystricomorphs on a system basis (chiefly chinchillas and guinea pigs).

Sciuromorph disease therapies

Tables 6.21 and 6.22 discuss common treatments for selected diseases of sciuromorphs (chiefly chipmunk) on a system basis.

Marsupial disease therapies

Tables 6.23 and 6.24 discuss common treatments for selected diseases of sugar gliders and Virginia opossums on a system basis.

Mustelid disease therapies

Tables 6.25–6.28 discuss common treatments for diseases of mustelids (chiefly the domestic ferret) on a system basis.

Table 6.16 Treatment of selected skin diseases in guinea pigs.

Diagnosis	Treatment
Mites	Ivermectin at 0.2 mg/kg is effective against *Trixicara caviae* (various products licensed under the SAES in the United Kingdom). Analgesics (e.g. meloxicam) and tranquilisers (e.g. diazepam) may be necessary in severe cases.
Lice	Fipronil sprayed on to a cloth and then wiped over the fur. Ivermectin may also be useful.
Cervical lymphadenitis	Surgical lancing of the abscess and treatment with antimicrobials (e.g. enrofloxacin) is advised.
Dermatophytosis	See dermatophytosis in Table 6.12.
Pododermatitis	See bacterial diseases in Table 6.9.

Table 6.17 Treatment of selected digestive, respiratory and urinary system diseases in guinea pigs.

Diagnosis	Treatment
Dental disease	This is similar to rabbits. Change the diet to increase, abrasive, grass-based foods. Burr molar spikes every 6–8 weeks under sedation. Treat oral infections based on culture and sensitivity +/– information.
Bacterial disease	As for hamsters and gerbils, it is based on culture and sensitivity. Enrofloxacin useful for *Salmonella* spp.
Parasitic disease	Nematodes may be treated with 0.2 mg/kg ivermectin. Coccidiosis requires oral sulfadimidine at 40 mg/kg, once daily for 5 days. *B. coli* require metronidazole orally but use with caution due to risk of liver damage.
Faecal impaction	Manual emptying of perianal skin folds daily and flushing with dilute chlorhexidine.
Respiratory disease	Enrofloxacin, doxycycline and sulphonamide drugs are useful. Mucolytics, e.g. oral bromhexine hydrochloride and nebulised acetyl cysteine, are useful. Nebulised antimicrobials also helpful. Neoplasia often so advanced by the time diagnosis is made, that treatment is not possible.
Chronic renal failure	See chronic renal disease of rabbits in Table 6.7.
Urolithiasis	Restriction of dry food to 15–20 g/day to reduce dietary calcium levels. Fresh vegetables and fluids to help flush through calcium crystals. Treat with antimicrobials if cystitis is suspected.

Table 6.18 Treatment of selected reproductive, ocular and musculoskeletal diseases in guinea pigs.

Diagnosis	Treatment
Cystic ovarian disease	See hamsters in Table 6.15.
Pregnancy toxaemia	Oral glucose gel, intravenous or intraperitoneal glucose-saline as a 5–7 mL bolus. Dexamethasone 0.2 mg/kg intramuscularly (but will cause abortion). To prevent, do not let sow become overweight or stressed.
Mastitis	Antimicrobials such as enrofloxacin or sulphonamides with fluid therapy and NSAID analgesia. Surgery may be necessary.

Diagnosis	Treatment
Hypovitaminosis C ('Scurvy')	Vitamin C parenterally at 50 mg/kg and 200 mg/L drinking water.
Fractures	Splinting with hexalite materials plus cage restriction and analgesia. Surgical fixation with external fixators. Methyl-prednisolone may be needed if spinal trauma is involved and treatment can be administered within 12 hours. Otherwise NSAID use is preferred.
Conjunctivitis	Chlortetracycline eye ointment for *Chlamydophila psittaci* conjunctivitis. See scurvy for vitamin C related problems.

Table 6.19 Treatment of selected skin and digestive system diseases in chinchillas.

Diagnosis	Treatment
Dermatophytosis	See dermatophytosis in Table 6.12.
Dental disease	As for rabbits – dental burring under sedation every 6–8 weeks, dietary change to grass-based products. Analgesia for root pain using meloxicam +/– tramadol orally. Use of prokinetics such as cisapride (0.5 mg/kg q12 hours), ranitidine (2–5 mg/kg q12 hours) and metoclopramide (0.5 mg/kg q8–12 hours). Use of antimicrobials based on culture and sensitivity testing although anaerobes are common and so oral metronidazole at 10–20 mg/kg q12 hours (some texts suggest metronidazole is hepatotoxic in chinchillas so beware its overuse).
Hypomotility disorder ('colic')	This is generally associated with digestive tract disease or pain and so the cause of the discomfort/disease needs to be determined to ensure proper treatment. Symptomatic treatment of hypomotility can include fluid therapy, analgesia (e.g. meloxicam) and prokinetics as outlined for dental disease.
Hepatic lipidosis	Reduce excess fats and soluble carbohydrates in diet. Fluid therapy and assisted nutrition/feeding (e.g. B vitamins, L-carnitine, inositol and milk thistle) extract to support hepatocyte function.
Bacterial diarrhoea	Antimicrobial treatment is based on culture and sensitivity results. Fluid therapy and analgesia as well as assist feeding may also be required.
Parasitic diarrhoea	Treatment of giardiasis with fenbendazole at 25 mg/kg orally once daily for 3 days. Some texts avoid metronidazole due to hepatotoxicity, but this author has used it for dental disease and giardiasis at 10–20 mg/kg orally twice daily for 7 days without any side effects.

Table 6.20 Treatment of selected cardiovascular, musculoskeletal, nervous and ocular diseases in chinchillas.

Diagnosis	Treatment
Congestive heart failure associated with dilated cardiomyopathy	Treatment is based on reducing fluid congestion with diuretics such as furosemide (1–4 mg/kg as required) and spironolactone (1–2 mg/kg q24 hours); reducing the afterload the heart has to work against with ACE inhibitors such as enalapril/benazepril; positive inotropes such as pimobenden. If atrial fibrillation is present, then digoxin has been used at 0.005–0.01 mg/kg orally q24–48 hours.
Fractures	Long bone fractures are best fixed with external fixation surgically. Smaller fractures may be splinted with human finger splints.
Seizures	Symptomatic treatment with 1–2 mg/kg diazepam intramuscularly. Heat stroke treated with cooled intravenous/peritoneal fluids. Listeriosis with oxytetracycline 10 mg/kg twice daily intramuscularly.
Conjunctivitis	Use of chlortetracycline eye ointments is recommended for *Chlamydophila psittaci*. Always check for dental disease in any case of epiphora as molar root elongation pressing on the globe is a common cause of epiphora in chinchillas.

Table 6.21 Treatment of selected skin, digestive and respiratory system diseases in chipmunks.

Diagnosis	Treatment
Mites	Ivermectin at 0.2 mg/kg is advised. In addition, for *Dermanyssus gallinae*, burn bedding and dust cage with bromcyclen powder.
Bacterial skin disease	Antimicrobials based on culture and sensitivity. Generally, enrofloxacin, tetracycline and sulphonamides are safe and effective.
Dental disease	Burring of incisor malocclusion with a slow speed dental drill every 4–6 weeks.
Diarrhoea	As for rats and mice.
Respiratory disease	Oxytetracycline at 22 mg/kg once daily for 5–7 days is useful for *Mycoplasma* spp. Enrofloxacin and doxycycline may also be used.

Table 6.22 Treatment of selected urogenital, musculoskeletal and nervous system diseases in chipmunks.

Diagnosis	Treatment
Urolithiasis	Surgical or manual removal of obstructing uroliths. Give meat-based foods temporarily to acidify urine and dissolve crystals, or increase seeds and fruits and reduce pelleted food.
Hypocalcaemic paralysis	100 mg/kg calcium gluconate intramuscularly. Prevention based on dietary supplementation. Beware that some of these cases are actually associated with spinal trauma and not hypocalcaemia, so a radiographic assessment is advisable.
Uterine infections	Based on culture and sensitivity results. Pyometra may require surgery after fluid stabilisation.
Mastitis	Enrofloxacin and oxytetracyclines may be useful with NSAID analgesia. Surgery may be required if abscessation is severe.
Fractures	Spinal trauma has a poor prognosis, but methyl prednisolone may be used peracutely. Minor fractures may respond to cage rest and infood NSAIDs. Long bone fractures will require fixation preferably with external or tie-in fixators.
Seizures	Removal from rooms with TV and computer screens. Use of 0.5–1 mg/kg diazepam intramuscularly may help.

Table 6.23 Treatment of selected skin, digestive and respiratory system diseases in sugar gliders and Virginia opossums.

Diagnosis	Treatment
Bacterial skin disease	Antimicrobials such as amoxicillin, cephalexin, enrofloxacin and TMP sulfonamides have all been used successfully against bacterial pyodermas in marsupials.
Fungal skin disease	See dermatophytosis in Table 6.12.
Parasitic skin disease	Ivermectin at 0.2 mg/kg for mites. Pyrethrin powders have been used against other ectoparasites topically.
Dental disease	Extraction of rotten teeth, scaling and polishing and antibiosis with potentiated amoxicillin is recommended.
Gastroenteritis	Bacterial disease may be treated with amoxicillin or enrofloxacin. Nematodes may be managed with ivermectin (0.2 mg/kg) or fenbendazole (20–50 mg/kg). Giardiasis has been treated with metronidazole.
Pneumonia	Bacterial pneumonia has been treated with fluoroquinolones such as enrofloxacin or penicillins.

Table 6.24 Treatment of selected cardiovascular, urogenital, musculoskeletal and neurological diseases in sugar gliders and Virginia opossums.

Diagnosis	Treatment
Cardiomyopathy	Treatment is similar to that in ferrets
Heartworm	Treatment and prevention is similar to that in ferrets – again beware of anaphylactic shock when treating.
Urolithiasis	Catheterisation of the urethra in males to relieve any blockages. Flushing of the bladder or cystotomy to remove larger uroliths.
Metabolic bone disease	Correction of the diet to increase calcium and vitamin D3/provision of ultra violet light in early stages. Calcitonin has been used once blood levels have been normalised to encourage calcium deposition in the bones. In later stages, the problem is not reversible.
Paresis/paralysis	Common sequel to metabolic bone disease, particularly in sugar gliders and so may not be treatable.

Table 6.25 Treatment of selected skin diseases in mustelids.

Diagnosis	Treatment
Mites	Ivermectin at 0.2 mg/kg once and repeated after 14 days. This author has found success in treating ear mites (*Otodectes cynotis*) using Advocate spot-on for small cats and ferrets® (Bayer Animal Health), although this product is not specifically licensed for this use in the United Kingdom.
Fleas	A licensed product containing imidacloprid and moxidectin (Advocate spot-on for small cats and ferrets®, Bayer Animal Health) exists in the United Kingdom for treating flea infestation and preventing heart worm disease (*Dirofilaria immitis* infection).
Bacterial disease	Based on culture and sensitivity with drugs such as enrofloxacin at 5–10 mg/kg (licensed UK product Baytril 2.5% oral solution®, Bayer Animal Health), potentiated sulphonamides at 15–30 mg/kg twice daily and potentiated amoxicillin at 10–20 mg/kg twice daily.
Dermatophytosis	See dermatophytosis in Table 6.12.
Neoplasia	Surgical excision where possible.
Hormonal skin disease	Testosterone or oestrogen-dependent alopecia – implantation with a gonadotrophin releasing hormone (GnRH) agonist (e.g. deslorelin (Suprelorin®, Virbac)). Neutering is no longer recommended due to the development of adrenal gland neoplasia and disease subsequently. Hyperadrenocorticism treatment is given in Table 6.28.

Table 6.26 Treatment of selected digestive system diseases in mustelids.

Diagnosis	Treatment
Dental disease	Extraction of rotten teeth, antibiosis with clindamycin at 5.5 mg/kg twice daily or potentiated amoxicillin is recommended. Encourage dry foods to prevent recurrence.
Gastric ulceration	Remove any gastric foreign bodies as these can result in gastric ulceration. Use cytoprotectants: cimetidine (10 mg/kg twice daily), sucralfate (100 mg/kg daily orally) and bismuth subsalicylate (1 mL/kg three times daily, orally). If *Helicobacter mustelae* is present, combined amoxicillin and metronidazole is advised but enrofloxacin at 4.25 mg/kg q12 hours with bismuth subcitrate (6 mg/kg q12 hours) for 14 days has also been used successfully (Johnson-Delaney, 2009).
Proliferative ileitis	Chloramphenicol is the antibiotic of choice.
Lymphoma	Chemotherapy with drugs such as vincristine, cyclophosphamide and prednisolone has been tried but prognosis is guarded and depends on numerous factors including age, lymphoma grading and type.

(continued)

Table 6.26 *(continued)*

Diagnosis	Treatment
Bacterial disease	This is based on culture and sensitivity results of faeces samples, but fluoroquinolones and potentiated amoxicillin are effective against a range of Gram-negative and anaerobic bacteria.
Parasitic disease	Giardiasis treatment is with metronidazole. Coccidiosis is with sulfadimidine. Nematode infestations may be treated with 0.2 mg/kg ivermectin or with oral fenbendazole (various products licensed under the SAES).
Liver disease	Lactulose at 1.5–3 mg/kg orally once daily may help. Supportive therapy with vitamin B supplements and reduced fat/high biological value proteins advised. Use of inositol, L-carnitine and extract of milk thistle may also be useful where hepatic lipidosis is present.

Table 6.27 Treatment of selected respiratory, cardiovascular and urinary system diseases in mustelids.

Diagnosis	Treatment
Canine distemper virus	There is no treatment. Prevention is by vaccination. No currently licensed ferret vaccine in the United Kingdom (although one exists in the USA). In the United Kingdom, canine distemper vaccines are used but care should be taken to choose a vaccine not raised in ferrets. Consultation with the canine vaccine manufacturer is advised for specific dosing.
Bacterial pneumonia	This is based on culture and sensitivity results, but fluoroquinolones and potentiated amoxicillin are effective against a wide range of Gram-negative and positive respiratory pathogens.
Congestive heart failure associated with dilated cardiomyopathy	Furosemide at 1–4 mg/kg in acute crisis is useful, intravenously or intramuscularly. ACE inhibitor enalapril at 0.5 mg/kg every 48 hours but watch for hypotensive effects. Pimobenden at 0.25 mg/kg q12 hours may be used as a positive inotrope. Digoxin may also be used in heart failure where atrial fibrillation occurs.
Lungworm and heartworm	These can be treated using avermectins such as ivermectin, selamectin or moxidectin. When treating cases of patent heartworm infection, massive die-offs of the nematode can result in anaphylaxis or vascular blockage. In ferrets, Advocate spot-on® (Bayer) has a license in the United Kingdom for preventing heartworm.
Urolithiasis	Surgery may be required to remove obstructions and/or bladder stones. Feeding an all-meat-based protein diet is essential to prevent formation. Treatment of any primary or secondary cystitis is based on culture and sensitivity results.
Chronic renal failure	This may be treated as in the domestic cat.

Table 6.28 Treatment of selected endocrine, reproductive and ocular diseases in mustelids.

Diagnosis	Treatment
Hyperadrenocorticism	Medical therapy can be ineffective as the tumour is adrenal based. However, recent work with gonadotrophin releasing hormone agonist (GnRH) deslorelin (Suprelorin®, Virbac) suggests that this implant may help in some cases to reduce tumour size and clinical effects. Otherwise treatment is surgical.
Insulinoma	Surgical excision of pancreatic neoplasm – but may be difficult due to their small size. Management with oral prednisolone (0.25–2 mg/kg q12 hours) with weekly monitoring of blood glucose levels. Diazoxide has been used where resistance to prednisolone is seen.
Diabetes mellitus	Tends to be rare but treatment is based on protamine zinc insulin at 1–2 units per ferret, and increasing by 0.5 units until blood glucose falls to 15 mmol/L or urine glucose to 0.5%. Twice daily dosing may be required.
Pregnancy toxaemia	40% glucose at 0.5–1 mL/kg by slow intravenous bolus. Bicarbonate supplement to fluids is advised to counteract acidosis. Dexamethasone may be required in severe cases but abortion will occur.

Diagnosis	Treatment
Uterine infections	Surgical spaying after fluid stabilisation and treatment with broad-spectrum antibiotics until culture and sensitivity results are available. This may lead to adrenal gland neoplasia in later life.
Mastitis	Broad-spectrum antibiotics and NSAIDs with fluid therapy advised. Surgical excision of abscesses may be needed.
Hyperoestroginism	Prevention based on implantation of GnRH agonist deslorelin (Suprelorin®, Virbac) at 5 months, or mating with an entire or vasectomised hob, or regular proligesterone treatment at the start of the season (50 mg/jill).
	If disease has developed then treat with blood transfusion if PCV < 20%, or in early stages stop oestrus with proligesterone or human chorionic gonadotrophin and then use GnRH implant.

References

Girling, S.J. (2003) Preliminary study into the possible use of benazepril on the management of renal disease in rabbits. *British Veterinary Zoological Society Proceedings*, Edinburgh Zoo, p. 44.

Harcourt-Brown, F.M. and Holloway, H.K.R. (2003) *Encephalitozoon cuniculi* infection in pet rabbits. *Veterinary Record*, **152**, 427–431.

Johnson-Delaney, C. (2009) Ferrets: digestive system disorders. *Manual of Rodents and Ferrets* (eds A. Meredith & C. Johnson-Delaney), pp. 275–281. BSAVA, Quedgeley, UK.

Suter, C., Muller-Doblies, U.U., Hatt, J.M. and Deplazes, P. (2001) Prevention and treatment of *Encephalitozoon cuniculi* infection in rabbits with fenbendazole. *Veterinary Record*, **148**, 478–480.

Further reading

Fraser, M.A. and Girling, S.J. (2009) *Rabbit Medicine and Surgery for Veterinary Nurses*. Blackwell-Wiley, Oxford.

Keeble, E. and Meredith, A. (2009) *Manual of Rodents and Ferrets*. BSAVA, Quedgeley, UK.

Meredith, A. and Johnson-Delaney, C. (2010) *Manual of Exotic Pets*, 5th edn. BSAVA, Quedgeley, UK.

Quesenberry, K.E. and Carpenter, J. (2003) *Ferrets, Rabbits and Rodents*, 2nd edn. W.B. Saunders, Philadelphia, PA.

Chapter 7 | Small Mammal Diagnostic Imaging

RADIOGRAPHY
Introduction
Physical restraint

In most cases, small mammals will not lie still long enough to allow radiography. Therefore, chemical restraint is preferred.

Chemical restraint

Sedation with drugs such as Hypnorm® or medetomidine/ketamine/butorphanol combinations or anaesthesia with sevoflurane/isoflurane is preferred. See anaesthesia chapter for further details.

Positioning

In the majority of cases, it is preferable to ensure that the patient is immobilised chemically when performing radiography to ensure proper positioning. Lateral and dorsoventral/ventrodorsal views are routine. Further oblique views may be useful when imaging structures such as the head, where right and left dental arcades may need to be viewed separately. In addition, rostro-caudal views of the head may be useful where visualisation of the temporomandibular joint or frontal sinuses is required.

Interpretation of rabbit radiographs
Thorax

Two views, a traditional right later and a dorsoventral view, are generally preferred (see Figures 7.1 and 7.2). The heart sits between the fourth and sixth rib spaces and appears large due to the small size of the thoracic cavity in relation to the overall body. Enlargement of the heart silhouette is common in rabbits and can be due to pericardial fat or disease such as valvular disease or cardiomyopathy. Pathological atherosclerosis and mineralisation of the blood vessels can be seen radiographically (Shell & Saunders, 1989). The thymus persists in the adult rabbit and thymic neoplasia can be seen as a precardiac mass.

Other causes of a precardiac shadow can include mediastinal abscesses and other forms of neoplasia.

The lungs show similar changes to dogs and cats when affected by infection. They are also one of the main sites of metastasis for certain neoplasms, for example uterine adenocarcinomas. Pleural effusions may also be seen in rabbits, with the characteristic rounding/blunting of the caudal lung lobe border and widened pleural space on dorsoventral views and may be seen in cases of congestive heart failure.

Abdomen

The caecum should always be full of ingesta, often with small volumes of gas in the healthy rabbit, and is positioned ventrally and to the right side. Excessive gas build-up such as that seen in mucoid enteropathy and penicillin toxicity where the whole of the stomach, small intestine, caecum and large intestine may be filled with fluid and gas (see Figure 7.3).

The liver is found completely underneath the caudal ribcage and is a flattened shadow cranio-caudally. A number of liver diseases may result in enlargement and extension of the liver beyond the ribcage (e.g. hepatic lipidosis, hepatic coccidiosis due to *Eimeria* stiediae).

The stomach should always contain food – but a small gas crescent dorsally may be seen. Excessive gas build-up in the stomach can indicate a blockage or stasis of the bowel. Stomach emptying and intestinal motility are difficult to assess in the rabbit due to the permanently full stomach. However, one study suggested that 32% of a liquid marker should reach the caecum in 1 hour and 80% by 12 hours in the healthy rabbit (Pickard & Stevens, 1972). Solid markers however reached the caecum within 4 hours.

The normal kidney shadow should be 1.4–2.2 times the length of the second lumbar vertebra with a mean of 1.8 times. Renal calculi are frequently seen and may be a cause of intense pain in rabbits (see Figures 7.4 and 7.5). Negative contrast

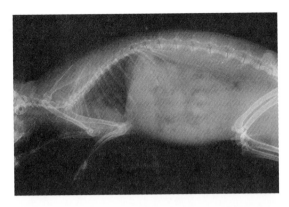

Figure 7.1 Lateral view of a normal rabbit. (Fraser and Girling, 2009)

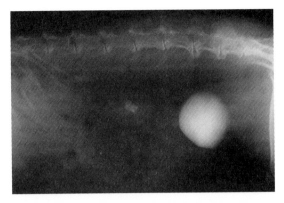

Figure 7.4 Lateral abdomen of a rabbit showing radiodense calculi in left kidney and radiodense silt in bladder. Note also spondylosis lesions in L5–6 and L6–7. (Fraser and Girling, 2009)

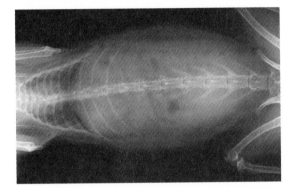

Figure 7.2 Dorsoventral view of a normal rabbit. (Fraser and Girling, 2009)

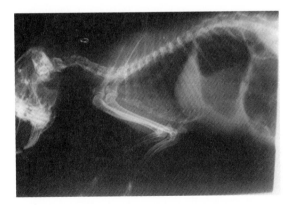

Figure 7.3 Gastric and intestinal bloat in a rabbit as a result of penicillin toxicity. Chest cavity is normal. The radiodense object over the neck is a staple in a skin wound. (Fraser and Girling, 2009)

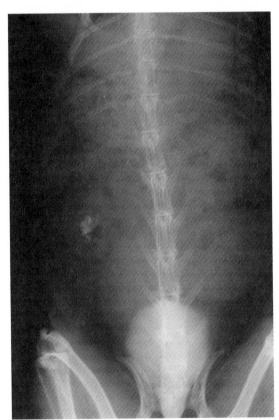

Figure 7.5 Dorsoventral view of the rabbit in Figure 7.4 showing multiple radiodense calculi in left kidney and radiodense silt in urinary bladder. (Fraser and Girling, 2009)

techniques after catheterisation of the bladder using air at 5–8 mL/kg body weight may be used in rabbits to outline the bladder lining. Double contrast techniques can be used with iodine at a rate of 2–3 mL/kg. Excretory urograms may be useful in assessing renal disease using 2 mL/kg of an intravenous iodine-based contrast media injected into a peripheral vein. In healthy rabbits, the presence of large amounts of calcium 'silt' may lead to a significant outline of the bladder.

The uterus may become enlarged due to neoplasia (e.g. uterine adenocarcinomas), pyometra or gravidity. The vagina may also become enlarged due to venous aneurysms.

In the male rabbit there is no *os penis*. The testes sit scrotally but can be retracted into the abdomen.

Head

Radiography is essential to assess dental disease which is common in rabbits (Harrenstein, 1999) (see Figure 7.6). Root elongation and lysis of the alveolar bone is often an early radiographic sign of abnormal dental wear (Redrobe, 2001). Irregular wear of the teeth and touching of the cheek teeth at rest are also indicators of dental disease.

Final stage of dental disease includes abscess formation and osteomyelitis. Oblique views of the head may allow examination of one dental arcade from the other.

Exophthalmos may be due to cheek–tooth abscess, retrobulbar neoplasia and cranial mediastinal masses such as thymic neoplasia; therefore, chest radiographs are also necessary.

Dacrocystitis may be associated with dental disease, often due to incisor root elongation or infection. Contrast studies of the nasolacrimal ducts may be performed using iodine-based contrast media injected into the ventral tear duct punctum and show the pinching of the duct around the roots of the incisor.

For otitis media causing vestibular disease, a dorsoventral square-on view of the skull is necessary (see Figure 7.7). Skull neoplasia has also been recorded in the rabbit (Weisbroth & Hurwitz, 1969).

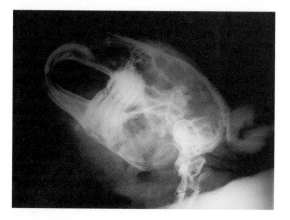

Figure 7.6 Lateral head of a rabbit showing cheek tooth and incisor malocclusion. Note contact of the occlusal surfaces of cheek teeth. Roots of cheek teeth projecting through ventral mandible and upper/lower incisors meeting end on. (Fraser and Girling, 2009)

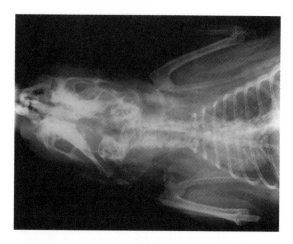

Figure 7.7 Dorsoventral view showing middle ear disease in a rabbit (worse in right middle ear), dental disease (flaring laterally of first cheek teeth) and enlarged heart. (Fraser and Girling, 2009)

Appendicular skeleton

Osteoarthritis is common in rabbits. Luxation of the elbow has also been observed. Neoplasia of the limb in the form of fibrosarcomas and osteosarcomas are also seen in rabbits. Hypertrophic osteopathy has also been reported associated with an intrathoracic neoplasm (DeSanto, 1997), as has a limb neurofibrosarcoma in association with a thymic neoplasm (Clippinger *et al.*, 1998).

Axial skeleton and ribs

The spine shows some breed variation in numbers of vertebrae with some individuals possessing 13 thoracic vertebrae (Kozma *et al.*, 1974). Fractures of the spine, associated often with metabolic bone disease, or luxations/subluxations of the vertebral joints are common.

Arthritis of the spine (spondylosis) and spinous process fractures are also common. In one study, three types of spinal lesions were observed in the rabbit nucleus pulposus of the intervertebral discs undergoing chondroid metaplasia, eventually involving the whole spinal column by 2 years of age; mineralisation with hydroxyapatite deposition in the nucleus pulposus of the discs radiographically, primarily in the thoracic segments (seen as young as 3 months of age) and finally, spondylosis in rabbits over 24 months, chiefly bridging those discs that did not show mineralisation (Green *et al.*, 1984).

Myelography has been described (Longley, 2005). The access point is L5/6 with 0.4 mL/kg of iodine-based contrast medium will extend the media from T2–L7. A 23G, 1¼-inch needle will allow access to the subarachnoid space.

Interpretation of rodent and marsupial radiographs

Imaging techniques in rodents and marsupials are the same as for other mammals. Their small size precludes the use of grids. The use of non-screen film may help in examining fine structures. In many cases, short exposure times are required due to the rapid rates of respiration, even when anaesthetised.

Anaesthesia or sedation is generally required in all cases to allow proper positioning. In all cases, several important features of rodents are visible on radiographs. The main problem is that the chest cavity is very small in relation to the abdominal cavity, making examination of the lung fields for minor abnormalities difficult (Girling, 2002) (see Figures 7.8a–7.8b). Generally though, when patients are presented, the pathology is advanced and it may be difficult to see any normal lung tissue! (see Figure 7.9). Heart disease is commonly seen in many

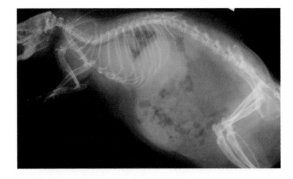

Figure 7.9 Lateral view of an adult (overweight) rat. Note the radiodense masses in the chest typical with mycoplasma pneumonia and lung consolidation. Note also the enlarged heart due to *cor pulmonale*.

small mammals (see Figure 7.10). Some species, such as rats, have open growth plates on many long bones, even as adults. Males of most rodents have an *os penis*, and extensive testicular tissue, which when retracted, may fill the caudal abdomen (see Figure 7.8a). In hind gut fermenters, such as the guinea pig and chinchilla, the capacious large intestine and caecum fills the abdomen making discernment of other structures difficult.

Dental disease is particularly common in Hystricomorphs such as chinchillas (see Figures 7.11 and 7.12), guinea pigs (see Figure 7.13) and degus.

Marsupials have an epipubic bone projecting cranially from the pubis and thought to support the ventral body wall and pouch. The sugar glider however does not possess this.

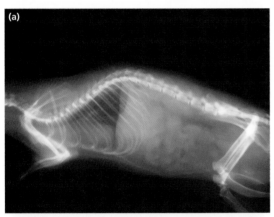

(a)

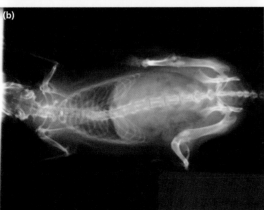

(b)

Figure 7.8 (**a** and **b**) Lateral and dorsoventral view of a normal healthy adult male rat. Note the small size of the chest, the open growth plates particularly on the proximal tibia and the ischial region of the pelvis and the presence of an *os penis*.

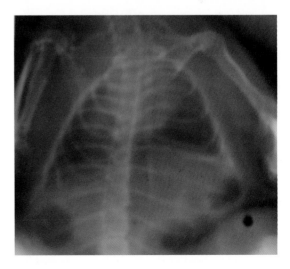

Figure 7.10 Dorsoventral view of a hamster's chest with cardiomegaly due to heart failure associated with bacterial endocarditis. This radiograph was taken using dental non-screen film to improve minor details.

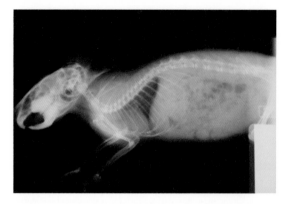

Figure 7.11 Lateral view of a chinchilla. Note the capacious intestinal mass full of ingesta, the small lung field size, which makes the heart look enlarged. The dentition of this chinchilla is near normal.

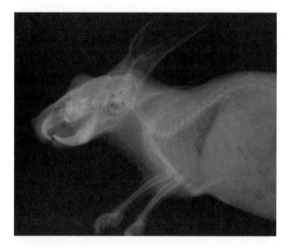

Figure 7.12 Lateral view of a chinchilla's head and thorax. Note the severe loss of cheek teeth.

Interpretation of ferret radiographs

Thoracic cavity

Heart

The heart is positioned more caudally than in the cat or dog and may be slightly elevated from the sternum due to fat deposition in the pericardiac ligament (Orcutt, 1998) (see Figures 7.14 and 7.15).

Cardiac enlargement due to cardiomyopathy and congestive heart failure is common in ferrets (see Figure 7.16). The size of the heart may be assessed using the modified vertebral heart score (VHS) that compares heart length along the long axis against its width on a right lateral plain radiograph and relating this to the length of the heart in

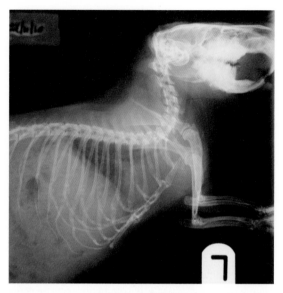

Figure 7.13 Lateral view of a guinea pig's head and thorax. Note the small lung field size that makes the heart look enlarged. Note also in this case the elongated cheek teeth whose roots are pushing into the nasal passages and through the ventral mandible and the incisors, which are meeting end on end instead of the maxillary incisors meeting rostral to the mandibular incisors.

thoracic vertebral units similar to that seen in the dog and cat. The following formula has been used to assess the heart of both male and female ferrets:

$$\frac{\text{RL LA (cm)} + \text{RL SA (cm)}}{\text{T5} - \text{T8 (cm)}}$$

where RL LA means right lateral long axis (base of heart to apex), RL SA means right lateral short axis (widest part of the heart) and T5–T8 means thoracic vertebra 5 to thoracic vertebra 8.

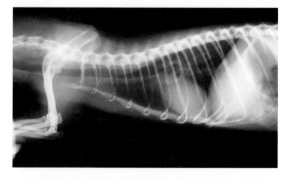

Figure 7.14 Lateral view of the thorax of a normal ferret. Note the apparently more caudal position of the heart and the narrow chest inlet which makes the trachea appear enlarged.

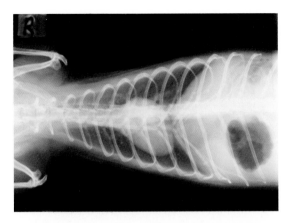

Figure 7.15 Dorsoventral view of the thorax of a normal ferret. Note the more transverse position of the heart. Note also in this case some gas in the stomach which in this case is due to pre-anaesthetic starvation.

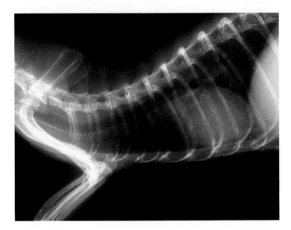

Figure 7.16 Lateral view of the thorax of a ferret with cardiomegaly.

The ratio was 1.35 (standard deviation 0.07) for males and a mean of 1.34 (standard deviation 0.06) for females (Stepien *et al.*, 1999).

Heartworm infestation may show a pleural effusion and cardiomegaly, principally the right side of the heart. In addition, the caudal vena cava is often noticeably dilated (Supakorndej *et al.*, 1995).

Lungs and other organs

Pneumonia produces a typically interstitial and then alveolar pattern similar to that seen in cats and dogs. Lung patterns around the perihilar region suggest lung oedema and congestive heart failure.

Pleural effusions may be seen due to a right-sided failure, for example thymic neoplasia, traumatic wounds and pleurisy or as with heartworm infestation. Soft tissue

mineralisation due to over-supplementation with calcium and vitamin D_3 can affect the primary vessels, and of course the kidneys.

The oesophagus

The oesophagus is not easily seen in the healthy ferret, but megaoesophagus has been reported. Contrast studies using barium sulphate are necessary to help define the oesophagus. A dose of 10–15 mL/kg orally and may be made more palatable by mixing it with a meat-based dog/cat food. Pollock (2007), however, describes that strawberry-flavoured barium sulphate is readily accepted by ferrets.

Abdominal cavity

Liver

The liver is normally completely covered by the caudal ribcage. Enlargement of the liver shadow has been associated with neoplasia (such as lymphoma, biliary cystadenoma, cholangiosarcomas and hepatocellular carcinomas), polycystic disease and infectious disease such as mycobacteriosis (Saunders & Thomsen, 2006).

Stomach and intestines

The stomach is on the left side dorsoventrally and immediately behind the dorsal part of the liver shadow on the lateral view. The cranial border of the stomach in a ventrodorsal radiograph extends to the 13th thoracic vertebra (Evans & An, 1998). Normally, the stomach has small amounts of gas present except in the case of an anaesthetic. Gastric bloat can be seen in recently weaned ferrets and can produce large amounts of gas (Fox, 1988). Other causes of gas in the stomach are usually due to ulceration of the stomach (e.g. foreign bodies, neoplasia and *Helicobacter mustelae* infections) or small intestinal foreign bodies.

The small intestine is much the same diameter throughout. There is no caecum.

Thickening of the small intestine may be seen due to neoplasia such as malignant lymphoma and inflammatory disease such as proliferative ileitis caused by the bacterium *Lawsonia intracellulare*. Alternatively, it may be more diffuse as in eosinophilic enteritis and inflammatory bowel disease.

Spleen

As mentioned, the normal spleen may appear larger in the ferret and so radiographic interpretation of disease in the spleen may be difficult. Gross splenic enlargement may occur due to neoplasia such as lymphoma (see Figure 7.17) or haemangiosarcomas.

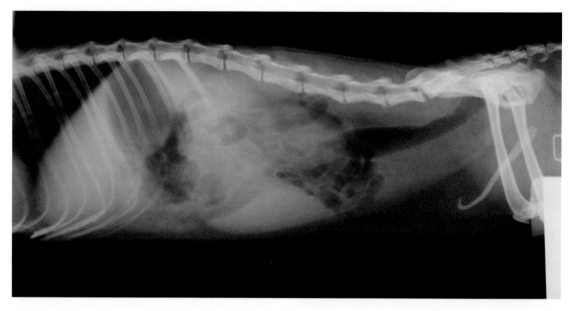

Figure 7.17 Lateral view of the abdomen of a ferret with an enlarged spleen due to early lymphoma.

Kidneys

The right kidney is in front of the left as in other mammals. Renal cysts are commonly seen in ferrets, although the genetically inherited polycystic kidney disease is less common (Orcutt, 2003).

Urinary bladder

Urolithiasis is common in ferrets and is more commonly seen in males due to the presence of the *os penis*.

Reproductive organs

The male ferret possesses a prostate which is at the neck of the urinary bladder and may be affected by adrenal gland neoplasia with the production of considerable cysts. The *os penis* is curved in the shape of the letter 'J'.

Radiography may of course be used to detect gravidity in the female – skeletal development occurs around day 29–30.

Contrast radiography of the gastrointestinal tract

The period of fasting for ferrets prior to radiography is around 3–4 hours – longer than this can cause problems. Positive contrast using barium sulphate mixed with meat-based food or strawberry-flavoured barium at 10–15 mL/kg. In cases of stomach/intestine perforation iodine-based products, for example iohexol, can be used. These should be diluted 1:1 with tap water and then administered at a rate of 10–15 mL/kg of this mixture orally or by stomach tube (Pollock, 2007).

Complete gastric emptying varies from conscious ferrets (75 +/− 54 minutes) to ferrets sedated with ketamine and diazepam (130 +/− 40 minutes) (Schwarz *et al.*, 2003). Normally, small intestinal width should not exceed 5–7 mm.

Contrast radiography of the urinary tract

After anaesthesia, catheterisation of the female ferret's bladder is possible, but difficult with the urethral opening positioned approximately 1 cm cranial to the clitoris on the ventral floor of the vestibule. The male ferret is more challenging due to the J-shaped *os penis* and the small diameter of the urethra. Orcutt (2003) suggests using a 22 gauge, 8-inch jugular catheter to catheterise male ferrets. However, if severe para-urethral/prostatic disease is present, the pressure on the urethra may still prevent passage of a catheter.

Pyelograms may be performed with a dose of 720 mg iodine/kg ferret of a non-ionic iodine-containing media, for example iohexol, intravenously via a peripheral vein (Orcutt, 2003). Non-ionic iodine media is preferable to ionic as it does not induce osmotic diuresis so making contrast studies clearer, and it induces less side-effects. The cephalic vein is perhaps the most easily accessed vessel.

Head

Dental disease is common and bisecting angle radiography as used in cats and dogs can help in the detection of periodontal disease and abscess formation.

Benign neoplasia of the skull such as osteomas have been described (Dernell *et al.*, 2001). However, more aggressive neoplasia has also been described including squamous cell carcinomas of the gums which may invade underlying bone producing radiolucent bony changes on radiography (De Voe *et al.*, 2002).

Axial and appendicular skeleton

The vertebral formula of the ferret is C7, T14–15, L5–7, S3, Cd18, and the dental formula is I 3/3 C 1/1 Pm 3/3 M 1/2 in the adult ferret. The growth plates particularly in the pelvis and long bones do not often close until the ferret is more that 7 months of age.

Spinal lesions are frequently reported in ferrets due to traumatic injuries creating in vertebral disc collapse or more commonly vertebral body fractures and neoplastic processes being seen (Ritzman & Knapp, 2002).

Chordomas, a tumour of the spinal cord, commonly affect the end of the spine but may also affect the cervical area (Li & Fox, 1998). Other neoplasms affecting the spine in ferrets include lymphoma and plasma cell myeloma, both of which can produce metastasise and produce lytic lesions (Li & Fox, 1998).

ULTRASONOGRAPHY

Physical/chemical restraint and positioning

A right lateral position, using a cut out imaging window in the table below, is useful for the examination of the heart and kidneys, but it can be stressful to some patients and may require prior sedation.

A standing position is often better tolerated in the conscious patient and allows easier access to organs such as the liver which sits underneath the ribcage.

Equipment for small mammals

Ultrasound unit

A sector probe transducer is preferred due to its smaller footprint. This is particularly important if trying to image the heart due to the narrow inter-rib spaces. 10 MHz probes may be useful for imaging structures such as the eye but otherwise 7.5 MHz are suitable. B mode ultrasound is mainly used to provide a two-dimensional real-time image of the organs being examined. M mode is useful when examining the heart to assess its contractility. Pulsed wave Doppler techniques for assessing blood flow direction and the measurement of ejection volumes with continuous

wave Doppler techniques are also extremely useful in assessing cardiac disease and may be used in the rabbit as with cats and dogs.

Additional equipment

The patient should be shaved and a coupling gel is applied a few minutes before imaging, as with any species, to allow it to soak into the outer layers of the skin. In some cases, a stand-off is required. Commercial stand-offs are superior to home-made ones as they do no create attenuation, resolution or distortion artefacts.

Rabbit ultrasound interpretation

Thorax

Echocardiography has been described in the rabbit (Tello de Meneses *et al.*, 1989; Marano *et al.*, 1997). Some injectable anaesthetics have an effect on cardiac function but isoflurane has less of an effect on reducing myocardial contractility than halothane, for example (Marano *et al.*, 1997). Marini *et al.* (1999) used ultrasonography to demonstrate myocardial fibrosis associated with ketamine/xylazine anaesthesia in rabbits.

Orcutt (2000) has shown the ultrasound problems associated with congestive heart failure. In addition, bacterial endocarditis has also been reported as has atherosclerosis and associated thrombi (Snyder *et al.*, 1976) (see Figure 7.18).

A prominent thymus and wide cranial mediastinum exist even in the adult rabbit and may be imaged through the heart.

Abdominal cavity

The urinary bladder is often used as an acoustic window to assess many of the caudal abdominal organs, such as the uterus and kidneys. However, calcium carbonate

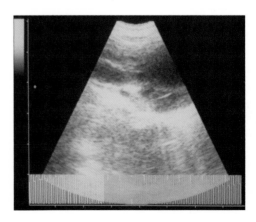

Figure 7.18 Aortic valve disease and atherosclerosis in a rabbit.

crystals may cause a scintillating snow-storm effect and reduce transmission of the ultrasound beam.

Examination of the liver, just caudal to the xiphoid is straightforward. Hepatic lipidosis can be diagnosed as an increase in echogenicity. The gall bladder is easily seen.

The normal kidney outline and internal structure is similar to that seen in the cat, although rabbits are unipapillate (see Figure 7.19). A decrease in renal size plus irregular surface is commonly seen in cases of chronic damage caused by *E. cuniculi*.

Adenocarcinomas of the uterus may be demonstrated with ultrasound (see Figure 7.20), which can also be used for pregnancy diagnosis and the presence of pyometra. Venous aneurysms within the vagina may also be seen.

Ocular ultrasound

The eye may also be imaged using a 10 MHz probe preferably with a stand-off. It can be useful to check for

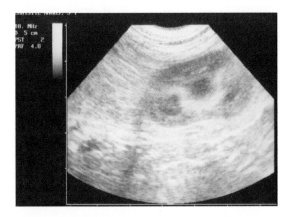

Figure 7.19 A normal rabbit kidney in longitudinal section.

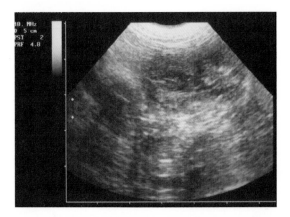

Figure 7.20 Uterine adenocarcinomas in the uterus of a rabbit.

lymphoma, ocular abscesses and uveitis lesions caused by lens rupture due to *Encephalitozoon cuniculi*. In addition, retrobulbar masses may be determined using ultrasonography (Redrobe, 2001).

Ferret ultrasound interpretation

Thoracic cavity

Echocardiography

Numerous authors have reported M mode and Doppler echocardiography in the ferret (Stepien *et al.*, 2000; Vastenburg *et al.*, 2004). The pulmonary artery (rather than the aorta) was recommended for measurement of volume flow in ferrets due to the difficulty in aligning the aortic outflow tract (Stepien *et al.*, 2000). Vastenburg *et al.* (2004) showed that mitral/pulmonary valve regurgitation is not significant.

Dilated cardiomyopathy and less commonly hypertrophic cardiomyopathy have been reported in ferrets. Valvular insufficiency is increasingly commonly diagnosed in older ferrets. Aortic regurgitation is a common incidental finding in ferrets with little significance (Petrie & Morrisey, 2004).

Dirofilaria immitis heartworm produces typically a right-sided heart failure with right ventricle, right atrial and caudal vena cava enlargement on echocardiography. The adult worms may be seen in the right ventricle, right atrium and pulmonary artery.

Abdominal cavity

Adrenal glands

Adrenal neoplasia has been detected using ultrasound. Average normal adrenal lengths vary from 5 to 13 mm and widths from 2 to 5 mm (Neuwirth *et al.*, 1997).

Kidneys

About 10–15% of ferrets undergoing a post-mortem report had a coincidental renal cyst (Orcutt, 2003). Polycystic disease including polycystic kidneys is unusual in ferrets and is differentiated from renal cysts by the presence of multiple irregular cysts in the kidneys and often the liver (Puerto *et al.*, 1998).

Spleen

The spleen can be one of the initial sites along with the thymus and liver for juvenile lymphoblastic leukaemia and haemangiosarcomas and so may show increased echogenicity and overall size.

Liver

Neoplasia of the liver is common in the ferret and includes juvenile lymphoblastic leukaemia, biliary cystadenoma, cholangiosarcoma and hepatocellular carcinoma. The normal liver has six lobes and a gall bladder.

Pancreas

Insulinomas are very small (1–2 mm) and so are often missed on ultrasound examination.

Intestines

Focal thickening of the ileum caused by the bacterium *Lawsonia intracellulare* and lymphoma which may affect the whole intestine may be seen on ultrasound. These are often focal. More diffuse areas, as in eosinophilic enteritis and inflammatory bowel disease with hyperechoic areas of gas, may also be seen.

Urinary bladder

Urolithiasis is common and may result in cystitis and bladder wall thickening. Para-urethral cysts are common in hyperadrenocorticism (adrenal gland disease). Neoplasia is uncommon but has been reported.

Prostate

The prostate is bilobed in the male ferret and sits at the neck of the urinary bladder. Hyperadrenocorticism is associated with the enlargement of the prostate and the development of large cysts, which are easily detectable using ultrasound.

Uterus

The non-gravid uterine body diameter has been quoted as 1.1–2.5 mm (An & Evans, 1988). Gravidity, cystic and neoplastic endometrial changes and pyometras may all be diagnosed with ultrasound. It may also be used to detect uterine stump hypertrophy in previously spayed ferrets suffering from hyperadrenocorticism.

Mesenteric lymph node

The mesenteric lymph node, situated at the junction of the cranial and caudal mesenteric veins, may be mistaken for one of the adrenal glands, but its mobile and more ventral position should aid in differentiating it. A technique to allow fine needle aspirate cytology of the mesenteric lymph node as an aide to detecting lymphoma has been described in the ferret (Paul-Murphy *et al.*, 1999).

Other organs

Ocular ultrasonography has been recorded. A 10 MHz transducer is required in B mode due to the short focal distances involved. However, despite this, a considerable amount of contact gel is required as a stand-off pad to avoid near-field artefacts. Normal values for the eye have been determined (Hernandez-Guerra *et al.*, 2007).

Other small mammal ultrasound interpretation

A 7.5 MHz probe is usually required. A stand-off may also be useful.

Cardiac disease, common in marsupials, chinchillas and guinea pigs, as well as hamsters, may be interpreted using ultrasonography using principles described above for rabbits (see Figure 7.21).

Pregnancy diagnosis may be made easily in hystricomorphs and it is an extremely useful tool to confirm the presence of cystic ovarian disease (see Figure 7.22).

In addition, renal structure may be examined where cystic disease of chronic failure and atrophy is suspected.

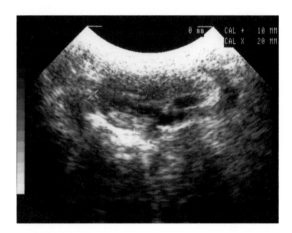

Figure 7.21 Long axis section through the heart of a hamster with bacterial endocarditis.

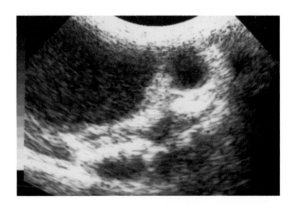

Figure 7.22 Large ovarian cysts in the abdomen of a gerbil.

MRI AND CT SCANNING OF SMALL MAMMALS

These techniques are becoming more commonplace in rabbits and small mammals.

Computed tomography (CT) scanning creates a cross-sectional image of the patient and is particularly good for assessing bony changes such as that seen with advanced dental disease as has been suggested in chinchillas (*Chinchilla laniger*) (Crossley *et al.*, 1998) and rabbits. In addition, other conditions affecting the head, such as neoplasms, sclerosis of the middle ear and turbinate atrophy and infection, are ideally suited to this modality. Anaesthesia must be used as the patient must be completely immobile while a rotating X-ray beam images the patient in segments.

Magnetic resonance imaging (MRI) is more useful for assessing soft tissue structures, such as aneurysms, tumours and organ enlargement. It also requires the patient to be anaesthetised and completely immobile. Lesions in organs such as the brain make ideal candidates for MRI, although spinal abscesses (Runge *et al.*, 1998) and pyelonephritis (Runge *et al.*, 1997) have been assessed in the rabbit using MRI.

References

An, N.Q. and Evans, H.E. (1988) Anatomy of the ferret. *Biology and Diseases of the Ferret* (ed G.J. Fox), 1st edn, pp. 15–65. Lea & Febiger, Philadelphia, PA.

Clippinger, T.L., Bennett, R.A., Alleman, A.R., Ginn, P.E. and Bellah, J.R. (1998) Removal of a thymoma via median sternotomy in a rabbit with recurrent appendicular neurofibrosarcoma. *Journal of the American Veterinary Medical Association*, **213**, 1140–1143.

Crossley, D.A., Jackson, A., Yates, J. and Boydell, I.P. (1998) Use of computed tomography to investigate cheek tooth abnormalities in chinchillas (*Chinchilla laniger*). *Journal of Small Animal Practice*, **39**, 385–389.

Dernell, W.S., Straw, R.C. and Withrow, S.J. (2001) Tumors of the skeletal system. *Small Animal Clinical Oncology* (eds S.J. Withrow & E.G. MacEwen), 3rd edn, pp. 406–454. WB Saunders, Philadelphia, PA.

DeSanto, J. (1997) Hypertrophic osteopathy associated with an intrathoracic neoplasm in a rabbit. *Journal of the American Veterinary Medical Association*, **210**, 1322–1323.

De Voe, R.S., Pack, L. and Greenacre, C.B. (2002) Radiographic and CT imaging of a skull associated osteoma in a ferret. *Veterinary Radiology and Ultrasound*, **43**(4), 346–348.

Evans, H.E. and An, N.Q. (1998) Anatomy of the ferret. *Biology and Diseases of the Ferret* (ed J.G. Fox), 2nd edn, pp. 19–70. Williams & Wilkins, Baltimore, MD.

Fox, J.G. (1988) Systemic diseases. *Biology and Diseases of the Ferret* (ed J.G. Fox), pp. 258–259. Lea & Febiger, Philadelphia, PA.

Girling, SJ (2002) Mammalian imaging and anatomy. *Manual of Exotic Pets* (eds A. Meredith & S. Redrobe), 4th edn, pp. 1–12. BSAVA, Quedgeley, UK.

Green, P.W., Fox, R.R. and Sokoloff, L. (1984) Spontaneous degenerative spinal disease in the laboratory rabbit. *Journal of Orthopaedic Research*, **2**, 161–168.

Harrenstein, L. (1999) Gastrointestinal diseases of pet rabbits. *Seminars in Avian and Exotic Pet Medicine*, **8**, 83–99.

Hernandez-Guerra, A.M., Rodilla, V. and Lopez-Murcia, M.M. (2007) Ocular biometry in the adult anesthetized ferret (*Mustela putorius furo*). *Veterinary Ophthalmology*, **10**(1), 50–52.

Kozma, C., Macklin, W., Cummins, L.M. and Mauer, R. (1974) The anatomy, physiology and biochemistry of the rabbit. *The Biology of the Laboratory Rabbit* (eds S.H. Weisbroth, R.E. Flatt & A.L. Kraus), pp. 50–69. Academic Press, London.

Li, X. and Fox, J.G. (1998) Neoplastic diseases. *Biology and Diseases of the Ferret* (ed J.G. Fox), 2nd edn, pp. 405–447. Williams & Wilkins, Baltimore, MD.

Longley, L. (2005) Epidural catheterisation in rabbits. *Proceedings of the British Veterinary Zoological Society Spring Meeting*, Chester, UK, 2005, pp. 56–57.

Marano, G., Formigari, R., Grigioni, M. and Vergari, A. (1997) Effects of isoflurane versus halothane on myocardial contractility in rabbits: Assessment with transthoracic two-dimensional echocardiography. *Laboratory Animal Science*, **31**, 144–150.

Marini, R.P., Li, X., Harpster, N.K. and Dangler, C. (1999) Cardiovascular pathology possibly associated with ketamine/xylazine anesthesia in Dutch belted rabbits. *Laboratory Animal Science*, **49**, 153–160.

Neuwirth, L., Collins, B. and Calderwood-Mays, M. (1997) Adrenal ultrasonography correlated with histopathology in ferrets. *Veterinary Radiology and Ultrasound*, **38**(1), 69–74.

Orcutt, C.J. (2000) Cardiac and respiratory disease in rabbits. *Proceedings of the British Veterinary Zoological Society Autumn Meeting*, RVC, London, pp. 68–73.

Orcutt, C.J. (1998) Emergency and critical care of ferrets. *Veterinary Clinics of North America: Exotic Animal Practice*, **1**(1), 99–126.

Orcutt, C.J. (2003) Ferret urogenital diseases. *Veterinary Clinics of North America: Exotic Animal Practice*, **6**(1), 113–138.

Paul-Murphy, J., O'Brien, T., Spaeth, A., Sullivan, L. and Dubielzig, R.R. (1999) Ultrasonography and fine needle aspirate cytology of the mesenteric lymph node in normal domestic ferrets (*Mustela putorius furo*). *Veterinary Radiology and Ultrasound*, **40**(3), 308–310.

Petrie, J-P. and Morrisey, J.K. (2004) Cardiovascular and other diseases. *Ferrets, Rabbits and Rodents: Clinical Medicine and Surgery* (eds K.E. Quesenberry & J.W. Carpenter), pp. 58–71. WB Saunders, Philadelphia, PA.

Pickard, D.W. and Stevens, C.E. (1972) Digesta flow through the rabbit large intestine. *American Journal of Physiology*, **222**, 1161–1166.

Pollock, C. (2007) Emergency medicine of the ferret. *Veterinary Clinics of North America: Exotic Animal Practice*, **10**(2), 463–500.

Puerto, D.A., Walker, L.M. and Saunders, M. (1998) Bilateral perinephric pseudocysts and polycystic kidneys in the ferret. *Veterinary Radiology and Ultrasound*, **39**(4), 309–312.

Redrobe, S. (2001) Imaging small mammals. *Seminars in Avian and Exotic Pet Medicine*, **10**, 187–197.

Ritzman, T.K. and Knapp, D. (2002) Ferret orthopedics. *Veterinary Clinics of North America: Exotic Animal Practice*, **5**(1), 129–155.

Runge, V.M., Timoney, J.F. and Williams, N.M. (1997) Magnetic resonance imaging of experimental pyelonephritis in rabbits. *Investigative Radiology*, **32**, 696–701.

Runge, V.M., Williams, N.M., Lee, C. and Timoney, J.F. (1998) MRI imaging in a spinal abscess model. Preliminary report. *Investigative Radiology*, **33**, 246–255.

Saunders, G.K. and Thomsen, B.V. (2006) Lymphoma and Mycobacterium avium infection in a ferret (*Mustela putorius furo*). *Journal of Veterinary Diagnostic Investigation*, **18**(5), 513–515.

Schwarz, L.A., Solano, M., Manning, A., Marini, R.P. and Fox, J.G. (2003) The normal upper gastrointestinal examination in the ferret. *Veterinary Radiology and Ultrasound*, **44**(2), 165–172.

Shell, L.G. and Saunders, G. (1989) Arteriosclerosis in a rabbit. *Journal of the American Veterinary Medical Association*, **194**, 679–680.

Snyder, S.B., Fox, J.G., Campbell, L.H. and Soave, O.A. (1976) Disseminated staphylococcal disease in laboratory rabbits (*Oryctolagus cuniculus*). *Laboratory Animal Science*, **26**, 86–88.

Stepien, R.L., Benson, K.G. and Forrest, L.J. (1999) Radiographic measurement of cardiac size in normal ferrets. *Veterinary Radiology and Ultrasound*, **40**(6), 606–610.

Stepien, R.L., Benson, K.G. and Wenholz, L.J. (2000) M-mode and Doppler echocardiographic findings in normal ferrets sedated with ketamine hydrochloride and midazolam. *Veterinary Radiology and Ultrasound*, **41**(5), 452–456.

Supakorndej, P., Lewis, R.E. and McCall, J.W. (1995) Radiographic and angiographic evaluations of ferrets experimentally infected with *Dirofilaria immitis*. *Veterinary Radiology and Ultrasound*, **36**(1), 23–29.

Tello de Meneses, R., Mesa, M.D. and Gonzalez, V. (1989) Echocardiographic assessment of cardiac function in the rabbit: a preliminary study. *Annals of Veterinary Research*, **20**, 175–185.

Vastenburg, M.H.A.C., Boroffka, S.A.E.B. and Schoemaker, N.J. (2004) Echocardiographic measurements in clinically healthy ferrets anesthetized with isoflurane. *Veterinary Radiology and Ultrasound*, **45**(3), 228–232.

Weisbroth, S.H. and Hurwitz, A. (1969) Spontaneous osteogenic sarcoma in *Oryctolagus cuniculus* with elevated serum alkaline phosphatase. *Laboratory Animal Care*, **19**, 263–265.

Further reading

Besso, J.G., Tidwell, A.S. and Gliatto, J.M. (2000) Retrospective study of the ultrasonographic features of adrenal lesions in 21 ferrets. *Veterinary Radiology and Ultrasound*, **41**(4), 345–352.

Fraser, M.A. and Girling, S.J. (2009) *Rabbit Medicine and Surgery for Veterinary Nurses*. Blackwell-Wiley, Oxford.

Girling, S.J. (2006) Diagnostic imaging. *Manual of Rabbits* (eds A. Meredith & P. Flecknall), 2nd edn, pp. 51–62. BSAVA, Quedgeley, UK.

Jensen, W., Myers, R. and Lin, C. (1985) Osteoma in a ferret. *Journal of the American Veterinary Medical Association*, **187**(12), 1375–1376.

Neuwirth, L., Isaza, R., Bellah, J., Ackerman, N. and Collins, B. (1993) Adrenal neoplasia in seven ferrets. *Veterinary Radiology and Ultrasound*, **34**(5), 340–346.

O'Brien, R.T, Paul-Murphy, J. and Dubielzig, R.R. (1996) Ultrasonography of adrenal glands in normal ferrets. *Veterinary Radiology and Ultrasound*, **37**(6), 445–448.

Silverman, S. (1993) Diagnostic imaging of exotic pets. *Veterinary Clinics of North America: Small Animal Practice*, **23**, 1287–1299.

Stefanacci, J.D. and Hoefer, H.L. (2004) Radiology and ultrasound. *Ferrets, Rabbits and Rodents, Clinical Medicine and Surgery* (eds K.E. Quesenberry & J.W. Carpenter), 2nd edn, pp. 395–413. WB Saunders, Philadelphia, PA.

Williams, J. (2002) Orthopaedic radiography in exotic animal practice. *Veterinary Clinics of North America: Exotic Animal Practice*, **5**(1), 1–22.

Chapter 8

Small Mammal Emergency and Critical Care Medicine

RABBIT EMERGENCY AND CRITICAL CARE MEDICINE

Introduction

Emergency medicine is a challenging discipline, and perhaps none more so than in some of the smaller patients that we deal with. Rabbits are often presented to veterinary practices and emergency clinics with acute ailments, many of which can lead rapidly to a life-threatening condition. Although specific information on emergency medication of the acutely collapsed rabbit is scarce, the medical approach should follow protocols already created for cats and dogs, but with some tailoring of the therapy based on the differing anatomy and biology of the rabbit. This chapter aims to provide clinicians with information on emergency therapy and stabilisation of the domestic rabbit.

As with other small mammals, emergency therapy in the rabbit should initially follow the 'ABC' (Airway, Breathing and Circulation) protocol already adopted for cats and dogs. However, there is increasing debate that the protocol should be CAB as the blood stream in acute cases has sufficient oxygen to keep organs functioning providing the circulation persists. It should be noted that the drugs listed below, unless stated, are not licensed for use in rabbits.

Emergency airway access and ventilation (A and B)

Should breathing stop, or hypoxia be detected, then emergency ventilation will be required. This is best achieved by immediate endotracheal intubation.

Intubation may be achieved blindly, with the rabbit in sternal recumbency. The rabbit's head is lifted and the ET tube is advanced slowly until breathing sounds are heard through the tube. The tube may then be quickly advanced on inspiration. If a transparent tube is used, then condensation from the rabbit's breath when the tube is over the glottis can be seen aiding intubation. If the rabbit has stopped breathing, then this technique becomes extremely difficult; therefore, a laryngoscope with a Wisconsin 0 paediatric blade can be used to visualise the glottis (Heard, 2004). This is best achieved with the rabbit in dorsal recumbency and the tongue pulled laterally. A guide wire may be inserted through the glottis first and the ET tube threaded over the top. Alternatively a fine endoscope or needlescope may be used as a guide wire instead, threading the ET over the scope prior to intubation. Once through the glottis, the ET tube may be advanced and the scope retracted easily.

Direct intubation itself may be difficult in the rabbit owing to the narrow oral cavity and relatively large size of the tongue caudally, or the presence of an obstruction such as a pharyngeal abscess or foreign body. In an emergency therefore it may be necessary to pass a long through-the-needle catheter into the tracheal lumen between two tracheal rings ventrally. A luer adaptor may be attached to allow connection to an anaesthetic circuit for oxygen administration. A tracheostomy may also be performed in the same way as for a cat or dog. The main difference is that some breeds of rabbit, particularly the doe, have large dew flaps with plentiful subcutaneous fat deposits which may make tracheostomy surgery challenging. Otherwise see below.

1. A longitudinal incision is made over the trachea caudal to the larynx, followed by blunt dissection onto the trachea itself.
2. A 180° ventral incision in between the tracheal rings 3–4 below the larynx is made and an ET tube inserted.
3. Incise the skin and subcutis – note the lack of extensive muscles. Incise between the tracheal rings.
4. Insert the ET tube.
5. Connect ET tube to anaesthetic circuit.

If intubation is not possible, then either a tight-fitting face mask connected to an anaesthetic circuit may be applied, and a high flow rate of oxygen (4–5 L), or an Ambu bag, to force ventilate the rabbit. Alternatively, moving the rabbit in a see-saw manner may aid ventilation by moving the abdominal viscera backwards and forwards onto the diaphragm and acting as a pump mechanism (Briscoe & Syring, 2004). This works on the basis that most of the impetus for inspiration comes from the flattening of the diaphragm rather than the outward movement of the ribcage.

Interestingly, end-tidal CO_2 levels may be used to monitor cardiac output during CPCR. A steady increase in end-tidal CO_2 is more likely to be associated with a successful outcome and conversely if the end-tidal CO_2 does not increase above 10 mm Hg after a resuscitation time of 15–20 minutes, then it is unlikely to be successful (Marino, 1997).

Cardiovascular support (C) and drugs (D)

In mammals <10 kg, direct cardiac massage by compressing the chest directly over the heart is most effective at increasing thoracic pressure and forcing blood through the arterial vasculature (Henrik, 1992). Heart compression rates of 100 beats per minute need to be achieved in rabbits; the technique recommended to maximise cardiovascular output is circumferential chest compression, as is used in human infants, where the chest is compressed over the heart from both sides at once (Costello, 2004).

If a cardiac beat is present or a beat is restarted, ECG leads should be applied to discern any dysrhythmias. The type of dysrhythmia reported in rabbits during resuscitation techniques has thus far been different from that reported in cats and dogs. The latter have been associated with electro-mechanical dissociation, whereas in rabbits, profound bradycardia, ventricular asystole and ventricular fibrillation have been reported (Rush & Wingfield, 1992). Adrenaline may be used, intratracheally if intubated, or intravenously if no cardiac beat is detected and no ECG trace. In the case of fine ventricular fibrillation, the use of adrenaline has been advocated to convert the electrical activity to coarse ventricular fibrillation which is easier to convert (DeFrancesco, 2000) – see Table 8.1 for dosages.

Conversion of coarse fibrillation is based on the use of cardiac massage as described above, or if the clinic has access to defibrillation devices then the use of these externally at 2–10 J/kg (starting at low energies and increasing if no response is achieved) may be performed (Costello, 2004). Greater success is achieved with defibrillation devices if three initial countershocks are applied at low energies.

Table 8.1 Emergency drugs used in rabbits.

Drug	Dosage and route
Adrenaline (1:1000 = 1 mg/mL)	0.2–1 mg/kg IV, intratracheally
Dexamethasone	2 mg/kg IV (use with caution)
Diazepam	1–3 mg/kg IV, IM
Doxapram	2–5 mg/kg SC, IV, PO q 15 min
Fluids	100 mL/kg per day maintenance
Furosemide	1–4 mg/kg IV, SC, IM
Glycopyrrolate	0.02 mg/kg SC, IM
Lidocaine	1–2 mg/kg IV; 2–4 mg/kg intratracheally
Midazolam	0.5–2 mg/kg IV, IM, intranasally

Source: Adapted from Kottwitz and Kelleher (2003).

If severe bradycardia is detected, glycopyrrolate should be used (see Table 8.1) in preference to atropine as 60% of domestic rabbits possess serum atropinesterases making atropine less effective (Okerman, 1994).

Lidocaine may be administered intratracheally or intravenously if ventricular arrhythmias such as ventricular premature complexes leading to ventricular tachycardia occur (see Table 8.1 for dose). However, lidocaine should not be used in cases of AV block or severe bradycardia (DeFrancesco, 2000), which are more commonly seen in rabbits.

Cardiomyopathy and valvular insufficiency with resultant congestive heart failure are also seen in rabbits as is atherosclerosis. Treatment of congestive heart failure initially depends on the use of diuretics such as furosemide at 1–4 mg/kg intravenously, repeated every 4–6 hours as required. ACE inhibitors have been used in rabbits but they are more susceptible to hypotensive side effects than cats or dogs. Therefore, reduced dosages and regular monitoring of the systolic blood pressure using non-invasive techniques devised for cats are advisable (Girling, 2003).

Diagnostic procedures

ECG (E)

As mentioned above, should cardiac arrest or arrhythmias be detected, ECG leads may be applied as in cats and dogs and the trace assessed. See Table 8.2 for some normal values for rabbits.

Table 8.2 Normal ECG values (lead II) for healthy rabbits.

Parameter	Normal result	Notes
P wave height	0.1–0.15 mV	Deflection is low or negative in lead I and always positive in leads II and III
P wave duration	0.03–0.04 s	
P-R interval	0.05–0.1 s	
QRS complex duration	0.015–0.04 s	
R wave amplitude	0.3–0.39 mV	
Q-T interval	0.08–0.16 s	Change of deflection of the T-wave from positive to negative or vice versa indicates myocardial hypoxia as with cats and dogs

Source: From Kozma *et al.* (1974) and Huston and Quesenberry (2004).

Radiography

This is essential where acute gastrointestinal signs are present, such as bloat or visceral pain, or where evidence of limb fractures, paresis or paralysis is present and should be performed when clinically safe to do so as part of a full clinical work-up. In this chapter there is not enough time to go into detail regarding diagnostic imaging but the following conditions may be associated with radiographically visible changes.

Abdominal pain may be associated with a number of conditions including renal calculi, obstructive and non-obstructive intestinal ileus and peritonitis. Spinal luxations, fractures and dislocations may also be identified radiographically. Gradation of severity may be made as with cats and dogs. Acute treatment with short-acting intravenous corticosteroids (e.g. dexamethasone, see Table 8.1) and immobilisation with analgesia are advised for spinal trauma with concurrent paresis or paralysis as for other small mammals. Surgery may then be performed for collapsed discs or fractures as for cats and dogs as required.

Ultrasound

This may be of use where renal, bladder, cardiac and hepatic diseases are concerned. Cardiomyopathies (dilated) and atherosclerosis have been reported. Hepatic lipidosis is common in rabbits. Urinary bladders often contain large amounts of silt which create a snow-storm effect.

Blood testing

Routine haematology and biochemistry assessment should be made – values may be found in standard rabbit textbooks. On a critical care level, blood lactate levels may also be measured in rabbits with levels above 10 mmol/L being viewed as abnormal (Lichtenberger & Ko, 2007).

Fluid therapy (F)

Hypovolemic shock

If the rabbit is dehydrated or hypovolemic, shock doses of fluids should be administered. It should be noted that fluids should be avoided post resuscitation in cases of cardiovascular arrest where there is no hypovolemia/dehydration prior to the arrest as these fluids may decrease myocardial perfusion pressures and diminish overall nutrient delivery through the cerebral and coronary vasculature (Cole *et al.*, 2002). Rabbits tend to more closely mimic cats in hypovolemic shock with the decompensatory stage being seen without compensatory shock, i.e. evidence of bradycardia, hypotension and hypothermia. In these cases a slow intravenous bolus of fluids such as hypertonic saline 7.2–7.5% at 3 mL/kg to draw fluid rapidly into the circulation is advised (Lichtenberger & Lennox, 2010). This can be maintained by follow-up administration of Hetastarch (3 mL/kg) over 10 minutes. The patient should be warmed, and crystalloids at 3–4 mL/kg/h should be administered. It is important to measure systolic blood pressure during this procedure. Once the rabbit has been warmed, the aim is to get the systolic blood pressure above 90 mm Hg. This may require further boluses of isotonic crystalloids (10 mL/kg) with Hetastarch (5 mL/kg). Once normovolaemia has been achieved, replacement of fluid deficits may be started (remember maintenance values for rabbits are 80–100 mL/kg per day).

General fluid administration

Oral

Not such a good route for seriously debilitated animals but useful for those with naso-oesophageal feeding tubes in place. Again it may be useful for mild cases of dehydration where owners wish to home treat their pet. This route though is restricted to small volumes with a maximum of 10 mL/kg at any one time administered. In practice it may be possible to administer much less than this.

Subcutaneous

The scruff area or lateral thorax makes ideal sites. This is a good technique for routine post-operative administration of fluids for longer recovery patients undergoing minor surgical procedures such as spaying or castration. It is possible to give a maximum of 30–60 mL split into two or more sites depending on the size of rabbit at one time.

Intraperitoneal

To perform this it is necessary to tilt the rabbit's head downwards whilst it is in dorsal recumbency to allow the gut contents to fall out of the injection zone. The needle is inserted in the caudal right quadrant of the ventral abdomen. It is inserted just through the abdominal wall and the plunger drawn back on the syringe to ensure that no puncture of the bladder or gut has occurred. A maximum volume of 20–30 mL may be given at one time depending on rabbit size. Previous notes regarding concurrent respiratory or cardiovascular disease should be considered. If positioned correctly, there should be no resistance to injection.

Intravenous

Venous access is relatively straightforward in the rabbit. The marginal ear vein, jugular vein, cephalic vein and lateral saphenous vein can all be used for intravenous catheter placement. Long-term (>2–3 days) use of the marginal ear vein may, however, cause sloughing of the ear tip, although in the author's experience this is relatively rare with careful venipuncture technique. Use of a topical local anaesthetic cream is recommended prior to placement. In addition, if a sedative such as Hypnorm® (VetaPharma UK Ltd.) is used (a fentanyl/fluanisone combination neuroleptanalgesic drug), peripheral vasodilation is common facilitating ear vein catheter placement. The fentanyl portion of this drug may be reversed using the partial opioid agonists – buprenorphine (0.01–0.05 mg/kg) or butorphanol (0.1–0.5 mg/kg). The jugular vein may be difficult to access, particularly in does where there is a pronounced ruff of skin and fat deposits. In addition it forms the main venous drainage for the eye, and thrombus formation may lead to periocular swelling. An Elizabethan collar can be used to prevent the rabbit from chewing or removing the catheter, although this will prevent caecotrophy and care should be taken to ensure the rabbit is still managing to eat, otherwise assisted feeding (see below) should be instituted.

Intraosseous

Intraosseous catheters may be placed into the proximal femur, in the trochanteric fossa, in a parallel direction to the long axis of the femur. Use an 18–23 gauge, 1–1.5 inch spinal or hypodermic needle. Analgesia should be employed (see Chapter 3) whenever placing an intraosseous catheter as should prophylactic antibiosis such as enrofloxacin (Baytril 2.5% Bayer – licensed for use in rabbits).

Intraosseous and intravenous fluid administration should be accurately titrated using syringe drivers rather than relying on drip sets since even a small error in fluid administration may be proportionally more significant considering the small size of many rabbits.

Other medications and supportive nutrition

Many rabbits presented as an acute emergency either have already or frequently go on to develop gastrointestinal stasis. Providing obstructive causes have been ruled out; the use of prokinetic medications, such as cisapride, metoclopramide and ranitidine, should be performed (see Table 8.3). Ranitidine acts to reduce acidity in the stomach, which is beneficial as many rabbits with gastrointestinal stasis have punctate ulceration of the stomach lining. In humans it also has prokinetic effects encouraging emptying of the stomach and some increased motility of the small intestine, which seems to be synergised by metoclopramide; this appears clinically to be the case in rabbits in this author's and others' opinion.

Assisted feeding should be carried out in conjunction with the use of prokinetics. This can start off with easily absorbed essential sugars and amino acids (e.g. Critical Care Formula®, Vetark Professional) either syringed into the mouth or delivered via a naso-oesophageal tube. As the rabbit improves clinically, this should be stepped up to use proprietary critical feeding formulas such as Science Recovery® and RecoveryPlus® (Supreme Petfoods) or Critical Care for Herbivores® (Oxbow Pet Products) or vegetable-based baby foods (lactose-free

Table 8.3 Gut motility enhancing drugs for rabbits.

Drug	Dose rate	Frequency of dosing and notes
Cisapride	0.5 mg/kg PO	12 hourly
Metoclopramide	0.5 mg/kg SC	8–12 hourly
Ranitidine	2–5 mg/kg PO	12 hourly (in combination with metoclopramide acts to promote motility as well as reducing acidity)

Note that none are licensed for use in rabbits.

varieties). The disadvantage of baby foods is that they do not contain fibre and thus have little or no prokinetic activity, although they do provide nutrients in an easily digestible form.

The levels of energy required for a debilitated rabbit should approach that calculated for growing-to-lactating rabbits using the formula – $MER = k \times (wt\ [kg])^{0.75}$, where $k = 200$ for growth and 300 for lactation (Carpenter & Kolmstetter, 2000). Therefore for debilitation, the following daily energy requirement may be used:

$$MER = 250 \times (wt\ [kg])^{0.75}$$

To re-populate the intestinal flora, transfaunation of caecotrophs from a healthy rabbit may aid the return of normal bowel function. The use of commercial probiotics designed for rabbits has also been advocated, and reduces the risk of transferring potential parasites and other agents to the debilitated patient.

Naso-oesophageal tube in rabbits

A naso-oesophageal tube (as the tubing must not allow reflux of acid stomach contents into the oesophagus) is placed after first spraying the nose with lidocaine spray and inserting the 3–4 French tube which has been pre-measured from the extended nose to the seventh rib. Sterile water should be flushed through the tube before and after feeding to ensure it is correctly placed and does not become blocked. The tube may then be glued, taped or sutured to the dorsal aspect of the head and a bung inserted when not in use. It may be necessary to put an Elizabethan collar on the rabbit to prevent removal.

EMERGENCY CARE OF OTHER SMALL MAMMALS
Emergency airway access and ventilation (A and B)

Providing a direct airway may be very difficult in rodents. In ferrets and omnivorous marsupials, intubation is similar to small cats. Access to the epiglottis is difficult owing to the nature of rodent anatomy, whereby the soft palate is locked around the epiglottis making its access via the mouth very difficult.

If the rodent is still breathing, placement in a small container and piping in oxygen may be all that is necessary.

If the small mammal is not breathing, then any of the following three techniques may be attempted.

1. Massage the chest of the small mammal gently with two fingers on either side of the chest with the rodent in sternal recumbency whilst the head of the rodent is placed into a face mask with 100% oxygen.
2. Place the small mammal in dorsal recumbency and grasp the trachea between the fingers of one hand. Pass a 23–25 gauge over the needle catheter between two cartilage rings 1 cm caudal to the larynx. Remove the stylet and leave the catheter in place. This may then be used to administer IPPV and 100% oxygen.
3. Place the small mammal in dorsal recumbency. Make a skin incision over the trachea caudal to the larynx and bluntly dissect down onto the trachea as with the rabbit. The trachea may then be incised between cartilage rings to insert a tube.

For IPPV, a rate of 20–30 breaths per minute with a pressure of 8–10 cm H_2O may be applied similar to rabbits.

Cardiovascular support (C)

As for rabbits, circumferential chest compressions should be instituted, but chest compression rates of 150+ beats per minute should be attempted where possible.

Drugs (D)

Similar drugs may be used for small mammals as are used for rabbits (see Table 8.4). Cardiac disease, specifically dilated cardiomyopathies and associated congestive heart failure, may be seen in guinea pigs and hamsters commonly. Hamsters are also prone to bacterial endocarditis.

Atropine may be used where bradycardia is seen as none of the species discussed here have serum atropinesterases.

Table 8.4 Emergency drugs used in small mammals.

Drug	Dosage and route
Epinephrine (1:1000 = 1 mg/mL)	0.2–1 mg/kg IV, intratracheally
Atropine	0.1–0.2 mg/kg SC, IM
Dexamethasone	0.5–2 mg/kg IV (use with caution)
Diazepam	3 mg/kg IV, IM
Doxapram	2–5 mg/kg SC, IV, PO q 15 min
Fluids	100 mL/kg per day maintenance
Furosemide	2–10 mg/kg PO, SC, IM
Glycopyrrolate	0.02 mg/kg SC, IM
Lidocaine	1–2 mg/kg IV; 2–4 mg/kg intratracheally
Midazolam	1–2 mg/kg IV, IM, intranasally

Gerbils are prone to epilepsy which is hereditary. This may be controlled using midazolam/diazepam.

Diagnostic procedures

ECG (E)

Most small mammals have such a fast heart rate and such a small cardiac mass that the ECG trace is difficult to determine. However, it is still often worth applying ECG leads should an arrhythmia be detected on auscultation or where cardiac disease is suspected. A trace speed of 50 mm/s should be used preferably with a 2 cm to 1 mV deflection if possible.

Radiography

This is of use where respiratory and cardiovascular diseases are concerned. Lung volumes are small in rodents, and clear lung fields are often difficult to visualise. However, lung tumours are common in rats and guinea pigs, and varying degrees of lung consolidation may be seen in cases of pneumonia, common in rats, mice and guinea pigs. Cardiomyopathies and heart failure are common in guinea pigs and hamsters.

Spinal fractures can be seen in any rodent, but are more commonly seen in guinea pigs and chipmunks, and collapsed spinal columns are common with nutritional hyperparathyroidism in sugar gliders.

Urinary bladder stones (calcium oxalate usually) are common in guinea pigs and hamsters, and calculi may also be seen in the kidneys.

Gastrointestinal bloat may be seen in chinchillas and guinea pigs associated with severe enteritis or inappropriate antibiotic administration.

Ultrasound

Polycystic ovarian disease is easily diagnosed using ultrasound in guinea pigs, gerbils and hamsters.

Cardiac disease may be diagnosed using the smaller 10 MHz or even 7.5 MHz frequency in larger individuals in the case of hamsters and guinea pigs where cardiac enlargement and valvular disease are common.

Fluid therapy (F)

Hypovolemic shock

As with rabbits, the rapid support of blood pressure in hypovolemic shock is essential. A bolus of isotonic fluids is administered (warmed to body temperature) at 10–15 mL/kg intravenously/intraosseously. If severe hypovolemia is present, then a bolus of hypertonic saline may be administered at 3–4 mL/kg intravenously/

intraosseously. This is followed by a bolus of a colloid, preferably Hetastarch at 5 mL/kg intravenously (or intraosseously) slowly over 5–10 minutes. Once blood pressure has risen above 50 mm Hg or more, then the patient may be warmed and further crystalloid fluids administered. Blood pressure may be measured in larger rodents using the same techniques as in rabbits. In small rodents, such as mice and rats, this may not be possible, so one cycle of crystalloid:colloid fluids should be administered to see if a response to treatment occurs. This may be repeated twice further, leaving an interval of 15–20 minutes between attempts. Warming is essential as the adrenergic receptors do not tend to respond to fluid therapy and catecholamines if the body temperature is less than 98°F (Lichtenberger, 2007).

General fluid therapy provision

See the section in Chapter 6.

Other medications and supportive nutrition

Herbivorous rodents, such as guinea pigs and chinchillas, often benefit from the use of prokinetics as rabbits. Dosages are similar. Small herbivores should avoid the same antibiotics that are harmful to rabbits. It is possible to safely use fluoroquinolones and trimethoprim sulphonamides in small herbivores at doses similar to that used in rabbits.

For nutritional support the same MER formula for rabbits may be used as for rodents. The value of k will change according to the species and has been estimated to be 300–450.

General notes on fluid therapy and blood transfusions

If small mammals are dehydrated or hypovolemic, shock doses of fluids should be administered. It should be noted that fluids should be avoided post resuscitation in cases of cardiovascular arrest where there is no hypovolemia or dehydration prior to the arrest as these fluids may decrease myocardial perfusion pressures and diminish overall nutrient delivery through the cerebral and coronary vasculature (Cole et al., 2002).

Maintenance values

Maintenance fluid rate for all small mammals is estimated to be at 80–100 mL/kg per day, i.e. twice that estimated for cats and dogs. The reason is their generally smaller sizes and higher metabolisms. This leads to greater glomerular filtration rates and insensible losses through the lungs, etc.

Calculation of fluid deficits

These may be calculated as for cats and dogs; however, it is worth noting that a lot of fluid intake normally is consumed as 'food', i.e. in the form of fresh vegetation. This is difficult to take into consideration, and therefore it is safer to assume that the debilitated small mammal will not be eating significant enough amounts for this to matter in the calculation.

As with cats and dogs, assume that 1% dehydration equates with needing to supply 10 mL/kg body weight fluid replacement in addition to the maintenance requirements.

Assumptions then have to be made on the degree of dehydration of the small mammal concerned, and this can be done clinically as follows:

3–5% dehydrated	Increased thirst, slight lethargy, tacky mucous membranes
7–10% dehydrated	Increased thirst leading to anorexia, dullness, tenting of the skin and slow return to normal, dry mucous membranes, 'dull corneas'
10–15% dehydrated	Dull-comatose, skin remains tented after pinching, desiccating mucous membranes

Alternatively we can rely on the PCV and total protein levels to assess dehydration if a blood sample can be taken (see Chapter 5).

Day 1: Maintenance fluid levels + 50% of calculated dehydration factor

Day 2: Maintenance fluid levels + 50% of calculated dehydration factor

Day 3: Maintenance fluid levels

If the dehydration levels are so severe that volumes are still too large at any one time, it may be necessary to take 72 hours to replace the calculated deficit rather than 48 hours.

In addition for those species which can vomit, such as ferrets, the levels of vomitus expelled should be considered. As with cats and dogs, assuming 2–4 mL/kg body weight per vomit is an acceptable level.

In other species where diarrhoea only is the norm, such as small herbivores, it is much more difficult to make estimations, although fluid losses may approach 100–150 mL/kg body weight per day.

Fluid types suitable for use

Crystalloids

The main rehydration fluid of choice is likely to be a lactated Ringer's compound. However, species such as guinea pigs are prone to ketosis, and a glucose saline isotonic/hypotonic fluid may be of use. Hypertonic saline is useful where severe hypovolemia is present as it can rapidly increase blood pressure. However, it should always be followed by isotonic/hypotonic fluids as it does not replace the overall fluid deficit, rather it relies on drawing fluid from the intra and extracellular space into the bloodstream.

Colloids

These may be used in small mammals as in cats and dogs.

Additives

Protein amino acid/B vitamin supplements

These are useful for nutritional support, e.g. Duphalyte® (Fort Dodge) at the rate of 1 mL/kg body weight per day. They are particularly good in cases where the patient is malnourished or has been suffering from a protein-losing enteropathy, such as cases of heavy parasitism, to help replace some of the compounds needed for replenishment. It is also a useful supplement for patients with hepatic diseases or severe exudative skin diseases such as heater burns.

Bicarbonate

This should be considered where metabolic acidosis exists such as in rabbits with hepatic lipidosis and secondary ketosis and guinea pigs with pregnancy ketosis. Calculations of replacements are same as for cats and dogs.

Electrolytes

Sodium and potassium levels should be monitored and corrected for deficits where found. In practice, potassium levels will often be depressed in cases of long-standing diarrhoea and elevated in cases of renal disease. The use of calcium gluconate when a patient has a high potassium level can help minimise hyperkalemia-associated arrhythmias.

Blood transfusions

Blood transfusions are sometimes performed if PCV levels start to drop below 20%. They are best performed by direct, same species-to-species transfers (i.e. a rat to a rat, and a guinea pig to a guinea pig). A healthy donor may have the equivalent of 1% of body weight removed as blood without any deleterious effects. This may be increased to 4% if required, although careful monitoring of the donor after this is needed. The sample is best taken directly into a pre-heparinised syringe (or use citrate acid dextrose if available at a rate of 1 mL of anticoagulant to 5–6 mL of blood) and immediately transferred in bolus fashion to the donor. Intravenous catheters are advised for the transfers as administration should be slow, giving 1 mL over a period of 5–6 minutes if possible, hence sedation or good restraint is required. Very little information is currently available about cross-matching blood groups of small mammals, although ferrets, it seems, do not have appreciably detectable groups. Intraosseous donations may be made if vascular access is not possible.

Oxyglobin® may be used at 4–10 mL/kg replacement for severe deficits and 1–2 mL/kg replacement for minor losses.

References

Briscoe, J.A. and Syring, R. (2004) Techniques for emergency airway and vascular access in special species. *Seminars in Avian and Exotic Pet Medicine*, **13**(3), 118–131.

Carpenter, J.W. and Kolmstetter, C.M. (2000) Feeding small exotic animals. *Hill's Nutrition III* (eds L.D. Lewis, M.L. Morris & M.S. Hand), pp. 943–960. Mark Mervis Institute, Marceline, MO.

Cole, S.G., Otto, C.M. and Hughes, D. (2002) Cardiopulmonary cerebral resuscitation in small animals: a clinical practice review. *Journal of Veterinary Emergency Critical Care*, **12**, 261–267.

Costello, M.F. (2004) Principals of cardiopulmonary cerebral resuscitation in special species. *Seminars in Avian and Exotic Pet Medicine*, **13**(3), 132–141.

DeFrancesco, T.C. (2000) Cardiac emergencies. *Kirk and Bistner's Handbook of Veterinary Procedures and Emergency Treatment* (eds S.I. Bistner, R.B. Ford & M.R. Raffe), pp. 54–61. WB Saunders, Philadelphia, PA.

Girling, S.J. (2003) Preliminary study into the possible use of benazepril in the management of renal disease in rabbits. *Proceedings of the British Veterinary Zoological Society*, Edinburgh, Scotland, p. 44.

Heard, D. (2004) Anesthesia, analgesia and sedation of small mammals. *Ferrets, Rabbits and Rodents: Clinical Medicine and Surgery* (eds K.E. Quesenberry & J.W. Carpenter), 2nd edn, pp. 356–369. WB Saunders, Philadelphia, PA.

Henrik, R.A. (1992) Basic life support and external cardiac compression in dogs and cats. *Journal of the American Veterinary Medical Association*, **200**, 1925–1931.

Huston, S.M. and Quesenberry, K.E. (2004) Cardiovascular and lymphoproliferative diseases. *Ferrets Rabbits and Rodents: Clinical Medicine and Surgery* (eds K.E. Quesenberry & J.W. Carpenter), 2nd edn, pp. 211–220. WB Saunders, St Louis, MO.

Kottwitz, J. and Kelleher, S. (2003) Emergency drugs: quick reference chart for exotic animals. *Exotic DVM*, **5.5** (November), 23–25.

Kozma, C., Macklin, W., Cummins, L.M. and Mauer, R. (1974) The anatomy, physiology and biochemistry of the rabbit. *The Biology of the Laboratory Rabbit* (eds S.H. Weisbroth, R.E. Flatt & A.L. Kraus), pp. 50–69. Academic Press, London.

Lichtenberger, M. (2007) Shock and CPCR in small mammals and birds. *Veterinary Clinics of North America: Exotic Animal Practice*, **10**(2), 275–291.

Lichtenberger, M. and Ko, J. (2007) Critical care monitoring. *Veterinary Clinics of North America: Exotic Animal Practice*, **10**(2), 317–344.

Lichtenberger, M. and Lennox, A. (2010) Updates and advanced therapies for gastrointestinal stasis in rabbits. *Veterinary Clinics of North America: Exotic Animal Practice*, **13**(3), 525–541.

Marino, P.R. (1997) Cardiac arrest. *The ICU Book* (ed. P.L. Marino), pp. 260–298. Lippincott Williams & Williams, Philadelphia, PA.

Okerman, L. (1994) Inherited conditions and congenital deformities. *Diseases of Domestic Rabbits*, 2nd edn, pp. 109–112. Blackwell Publishing, Oxford.

Rush, J.E. and Wingfield, W.E. (1992) Recognition and frequency of dysrhythmias during cardiopulmonary arrest. *Journal of the American Veterinary Medical Association*, **200**, 1932–1937.

Further reading

Kelleher, S. (2006) Rabbit cardiology cases. *Proceedings of the British Veterinary Zoological Society*, Bristol, November, pp. 17–18.

Part II Avian Species

Chapter 9

Basic Avian Anatomy and Physiology

Classification

Birds are classified into many different family groups according to a number of physical, anatomical and evolutionary factors. It is useful to know to which group a bird belongs as this gives an indication of the other birds it is related to. This is of some help when faced with a species which you have not seen before.

Table 9.1 contains some of the more commonly encountered family groups of birds seen in general and avian-orientated practices.

The Psittaciformes are among the most colourful of birds kept as pets.

Nervous system

The avian brain is extremely smooth, lacking the many gyri (the ridges in the brain) seen in mammals (Figure 9.1). Sight appears to be the dominant sense in most birds. Two large optic lobes lie between the cerebral hemispheres and the cerebellum, and it is here where the optic nerves communicate and disseminate information. There is no corpus callosum, the cerebral cortex is generally very thin but the corpus striatum is well developed and is thought to be the site of mental association in birds. An important feature of the bird's brain is the pineal body which sits in the diencephalon, cranial to the cerebellum in midline dorsally. The pineal body has secretory cells similar to photoreceptors and so will respond to light. They are linked also via the cranial cervical ganglia to the optic nerve. The pineal body is responsible for regulating many seasonal effects such as reproduction and migration as well as circadian rhythms. It has a direct effect via hormone secretion onto the hypothalamus.

The avian nervous system is not dissimilar to that seen in its mammalian counterpart. Birds possess 12 cranial nerves (CN), the same number as in cats and dogs. In birds, the optic nerve (CN II) is the largest cranial nerve, being almost half the diameter of the spinal column. It passes through the calvarium via a single hole rather than through multiple smaller ones associated with the cribriform plate of mammals. The other 11 cranial nerves have similar functions as seen in mammals, and the reader is referred to more in-depth anatomy texts for more information (King & McLelland, 1975; Bennett, 1994).

Each of the wings has a nervous supply from a brachial plexus derived from the spinal nerves in the caudal cervical area. There are three nerve plexuses in the lumbosacral region: lumbar, ischiatic and pudendal. The lumbar plexus derives from the last two lumbar and the first one to two sacral spinal nerve roots. Like the other lumbosacral plexuses, it lies in a hollow of the pelvis, dorsal to the cranial kidney area. It supplies the body wall and upper leg muscles and gives rise to the obturator, femoral, cranial gluteal and saphenous nerves. Unlike dogs and cats, birds have an ischiatic plexus which is derived from four to seven spinal nerves in the sacral area and which is situated in a hollow of the pelvis dorsal to the mid-kidney structure. It gives rise to the principal nervous supply for the hindlimbs – the ischiatic nerve which is the largest peripheral nerve in the body and the caudal gluteal nerve. Finally, a pudendal plexus forms in a hollow of the pelvis dorsal to the caudal kidney area from five coccygeal spinal nerves and innervates the tail and cloacal area.

Musculoskeletal system

Most birds have the power of flight. The dense, cumbersome bones of the earthbound mammal would require too much effort to lift into the air. Birds have therefore adapted their skeletal structure, simplifying the number of bones by fusing some together, and generally lightening the whole structure by creating air spaces within many of the bones.

To further lighten the skeleton, several of the larger bones, and even some of the vertebrae in the spine, are connected directly or indirectly to the airways, and are

Table 9.1 Avian family groups commonly encountered in veterinary practice.

Order	Common species
Psittaciformes	This is the order of birds which includes those we know as 'parrots'. This includes the budgerigar, the amazons, the macaws, cockatiels, African grey parrots, cockatoos, parakeets and others.
Passeriformes	This is the largest order of birds and includes the canary, the finch family, birds of paradise, the mynah birds, ornamental starlings, sparrows and others.
Anseriformes	This order includes • The family Anatidae, subfamily Anatinae, for example the mallard duck, shoveller, eider ducks and shelducks • The family Anatidae, subfamily Anserinae, Tribe Anserini (swan and true geese), for example the mute, Whooper's and Bewick's swans, barnacle and greylag geese
Piciformes	This order includes the family Rhamphastidae such as toucan, toucanette and hornbills.
Strigiformes	This covers the owl families.
Falconiformes	This order covers • The Falconidae family for example the peregrine falcon, the saker, the llanner, the gyrfalcon • The Accipitridae family such as the buzzards (common, rough-legged and honey), the sparrowhawk, goshawk, golden eagle

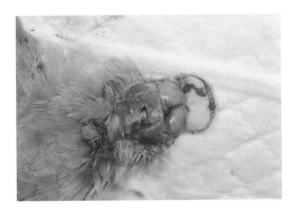

Figure 9.1 Dorsal aspect of avian cerebral hemispheres showing lack of gyri.

said to be pneumonised. This replaces the thick medullary cavity or bone marrow present in the centre of mammalian bones, and produces a light, trabecular structure. Whilst light, the structure is nevertheless extremely strong.

Figure 9.2 shows a generalised avian skeleton.

Skull
Beak
The beak, or bill, is the principal feature of the avian skull. It has been modified into a bewildering number of shapes and sizes, depending mainly on the diet to which the bird has become adapted. In all cases it is composed of an upper (maxillary) and lower (mandibular) beak which are covered in a layer of keratin, a tough protein compound

similar to that which forms the exoskeleton of insects. This keratin layer is known as the rhamphotheca. It is further classified so that the maxillary layer is referred to as the rhinotheca, and the mandibular layer as the gnatotheca. The rhinotheca and gnatotheca grow from a plate at the base of the respective sides of the beak, the rate of replacement depending upon the type of food eaten and the abrasion the beak receives.

In Psittaciformes (Table 9.1), the upper beak is powerfully developed and ends in a sharp point overhanging the broader, stouter lower beak. The tremendous power in a parrot's beak is due to a synovial joint or hinge mechanism, known as the kinetic joint, which joins the beak to the skull. The parrot's lower beak has a series of pressure sensors at its tip, which allow it to test the consistency and structure of objects grasped.

In raptors, the upper beak is extremely sharp and pointed, but lacks the kinetic joint attachment so it cannot produce such powerful downward force. Instead, it is used as a ripping instrument.

In Anseriformes (the duck family), the beak is flattened and may have fine serrations at the edges which allow the bird to filter fine particles from the water. Ducks such as mallards and shovellers have this type of beak. These serrations may be further developed to a jagged edge (e.g. in the aptly named sawbill family) which allows the bird to grip slippery food, such as fish. Anseriformes also have nerve endings in a plate at the tips of their beaks (known as the 'nail') which allow them to find food hidden in mud.

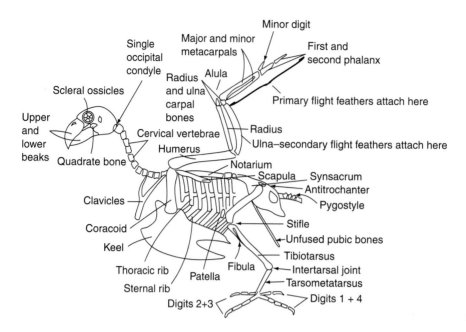

Figure 9.2 Avian skeleton.

In all birds there is a series of smaller bones behind the lower and upper beaks which allow them to move the beak independently of the skull. These include the palatine, quadrate and pterygoid bones and the jugal arches. Their exact movements are beyond this text to describe, but many of the references at the end of this chapter give good accounts of their function.

Nostrils

The nostrils, or nares, lie at the base of the upper beak in most birds and are often surrounded by an area of featherless skin known as the cere. This may be highly coloured in some species, such as the budgerigar, where they may be used to identify the sex of the bird. In many Anseriformes the nares lie more towards the tip of the beak. The nares themselves are merely openings into the sinus chambers, which in turn connect with a branching network of bony chambers throughout the bird's head. These sinuses vary according to the species, but the majority of avian patients have an infraorbital sinus. This sits below the eyes, and is often involved in sinus and ocular infections. It differs from sinuses seen in most mammals in that the lateral wall has no bone, being covered by soft tissue only. This means any infraorbital sinus infection often results in swelling on the face of the bird ventral to the eye. These sinuses also communicate with head and neck air sacs. The function of these air sacs is not clear, but they may help with voice resonance. When a bird suffers from sinus infections, the narrow inlets to these sinuses may become partially blocked and act as one-way valves, allowing air into the sacs but not out. The sacs may then overinflate, and soft swellings are then commonly seen over the back or nape of the bird's head.

The sinuses and external nares communicate with the oropharynx via the choanal slit. This is a narrow opening in the midline of the hard palate and is sited immediately over the glottis when the beak is closed, allowing the bird to breathe through its nostrils. It is often the area chosen for taking samples when trying to isolate infectious agents for upper airway disease in birds.

The skull of the avian patient connects to the atlas (or first spinal vertebra) via only one occipital condyle at the base of the skull, unlike the mammalian two. There are also a large number of highly mobile cervical vertebrae. These two factors make the avian head extremely agile. However, the atlanto-occipital joint is also a weak point, making dislocation at that site very easy.

Vertebral column

Cervical vertebrae

The cervical vertebrae (Figure 9.2) are independently mobile in the avian patient, as they are in the mammalian patient, and vary in number depending on the species between 11 and 25. They are generally box-like in form.

Thoracic, lumbar and sacral vertebrae

The thoracic vertebrae (Figure 9.2) are fused in raptors, pigeons and many other species to form a single bone known as the notarium. In other species they have some limited mobility. There are then two intervertebral joints between the notarium and the fused lumbar and sacral vertebrae. These fused vertebrae are known as the synsacrum. The synsacrum fuses with the pelvis itself to form a dorsal shield of bone over the caudal aspect of the bird.

Coccygeal vertebrae

The majority of the caudal coccygeal vertebrae (Figure 9.2) are usually fused into a single structure known as the pygostyle – which forms the 'parsons nose' part of the chicken!

Pelvis

The roof of the pelvis is formed by the synsacrum (Figure 9.2). The two 'sides' of the pelvis are reduced in size compared with mammals but consist of the iliac and ischial bones, with the acetabulum being created where they meet. The acetabulum in birds is not a complete bony socket as it is in mammals, but a fibrous sheet. There is a ridge on the lateral pelvis known as the antitrochanter, which articulates with the greater trochanter of the femur. The function of this ridge is to prevent the limb from being abducted when perching. The pubic bones of the pelvis do not fuse in the ventral midline as in mammals. Instead they form fine long bones which extend caudally towards the vent. They provide support for the skin covering the caudal abdomen and enough space for the passage of eggs in the female bird.

Ribcage

Psittaciformes have eight pairs of ribs (Figure 9.2). Each rib has a dorsal segment known as the thoracic rib, and a ventral segment, or sternal rib. These ribs point backwards and rigidly connect the thoracic vertebrae dorsally and the keel, or sternum, ventrally.

Sternum

The sternal vertebrae are fused in birds to form the keel. The keel has a midline ridge which divides the pectoral muscles into right and left sides. The ridge may be a deep structure, as is seen in pigeons, raptors and Psittaciformes, allowing large pectoral muscles to attach for strong flight. Alternatively, the keel may be flattened, as with Anseriformes, to provide a boat-like structure more suited to floating.

Wings

The shoulder joint is formed by the meeting of three bones: the humerus, the scapula (which is more tubular than the flattened mammalian one) and a third bone known as the coracoid (Figure 9.2). This latter bone forms a strut propping the shoulder joint against the sternum. The supracoracoid muscle attaches to the keel, then passes through the foramen, or opening, formed at the meeting point of these bones, and so reaches the dorsal aspect of the humerus where it attaches. Contraction of this muscle, along with some elastic tissues which are also present, helps to raise the wing. The pectoral muscles attach from the keel onto the humerus to pull the wing downwards. The fused clavicles, or wishbone (often referred to as the furcula), articulate with the coracoid bone and provides a degree of spring to the flapping of the wings. The humerus is pneumonised, which means that it cannot be used for intraosseous fluid therapy. This is also an important point to consider when repairing fractures.

The humerus articulates with the radius and ulna at the elbow joint. The radius is the smaller of these two bones and lies cranially. The ulna provides the source of attachment for the secondary flight feathers, which insert directly into the periosteum of this bone (Figure 9.3). The ulna is often used for intraosseous fluid administration in birds.

The radius and ulna articulate with one radial carpal bone and one ulnar carpal bone, respectively. These in turn articulate with three metacarpal bones. The first metacarpal bone is the equivalent of the avian 'thumb'. It is known as the alula, or 'bastard wing', and forms a feathery projection from the cranial aspect of the carpometacarpal joint. The remaining two metacarpal bones are known as the major and minor metacarpal bones, and articulate with the first phalanx cranially and the minor digit caudally. The first phalanx then articulates with the second phalanx, forming the wing tip. The primary

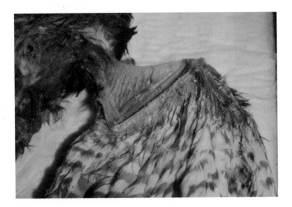

Figure 9.3 Ventral aspect of a kestrel's (*Falco tinnunculus*) wing with covert feathers removed showing the attachment of the primaries to the manus and the secondaries to the ulna.

feathers attach to the periosteum of the phalanges and minor metacarpal bones (Figure 9.3).

The area of the wing is enlarged by thin sheets of elastic tissue which span from one joint surface to another. The largest extends from the shoulder to the carpal joint cranially and is known as the propatagium or 'wing web' (Figure 9.4). This can be used in some species, such as pigeons, for vaccine administration.

Pelvic limb

The acetabulum of the pelvis holds the femoral head (Figure 9.2). The limb may be locked, and prevented from being abducted, by the greater trochanter of the femur engaging with the antitrochanteric ridge on the pelvis. The femur is pneumonised in many birds. At the stifle joint, the femur articulates with the patella and the tibiotarsal bone. The tibiotarsal bone is so called because it is formed from the fusion of the tibia and the proximal row of tarsal bones, and may also be used for intraosseous fluid administration. On the lateral aspect of the proximal tibiotarsus is the much reduced fibula.

Distally, the tibiotarsal bone articulates with the tarsometatarsal bone. This bone is formed by the fusion of the distal row of tarsal bones with the solitary metatarsal bone. The joint between the tibiotarsus and the tarsometatarsus is known as the intertarsal, or suffrago, joint. The tarsometatarsus then articulates with the phalanges.

In Psittaciformes, two digits point forwards (the second and third) and two backwards (the first and fourth), creating a zygodactyl limb. The first digit has two phalanges, the second digit has three phalanges, the third has four phalanges and the fourth has five phalanges. In perching birds (Passeriformes) and raptors, the second, third and fourth digits point forwards and the first points backwards creating an anisodactyl limb. Some species, such as the osprey (*Pandion haliaetus*), may move the fourth digit to face forwards or backwards to aid capturing its prey, creating a semi-zygodactyl limb.

Special senses

Eye

The avian eye is unique in that it contains a series of small bones. These are known as the scleral ossicles (Figure 9.2). They form a ring-shaped structure which supports the front of the eye. The avian eye also differs from the mammalian eye in that it is not a globe, but pear-shaped, with the narrower end outermost.

The avian eye is large in proportion to the overall size of the skull, with only a paper-thin bony septum separating the right and left orbits. Birds have a mobile, translucent third eyelid, and upper and lower eyelids, the lower of which is more mobile than the upper. Two tear-producing glands commonly exist: the third eyelid, or Harderian gland, which is located at the base of the third eyelid, and the lacrimal gland situated caudolaterally, as in mammals.

The colour of the iris may change with age in some parrots, for example the African grey parrot has a dark grey iris until 4–5 months of age, when it turns yellow-grey, and then silver as it continues to age. In others the iris may be used as an indicator of the sex of the bird: in large cockatoos, for example, the female has a bright, red-brown iris, whereas the male's is a dark, brown-black.

The avian retina is thick and possesses no visible surface blood vessels, unlike that of mammals. To provide nutrition to the retina, birds possess a pleated and folded vascular structure called the pecten oculi, which is found at the point where the optic nerve enters the eye. It contracts intermittently, expelling nutrients into the vitreous humour.

Finally, the avian iris has skeletal-muscle fibres within it, unlike mammals which possess only smooth-muscle fibres. This means the avian patient can constrict and dilate its pupil at will, so reducing the value of the pupillary light reflex as a tool in determining ocular function. Because the two optic nerves are completely separated from each other, the consensual light reflex is also a poor indicator of cerebral function.

Ear

There is no pinna in birds, although some species, such as the long- and short-eared owls, have feathers in this area. There is a short, horizontal external canal, covered by feathers, which is located caudolateral to the ocular orbit.

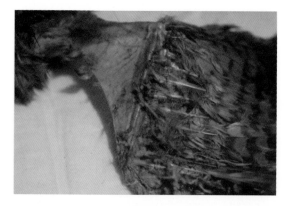

Figure 9.4 Dorsal aspect of a kestrel's (*Falco tinnunculus*) wing with covert feathers removed showing the elastic sheet of the propatagium bridging the elbow joint.

The tympanic membrane may be clearly seen. The middle ear connects to the oropharynx via the Eustachian canal. The mammalian aural ossicles are replaced in the bird by a lateral, extra columella cartilage and a medial columella bone which transmit sound waves to the inner ear.

The inner ear contains the cochlea and the semicircular canals, which fulfil the same functions as in mammals.

Respiratory anatomy

Upper respiratory system

The nares open into the nasal passages, which in turn communicate with the glottis of the larynx via a midline aperture in the hard palate which forms the roof of the caudal mouth. This aperture is called the choanal slit. The sinus system and cervicocephalic air sacs have been previously mentioned.

Larynx

Birds have a reduced laryngeal structure, lacking an epiglottis, the thyroid cartilage, and the vocal folds seen in cats and dogs. The main structure is the glottis, which protects the entrance to the trachea. External muscles pull the glottis and trachea forwards so that it communicates directly with the choanal slit, allowing the bird to breathe through its nostrils. The glottis is held closed when at rest, only opening on inspiration and expiration.

Trachea

The trachea of avian species differs from the mammalian trachea in that its cartilage rings are complete, signet-ring-shaped circles, interlocking one on top of the other, rather than the C-shaped rings of the mammalian trachea. In Psittaciformes and diurnal raptors, the shape of these cartilage rings is slightly flattened in a dorsoventral direction, whereas in most Passeriformes they are round.

In some species, such as the Whooper's swan and the guinea fowl, the trachea forms a series of loops and coils at the thoracic inlet. Other species, such as the emu, have a midline ventral split in the trachea three quarters of the distance between the head and the thoracic inlet. The tracheal lining mucosa projects through this slit to form a tracheal sac. This improves vocal resonance. In male ducks, such as mallards, there is a swelling in the last portion of the trachea, often just inside the thorax, known as the tracheal bulla.

Syrinx

Before the trachea divides into the two main bronchi, there is a structure known as the syrinx (Figure 9.6).

This is where the bird produces most of its voice. It is composed of a series of muscles and two membranes which can be vibrated, independently of inspiration or expiration.

Lower respiratory system

Lungs

The lungs of avian species are rigid in structure and do not inflate or deflate significantly. They are flattened in shape and firmly attached to the ventral aspect of the thoracic vertebrae and vertebral ribs. There is no diaphragm in birds, and the common body cavity is referred to as the coelom.

The paired bronchi are supported by C-shaped rings of cartilage, unlike the trachea. The primary bronchi supply each of the two lungs, and rapidly divide into secondary and tertiary bronchi, or parabronchi. There are four main groups of secondary bronchi supplying the lung but their role in gas exchange is minimal. The tertiary bronchi, however, do play a role in gas exchange, as their walls are filled with membranes capable of gaseous exchange. These areas appear as small pits, or atria, to which are connected even finer tubes known as air capillaries. These intertwine with each other to form a three-dimensional mesh interwoven with the blood capillary beds. These air capillaries vary in size but average around 3–5 mm in diameter. This extremely small diameter produces very high forces of attraction between their walls when fluid secretions are present, resulting in rapid blocking of the respiratory surfaces. To stop this from occurring, there are cells within the parabronchi which secrete surfactant, to ensure the airways stay open.

The lung structure may be further classified by the direction of airflow within it into the neopulmonic lung and the paleopulmonic lung. These will be mentioned later on when discussing respiratory physiology.

Air sacs

The final part of the avian lower respiratory system is composed of the air sacs (see Figure 9.5). These are balloon-like sacs which act as bellows, pumping the air into and out of the rigid avian lungs in response to movements of the body wall and sternum. The air-sac walls are very thin and composed of simple squamous epithelium which covers a layer of poorly vascularised elastic connective tissue.

In the majority of birds there are nine air sacs. One of these is the separate air sac already mentioned, the cervicocephalic air sac, which does not communicate with

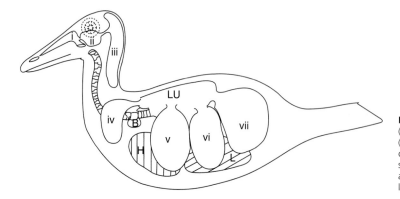

Figure 9.5 Avian air-sac system in a duck: (a) nasal passages; (b) infra-orbital sinus; (c) cervicocephalic air sacs (single); (d) clavicular air sacs; (e) cranial thoracic air sacs; (f) caudal thoracic air sacs; and (g) abdominal air sacs. H, heart; L, liver; Lu, lungs; B, syringeal bulla (male ducks).

the lungs at all. The other eight all communicate with the lungs via a secondary bronchus (except the abdominal air sacs which connect to the primary bronchus on each side). Figure 9.5 shows the air sac system of a duck.

In addition to the separate cervicocephalic air sac, the other standard eight air sacs are

1. A single cervical air sac which lies between the lungs and the dorsal oesophagus and communicates with air spaces within the cervical vertebrae.
2. A single clavicular air sac which has two diverticuli, one of which involves the heart and, cranial to this, the thorax. The other extends around the bones and muscles of the pectoral girdle and crop. This air sac communicates with the air spaces within the medullary cavity of the humeri, scapulae and sternum.
3. The paired cranial thoracic air sacs lie dorsolaterally in the chest, ventral to the lung field and immediately caudal to the heart.
4. The paired caudal thoracic air sacs lie immediately caudal to the cranial air sacs. These are again positioned dorsolaterally within the chest and tend to be slightly smaller than the cranial ones.

5. The paired abdominal air sacs lie caudal to the caudal thoracic air sacs. They touch the caudal aspect of each lung field before spreading caudally into and around the gut. These communicate with the air spaces in the medullary cavities of the notarium, synsacrum, pelvis and femurs.

Respiratory physiology
Respiratory cycle

The downward movement of the sternum and the cranial and lateral movement of the ribs create negative pressure in the coelom and so inflate the air sacs and draw air through the lungs. There are two portions to the avian lung, known as the neopulmonic and paleopulmonic sections. The neopulmonic part of the lung is caudolateral and is absent in certain species, such as penguins. It differs from the paleopulmonic lung in that air passes through the paleopulmonic section of the lung in one direction only, whereas the neopulmonic lung receives air on inspiration and expiration. The avian cycle of inspiration and expiration is given in Box 9.1.

Box 9.1 Avian respiratory cycle	
Inspiration	Fresh air and the air in the dead space of the trachea and the primary bronchi move into the secondary and tertiary bronchi, where gas exchange can begin. In addition some of this air travels through the neopulmonic tertiary bronchi into the caudal thoracic and abdominal air sacs where it takes no part in respiration.
Expiration	The caudal thoracic and abdominal air sacs contract and expel their air back through the neopulmonic part of the lung and into part of the paleopulmonic lung where gas exchange occurs.
Second inspiration	The air expelled during expiration through the neopulmonic and paleopulmonic lung continues to move cranially into the cervical, clavicular and cranial thoracic air sacs.
Second expiration	The air in the clavicular, cervical and cranial thoracic air sacs is expelled through secondary bronchi to the primary bronchi and so out of the body.

It can be seen that the avian respiratory system is extremely efficient at extracting oxygen from the air. For one thing, the whole cycle occurs over two inspirations and expirations, allowing oxygen to be extracted on both inspiration and expiration. In addition, the air flow through the parabronchial tubes is at right angles to the accompanying blood flow. This creates a cross-current system, wherein oxygen in the airway is always at a higher concentration than its accompanying blood vessel, so encouraging the movement of oxygen from airway to bloodstream.

Physiological control of respiration

This is in many ways similar to mammalian respiratory control. Carotid body chemoreceptors in the carotid arteries monitor the partial pressure of oxygen in the blood, whilst carbon dioxide sensitive receptors in the paleopulmonic parabronchi of the airways stimulate respiration once the airway partial pressure of carbon dioxide reaches a critical threshold. Some anaesthetic gases, such as halothane, can depress the function of these carbon dioxide receptors, creating apnoea in the patient.

Digestive system

Oral cavity

The functions of this part of the digestive system are prehension, mastication and manipulation of food into the oesophagus, just as other mammals use their teeth, lips and tongue. The avian oral cavity differs from the mammalian in that it possesses relatively few taste buds and produces little saliva during the mastication process.

Tongue

The avian tongue may be relatively immobile and strap-like, as in Passeriformes (perching birds such as the canary, finch and songbird families), or it may be highly muscular and mobile as in the Psittaciformes family. Alternatively, it may be extensible and specialised as is found in the hummingbirds and, to a lesser extent, in the nectar-eating parrots, the lories and lorikeets which have a fringed tongue for pollen and nectar feeding.

Oesophagus and crop

The oesophagus is a muscular tube connecting the oral cavity to the first stomach (Figure 9.6). As in the lower digestive system, a series of peristaltic waves pass along the oesophagus when food is present, pushing the bolus of food towards the stomach. The oesophagus runs to the right of the trachea in the neck and is lined with many salivary glands. Some fish-eating species of birds have a series of hooks and papillae, directed caudally to force slippery food items to travel in one direction only.

Along its route, usually at the thoracic inlet, some species have a diverticulum of the oesophagus, known as the crop. This is an expansible sac acting as a storage chamber for food. It has no digestive-enzyme secreting properties, although in some species, such as pigeons, a form of lipid 'milk' is produced from the lining of the crop, which acts as a source of nutrition for the young. This crop 'milk' is really composed of exfoliated lining cells filled with lipid.

Some species, such as a few grain-eating finches, penguins, gulls, toucans, ducks and geese, do not have a specific crop, but instead have a much more distensible oesophagus, which can be used in the same way. The crop empties into the thoracic portion of the oesophagus, which passes dorsally over the heart before entering the proventriculus or true stomach.

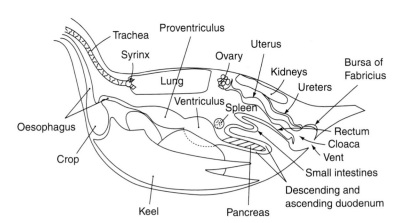

Figure 9.6 Generalised view of the internal organs of a female bird.

PART II: AVIAN SPECIES

Avian 'stomachs'

Birds have two stomachs (Figure 9.6). The first of these is the 'true' stomach, known as the proventriculus. This organ is responsible for the secretion of the digestive enzyme pepsin and hydrochloric acid. Unlike mammals, the secretion of these two substances occurs from the same compound gland, rather than two separate ones. Other glands are present which secrete a protective mucus. The sac-like proventriculus empties into the more circular ventriculus, also known as the gizzard or grinding stomach. There is often movement of food backwards and forwards between proventriculus and gizzard to mix and digest food thoroughly before passing it on to the rest of the gut.

In seed-eating species, the gizzard is larger than the proventriculus and very muscular. In nectar-eating species, such as the lories and lorikeet family of parrots, and other species, such as hummingbirds and raptors, the gizzard is much smaller. The mucosa of the gizzard is lined with deep tubular glands. These glands secrete a protein substance which, in conjunction with cells shed from the inside of the gizzard, forms a tough sheet-like layer known as the koilin or cuticle. This layer becomes heavily stained with bile refluxing into the gizzard from the duodenum (see Figure 9.7). Its function appears protective and it is periodically replaced. Some species of raptors will regurgitate the koilin as a neat package when expelling waste fur and bones from prey which has been consumed.

The gizzard itself is constructed of two pairs of muscles, one pair of smaller muscles and one larger pair, forming an asymmetric structure. Each muscle bundle is separated

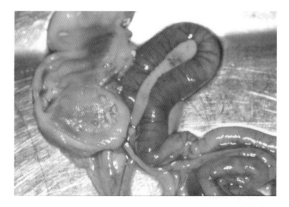

Figure 9.7 View of the opened gizzard (ventriculus) and associated digestive tract from a psittacine bird. Note the bile staining of the koilin lining of the opened gizzard and the loop of the duodenum to the upper right with a lobe of pancreas between the ascending and descending loop.

from its neighbour by a sheet of tendinous tissue. The gizzard lies on the left side of the avian coelomic cavity, caudally, and empties into the duodenum. Food outflow from the gizzard is regulated by a fold-like sphincter.

Grit particles may be consumed by the bird and lodge in the gizzard and act as an abrasive source for food grinding. This is important for seed eating, or granivorous, birds which do not remove the outer husks with their beaks, for example pigeons and gamebirds.

Small intestine

The first part of the small intestine is the duodenum. It forms a descending and then an ascending limb which are adherent to each other, but separated by the pancreas (Figure 9.6). The duodenum has separate openings into it from the liver biliary system and the pancreatic ducts.

The proximal duodenum contains many mucus-secreting goblet cells which serve to protect its lining from the acidic food mixture leaving the gizzard. As in the mammalian duodenum, the avian duodenum is covered with a thick carpet of villi, which increases its absorptive area. The small intestinal brush border cells secrete some disaccharidase and monosaccharidase enzymes to further digest food. There is no evidence of the enzyme lactase in birds, so the feeding of milk-sugar or lactose-containing foods is not recommended. The jejunum and ileum are very small in avian patients, and difficult to define.

Large intestine

The large intestine is frequently referred to as the 'rectum' in birds because of its small size. It is smaller in diameter than the small intestine (Figure 9.6). The rectum is responsible for the absorption of water and some electrolytes.

At the junction of the ileum and rectum are the caeca. These may be absent in most Psittaciformes or reduced in many Passeriformes to one or two lymphoid deposits. In some other species such as the duck family or the domestic fowl the caeca may be relatively large. Other examples of species with large caeca are ratites, such as the ostrich or emu, willow grouse and red grouse, which live off twigs and shoots such as heather. The caeca in these species often act as fermenting chambers for the microbial digestion of cellulose and hemicellulose present in these tougher vegetable foods. The rectum empties directly into the most cranial part of the cloaca known as the coprodeum.

Cloaca

This is the communal chamber into which the digestive, urinary and reproductive systems empty (Figure 9.6). The most cranial segment is the coprodeum which receives faeces from the rectum.

The coprodeum is separated by a mucosal fold from the next chamber of the cloaca, known as the urodeum. The urodeum receives the urinary waste from the ureters, and the reproductive tract opens into it as well. The mucosal fold may be everted or pushed out through the vent, ensuring that the faeces do not contaminate the urodeum and therefore the reproductive system. This fold can also close off the coprodeum from the urodeum completely when the male ejaculates, or when the female is egg laying, so as to prevent faecal contamination of semen or egg.

The last chamber of the cloaca before the vent is the proctodeum. The proctodeum is connected to the bursa of Fabricius which is the germinal centre for the B lymphocyte line of the immune system (see the Lymphatic System section).

Gastrointestinal tract innervation

The intestines and avian stomachs are supplied by branches of the tenth cranial nerve, the vagus, which also carries branches of the parasympathetic nervous system. The sympathetic nervous system also contributes to gut innervation, mainly via the intestinal nerve, which is a large plexus of sympathetic nerves that is close to the cranial and caudal mesenteric arteries and supplies the small and large intestines.

Liver

The liver is bilobed and lies caudal to the heart, ventral to the proventriculus and cranial to the gizzard (Figure 9.6). The liver produces bile salts and bile acids, which are excreted into the duodenum via bile canaliculi and bile ducts and aid in the emulsification of fats in the small intestine.

Some species have a gall bladder, but many parrots and pigeons do not possess one. In those species with a gall bladder, it tends to receive bile only from the right lobe of the liver, the left lobe draining directly into the duodenum.

The main bile pigment in birds is biliverdin. This means that measurement of total bilirubin levels is of no clinical use in birds for assessing liver disease. It does mean that liver inflammation may often be indicated by the presence of biliverdin pigments in the urate portion of the droppings. These pigments turn the urates mustard-yellow or lime-green. Starved blood bile acid levels are therefore preferred as indicators of liver function.

Pancreas

The pancreas lies mainly between the descending and ascending loops of the duodenum (Figure 9.6). It has three lobes: dorsal, ventral and splenic. The gland is tubuloacinar in structure, similar to that of mammals, and is responsible for the secretion of the enzymes: amylase, lipase, trypsin, chymotrypsin, carboxypeptidases, ribonucleases, deoxyribonucleases and elastases. As in mammals, it is also responsible for the production of bicarbonate ions which help neutralise the hydrochloric acid from the stomachs. The pancreas also produces the endocrine chemicals: insulin and glucagon.

Urinary anatomy

Kidney

The kidneys are paired structures found within the pelvis. They are tightly adhered to the backbone in the lumbosacral area (Figure 9.6). Each kidney is divided into cranial, middle and caudal lobes (Figure 9.8).

Nephron

The nephron is the functional unit of the kidney, as it is in mammals; however, there are two types in birds. One is the cortical form of nephron which lacks a loop of Henle. It makes up 70–90% of the nephrons, depending on the species, and is found only in the outer cortex of the kidney. It can only produce isotonic urine. The other

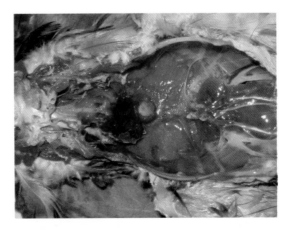

Figure 9.8 Ventral aspect of African grey parrot's (*Psittacus erithacus*) kidneys (far right of picture) showing vascular supply and three-lobed appearance.

is known as the medullary nephron, which accounts for the other 10–30%. This has a loop of Henle, which, like its mammalian counterpart, dips into the inner medullary region of the kidney and can produce mildly hypertonic urine. Irrespective of the type of nephron, they both start with a Bowman's capsule and a glomerulus. Both types of nephrons empty into the collecting ducts, with the duct tubes becoming fewer and fewer and their diameter becoming larger and larger until they empty into the ureter.

Ureters

Each kidney has a ureter which arises from its cranial lobe. The ureter then passes caudally, on the ventral surface of the middle and caudal renal lobes, receiving branches from the amalgamation of the collecting ducts. Each ureter continues caudally and finally empties into the urodeum segment of the cloaca, on its dorsal surface. Birds do not have a urinary bladder or urethra.

Renal blood supply

Each kidney in the avian patient is supplied by three renal arteries, the cranial, middle and caudal renal arteries, which supply the cranial, middle and caudal renal lobes, respectively.

In addition to this arrangement, the avian kidney also receives blood from the renal portal system. The renal portal veins form a ring of vessels surrounding the kidneys and connect with the vertebral sinus cranially and the caudal mesenteric vein caudally. Within the common iliac vein, draining the hindlimb and anastomosing with the renal portal veins, is a valve. This renal portal valve can divert blood in a number of directions. For instance

- It can allow blood through from the leg and so on into the caudal vena cava, bypassing the kidneys altogether.
- It could shut and so divert blood from the hindlimb into the kidney tissues. (This is of importance theoretically when administering potentially nephrotoxic drugs or drugs which are excreted by the kidneys, into the hindlimbs of birds.)
- The blood could equally be shunted towards the liver via the caudal mesenteric vein or into the internal vertebral venous sinus within the spinal canal. The blood flow is therefore complex and may alter almost at will.

Renal physiology

The anatomy of the cortical nephrons is significant because they do not have a loop of Henle, and so there is no counter-current multiplier system by which the urine

may be made more concentrated than the plasma. Therefore, most of the urine produced by birds is isosmotic, that is it is of the same concentration as the extracellular fluid.

The rennin–angiotensin system present in mammals is also present in birds and functions primarily to control sodium balance. It does this by causing the release of aldosterone from the adrenal glands or by altering the resistance of the afferent and efferent glomerular arterioles. This causes an alteration of the volume of the filtrate produced.

In mammals, when an animal becomes dehydrated, antidiuretic hormone (also known as arginine vasopressin) is released from the posterior pituitary. This causes the opening of channels in the renal collecting ducts for further absorption of water. In birds the chemical released is arginine vasotocin (AVT). This chemical works on several areas of the bird's body as, unlike mammals, birds do not rely solely on the kidneys for water conservation. This is because of their poor ability to produce concentrated, hypertonic urine. AVT therefore has more of an effect on the blood flow through the glomeruli rather than on the glomeruli themselves. By reducing this, it reduces the amount of filtrate produced and so conserves water.

To remove the salts which build up during dehydration, many species of birds have salt glands which excrete concentrated sodium chloride from the body. They are present in their nostrils and are also influenced, positively this time, by AVT.

Finally, some fluid is reabsorbed in the avian rectum as urine enters the urodeum of the cloaca and may then be refluxed back through the coprodeum and into the rectum.

Cardiovascular system

Heart

The avian heart has four chambers and is larger in proportion to the rest of its body than its mammalian counterpart, averaging 1–1.5% body weight as compared to 0.5% body weight on average in mammals (Figure 9.9).

The sinus venosus, which forms part of the wall of the mammalian right atrium, is actually a separate chamber in the bird, into which the caudal vena cava and the right cranial vena cava empty. The left vena cava empties nearby but is separated from the other two vessels by a septum. There are also sinoatrial valves separating the caudal vena cava entrance and the right cranial vena cava from the rest of the right atrium.

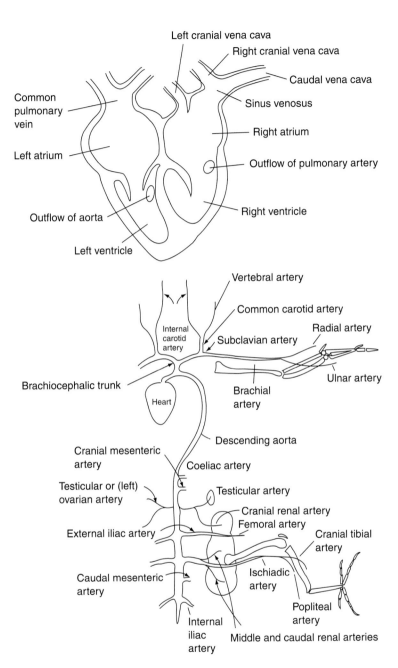

Left cranial vena cava

Right cranial vena cava

Caudal vena cava

Common pulmonary vein

Sinus venosus

Right atrium

Left atrium

Outflow of pulmonary artery

Outflow of aorta

Right ventricle

Left ventricle

Vertebral artery

Common carotid artery

Internal carotid artery

Radial artery

Subclavian artery

Brachiocephalic trunk

Ulnar artery

Heart

Brachial artery

Descending aorta

Cranial mesenteric artery

Coeliac artery

Testicular or (left) ovarian artery

Testicular artery

Cranial renal artery

Femoral artery

External iliac artery

Cranial tibial artery

Caudal mesenteric artery

Ischiadic artery

Internal iliac artery

Popliteal artery

Middle and caudal renal arteries

Figure 9.9 Dorsal view of avian heart and circulation.

PART II: AVIAN SPECIES

The two atria are separated from the ventricles by atrio-ventricular (AV) valves. The right AV valve has only one muscular flap with no chordae tendineae. The left AV valve is much the same as in cats and dogs as it has two valves. In some birds there may be three.

There are two coronary arteries supplying blood to the myocardium, and four major coronary veins as opposed to the single mammalian coronary vein.

Blood vessels

The avian patient differs from the mammalian in that the aorta curves to the right side of the chest rather than the left (Figure 9.9).

The avian 'abdominal' contents are supplied with the same coeliac, cranial and caudal mesenteric arteries as the mammalian. The main difference is that three arteries supply the kidneys. In the case of reproductive organs, the testes are supplied by arteries arising from the cranial renal arteries, whilst the left ovary is supplied by an artery branching off from the left cranial renal artery. (There is often only one ovary – see the Reproductive System section.)

The legs are supplied by a femoral artery arising from the external iliac artery. However, the leg is also supplied by a larger vessel than the femoral artery, known as the ischiatic artery. This arises from a common vessel offshoot of the aorta which also creates the middle and caudal renal arteries, and so passes through and over the kidney structure. It continues down the leg, changing into the popliteal and cranial tibial arteries.

The head is supplied with blood chiefly by the left and right carotid arteries which arise from the left and right brachiocephalic arteries. The wings are supplied from the subclavian arteries which also supply the pectoral muscles forming the breast. The subclavian artery gives rise to the brachial artery which supplies the humeral region. The brachial artery then gives rise to the radial and ulnar arteries to supply the rest of the more distal wing.

The head is drained chiefly by the right and left external jugular veins. In the majority of avian species, the right jugular vein is much larger than the left.

The abdominal contents of the bird are drained through a series of vessels. The main vessel returning to the heart is the caudal vena cava which is supplied by two large hepatic veins and many minor ones. The liver is supplied by two hepatic portal veins from the intestines as opposed to the one vessel in the mammal system. The caudal vena cava also receives blood from the common iliac vein and the two testicular or one ovarian vein depending on the sex of the bird.

The common iliac vein receives supplies from the caudal and cranial renal veins and from the structure known as the renal portal circulation.

The majority of the blood from the legs is drained first by the tibial vein, then into the popliteal vein, then femoral vein and finally the external iliac vein which itself empties into the common iliac vein.

The wing is drained by the radial and ulnar veins which converge to form the brachial vein. This runs alongside the humerus on its caudoventral aspect and can be used for intravenous injections in many species. The brachial vein runs into the subclavian vein and so on into the left or right cranial vena cava.

Lymphatic system
Spleen
The avian spleen is spherical in many species of Psittaciformes, but may be more strap-like in other species, and sits adjacent to the proventriculus. It has white and red pulp areas, as in mammals, and acts to remove old red blood cells, as well as functions as part of the immune system and in cell production. It is particularly important in systemic infectious diseases, such as psittacosis, where due to antigenic stimulation it may increase tenfold in size.

Thymus
The thymus is composed of a series of islands of lymphoid tissue strung out along the neck and thoracic inlet. It is responsible for the production of T-lymphocytes which are necessary for cellular immunity. As with mammals, the thymus decreases in size with age but may still be present in the adult bird.

Lymph nodes
These do not occur as recognisable organs in birds except in some waterfowl such as ducks and geese. These waterfowl have two main nodes, one near to the gonads and kidneys and one near to the thoracic inlet.

In other species, lymphatic tissue is present in accumulated areas within the internal body organs such as the kidneys, liver, digestive system, pancreas and lungs.

Bursa of Fabricius
This is a structure unique to birds. It is situated in the dorsal wall of the proctodeum segment of the cloaca. It is where the avian B-lymphocyte population, responsible for humoral or antibody immunity, is produced. The bursa, as does the thymus, decreases in size with age and usually disappears altogether in the adult bird.

Reproductive anatomy
Male
Testes
There are two testes, both of which, unlike in mammals, sit entirely within the abdominal or coelomic cavity. They are positioned cranial to the kidneys and are tightly adherent to the dorsum of the body wall either side of the midline.

The testes often enlarge during the reproductive season, most noticeably in species such as the pigeon and dove family (Columbiformes), where the testes may enlarge by up to 20 times their out-of-season size. From each testis runs a single vas deferens or spermatic cord which traverses the ventral surface of the kidney before entering the urodeum section of the cloaca.

Phallus

There is no phallus in many species of birds. Instead the semen is transferred by the apposition of the male cloacal vent to female cloacal vent.

Some species do have a phallus, including the Anseriformes, or duck, goose and swan family, as well as the ratite (ostrich, cassoary, emu and rhea) family and the domestic chicken.

The phallus lies in its dormant state on the ventral aspect of the cloaca. When aroused it engorges with blood and everts through the vent to curve in a ventral and cranial direction. Along the dorsal surface of the erect phallus runs the seminal groove. The semen drops from the vas deferens openings in the cloaca into the groove, which then guides the sperm into the female cloaca. The phallus therefore plays no part in the process of urination, unlike its mammalian counterpart.

Female

Ovary

There is only one ovary, the left, in most species (Figure 9.10). One or two species have two ovaries, the kiwi and many hawks for example. The ovary is cranial to the left kidney, suspended from the dorsal body wall by a mesentery containing numerous short ovarian arteries derived from the aorta. For this reason, when speying an avian patient, only the uterus is removed, leaving the ovary intact.

Infundibulum

From this one ovary arises a one-sided reproductive system. Adjacent to the ovary is the fimbria or funnel part of the infundibulum. This 'catches' the oocyst when it is shed into the reproductive tract. Attached immediately to the funnel is the tubular part of the infundibulum, which is also known as the chalaziferous region.

Magnum

Joining onto the infundibulum is the magnum portion of the reproductive system. This is highly coiled and much larger in diameter than the infundibulum, with many folds to its lining. There are multiple ducts leading to the lumen of the magnum, with the most caudal portion containing mucus glands as well.

Attached to the caudal portion of the magnum is the isthmus, which is narrower in diameter and less coiled, but with more prominent longitudinal folds.

Uterus

Attached to the caudal portion of the isthmus is the shell gland or uterus. This is a short portion of the tract with many leaf-like folds. It empties into the S-shaped vagina, from which it is separated by a muscular sphincter.

Reproductive physiology

Male

The male avian testes are primarily composed of seminiferous tubules. In between these are the interstitial, or Leydig, cells which are the main source of androgens, such as testosterone, in the male bird. The seminiferous tubules are similar to their mammalian counterparts and contain the Sertoli cells in which the spermatozoa are nourished and develop.

In perching birds (Passeriformes) each vas deferens forms an enlarged area just before entering the urodeum, known as the seminal glomus. The two glomi become so swollen during the breeding season as to form one mass, known as the cloacal promontory, which acts as the storage chamber for sperm. These can be used to sex many species of Passeriformes.

In general, the testes will enlarge during the reproductive season, with sperm production ceasing during the winter months. In many birds the left testis is larger than the right, following a pattern similar to that of the female gonad. The colour of the testes may also change during the breeding season, going from a yellow, or in some instances blackened, colour to a grey or white as they enlarge with spermatozoa.

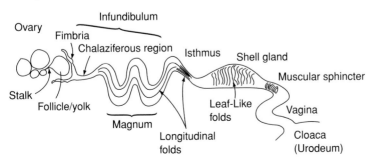

Figure 9.10 Avian female reproductive tract.

Female

In the ovary, folliculogenesis (production of the oocyte and its yolk) is similar to that seen in mammals. The cycle is as follows:

1. Each follicle starts with the oocyte. The oocyte obtains its 'yolk' of lipids and proteins from the liver via the bloodstream in response to follicle-stimulating hormone which is secreted by the anterior pituitary.
2. Over the surface of the follicle lies a white band known as the stigma which splits, shedding the oocyst from the follicle into the infundibulum. This occurs as a result of the release of luteinising hormone from the anterior pituitary.
3. The corpus haemorrhagicum and corpus luteum, which are seen in mammals, are absent in birds, although some progesterone hormone production may occur from remaining cells.
4. The ovum is fertilised in the infundibulum (assuming a successful mating) 15–20 minutes after ovulation. The fertilised ovum moves through the tubular portion of the infundibulum (the chalaziferous portion). Here the chalazion, or egg yolk supporting membrane, is deposited around the egg yolk. This is a dense layer of albumen or inner egg white. The ovum moves on into the magnum where the bulk of the egg white (albumen) is deposited. After this the egg moves into the isthmus gaining the tough shell membranes. Finally it moves into the uterus or shell gland where the mineralised shell is deposited. It is also here that 'plumping' occurs. This is when the bulk of the water content is added, mainly to the albumen portion of the egg. When the egg is ready, the uterine or vaginal sphincter opens, allowing the egg to move into the vagina.
5. The vagina acts as the main storage site for spermatozoa immediately after copulation and it is where the sperm mature. It is also responsible for the deposition of the outer egg surface (cuticle) providing a microporous, protective breathing membrane on the egg's surface. When the egg is ready, the vagina expels it by muscular contractions.

Sex determination and identification

In the majority of species of birds, sexual identity is chromosomally (i.e. genetically) determined.

Sex identification may be performed in three main ways:

1. Some species show sexual dimorphism. That is the two sexes appear physically different. For example
   - When sexually mature, the male budgerigar (in 95% of cases) has a blue cere, and the female a brown one.
   - Male cockatiels have a solid-coloured underside to their tails and a vivid orange cheek patch, whereas females have horizontal light and dark bars to the underside of the tail and a paler cheek patch. (Problems do arise in these two species when dilute colour variants (known as lutinos) and albino birds appear as there is often no pigmentation in the cere in these species.)
   - In some species the two sexes have totally different body feather colours. For example, the male eclectus parrot is a vivid green with a yellow beak, whereas the female is red and deep blue with a black beak.
   - Male large species cockatoos have a dark brown iris and the females a red-brown one.
   - Male canaries will sing during the breeding season.
   - Many male songbirds are more highly coloured than the female. This is also true of many waterfowl, for example many ducks.
   - In raptors there may be a wide variation in colours and sizes between the sexes. In most raptors, the female is larger than the male bird, often as much as double the size.

   In sexually monomorphic species, such as African grey parrots, many macaws and Amazons, identifying the sex of the bird has to be done by surgical sexing or DNA sexing, as there is no obvious reliable external difference between the sexes.
2. Surgical sexing involves anaesthetising the bird and passing a fine rigid endoscope through the flank of the patient in order to examine the internal gonad(s) visually. There are risks to such a procedure, which is why the process has been largely replaced by DNA sexing.
3. DNA sexing requires either a sample of the patient's blood or the pulp from a freshly plucked body feather. This is submitted to the laboratory to determine if the DNA is that of a male or female bird. In birds the female is the heterogametic sex, having sex chromosomes known as YZ; the male is homogametic for the sex chromosomes, being ZZ. This is the reverse of the situation in mammals where females are homogametic. In mammals, the sex chromosomes are referred to as X and Y.

Skin and feathers

Skin

Avian skin is much thinner than that of mammals, and has little or no hypodermis. This means that in general it is poorly or loosely attached to the underlying structures.

However, in regions such as the lower legs, the skin adheres directly to the bone.

The skin has an outer epidermal layer which is composed of three main layers – from inside to out: the germinatory layer; the maturation layer and the cornified layer.

The dermis is much reduced compared to mammals. It forms very little in the way of a substantial structure but it does give the skin some elasticity, although nowhere near as much as mammalian skin.

There are no sweat glands in avian skin. A bird regulates its temperature by panting, known as gular fluttering, and by altering feather alignment to allow heat either to escape or to be trapped against the body surface.

Claws

The tip of each toe is supplied with a claw, formed of a keratinous material similar to the beak. These may be adapted to form the basic perching claws of the Passeriformes, the multipurpose perching and grasping claws of Psittaciformes or the ripping and prey-capture implements of the raptor family.

The members of ratite family also have varying numbers of claws on their wing digits, and some falcons, such as the kestrel and peregrine falcon, have a claw on the first digit or alula of the wing.

Preen (uropygial) gland

The uropygial gland is situated over the synsacrum at the base of the tail. It is a highly developed structure in most waterfowl, as it is responsible for producing oil to waterproof the feathers. The oil produced from the preen gland may also act as a source of vitamin D for the bird. It has a bilobed structure with two tubular exits, one for each lobe. The preen gland is also present in many other species, but is absent in some parrots, Amazons for example, pigeons and some of the ratites.

Feathers

Feathers are unique to the class Aves (Figure 9.11). They are arranged in a set pattern over the surface of the body, with some tracts of skin being completely devoid of feather follicles. These areas of skin without follicles are known as apterylae, whilst other areas have rows of feather tracts known as pterylae.

There are six types of feathers in most species. These are known as
1. The contour or flight feathers
2. The down feathers
3. The powder feathers
4. The semi-plume feathers
5. The filoplume feathers
6. The bristle feathers

Contour feathers

These form the flight feathers on wings and tail, and the main feathers outlining the body. The flight feathers are subdivided into primaries and secondaries, depending on whether they are derived from the 'hand' or manus (the carpus and digits) of the wing (the primaries) or the ulna or antebrachium of the wing (the secondaries). There are also contour feathers forming the tail, known as the rectrices. (The primaries and secondaries combined are referred to as the remiges.)

The remiges attach directly onto the periosteum of the relevant wing bone and so are deeply attached. In addition they are covered at their bases by smaller feathers on the dorsal aspect of the wing known as covert feathers (Figure 9.12).

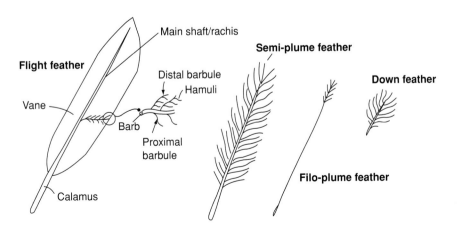

Figure 9.11 Avian plumage.

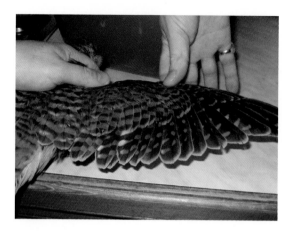

Figure 9.12 Dorsal aspect of a Kestrel's (*Falco tinnunculus*) wing showing the primary, secondary and covert feathers.

The structure of the contour feather is the classical quill shape. It is supported by the main shaft of the feather which is embedded in the follicle. The part of the shaft to which the vane of the feather is attached is known as the rachis. The vane is formed from parallel side branches set at 45° to the rachis, which are known as barbs. From the barbs arise distal and proximal barbules, each of which has its own smaller hooks known as hamuli. These form interconnections with other barbules, and this allows the feather to form a solid but ultra-light structure.

The part of the shaft which is devoid of the feather vane is known as the calamus. This is the part which is inserted into the follicle and which, in the immature growing feather, is filled with nerves and blood vessels. This is known as the feather pulp. It is this area which, when emerging through the skin, is at risk of being damaged by the bird. It can then bleed profusely, giving the young feather its alternative name of 'blood feather'.

Down feathers

The down feathers provide an insulating layer below the contour feathers of the adult bird. They are also the main feather of the chick. They are much shorter in length than the contour feathers and have a 'fluffy' look, as there are no barbules to interlock the vane structure.

Powder feathers

As their name suggests, the powder feathers produce a fine white powder which is shed over the surface of the bird. This appears to act as a semi-waterproof covering. Some species produce more powder than others, African grey parrots and cockatoos, for example. This powder may cause irritation to the airways of species which are

relatively powder-free, such as Amazon parrots. This is a good reason for not mixing these species together in the same aviary or cage.

Many viral and bacterial agents may infect the powder feathers. The infection is then spread when the powder is shed. Examples of these organisms are *Chlamydophila psittaci*, the cause of psittacosis, psittacine beak and feather disease virus (a circovirus), and the gamma herpes virus which causes Marek's disease. Other feather follicles may also be affected.

Semi-plume feathers

The semi-plume feathers have long shafts, but like the down feathers, they have no barbules. This gives them a 'fluffy' appearance. They are situated below the contour feathers and are thought to provide insulation.

Filoplume feathers

The filoplume feathers are situated close to the contour feathers and possess long, fine, bare shafts which end in a clump of barbs. Their roots are surrounded with sensory nerve endings. It is thought that these feathers are responsible for sensing the positions of the adjacent contour feathers. This allows the bird to make accurate alterations of flight and body feather positions.

Bristle feathers

These are similar to the filoplumes in that they have bare shafts with a few barbs at the tip. They are, however, shorter and found around the beak and eyes, and again seem to have a sensory, tactile function.

Blood feathers and pin feathers

The blood feather is the young immature feather as it emerges from the follicle. It is so named because it possesses a plentiful blood supply.

At this stage, the feather is protected by an outer keratin sheath, which gives it its other name of 'pin' feather. As the feather develops inside this sheath, it is surrounded by a blood supply. As the vane forms, the blood supply retracts to the base of the feather below the skin surface. At this point, the sheath should split and allow the feather to unfurl. If the sheath is damaged prior to retraction of the blood supply, then profuse bleeding will occur.

In some birds the sheath is retained long after the blood supply has regressed, and this gives the appearance of multiple, white pin-like structures over the plumage. This can be a sign of general debilitation or of a nutritional deficiency.

Moulting

Moulting occurs in most birds once a year, usually just after the breeding season in the late spring/early summer. Some species will moult more frequently, having a winter and a summer plumage which allows them to blend in with their surroundings. Many eagles and large Psittaciformes kept indoors though will moult every 2 years.

In general the stimulus for moulting seems to be a combination of diurnal rhythms and temperature changes. The new feather forms at the base of the old, and, like a permanent tooth pushing out a deciduous one, it dislodges the existing feather and grows in behind it.

Most species do this gradually, taking several weeks to moult all of the feathers fully. Some though, such as some ducks, become completely flightless due to the loss of all of their flight feathers at once.

Immature birds will often go through three to five rapid moults in their first year or so of life as the initial down feathers give way to more and more contour feathers and adult plumage.

Haematology: an overview

The cells in a bird's bloodstream are significantly different from those in mammals. There are five main differences:

1. The avian erythrocyte is nucleated and oval in shape. This contrasts with the mammalian anucleate, biconcave structure.
2. Heterophils replace the mammalian neutrophil. Their function is similar, as the first line of defence against viral and bacterial infections. Heterophils, however, are a rounded cell with a colourless-to-pale-pink cytoplasm and a multiple-lobed nucleus (averaging two to three lobes). They possess brick red, cigar-shaped-to-oval granules, and during infection these may appear to disintegrate, with the cytoplasm becoming vacuolated or foamy. This effect is useful in assessing the presence of infection, and these cells are referred to as 'toxic' heterophils. Excessive heterophil counts ($>30 \times 10^9$/L) are associated with diseases such as psittacosis, aspergillosis, avian tuberculosis or egg yolk peritonitis.
3. The basophil, lymphocyte and monocyte are basically similar to those in mammals and have broadly the same functions.
4. The eosinophil has a clear blue cytoplasm with a bi-lobed nucleus which stains more intensely than the heterophil. It has round, bright red staining granules. It is more commonly seen in increased numbers in parasitic conditions, such as intestinal ascarid (roundworm) infestations. It may appear more basophilic in some species, such as African grey parrots.
5. The thrombocyte (platelet) is nucleated, unlike the mammalian anucleated form.

Avian blood samples for haematological analysis may be taken into potassium EDTA tubes except in a few species. Examples of these exceptions are members of the crow, crane, flamingo and penguin families in which the erythrocytes will haemolyse. In these species heparin should be used for haematology. A fresh smear for the differential white cell count should also be made. This is because heparin samples yield inferior staining results.

Blood sampling for biochemistry testing in avian patients is best performed in heparin anticoagulant tubes.

References

Bennett, R.A. (1994) Neurology. *Avian Medicine: Principles and Application* (eds B.W. Ritchie, G.J. Harrison & L.R. Harrison), 1st edn, pp. 723–747. Wingers Publishing, Lake Worth, FL.

King, A.S. and McLelland, J. (1975) *Outlines of Avian Anatomy*. Bailliere and Tindall, London.

Further reading

Braun, E.J. (1998) Comparative renal function in reptiles, birds and mammals. *Seminars in Avian and Exotic Pet Medicine*, **7**(2), 62–71.

Heard, D.J. (1997) Avian respiratory anatomy and physiology. *Seminars in Avian and Exotic Pet Medicine*, **6**(4), 172–179.

Klasing, K.C. (1999) Avian gastrointestinal anatomy and physiology. *Seminars in Avian and Exotic Pet Medicine*, **8**(2), 42–50.

Ritchie, B., Harrison, G. and Harrison, L. (1994) *Avian Medicine: Principles and Applications*. Wingers Publishing, Lake Worth, FL.

Stormy-Hudelson, K. (1996) A review of mechanisms of avian reproduction and their clinical applications. *Seminars in Avian and Exotic Pet Medicine*, **5**(4), 189–190.

PART II: AVIAN SPECIES

Chapter 10   Avian Housing and Husbandry

Cage requirements for Psittaciformes and Passeriformes

The advice given in the Wildlife and Countryside Act 1981 (as amended in 2000) is that the cage should be sufficiently large enough for the bird to be able to stretch its wings in all three dimensions. This is a bare minimum requirement, and the cage sizes should be as large as is feasibly and financially possible.

Cages to avoid

It is worthwhile avoiding certain cage types:

- 'Hamster' style cages which are wider than they are high. Birds enjoy freedom of movement in a vertical plane and feel more at ease when caged accordingly.
- Tall, narrow cages which prevent lateral flight and movement.
- Cages coated in plastic which may be chewed off, as many plastics contain zinc and other compounds which may be toxic.
- Cages which have a poor metallic finish. Many cages are made of zinc alloys, and if the finish of the wire surface is poor, the zinc may become available to the bird. As parrots in particular use their beaks to manoeuvre themselves around the cage, the tendency is to swallow the zinc dust coating the wire. The zinc builds up in the bird's body over a number of weeks and can lead to kidney and liver damage and, in severe cases, death.
- Cages with very small doors on them, which makes catching the bird difficult.

The preferred construction material for cages for Psittaciformes and Passeriformes is stainless steel. This is non-toxic and easy to keep clean. Unfortunately, stainless steel cages are heavier and can be more expensive to buy.

Cage 'furniture'

Various items are necessary to provide for basic needs and to improve welfare. Consideration should be given to the type and position of perches, food and water bowls, floor coverings and toys.

Perches

Perches should be made of various different diameters, in order to provide exercise for the bird's feet and to prevent pressure sores from forming. The presence of single-diameter sized perches will lead to pressure being applied to the same parts of the bird's feet continuously. This causes reduced blood circulation and results in corns and ulcers. If not corrected, it will ultimately lead to deep foot infections, referred to as bumblefoot. The perches are best made of hardwood branches, such as beech, mahogany, and witch-hazel, which are relatively smooth and non-toxic. It is important to avoid using branches from trees such as ornamental cherries and laburnum, which are found in many gardens, as these are poisonous. If using branches collected from hedgerows, it is important to clean them to prevent contamination and disease transmission from wild birds. They should be cleaned in dilute bleach or an avian-safe disinfectant and then dried before placing them in the cage. Concrete perches should be avoided as some parrots in particular have been known to eat these, causing gastrointestinal problems or mineral over-supplementation leading to kidney problems.

Perches should never be covered with sandpaper. This does not keep their nails short, but does lead to foot abrasions which become seriously infected, resulting in conditions such as bumblefoot.

Perches should be positioned so as not to allow the bird to foul the food and water bowls and should not be stacked on top of one another as this allows any other bird in the cage to defaecate onto the one below!

Food and water bowls

Food and water bowls should not be made of metal alloys as most are galvanised with zinc or have soldered edges, which contain lead. Both lead and zinc are highly toxic to any cage bird. Plastic or ceramic bowls are therefore preferred. Alternatively, single-pressed (i.e. no soldered seams) stainless steel food bowls can be used instead.

Veterinary Nursing of Exotic Pets, Second Edition. Edited by Simon J. Girling. © 2013 John Wiley & Sons, Ltd. Published 2013 by John Wiley & Sons, Ltd.

Floor coverings

Sawdust, shavings and bark chips should be avoided as these are difficult to keep clean and are often consumed by the cage bird. Newspaper, kitchen towel paper, and the sandpaper sold in many pet shops are better options. However, certain ground-dwelling species, such as quail, may benefit from bark chippings as a floor covering because it allows natural foraging activity. Whatever the floor covering used, it should be changed regularly, at least twice-weekly. Newspaper or other paper coverings have the advantage that they are easy to remove, so it is easier to maintain hygiene standards, and the droppings may be observed for any changes from normal.

Toys

Passeriformes, the perching birds such as canaries, finches and mynah birds, are generally less interested in toys, although providing their food in novel forms can lead to a better quality of life. Psittaciformes, on the other hand, are much more intelligent birds. On average the larger parrots have a mentality of the typical 2-year-old human, and so benefit from toys and mental stimulation. Toys offered should of course be safe, attractive, and of a size and number appropriate to the space allowed.

Some toys are harmful and should be avoided. These include the following:

- *Open chain links:* A bird's foot can easily become caught in one of these, particularly if the bird has an identification ring on its leg.
- *Bells with clappers in them:* Birds, particularly parrots, will remove and often swallow these. The clappers are frequently made of a lead alloy, which is potentially dangerous as birds are very susceptible to lead and other heavy metal poisons.
- *Human mirrors:* These have various lead oxides as their backing and so present another source of lead poisoning. Polished, stainless steel mirrors are better.
- *Plastic children's toys:* The plastics are often too soft, and so are easily broken up and swallowed, sometimes leading to gut impaction. Some toys contain zinc, which is toxic.
- *Toxic plants:* Many tropical houseplants, such as spider plants and cheese plants, are poisonous.

Some toys which may be safely offered include:

- Whole vegetables, such as apples, pears, broccoli, beetroot or carrots.
- Pine cones and clean hardwood branches such as beech or mahogany (cockatoos and macaws particularly love to strip bark from these). Edible fruit trees such as apple trees and grape vines may also be used. It is essential that these are well cleaned and have not been sprayed with fertilisers/pesticides/fungicides first!
- Rye grass growing in a shallow dish may be particularly well accepted by smaller Psittaciformes and many Passeriformes, such as canaries.
- Placing favourite food items inside hollowed-out pieces of wood – so the bird has to pick the food out – can keep a bird occupied for hours.
- Thick ropes and closed chains may be used to suspend toys. However, no bird should be left unattended with these as they can easily become entangled.

Positioning of the cage

Correct positioning of the cage is vitally important. Wrong positioning can lead to a permanently stressed bird. Severe illness or even death may result from an incorrectly placed cage.

Birds of the Psittaciformes and Passeriformes families are prey animals rather than predators and are therefore constantly on the look-out for potential predators. If left to their own devices, they will position themselves in such a way as to minimise risk. This means achieving some height (to avoid ground-based predators) and getting themselves into a position where a predator can only approach from one or two sides.

Therefore, some perches should be at eye level to achieve a little height. It is important not to place the bird too far above this as the bird may then start to feel dominant to its owner and may become increasingly difficult to catch. To minimise fear of predator attack, the cage should be placed in a corner of the room, rather than in its centre. For greater security, three of the four sides may be 'blocked off', for example by a wall or with a towel.

The positioning should also allow direct sunlight to fall on the cage for some part of the day, although the bird should not be in direct sunlight continuously as this will lead to heat stress. Day length should mimic that of the bird's native habitat, which often means a 12- to 14-hour day followed by a 10- to 12-hour period of darkness, and cages may be covered to provide the correct number of hours of darkness. Towels are often used to cover the cage, for this purpose, but it is important to ensure that ventilation remains adequate.

Room temperature is also important. Smaller cage birds have a large body surface area in relation to their size and therefore lose heat rapidly. A comfortable room temperature should be maintained day and night for most species. This should be 16–20°C for most commonly kept Psittaciformes and Passeriformes. It is especially important to maintain room temperature for young birds.

The room chosen for the bird is also important. For example, the bird should not be placed in the kitchen. Many birds are potential carriers of zoonotic diseases which are more easily transmitted by close proximity to food preparation areas. In addition, many fumes produced by cooking can be life-threatening to birds. Some of these toxic fumes include:

- Fumes from overheated Teflon®-coated pans. These are lethal to birds within minutes but are completely undetectable to the human sense of smell.
- Fumes from frying fats can cause serious lung oedema and death within minutes.

With no antidote to even mild exposure to these hazards, they must simply be avoided. Supportive therapy will be discussed later on in the book.

Nor should birds be placed in bedrooms because the owner may be exposed to dander and faecal matter. This can cause allergic or anaphylactic reactions and poses a risk of zoonotic diseases which many birds carry. In addition bedrooms are often the coldest rooms in the house and so not suitable for a bird. If a bird is to be housed indoors, choose the living room or assign it a special room of its own.

Outdoor enclosures – aviary flights

One problem that occurs with indoor housing of cage birds is the lack of exposure to the ultraviolet spectrum of the sun's radiation. Ultraviolet light is required for vitamin D synthesis (Figure 10.1). Some evidence also suggests that ultraviolet light exposure is necessary for normal circadian rhythms to be set and to reduce stress and mental health problems which may lead to feather plucking and generalised illness. Specific ultraviolet lamps are now being sold for birds, which are kept indoors. However, it is becoming increasingly common to encourage owners to provide some form of outdoor enclosure for their pet birds for all or part of the year.

Exposure to the changing daylight lengths is required for setting the diurnal and seasonal body clock of the bird. Another advantage of an outdoor enclosure is that it can be made sufficiently large to allow the bird(s) room to fly and exhibit other natural display activities. These outdoor enclosures are often referred to as aviary flights by owners and breeders and may be used to house several members of the same species or even mixed species exhibits.

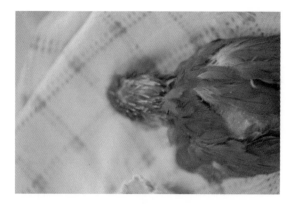

Figure 10.1 Multiple retained feather sheaths may suggest a nutritional disease or environmental problem. The latter may include a lack of exposure to ultraviolet light and low environmental humidity.

Aviary flight construction

Construction

Aviary flights are generally constructed of wood and stainless steel. The flight flooring is made of solid concrete. This is preferable to a soil covering which can allow the build-up of pathogens and can be extremely difficult to clean. The rest of the flight is usually based on four stainless steel mesh sides supported by a hardwood or stainless steel frame. The roof is also of wire mesh, or clear corrugated plastic, and some form of nest box or enclosed roosting area, for breeding and extra protection during bad weather, is provided. Many of these flights are attached to the sides of houses, providing a solid wall to one side and the additional protection that the heat and eaves of the house offer.

Any wire mesh used to form the sides of the aviary flight should ideally be made from stainless steel, rather than a galvanised alloy to avoid the risk of zinc poisoning. The size of the mesh depends on the size of the species kept.

If wood is used, it should preferably be hardwood and must not have been treated with any potentially harmful wood preservatives, such as creosote.

It is sensible to provide a double-door system to gain entry to the aviary flight. Usually one door gives access to a corridor, from which each aviary flight has a door branching off. This helps to minimise the risk of a bird escaping during entering or exiting.

Another potential hazard of outdoor flights is the risk of rodent and wild bird access to the system. This can cause fouling of food and water bowl contents as well as the transmission of diseases. Care should be taken to ensure that the wire mesh is regularly inspected for signs of damage and that the food and water bowls are placed in a part of the cage with a solid roof over them to minimise faecal contamination by wild birds.

Positioning

Protection from the prevailing wind direction is important to prevent chilling. Equally important is to ensure that the nest or roosting box is not in direct sunlight all day. Temperatures will soar during the summer, leading to hyperthermia of adults and chicks alike. It is also useful to provide an area in the flight that protects from wind in the winter and provides shade in the summer. This allows the bird to alter its own microclimate at will, minimising environmental stresses.

Nest box

The nest or roosting box should be large enough to accommodate all birds housed in the flight and should be cleaned out regularly during the non-breeding season. During the breeding season, if breeding pairs are kept, the box should not be disturbed at all to avoid stress and mis-mothering of the eggs or young. It is also important to provide additional nest boxes if multiple pairs of breeding adults are kept together, so as to prevent intra- and inter-species aggression. The nest boxes should be waterproofed and positioned out of the prevailing wind and direct sunlight. They are generally constructed of marine plywood. This can lead to chewing of the boxes by the larger parrot species, and so some breeders coat the inside and outside of the box with stainless steel wire. Care should be taken of the material used for this, and the wire should not have sharp edges which may harm chicks inside the box.

Perches

Within the flight, perches made of hardwood should be provided. These should be of differing diameters, as discussed earlier, and be sufficient to provide all flight occupants with a perch. Food bowls may be clipped to the mesh sides of the flight or placed in an alcove recessed into one of the walls. Food and water bowls should not be placed in the roost or nest boxes, as fouling of the water and fights are much more likely to occur. Again, multiple tiering of perches, especially over food and water bowls, is to be avoided as it may lead to widespread contamination of food and water.

Substrate

If mixed-species aviary flights are used, ground-dwelling species, such as quail, are often included. In these cases some form of flooring substrate is required, with bark chips or peat being the most popular. Care should be taken in these cases to ensure that the flooring is kept very clean and that any Psittaciformes present do not start eating large quantities of substrate.

Raptors
Cage requirements

The cage requirements for raptors are different from those of Psittaciformes and Passeriformes. This is due to both the different environmental requirements of raptors and the reasons for which they are being kept. For example, many trained raptors are kept tethered for much of their lives, although there is a growing trend to keep them loose in an outside aviary system.

It is still necessary though for working raptors to be tethered for 2–4 weeks during their training period. The tethering device is the jess, a leather strap which is attached to each leg via an anklet at the tarsometatarsal area just above the foot. Each jess is the same length and is attached to a metallic swivel that allows rotation. This swivel is then attached to a leash. The leash may then be used to tether the bird to a perch, which is usually positioned close to the ground. It is important to keep the leash relatively short to prevent the bird reaching sufficient flight velocity before the leash becomes taut as this can seriously damage its legs.

Cage or shelter designs

Cages are generally sited outdoors and vary to suit the particular raptor and the presence or absence of tethering.

As with Psittaciformes and Passeriformes, the cage design should provide protection from the weather as well as from rodents and other potential pests and predators.

Tethered raptors

Raptors should only be kept tethered during the summer months as, by the very nature of tethering, the bird cannot move around or achieve shelter and so may die from exposure during the colder months or suffer frostbite.

During the summer months, this form of housing for a tethered raptor is known as a weathering (Figure 10.2). This is a three-sided, solid wooden construction, with a solid roof and open at the front. The perch is placed centrally on a floor covered with sand or gravel. Recommended dimensions for these shelters are 2.5 m × 2.0 m for Falconidae and 3.5 m × 2.5 m for hawks and eagles (Forbes & Parry-Jones, 1996).

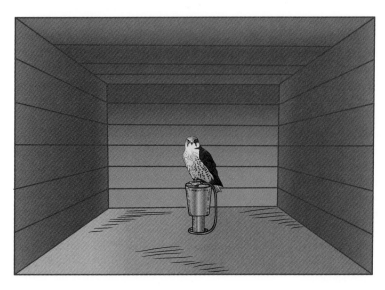

Figure 10.2 Basic layout of a weathering for raptors: a three-sided and roofed building, usually of wood, with a gravel floor and open at the front. The bird is tethered to a perch in the centre.

This form of shelter is prone to two major problems. One is that during the summer, the weathering may become extremely hot, and so adequate shade must be provided to prevent heat stroke. Dehydration may also be a problem as most raptors (particularly Falconidae) obtain their water from their food and will not drink free water. The second problem is the risk of predation due to the open housing and the restrained, low position of the bird.

Aviary flights

These are often built along similar designs to the Psittaciformes and Passeriformes styles already mentioned. There is a major difference, though, in that raptors do not socialise well with other raptors, and so aviaries tend to contain individuals or a breeding pair and no others.

One of the more successful designs is a pattern similar to the weathering, except the front is covered with a wire mesh rather than being open. Roofing materials which have been found to minimise overheating during the summer, but are waterproof, include the compound Eternit®, which is a type of concrete matting (Forbes & Parry-Jones, 1996).

As with the aviary flights already mentioned, it is advisable to have a double-door system so as to avoid escapees. Food is often provided on a feeding block mounted on one side of the aviary, off the ground. It is accessed either directly from inside the aviary or from outside the aviary via an access hatch. Feeding frequency is generally geared to the appetite of the individual bird, but care must be taken as overfeeding non-working raptors with fatty prey such as laboratory rats can lead to atherosclerosis and obesity.

Water should be provided fresh each day, even for those species which do not routinely drink. Many free flight aviaries also provide some form of shallow bathing area, which should be kept scrupulously clean on a daily basis.

The floor should be of solid concrete, with excellent drainage to minimise the build-up of potential pathogens.

Perches

These depend on whether the bird is tethered or free flying. In tethered situations there are two types of perches (Figure 10.3).

The first is the block perch, which is mainly used for falcons. As its name suggests, it comprises a block of flat wood, mounted on a short pole (usually 30–60 cm long). The block is often padded with a material such as Astroturf® to provide cushioning for the feet. This is to prevent bumblefoot or deep-seated foot infections. Raptors, particularly falcons, will remain motionless on block perches for hours at a time, putting continuous pressure on the same parts of the sole of the feet. This causes reduced blood supply and necrosis of small areas of skin which may become secondarily infected leading to infection (bumblefoot – see Figure 10.4).

The second type of perch for tethered raptors is the bow perch. This is a curved rod, usually of tubular iron or steel with padding wound around the highest point of the curve for the bird to grasp. This is the commonest perch offered to the larger raptors such as hawks and eagles.

In both cases the length of the leash should not be so long as to allow the bird sufficient speed off the perch to

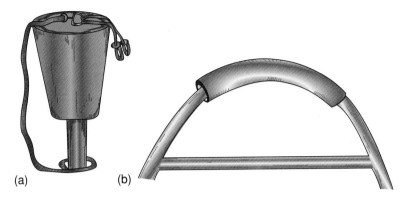

Figure 10.3 (a) A block perch for falcons, with tether, metal swivel and jesses. **(b)** A bow perch for hawks with padding to prevent bumblefoot.

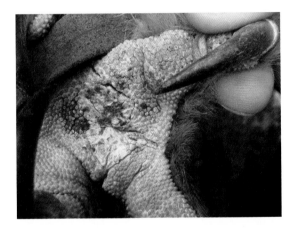

Figure 10.4 Bumblefoot in an Eagle owl (*Bubo bubo*).

be violently jerked backwards when it becomes taut but neither should it be so short that if the bird should lose its footing, it becomes suspended in mid-air by its legs.

Hacking boxes

These are carry boxes to move birds of prey around from place to place. They are a simple box design, often made of wood or plastic, with a perch and a front opening door. The raptor is placed into the box, and a leash and swivel are attached to its jesses which then exits the box so the falconer can control the bird by grasping this leash before the door is opened (see Figure 10.5).

Columbiformes

Shelter requirements

There is a huge variation in the forms of housing offered to doves and pigeons in the United Kingdom. To a large extent, it depends on the reason for which the bird is being kept. Ornamental doves and pigeons are often kept

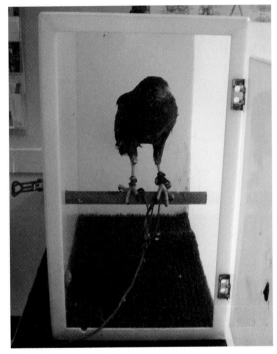

Figure 10.5 A hacking box containing a Harris hawk (*Parabuteo unicinctus*). Note the leash attached to the jesses that trails outside the box and the Astroturf® covering the floor of the box.

in dovecotes or dove lofts, many of which are hundreds of years old. Conversely the more athletic racing pigeons are housed mostly in lofts specifically designed for the purpose and divided into breeding quarters, roosting areas and traps for racing.

Racing pigeons

A loft design will depend largely on the individual owner's preference and space available. It is recommended that the minimum space requirement in the loft area be 0.25 m² per bird with head room of around 2 m for the younger stock. This requirement should be doubled for adult individuals (Harper, 1996).

The provision of wooden doweling perches is standard. It is recommended that 20–25% more perching space than there are birds be provided to avoid overcrowding stresses (Harper, 1996). The perches should be arranged side by side rather than stacked vertically. This is because, as with all birds, the dominant individuals take the highest perches leading to soiling of birds below.

Within the loft system, an owner may house his or her pigeons in several different ways.

Racing loft – natural loft system: In the natural loft system, both male and female pigeons are housed together during the reproductive season. Each pair has its own nest box and perch but can mix with the other pairs in a communal area. As its name suggests, this system is the most natural, but it may be more stressful for the birds, demanding that they race and rear their young at the same time.

Racing loft – widowhood loft system: The widowhood loft houses only the males. The hen birds are housed in an adjacent loft, and this provides an additional incentive for the males to race back! To reduce fighting, it is necessary to provide more room per bird, and each bird often has a double-sized nest box as well as individual feeding stations. The racing season in the United Kingdom is from April to July for the older birds and July to September for the younger ones. The females are allowed into the widowhood loft just before the males to allow rearing of a single chick. After this the hens are removed and the males fed to fitness for racing.

Young loft: The young loft is used to house that year's young and so will have differing populations of pigeons throughout the year. Depending on the breeding success of the year, overcrowding can occur and the diseases and stress that go with it.

Anseriformes
Shelter requirements

The Anseriformes order is a large one but there is a common requirement for all the species and that is the need for open water. The form in which it is presented, however, depends on the species. The swan family will benefit from deeper water in which they can swim and dabble than the duck family.

The type of species kept also determines the nature of the enclosure. For example, geese enjoy areas of open grassland to graze. However, they are inclined to turn grass around a pond into a mud-bath. This can lead to the rapid spread of pathogens, such as avian tuberculosis (*Mycobacterium avium*). Because of this, many waterfowl keepers will concrete the edges of ponds or place obstacles around them to prevent such damage occurring.

Other factors must be taken into account when providing ponds. One is the high incidence of bumblefoot or pedal dermatitis and abscessation, which is made worse if the standing surfaces surrounding the pond are rough and muddy. A smooth concrete finish is therefore preferred.

Any pond should also contain an island at its centre. This is useful to encourage nesting, as waterfowl feel more secure from predation on such islands.

Maintenance of water quality

Maintaining good water quality can be one of the most difficult aspects of keeping waterfowl. With large stocking densities or with muddied margins to the water area, the water itself can be rapidly turned into a murky breeding ground for bacteria and parasites. It is important to prevent stagnation of the water, which means the standing water must move out of the pond, to be replaced by fresh water. Ideally this should be achieved by using natural resources such as local streams, but in some cases water has to be piped in and out to achieve it.

Other methods of water purification include the planting of certain marginal bog plants, which can also provide cover for waterfowl and enhance the look of a pond. A specific reed type (*Phragmites australis*) has been used for this.

Mixing species

Many waterfowl keepers will wish to keep several different species together. There are some species which cannot be kept in the same water. Examples include mixing freshwater species and salt-water species. Salt-water birds can be kept on freshwater, but they do need very deep water levels to enable them to dive properly.

Other combinations to avoid include:
- Mixing together more than one pair of trumpeter swans
- Mixing of Hawaiian geese with Canada geese
- Mixing of a pair of Bewick's swans with a pair of whistling swans (Forbes & Richardson, 1996).

It is generally advisable to keep any swan or shelduck as a single pair on smaller ponds as multiple pairs will always fight in the nesting season.

Other considerations

One of the main concerns of any waterfowl keeper is the loss of birds to wild predators, such as foxes, cats, weasels, stoats and mink. The provision of an island in the centre of an expanse of water is one of the most useful preventive measures. Other measures include the erection of fox-proof fencing or the setting of live traps for mink, weasels and stoats. It is worthwhile noting that if non-native species of birds are allowed to escape, the owner could be in contravention of the Wildlife and Countryside Act 1981, which expressly forbids the release of non-native species into the wild in the United Kingdom.

Quarantine

Birds are highly susceptible to viral diseases, and many small Psittaciformes may carry *Chlamydophila psittaci* without showing clinical signs. For this reason it is important to consider quarantining any new bird addition before adding it to your collection. Periods of quarantine suggested have varied from 4 weeks to 6 months. Testing for important diseases where possible should be undertaken within this period.

The new bird(s) should be housed preferably not only in a separate cage/aviary but in a separate air space as many diseases such as psittacosis and Bornaviruses may spread through the aerosol route. Separate utensils should be used, and the quarantined birds should be cleaned out and fed last to avoid cross-contamination. Disinfection is important to avoid potential spread of diseases. Typical disinfectants suitable for birds include quaternary ammonium compound based products, such as Ark-Klens® (Vetark Professional Ltd) and F10® (Health and Hygiene Pty) as well as sulphur-based compounds such as Virkon-S® (Dupont Animal Health).

Hospitalised birds

The guidelines given above should be applied as much as possible for any hospitalised bird. Raptors may be brought in on their mobile block or bow perch and tethered inside a standard veterinary kennel unit which is sufficiently large enough to allow them to stretch their wings in all three dimensions. Parrot minimum cage sizes should be similarly assessed, but often they can be housed in their own cages within the veterinary practice to maintain some degree of familiarity. For longer periods of treatment, larger spaces should be provided to encourage exercise.

It is important to site birds away from areas of noise and from potential predators (e.g. cats), which may stress the patient. If the bird is feather plucking, then every attempt to maintain environmental temperatures above 20°C should be made to avoid chilling. Dimming lights may also help reduce stress as may providing some low-level background noise such as a radio – particularly for prey species such as Psittaciformes and Passeriformes.

Waterfowl may be kept out of water for a few days, but if longer periods are anticipated then attempts should be made to provide water for swimming and to encourage preening and dabbling behaviour.

It is vitally important that any practice-owned bird cage is cleansed thoroughly between patients to avoid spread of diseases. The use of povidone iodine based cleansing agents such as Tamodine-E (Vetark Professional Ltd) or quaternary ammonium compounds such as F10® (Health and Hygiene Pty) or sulphur compounds such as Virkon-S® (Dupont Animal Health) should be considered.

References

Forbes, N.A. and Parry-Jones, J. (1996) Management and husbandry (raptors). *Manual of Raptors, Pigeons and Waterfowl* (eds P.H. Benyon, N.A. Forbes & N.H. Harcourt-Brown), pp. 116–128. BSAVA, Cheltenham, UK.

Forbes, N.A. and Richardson, T. (1996) Husbandry and nutrition (waterfowl). *Manual of Raptors, Pigeons and Waterfowl* (eds P.H. Benyon, N.A. Forbes & N.H. Harcourt-Brown), pp. 289–298. BSAVA, Cheltenham, UK.

Harper, F.D.W. (1996) Husbandry and nutrition (pigeons). *Manual of Raptors, Pigeons and Waterfowl* (eds P.H. Benyon, N.A. Forbes & N.H. Harcourt-Brown), pp. 233–236. BSAVA, Cheltenham, UK.

Further reading

Chitty, J.C. and Harcourt-Brown, N. (2005) *Manual of Psittacine Birds*, 2nd edn. BSAVA, Quedgeley, UK.

Chitty, J.C. and Lierz, M. (2008) *Manual of Raptors, Pigeons and Passerine Birds*. BSAVA, Quedgeley, UK.

Handling the avian patient

Is there a need to restrain the avian patient?

This may seem a basic point, but it is sometimes necessary to be sure that restraint is required. A decision on whether the bird in question is safe to restrain has to be made.

Points which need to be considered include

- Is the bird in respiratory distress, and is the stress of handling going to exacerbate this?
- Is the bird easily accessible, allowing quick, stress-free and safe capture?
- Does the bird require medication via the oral or injectable route, or can it be medicated via nebulisation, food or drinking water?
- Does the bird require an in-depth physical examination at close quarters, or is cage observation enough?

If the decision is reached that restraint is necessary, it should be remembered that many avian patients are highly stressed individuals, so any restraint should involve minimal periods of handling and captivity.

Techniques useful in handling avian patients

The majority of avian patients seen in practice (with the exception of the owl family, Strigiformes) are diurnal, so reduced or dimmed lighting usually has a calming effect. This can be used to the handler's advantage when catching a flighty or stressed bird.

In the case of Passeriformes and Psittaciformes, turning down the room lights or drawing the curtains or blinds in order to dim the room is enough. For birds of prey, there may well be access to the practice's or the bird's own hoods. These are leather caps which slot over the head and draw tight around the neck, leaving the beak free but completely covering the eyes. They are used to calm some raptors when on the wrist or during handling or transporting.

It is also advisable to keep noise levels down when handling avian patients as their sense of hearing is their next best sense after sight. With these two factors borne in mind, stress and time for capture can be greatly reduced.

Prior to approaching the capture of the avian patient, all items of cage furniture or other obstacles, such as toys, water bowls, food bowls, perches, should be removed from the cage or box. This helps to avoid self-trauma and reduces the time needed to capture the patient.

Once you have made these initial arrangements, you can then confidently approach the avian patient.

Equipment used in avian handling

Birds of prey

Leather gauntlets are a must for restraint of all birds of prey as their talons, and the power of the grasp of each foot, can be extremely strong. The feet of birds of prey and not the beak (unless dealing with the larger eagles where the beak is also a formidable weapon) represent the major danger to the handler. It is important to note that when the bird of prey is positioned on the gauntleted hand the wrist of this hand (traditionally the left hand in European falconers) is kept above the height of the elbow. If not, the bird has a tendency to walk up the arm of the handler with potentially serious and painful results! The type of gauntlet should be either a specific falconer's gauntlet or one of the heavy-duty leather pruning gauntlets available from garden centres. The larger the bird of prey generally the larger and thicker the gauntlet required. To handle a bird of prey, the following steps should be taken:

- First, place the gauntleted hand into the cage or box or beside the bird's perch.
- Grasp the jesses (these are the leather straps which are attached to the anklets) with the thumb and forefinger of the gauntleted hand and encourage the bird to step up onto the glove. Most birds prefer to step up, so always position your hand slightly above the perch.
- Once the bird is on the hand, retain hold of the jesses between thumb and forefinger close to the bird's leg and loop the end of the jesses through the third and fourth fingers. In birds where a hood can be used, such as many of the falcons, then slip the hood over the bird's head.

Veterinary Nursing of Exotic Pets, Second Edition. Edited by Simon J. Girling. © 2013 John Wiley & Sons, Ltd. Published 2013 by John Wiley & Sons, Ltd.

The bird of prey may then be safely examined 'on the hand' and frequently is docile enough to allow manipulation of wings and beak, for small injections to be administered or for oral dosing.

If the bird of prey does not have jesses on but is trained to perch on the hand, it may well step up onto the gauntlet of its own accord. If not, then it is advisable to have the room darkened for Falconiformes. Alternatively, a blue or red light source could be used. This allows the handler to see the bird but prevents the bird of prey seeing normally as their sight is limited in these light spectra.

You must then 'cast' the bird by grasping it from behind, ensuring that you are aware of where its head and feet are.

In order to cast the bird of prey for a closer examination, the bird may be approached once on the fist by a second handler from behind with a thick towel, ensuring that you are aware of where the bird's head is. The towel is draped over the wings and the hands are quickly slipped down to grasp the legs just above the feet to prevent the bird footing (grasping) either itself or you. The bird's dorsum may then be brought against the handler's ventrum and another person can then examine the bird more closely. It is vitally important that the handler keeps the feet separate to prevent the raptor from grasping one foot with its other foot, thus avoiding puncture wounds and infection which can have serious consequences. If the raptor is loose in its aviary, then it is advisable to use nets and towels.

Finally, it is important to remember that the majority of birds of prey are regularly flown, so it is vital to preserve the integrity of their flight and tail feathers. A falconer may not thank you for saving his or her bird's life if they then cannot fly that bird until after the feathers have been replaced at the next moult – usually the following autumn.

Parrots and other cage birds

All of these birds will benefit from the use of subdued or blue or red light to calm the bird and to allow it to be restrained with minimal fuss.

Psittaciformes' main weapon is its beak and powerful bite. (The hyacinth macaw, the largest in the family, can easily crack the largest Brazil nuts, and so even sever a finger.)

Passeriformes' main weapon may be its beak, although this is less damaging as a biting weapon. It may still be a sharp stabbing weapon in the case of starlings and mynahs.

Heavy gauntlets are not recommended for restraint of either family group as they do not allow for accurate judgement of grip on the patient. Instead, dish or bath towels for the larger species and paper towels for the smaller ones are advised. These provide some protection

from being bitten without masking the true strength of the handler's grasp. This is very important because birds do not have a diaphragm and so rely solely on the outward movement of their ribcage for inspiration. Restriction of this with too tight a grip can be fatal.

Before attempting to restrain the patient, its cage should be cleared of all obstacles which may hinder capture or result in injury of the patient. The towel and hand are then introduced into the cage, and the bird is firmly but gently grasped from behind. First grasp the head. Position the thumb and forefinger beneath the lower beak, pushing it upwards and preventing the bird from biting. Then use the rest of the towel to wrap around the bird, gently restraining its wing movements. This will avoid excessive struggling and wing trauma (Figure 11.1). The patient may then be cocooned in the towel with the head still held extended from behind through the towel and the rest loosely wrapped around the bird's body. Individual limbs may then be drawn from the towel one at a time for examination, or the body accessed for medicating.

The towel technique is also better than gloves alone because the towel presents a larger surface area for the bird to try to evade. The bird is then less likely to try to bolt for freedom, whereas a bare hand is a much smaller target and encourages escape attempts.

For smaller cage birds, a piece of paper towel may be used and the bird transferred to a latex gloved hand.

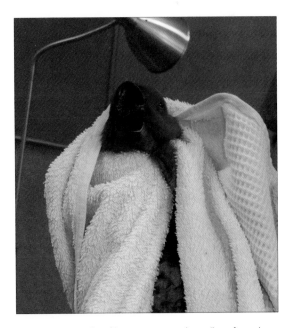

Figure 11.1 Restraint of larger parrots may be easily performed with a towel.

PART II: AVIAN SPECIES

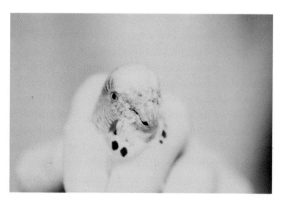

Figure 11.2 Smaller Psittaciformes such as this budgerigar (*Melopsittacus undulatus*) may be restrained with one hand. Note the scaly beak infection.

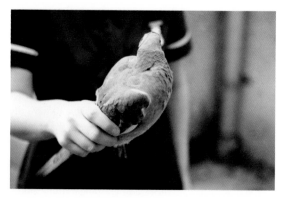

Figure 11.3 Restraint of a pigeon.

The neck of the bird should be held between the index and middle fingers. You can then use your thumb and forefinger to manipulate the legs or wings. The rest of the hand should gently cup the bird's body to discourage struggling (Figure 11.2). It is still necessary to be cautious with this approach to prevent over-constraining the patient as this could cause physical harm.

In the case of particularly aggressive parrots, which are very difficult to handle, leather gauntlets may be used. Extreme care should be exercised as too strong a grasp around the bird's body could prove fatal.

Other avian species

Toucans and hornbills: These have an extremely impressive beak, with a serrated edge to the upper bill. Providing the head is initially controlled using the towel technique previously described for parrots, an elastic band or tape may be fastened around the bill to prevent biting. The handler still needs to be careful of stabbing manoeuvres, and it is a good idea to work with a second handler who is solely responsible for containing the beak. Otherwise, restraint is the same as for the Passeriformes.

Columbiformes: These are restrained in a manner similar to the Psittaciformes (Figure 11.3). The following approach may be used, with the bird's wings and feet cupped in one hand from the dorsum, while resting the sternum in the other hand.

Waterfowl: Restraint of these species is relatively straightforward but may become hazardous with the larger swan and goose family. The first priority is capturing the head. This can be done by grasping the waterfowl around the upper neck from behind. It is important to ensure that the

handler's fingers curl around the neck and under the bill, while the thumb supports the back of the neck and the potentially weak area of the atlanto-occipital joint. Failing this, a swan's or shepherd's crook, or other smooth metal, or a wooden pole with a hook attached, can be used to catch the neck – again high up under the bill. Care should be exercised with these 'swan hooks' as overzealous handling can lead to neck trauma.

Having restrained the head and beak, it is essential that you control the powerful wings by using a towel, thrown or draped over the patient's back and loosely wrapped under the sternum. Many institutions have access to more specialised goose or swan cradle bags which wrap around the body, containing the wings but allowing the feet, head and neck to remain free.

The waterfowl may now be safely carried or restrained by tucking its body (contained within the towel or restraint bag) under one arm and holding this close to the torso. With the other hand, the handler may hold the neck loosely from behind, just below the beak.

Capturing escaped avian patients

Where a bird is loose, a number of methods can be used to capture it. Darkening the room and reducing its area, if possible, are both helpful to calm and confine the bird.

In the case of larger parrots, the use of a heavy bath towel thrown over the bird can confine it long enough to allow the handler to restrain the head from behind and then wrap the patient in the towel.

For very small birds, a fine aviary or butterfly net is extremely useful to catch the bird safely either in mid-flight or against the side of the cage or room. The mesh should be fine enough to ensure that no limbs or feathers will become entangled within it. The mesh is best made of a dark or black material to restrict light and calm the bird.

It is important to ensure that the patient is rapidly transferred from the net into the handler's hands or a container as this is the most stressful period of the capture, and the inability to see whether the patient is in respiratory distress can lead to fatalities.

To recapture escaped raptors, a lure, baited with prey, can be used. Most raptors will remain within the area of their release for several days, and many captive-reared birds will not be able to kill prey for themselves. They will then become hungry and will often look for their handler to offer prey, either on the glove, if they are trained birds, or within the vicinity of their cage, if they are non-trained exhibit or breeding birds. Patience and persistence are two essential virtues when trying to recapture escaped raptors!

Aspects of chemical restraint
Assessment of the patient's status

All methods of chemical restraint require that the patient is first restrained manually, even though it may be for a short period, while the medication is being administered. The aim is to keep the period of manual restraint to a minimum, in order to reduce stress.

Before any form of chemical immobilisation can be used, an assessment of the patient's status must be made. The following points need to be considered:

- Is the procedure to be performed necessary for life-saving medication or treatment, or can it be postponed if the patient's health is sub-optimal?
- Is the patient's condition likely to be worsened by the anaesthetic drugs used?

Implications of avian respiratory anatomy and physiology

There are three main differences between avian and mammalian anatomy and physiology, which are important when considering restraint:

1. Absence of a complete larynx. The bird does have a glottis, but there are no vocal cords or epiglottis to worry about on intubation. The majority of the vocal sounds a bird makes come from the syrinx, which lies at the bifurcation of the trachea into the bronchi.
2. Presence of complete cartilaginous rings supporting the trachea. This is important for two reasons.
   - It is difficult to suffocate the bird by constricting the neck.
   - There is no 'give' to the trachea, and so inflatable cuffs on endotracheal tubes should not, if at all

possible, be inflated as this will cause pressure necrosis in the lining of the trachea. In some cases, such as when flushing out the crop or proventriculus of the bird to remove foreign bodies, it may be necessary to inflate the cuff in order to prevent inhalation pneumonia. This must be performed with great care.
3. Avian lungs are semi-rigid structures. It is the air sac system that is responsible for the movement of air through the lungs, in combination with the lateral movement of the chest wall. Therefore, if there is any form of restriction to the outward movement of chest and keel, ventilation will be reduced, leading to hypoxia.

Pre-anaesthetic preparation
Blood testing

It may be advisable to run biochemistry and haematology tests on avian patients prior to administering anaesthetics, particularly in older and obviously unwell individuals. Blood may be taken from the following vessels:

- The right jugular vein in nearly all species (it is significantly larger than the left) (see Figure 11.4).
- In the larger species the brachial vein, which runs cranially on the ventral aspect of the humerus (see Figure 11.5).
- In many waterfowl, long-legged birds and raptors, the medial metatarsal vein, which runs, as its name suggests, along the medial aspect of the metatarsal area (see Figure 11.6).

Fasting

Because of the high metabolic rate of avian patients, extended fasting may be detrimental to their health and their ability to recover from anaesthesia. This is because

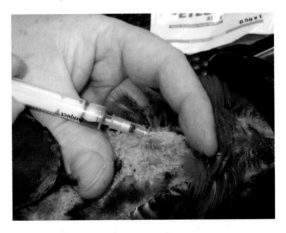

Figure 11.4 The right jugular vein is the largest accessible vein in most birds.

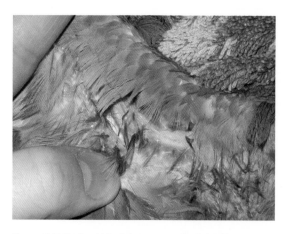

Figure 11.5 The brachial vein is easy to see but is fragile and 'blows' easily.

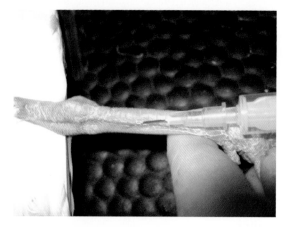

Figure 11.6 The medial metatarsal vein is easy to access in waterfowl and long-legged birds.

hepatic glycogen stores, which provide the most rapid form of stored energy, can be quickly depleted. Birds larger than 300 g bodyweight, which have larger glycogen stress, are slightly less likely to become hypoglycaemic with fasting.

The purpose of fasting is to ensure emptying of the crop. Fasting prevents passive reflux of fluid or food material during the anaesthetic which may then be inhaled, obstructing the airway or causing pneumonia.

Ideally, most birds are fasted between 1 and 3 hours depending on their body size. The smallest have the shortest period of fasting, often amounting to just 1–2 hours at most. Birds weighing over 300 g may be able to tolerate an overnight fast of 8–10 hours, assuming good health and body condition, and this may be necessary particularly if surgery on the gastrointestinal system or crop is intended. Whatever the period of fasting, water should only be withheld for 1 hour prior to anaesthesia.

Pre-anaesthetic medications

Pre-anaesthetic medications are infrequently used in birds. Of those used, fluid therapy is the most important. Whether it is crystalloid or colloid, pre-, intra- and post-operative fluids can make the difference between successful surgery and failure. Fluid therapy is covered in more detail in Chapter 14.

Antimuscarinic premedicants

Atropine and glycopyrrolate have been used as pre-anaesthetic medicants to reduce vagally induced brady-cardia and oral secretions which may block endotracheal tubes. They both, however, may have unwanted side effects. The two main side effects are

- Causing unacceptably high heart rates, increasing myocardial oxygen demand and so increasing the risk of cardiac hypoxia and arrest.
- Making oral or respiratory secretions so thick and tenacious that they make endotracheal tube blockage even more likely.

Benzodiazepine premedicants

Diazepam or midazolam may be used in waterfowl as these species may exhibit periods of apnoea during mask induction of anaesthesia. This is a stress response (often referred to slightly inaccurately as a 'diving response') mediated by the trigeminal receptors in the beak and nares. When this response is triggered, the breath is held and the blood flow is preferentially diverted to the kidneys, heart and brain.

Induction of anaesthesia

Anaesthesia may be induced with two main categories of drugs: injectable anaesthetics and inhalational anaesthetics.

Injectable agents

Advantages of injectable anaesthetics include

- Ease of administration (most birds have a good pectoral muscle mass for intramuscular injections)
- Rapid induction
- Low cost
- Good availability

Disadvantages include

- Recovery is often dependent on organ metabolism.
- Reversal of medications in emergency situations is potentially difficult.
- Prolonged and sometimes traumatic recovery periods may ensue.

- Muscle necrosis at injection sites and lack of adequate muscle relaxation may occur with some medications.

The following are some of the injectable anaesthetics more commonly used in avian practice.

Ketamine and ketamine combination anaesthesia: When used alone, ketamine produces inadequate anaesthesia and recoveries are often traumatic, with the patient flapping wildly. Doses of 20–50 mg/kg are quoted (Forbes & Lawton, 1996). However, combining it with the benzodiazepines, diazepam (0.5–2 mg/kg) or midazolam (0.2 mg/kg) (Curro, 1998) helps with muscle relaxation and sedation, reduces flapping on recovery and allows the dose of ketamine to be reduced to around 10–20 mg/kg.

Ketamine may also be combined with xylazine (1–2.2 mg/kg) (Forbes & Lawton, 1996) or medetomidine (60–85 mg/kg) (Forbes & Lawton, 1996). This improves recovery, sedation and analgesia and again allows reduction of the ketamine dosage to 10–20 mg/kg depending on the species and procedure. The medetomidine may be reversed with atipamezole (the same volume as medetomidine is given). However, the alpha-2 drugs such as medetomidine have severe cardiopulmonary depressive effects and may compromise blood flow to the kidneys, risking renal damage. Sun-conures have been noted to be particularly intolerant of ketamine–alpha-2 combinations (Rosskopf *et al.*, 1989).

The combined medications are usually given intramuscularly. Induction will take on average 5–10 minutes, but complete recovery may take 2–4 hours or more and is dose dependent.

It is also worth noting that ketamine is actively excreted from the proximal tubule of the kidneys, and so any kidney damage can lead to a prolonged recovery when using this drug.

Propofol: Propofol is given intravenously, preferably via a jugular, medial metatarsal or brachial vein catheter. It produces profound apnoea and is rarely used as an induction or anaesthetic agent in birds.

Inhalation agents

Nitrous oxide: This is rarely used in avian anaesthesia. It has good analgesic properties, but accumulates in large, hollow organs. There is some thought that it may therefore accumulate in the air sacs and may considerably prolong anaesthetic recovery times. Recent evidence disputes this, but it cannot be used on its own for anaesthesia. It must be used in combination with halothane or isoflurane to allow a surgical plane of anaesthesia to be reached.

Isoflurane: Isoflurane is the anaesthetic of choice for the avian patient. It is also licensed for use in avian species in the United Kingdom. Induction may be achieved by face mask at 4–5% concentration, reducing to 1.25–2% for maintenance, preferably via endotracheal tubing inserted into the trachea or an air sac. If using a mask for maintenance, an increase in gas concentration of 25–30% is required.

Advantages of isoflurane include

- Low blood solubility and minimal metabolism of the drug by the bird (<0.2%). This means that the drug does not accumulate in the bloodstream and is rapidly excreted by the patient, allowing rapid changes in anaesthetic depth.
- Minimal cardiopulmonary effects at sedative or light anaesthesia levels.
- Little or no tendency to cause cardiac arrhythmia.
- Unlike halothane, isoflurane does not require metabolism in the liver, making it suitable for sick avian cases.
- Cardiovascular arrest does not occur at the same time as respiratory arrest, allowing time for resuscitation.
- Isoflurane has a minimum alveolar concentration (MAC) (i.e. the concentration that produces no response in 50% of cases exposed to a noxious stimulus) of 1.44% in cockatoos (Curro *et al.*, 1994).

Sevoflurane: Like isoflurane, it requires little or no organ metabolism and is very safe. Slightly higher percentages are required to induce and maintain the patient, but low blood solubility does allow rapid changes in anaesthesia levels (Greenacre, 1997). It also depresses plasma ionised calcium levels significantly, and so care should be taken when using in African Grey parrots which are prone to hypocalcaemia.

Maintenance of anaesthesia

For prolonged anaesthetic procedures, gaseous maintenance is required. Isoflurane and sevoflurane are currently the agents of choice.

For avian patients larger than 100 g, it is advisable to intubate the bird for more effective control of rate and depth of anaesthesia. Its respiratory depressive effects are also dose dependent. This means that with prolonged procedures, the patient may become apnoeic and require either manual or positive pressure ventilation. This can be more of a risk with some species, such as the African grey parrot, than with others.

Endotracheal intubation

The beak must be held open by using an avian gag or by attaching short lengths of bandage to the upper and lower beaks. One handler can then use them to hold the beak open, while a second intubates the bird (see Figure 11.7). The glottis will be easily visible at the base of the tongue, in the midline. Intubation can be made easier if the tongue is grasped with atraumatic forceps, enabling it and the glottis to be pulled forward. Sizes of tube vary but would be typically a 3–3.5 F for a Grey parrot and up to a 4–5 F for a larger Macaw. The smaller tubes will block more easily with respiratory secretions, and the use of parasympatholytics does not stop this. Indications of tube blockage include apnoea and initially increased expiratory phase of respiration. Such cases should be extubated and the tube checked for mucus plugs.

It is better not to inflate the cuff on endotracheal tubes because of the risk of causing severe damage to the lining of the rigid avian trachea. It is therefore essential to use a well-fitting tube. If positive pressure is required, the very smallest inflation of the cuff may be used – enough to prevent air escaping when ventilated but not enough to traumatise the tracheal rings.

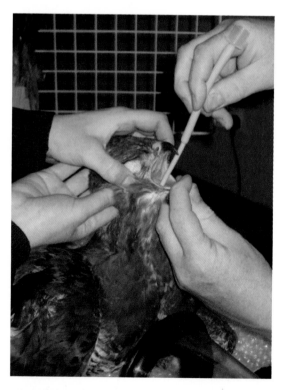

Figure 11.7 Intubation of a Buzzard using a 'Coles' endotracheal tube which is tapered at the tip to make intubation easier.

Anaesthetic circuits

Anaesthetic circuits used must be non-rebreathing and minimise dead space as many avian patients are much smaller than the more routinely seen cats and dogs. Modified Bain circuits or Mapleson C circuits are useful for these reasons. Even the Ayres T-piece may be used for larger parrots and waterfowl. In any instance a 0.25–0.5 L rebreathing bag is frequently necessary.

Air sac catheterisation

In an airway obstruction, or if head or oral surgery is required, it may be necessary to deliver the inhalant gases via a tube placed directly into one of the air sacs. This is possible because many of the avian air sacs are very close to the skin's surface. These structures take no part in gaseous exchange, simply shunting the air back and forth through the rigid lung structure, but, as birds extract oxygen from the air on expiration as well as inspiration, it does not matter which direction the oxygen and gases are introduced into the respiratory system.

Air sacs which may be catheterised include the clavicular air sacs and the abdominal or caudal thoracic air sacs. A small stab incision is made in the skin over the air sac. The underlying muscle is bluntly dissected with a pair of haemostats, and the endotracheal tube may then be inserted to a depth of 4–5 mm and sutured in place. The clavicular air sacs lie at the thoracic inlet, just dorsal to the clavicles. The caudal thoracic air sacs may be entered between the sixth and seventh ribs in Psittaciformes. The abdominal air sacs may be entered by raising the leg cranially so that the femur crosses the last ribs, incising just caudal to the stifle.

Monitoring of anaesthesia

Monitoring of anaesthesia is crucial. The depth of anaesthesia should be adequate enough for the procedure required, while cardiovascular and respiratory parameters should remain constant. The following points should be considered:

- During the initial stages of anaesthesia (stages 1 and 2), the respiratory rate will be shallow and erratic. The patient will be lethargic and have drooping eyelids, a lowered head and ruffled feathers.
- As the depth increases, palpebral, corneal, pedal and cere reflexes will remain, but all voluntary movement ceases.
- As the next stage of anaesthesia (stage 3) is reached, the respiration rate becomes regular, and the depth of breathing is increased. The corneal and pedal reflexes are slow and the palpebral reflex disappears. This is the

light plane of anaesthesia required for minor procedures. The depth at which the pedal reflex is lost but the corneal reflex is retained will allow most surgical procedures to be performed.

• As anaesthesia is allowed to deepen, respiratory rate and tidal volume will continue to decrease, until, if allowed, respiratory arrest will occur. Therefore, monitoring of the rebreathing bag, for rate and depth of respiration, can provide valuable information.

One study indicated that the ideal anaesthetic depth occurred when the patient's eyelids were completely closed, pupils were mydriatic, pupillary light reflex was delayed, corneal reflex resulted in slow movement of the third eyelid across the eye, all muscles were relaxed and all pain reflexes were absent (Korbel et al., 1993).

Equipment used for monitoring anaesthesia

A stethoscope may be used to monitor the heart rate externally, or, during anaesthesia, an oesophageal stethoscope may be inserted.

ECG leads may be attached using adhesive pads or fine needles to the avian skin rather than the more cumbersome and traumatic alligator clips. These leads may be attached to the wing web (propatagium) and the folds of skin connecting the legs to the body wall cranially. The avian ECG differs somewhat from its mammalian counterpart due to a much larger RS wave than Q. Readers are advised to consult standard texts for further information on the ECG trace for avian patients (Lumeij & Richie, 1994; Oglesbee et al., 2001). An example of a lead II normal ECG wave in a bird is shown in Chapter 16.

Respiratory flow monitors can be used if endotracheal tubes are involved, although the very low flow rates of some smaller avian species may not register on machines designed with cats and dogs in mind.

Capnography may be used in birds. Side stream tends to be preferred owing to many patients' small size. An end-tidal CO_2 level of 30–45 mm Hg indicates adequate ventilation in an African Grey Parrot (Edling et al., 2001). The advantage of capnography is that it can then be used to indicate the rate and depth of respiration required when performing IPPV.

Doppler flow recorders can be useful to assess peripheral perfusion and rate and rhythm of pulse. The medial metatarsal vessels (which as their name suggests run up the medial aspect of the lower leg) can be readily used for this technique.

Pulse oximeters may also be used to measure the relative saturation of the haemoglobin with oxygen. Reflector probe attachments are the best and may be used cloacally or orally. However, care should be taken in interpreting results due to the difference in haemoglobin format in birds from mammals, and their main use is in monitoring trends rather than relying on their accuracy in birds. In addition, many birds can be hypercapnic despite being well oxygenated, so monitoring end-tidal CO_2 is suggested as more accurate for assessing avian ventilation (Edling et al., 2001).

Again, it is important to find an oximeter which can read the higher heart rates of even anaesthetised birds as these will be greater than those of cats or dogs. Indeed, no pulse oximeters currently available commercially will read heart rates of birds less than 150 g accurately.

Additional supportive therapy

Recumbency

It is important that the ribcage is unrestricted, otherwise hypoxia will develop. Common positions for surgery include lateral or dorsal recumbency.

Dorsal recumbency may be a problem in larger animals of any species when the larger body organs may press on the lungs. This is exacerbated in birds because of the lack of a diaphragm and presence of thin-walled air sacs. Some really large species also have a problem with ventral recumbency due to the weight of the bird pressing on the keel or sternum. However, the smaller species generally do not suffer as severely from this problem and may be positioned according to need.

Intermittent positive pressure ventilation and resuscitation techniques

If a bird's respiratory rate becomes depressed below 3–4 breaths per minute, then it should be given respiratory assistance. The usual anaesthetic checklist should be checked – flow rates, patency of endotracheal tubing, anaesthetic gas levels, etc., and the emergency ABC (Airway, Breathing, Cardiovascular) protocol initiated if apnoeic. In general, the percentage of anaesthetic gas delivered should be reduced or the anaesthetic ceased during periods of apnoea, and respiratory support started.

If the avian patient is still breathing, even sporadically, then positive pressure ventilation with 100% oxygen should be used at a rate of 2–3 times per minute. This is best done with a mechanical ventilator unit, operating at 10–15 cm of water (see Figure 11.8). If using manual 'bagging' techniques, then the gentlest of touches on the rebreathing bag – enough just to allow the bird's ribcage to rise – should be used. If the bird is

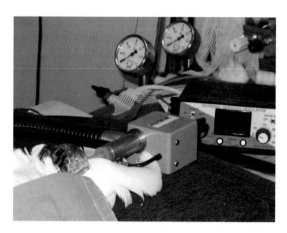

Figure 11.8 A cockatoo attached to a small animal ventilator after intubation.

totally apnoeic, then a rate of 10–15 breaths per minute should be started.

Doxapram may be used orally or by injection to stimulate the central nervous system respiration centres. Doses of 10 mg/kg by injection or 0.5 mg orally are useful.

If the bird is being maintained on a mask rather than being intubated, it is possible to carry out mechanical ventilation by grasping the uppermost wing at the carpus, and gently but firmly moving it in and out at 90° to the chest wall. This will simulate muscular movement of the ribcage and so allow air to move back and forth through the air sacs and lungs. Alternatively, the sternum may be pushed towards the spine. This can also be useful for cardiac massage in cases of cardiac arrest.

Cardiac arrest frequently and rapidly follows apnoea, and it is then extremely difficult to revive an avian patient. Adrenaline may be given at 1000 units/kg body weight – preferably via endotracheal tubing or directly through the glottis into the trachea. Alternatively, it may be administered intravenously via either the right jugular vein or the brachial wing vein, but generally there is a poor success rate.

The likelihood of apnoea occurring depends upon the type of anaesthetic used. Xylazine is notorious as a deep respiratory depressant (Curro, 1998). Isoflurane will also produce respiratory depression in African grey parrots, even at the lowest surgical levels (Forbes & Lawton, 1996).

Maintenance of body temperature

Maintaining the body temperature is important for the successful outcome of any anaesthetic procedure. The large body surface to volume ratio of birds results in loss of body heat at a faster rate than dogs and cats.

Minimising the risk of hypothermia
To minimise hypothermia a series of procedures can be used:

- The surgical field should receive minimal plucking of feathers and minimal soaking with surgical antiseptic solutions. (Avian skin has low levels of bacteria and fungi in comparison to mammals.)
- The patient should be covered with surgical drapes, preferably clear drapes.
- The patient may be placed onto a circulating warm water or hot air blanket.
- Warm water filled latex gloves may be placed close to the patient. These should not be allowed to come into direct contact with the bird, as when too hot they may scald, and as they cool they may actually draw heat away from the patient.

Although it is important to prevent hypothermia, care should also be taken not to induce hyperthermia. During the operation, cloacal temperature can be measured directly. It may be necessary to use an electronic probe as most mercury-based thermometers do not register temperatures as high as the core body temperature of birds.

Fluid therapy and blood transfusions

Healthy, anaesthetised birds should receive replacement fluids at 10 mL/kg/h for the first 2 hours, and then 5–8 mL/kg/h thereafter to prevent overhydration (Curro, 1998).

If blood loss occurs during surgery, then the replacement volume of crystalloid fluid should be three times the blood loss volume. However, if the volume of blood lost is greater than 30% of the normal total blood volume, then a blood transfusion should be considered. Other indicators for blood transfusions are a total plasma protein level below 25 g/L and/or a packed cell volume (PCV) below 15%.

Blood donors should at least be of the same avian family – for instance parrot to parrot, and preferably the same species, for example, one budgerigar to another budgerigar. It is useful to remember that on average one drop of blood is roughly equivalent to 0.05 mL, and that the estimated blood volume of an avian patient is 10% of its body weight in grams. This means, for instance, that a healthy 500 g African grey parrot would have roughly 50 mL of blood circulating in its body. However, it is equally worrying to note that a 40 g budgerigar will only have 4 mL of blood, and thus the loss of 25% of its blood volume will occur with just 20 drops of blood (1 mL).

Routes of administration of fluids will depend on the surgical procedure and the health status of the patient.

Subcutaneous routes are frequently used for healthy birds undergoing minor or routine surgery. Areas that can be used for this purpose include the interscapular area, the axillae, and the fold of inguinal skin which lies cranial to each leg.

For more serious cases, the intraosseous and intravenous routes should be used (see Chapter 14).

Post-operative recovery

Recovery should always involve ventilation with 100% oxygen. The endotracheal tube should be removed once the bird starts to cough or swallow. It is important to note that practically all patients will appear disorientated and will attempt to flap their wings during recovery. Every attempt should be made to constrain them gently (without restricting respiration) to ensure that they do not damage their wings or feathers. This can best be achieved by lightly wrapping them in a towel.

With isoflurane anaesthesia, recovery is complete in 5–10 minutes, and the patient is often then able to perch. However, if ketamine is used, recovery may take much longer – anything up to 3–4 hours. During any recovery the environmental temperature should be kept between 25°C and 30°C to prevent hypothermia developing. It also helps to keep the recovery area quiet and dimly lit to ensure minimal adverse stimulation.

The patient should be encouraged to take food as soon as it is able. This is to minimise the deleterious effects of hypoglycaemia seen in these high metabolic rate species.

Analgesia

Pain assessment in birds

Pain assessment in many birds is difficult as many are prey species and so, like small herbivores, will not demonstrate pain and often become immobile when watched. Feather grooming may cease with mild pain, but will increase and move to feather chewing or plucking with more serious pain. In social species of birds, pain will often result in that individual isolating itself from the group. Others may sleep more and become less interactive with their owners, or become more aggressive or demonstrate inappropriate aggression towards cage mates, owners or handlers.

Analgesics used in birds

Butorphanol: Butorphanol, at a dose of 3–4 mg/kg (Bauck, 1990) or at 1 mg/kg intramuscularly (IM) or 0.02–0.04 mg/kg intravenously (IV), reduced the amount of isoflurane required during anaesthesia (Curro *et al.*, 1994). However, it did not produce the same results in Blue-fronted Amazon parrots, indicating species variability at this dosage. It has been used at 2 mg/kg IM as a single injection in Hispaniolan Amazon Parrots as pre-emptive, pre-operative analgesia, where sevoflurane has been used for endoscopy and shown to be both safe and effective (Klaphke *et al.*, 2006). Butorphanol had less than 10% bioavailability when given orally at 5 mg/kg in Hispaniolan Amazon Parrots, and so the oral route is not recommended (Sanchez-Migallon *et al.*, 2008). Adverse effects such as dysphoria have not been reported in birds. Dosage frequency appears to be as frequent as 2 hours in birds.

Butorphanol does, however, cause some respiratory depression. It also requires metabolism by the liver for excretion. However, these disadvantages are much reduced in comparison with many other opioid analgesics.

Buprenorphine: Work in pigeons has shown predominant kappa opioid receptors in the central nervous system (Mansour *et al.*, 1988). Buprenorphine does not appear to be effective at 0.1 mg/kg in African grey parrots when tested, and it was shown that the drug did not reach plasma levels known to be effective in humans at this dosage (Paul-Murphy *et al.*, 1999, 2004). However, dosages of 0.25–0.5 mg/kg in pigeons increased the latency period for withdrawal from noxious electrical stimuli from 2 to 5 hours (Gaggermeier *et al.*, 2003). It is postulated that birds may not possess distinct mu and kappa receptors or that the two receptors in birds have similar functions.

Opioids do, however, have some respiratory suppression side effects and will require some liver metabolism to excrete, but these are much reduced in comparison with other opioid analgesics.

Nalbuphine hydrochloride: This predominant kappa receptor active opioid (some partial mu activity) was shown to have little respiratory depression, good bioavailability after intramuscular dosage and had little sedative effects, but it did increase threshold values of thermal foot withdrawal in Hispaniolan Amazon parrots for up to 3 hours when dosed at 12.5 mg/kg (Keller *et al.*, 2009). Increased dosage of nalbuphine did not increase analgesia.

NSAIDs: Cyclo-oxygenase (COX) has been demonstrated in chickens (Mathonnet *et al.*, 2001). Therefore, it is assumed that COX receptors are present in other birds. The distribution of COX-1 and COX-2 enzymes varies between species, and both enzymes appear important in pain pathways.

NSAIDs which have been used and shown to have beneficial effects include meloxicam (0.1–1 mg/kg q12–24h). As with all NSAIDs, particular care should be taken with patients with gastrointestinal or renal disease just as you would with mammalian patients. Avian patients, due to their kidney structure, are more sensitive to some of these side effects. The recent mass mortalities due to the use of the NSAID diclofenac acid in Indian white backed vultures, which has seen a 95% population decline, are an example of the potential toxic effects of some NSAIDs in birds. Concurrent fluid therapy is therefore often advised when using NSAIDs, with or without gastrointestinal protectants such as sucralfate and ranitidine. There appears to be a wide variation in dosage within birds for meloxicam with Budgerigars receiving 0.1 mg/kg q24h for 7 days showing signs of glomerular congestion (Pereira & Werther, 2007) and Hispaniolan Amazon parrots showing improved weight bearing on arthritic limb at 1 mg/kg IM q12h (Cole et al., 2009). A pharmacokinetic study carried out by Wilson et al. (2005) suggested 0.5 mg/kg per os q12h was required to maintain serum levels in ring-necked parakeets (*Psittacula krameri*). It is therefore apparent that birds often metabolise NSAIDs rapidly but there is considerable species variation.

Carprofen has also been widely used but its dosage is difficult to elucidate. Extremely high doses (30 mg/kg) had to be administered to provide analgesia in chickens with experimentally induced arthritis (Hocking et al., 2005). In a study in Hispaniolan Amazon parrots, a dose of 3 mg/kg produced an improvement in lameness of an arthritic limb within 2 hours but wore off before the 12-hour dosage interval used in mammals (Paul-Murphy et al., 2009).

It is important to point out, however, that NSAIDs can cause unwanted gastrointestinal and renal side effects, just as is the case in mammalian patients. Because of their kidney structure, avian patients are more sensitive to some of these renal side effects. Concurrent fluid therapy is therefore advised when using NSAIDs, as is the use of gastrointestinal protectants such as sucralfate and cimetidine.

Other analgesics: Tramadol has been used in bald eagles at 11 mg/kg q12h and achieved plasma concentration equivalent to that required in humans for analgesia. Its oral bioavailability in birds is higher than that observed in humans or dogs (mean 97.94%) and its t1/2 in bald eagles was two times that reported in dogs but half as long as that in humans (Souza et al., 2009).

Gabapentin (a gamma-aminobutyric acid analogue) has been used in multimodal analgesia in birds. It is believed to work via N-type calcium ion voltage-gated channels. It was shown to relieve self-mutilation in three studies (Doneley, 2007; Siperstein, 2007; Shaver et al., 2009).

It is worth remembering that drugs such as ketamine and the alpha-2 adrenergic drugs have analgesic properties as well.

Local anaesthesia: Local anaesthetics may be used as ring blocks around amputations to reduce the chances of post-operative self-mutilation. Doses should not exceed 4 mg/kg of lidocaine and should be diluted to at least 1:10.

Bupivicaine has also been used, but there are concerns that its toxic effects take longer to resolve in birds than in mammals. In ducks (*Anas platyrhynchos*) a dose of 2 mg/kg bupivicaine subcutaneously showed a faster uptake versus elimination rate, but evidence of sequestration and redistribution of bupivicaine suggested by increases in plasma concentrations 6 and 12 hours after dosing suggests that toxicity may be delayed (Machin & Livingstone, 2001). Bupivicaine has also been used as intra-articular injections in chickens with osteoarthritis and showed improved analgesia (Hocking et al., 1997) and has been mixed 1:1 with dimethyl sulfoxide and applied to beak amputations in chickens where an increase in feed consumption was observed (Glatz et al., 1992).

References

Bauck, L. (1990) Analgesics in avian medicine. *Proceedings of the Association of Avian Veterinarians*, pp. 239–244.

Cole, G.A., Paul-Murphy, J., Krugner-Higby, L., et al. (2009) Analgesic effects of intramuscular administration of meloxicam in Hispaniolan Amazon parrots (*Amazona ventralis*) with experimentally induced arthritis. *American Journal of Veterinary Research*, **70**, 1471–1476.

Curro, T.G. (1998) Anaesthesia of pet birds. *Seminars in Avian and Exotic Pet Medicine*, **7**(1), 10–21.

Curro, T.G., Brunson, D.B. and Paul-Murphy, J. (1994) Determination of the ED50 of isoflurane and evaluation of the isoflurane-sparing effect of butorphanol in cockatoos (*Cacatua* spp.). *Veterinary Surgery*, **23**, 429–433.

Doneley, B. (2007) The use of gabapentin to treat presumed neuralgia in a little corella (*Cacatua sanguinea*). *Proceedings of the Australian Association of Avian Veterinarians Conference*, pp. 169–172.

Edling, T.M., Degernes, L., Flammer, K. and Horne, W.B. (2001) Capnographic monitoring of African Grey Parrots during positive pressure ventilation. *Journal of the American Veterinary Medical Association*, **219**, 1714–1717.

Forbes, N.A. and Lawton, M.P.C. (1996) Formulary. *Manual of Psittacine Birds* (ed. P.H. Beynon), BSAVA, Cheltenham, UK.

Gaggermeier, B., Henke, J. and Schatzmann, U. (2003) Investigations on analgesia in domestic pigeons (*C. livia*, Gmel., 1789, var dom.) using buprenorphine and butorphanol. *Proceedings of the European Association of Avian Veterinarians*, pp. 70–73.

Glatz, P.C., Murphy, L.B. and Preston, A.P. (1992) Analgesic therapy in beak-trimmed chickens. *Australian Veterinary Journal*, **69**, 18.

Greenacre, C.B. (1997) Comparison of sevoflurane to isoflurane in Psittaciformes. *Proceedings of the Association of Avian Veterinarians*, pp. 123–124.

Hocking, P.M., Gentle, M.J., Bernard, R. and Dunn, L.N. (1997) Evaluation of a protocol for determining the effectiveness of pretreatment with local analgesics for reducing experimentally induced articular pain in domestic fowl. *Research in Veterinary Science*, **63**(3), 263–267.

Hocking, P.M., Robertson, G.W. and Gentle, M.J. (2005) Effects of non-steroidal anti-inflammatory drugs on pain-related behaviour in a model of articular pain in the domestic fowl. *Research in Veterinary Science*, **78**, 69–75.

Keller, D., Sanchez-Migallon, G.D., Klauer, J., *et al.* (2009) Pharmacokinetics of nalbuphine HCL in Hispaniolan Amazon parrots (*Amazona ventralis*). *Proceedings of the American Association of Zoo Veterinarians Conference*, p. 106.

Klaphke, E., Schumacher, J., Greenacre, C., *et al.* (2006) Comparative anesthetic and cardiopulmonary effects of pre-versus postoperative butorphanol administration in Hispaniolan Amazon Parrots (*Amazona ventralis*) anesthetized with sevoflurane. *Journal of Avian Medicine and Surgery*, **20**, 2–7.

Korbel, R., Milovanovic, A., Erhardt, W., *et al.* (1993) Aerosacular perfusion with isoflurane – an anesthetic procedure for head surgery in birds. *Proceedings of the 2nd Annual Conference of the European Association of Avian Veterinarians*, pp. 9–37.

Lumeij, J.T. and Richie, B. (1994) Cardiology. *Avian Medicine: Principles and Applications* (eds B. Richie, G. Harrison & L. Harrison), pp. 697–711. Wingers Publishing, Lake Worth, FL.

Machin, K.L and Livingstone, A. (2001) Plasma bupivicaine levels in mallard ducks (*Anas platyrhynchos*) following a single subcutaneous dose. *Proceedings of the American Association of Zoo Veterinarians Conference*, pp. 159–163.

Mansour, A., Khachaturian, L.M.E., Akil, H. and Watson, S.J. (1988) Anatomy of CNS opioid receptors. *Trends in Neuroscience*, **11**, 301–314.

Mathonnet, M., Lalloue, F., Danty, E., *et al.* (2001) Cyclooxygenase 2 tissue distribution and developmental pattern of expression in the chicken. *Clinical Experimental Pharmacological Physiology*, **28**, 425–432.

Oglesbee, B.L., Hamlin, R.L. and Hartman, S.P. (2001) Electrocardiographic reference values for macaws (*Ara*

species) and cockatoos (*Cacatua* species). *Journal of Avian Medicine and Surgery*, **15**(1), 17–22.

Paul-Murphy, J., Brunson, D.B. and Miletic, V. (1999) Analgesic effects of butorphanol and buprenorphine in conscious African grey parrots (*Psittacus erithacus erithacus* and *Psittacus erithacus timneh*). *American Journal of Veterinary Research*, **60**, 1218–1221.

Paul-Murphy, J., Hess, J. & Fialkowski, J.P. (2004) Pharmacokinetic properties of a single intramuscular dose of buprenorphine in African grey parrots (*Psittacus erithacus erithacus*). *Journal of Avian Medicine and Surgery*, **18**, 224–228.

Paul-Murphy, J.R., Sladky, K.K., Krugner-Higby, L.A., *et al.* (2009) Analgesic effects of carprofen and liposome-encapsulated butorphanol tartrate in Hispaniolan parrots (*Amazona ventralis*) with experimentally induced arthritis. *American Journal of Veterinary Research*, **70**(10), 1201–1210.

Pereira, M.E. and Werther, K. (2007) Evaluation of the renal effects of flunixin meglumine, ketoprofen and meloxicam in budgerigars (*Melospittacus undulatus*). *Veterinary Record*, **160**, 844–846.

Rosskopf, W.J., Woerpel, R.W. and Reed, S. (1989) Avian anaesthesia administration. *Proceedings of the American Animal Hospital Association*, pp. 449–457.

Sanchez-Migallon, G.D., Paul-Murphy, J., Barker, S., *et al.* (2008) Plasma concentrations of butorphanol in Hispaniolan Amazon parrots (*Amazona ventralis*) after intravenous and oral administration. *Proceedings of the Annual Conference of the Association of Avian Veterinarians*, pp. 23–24.

Shaver, S.L., Robinson, N.G., Wright, B.D., *et al.* (2009) A multimodal approach to management of suspected neuropathic pain in a prairie falcon (*Falco mexicanus*). *Journal of Avian Medicine and Surgery*, **23**, 209–213.

Siperstein, L.J. (2007) Use of neurontin (gabapentin) to treat leg twitching/foot mutilation in a Senegal parrot. *Proceedings of the Association of Avian Veterinarians Conference*, p. 335.

Souza, M.J., Sanchez-Migallon, G.D., Paul-Murphy, J., *et al.* (2009) Pharmacokinetics of intravenous and oral tramadol in the bald eagle (*Haliaeetus leucocephalus*). *Journal of Avian Medicine and Surgery*, **23**, 247–252.

Wilson, G.H., Hernandez-Divers, S., Budsberg, S.C., Latimer, S., Grant, K. and Perthel, M. (2005) Pharmacokinetics and use of meloxicam in psittacine birds. *Proceedings of the 8th European Association of Avian Veterinarians,* Arles, pp. 230–232.

Further reading

Taylor, M. (1988) General cautions with isoflurane. *Association of Avian Veterinarians Today*, **2**, 96–97.

Classification of birds according to diet

Dietary preferences may be used to help classify avian species into groups, which often possess similar physical characteristics dictated by these preferences.

There are two main categories of cage and aviary birds:

- Hardbills are predominantly members of the parrot and finch families. They will eat a variety of foods, both fruit and vegetable, and also seeds and nuts. To cope with these, the parrot family has developed a powerful crushing beak, the upper part of which has a synovial joint at its connection with the skull that allows even greater pressures to be generated.
- Softbills comes from a variety of species, from the insectivorous birds, such as wild blackbirds and starlings, to the nectivorous hummingbirds and the omnivorous toucans.

In addition, there is the raptor family, which contains the main species of birds of prey, including owls, falcons, eagles and buzzards, all of which possess a sharp hooked beak used as a ripping tool for tearing prey.

In all of these cases, the individual species have become highly evolved to handle certain types of food. We also know that many of these creatures in the wild have a changing food supply throughout the year, so what may form a staple diet in the summer does not necessarily apply in the winter.

General nutritional requirements

Water

Water is a necessity. However, just as important as providing it is maintaining its quality. Many birds will dunk their food in water, and indeed, if the water feeders are poorly situated, at low levels, may defaecate in the water bowls. This can lead to massive bacterial population explosions and gastroenteritis, sour crop and other health problems.

The quality of water that comes from the tap is also important. Many older buildings may have appreciable levels of lead in their water source. This can produce problems for humans at higher levels, but even low levels of lead can build up in a bird's body over a period of weeks, causing lead poisoning. This is an insidious disease and results in the gradual weight loss, with chronic bone marrow and immune system suppression as well as liver and kidney damage. Safe levels reported for humans of <50 mg/mL of water are acceptable for birds.

Problems can also arise when mineral and vitamin supplements are administered in the drinking water. The enriched water will allow rapid bacterial growth over a 24-hour period, requiring owners to be rigorous about bowl hygiene if they are giving their bird any of these 'tonics'.

The amount of water consumed by individual birds will depend on the diet being offered. On dry biscuit or seed-based diets, water consumption will be higher than for birds which consume large amounts of fruit and vegetables – even so, a budgerigar, e.g. may only consume 5–10 mL of water in a 24-hour period.

Maintenance energy requirements

It is extremely difficult to determine the basal metabolic rate (BMR) of avian patients, as this term covers the energy expenditure when at complete rest in a thermoneutral environment after a period of sleep. Therefore, the more useful concept of maintenance energy requirement (MER) is used in birds. This is the energy usage in a moderately active adult bird in a thermoneutral environment. This can still be difficult to calculate with accuracy; however, studies of the budgerigar, e.g. have revealed that current MER levels are 30 kJ per day for an adult bird.

There are times in a bird's life when this will vary. For instance, this requirement will be more than doubled in active egg-laying females, during heavy moults or during disease or growth. A formula has been devised to calculate MER. MER is dependent on the BMR and may be calculated from it by the following formula:

$$MER = 1.5 \times BMR$$

and

$$BMR = k \times [weight(kg)]^{0.75}$$

The constant, k, varies with family groups, and has been estimated at 78 for non-passerine (i.e. non-perching birds such as parrots) and 129 for passerines (perching birds such as finches, canaries).

The MER of a bird gives a guide to what a bird must consume per day in order to continue to maintain good health and body weight. If the foods offered are so low in kilojoules or calories that the bird has to eat more of it than will fit into its digestive system in 24 hours, the bird will rapidly lose condition. However, many pet birds will continue to eat until their digestive tracts are full, so if all they are offered is the high oilseed types then they will rapidly achieve their MER and then exceed it. This will lead to obesity.

Oilseeds, such as rapeseed or sunflower seeds, which have an energy content of 25 MJ/kg weight, have a high energy density, whereas carbohydrate-based seeds, such as millet, have a low energy density of 17 MJ/kg weight (Harper & Skinner, 1998). This means that the bird has to consume more of the carbohydrate based seeds to gain the same energy dose. In general, though, carbohydrates are the most important source of energy for the body, as they are the only source of energy the brain can use (Brue, 1994).

Protein and amino acids

Proteins are assembled from groups of up to 22 amino acids. In general terms, it seems that for humans and birds, ten amino acids are essential and therefore must be provided in the diet. The others may be manufactured from these ten. The essential amino acids are shown below:

- leucine
- lysine
- methionine
- phenylalanine
- threonine
- tryptophan
- isoleucine
- valine
- arginine
- histidine

In addition, it is known that if a diet is low in the amino acids methionine or arginine, an extra supplement of the amino acid glycine is required.

Proteins are assessed on their ability to provide these essential amino acids, with poor proteins supplying only non-essential ones. This is quantified by the term biological value. Foodstuff of high biological value contains more of the essential amino acids. For companion birds,

levels of 10–13% protein content in the diet have been shown to be adequate (Harper & Skinner, 1998). Most of this protein in cage birds seems to come from seeds. Some seeds are very high providers of certain amino acids. Sunflower seeds, white millet and rapeseed, e.g. provide high levels of the sulphur-containing amino acids methionine and cystine. These amino acids are useful during moulting when new feathers are being produced rapidly.

Deficiencies in certain amino acids have been shown to cause certain diseases (Figure 12.1). For example a deficiency in lysine has been shown to cause depigmentation of wing feathers and a lack of arginine is associated with feather picking. In some species of birds, e.g. the carnivorous raptors, a deficiency in essential amino acids is extremely rare.

Fats and essential fatty acids

Fats provide high concentrations of energy as well as supplying the bird with essential fatty acids (EFAs). The latter are required for cellular integrity and are used as the building blocks for internal chemicals. These internal chemicals, such as prostaglandins, play an important part in reproduction and inflammation. Fats also provide a carrier mechanism for the absorption of fat-soluble vitamins, such as vitamins A, D, E and K.

The primary EFA for birds is linoleic acid, as it is for mammals (Brue, 1994). The absolute dietary requirement of this fatty acid is 1% of the diet. If the diet becomes deficient in this EFA, there will be a rapid decline in cell structure. This is shown clinically by the skin becoming flaky, dry and prone to recurrent infection. Linoleic acid deficiency also leads to fluid loss through the skin, which in turn leads to polydipsia. It is, however, unlikely that

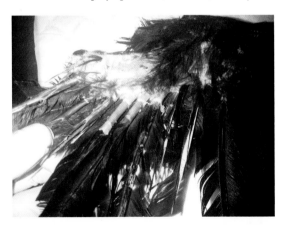

Figure 12.1 Amino acid deficiencies may lead to feather growth abnormalities.

any seed-eating bird will be deficient in linoleic acid, as it is widely found in sunflower seeds and safflower seeds amongst others.

Another EFA which is thought to be important for birds is alpha-linolenic acid, which is necessary for some prostaglandin and eicosanoid production.

The problem of overconsumption of fats in cage birds which are not exercising regularly is well known, and high-fat oil seeds are prime culprits for this (Figure 12.2). The same applies to under-worked raptors fed overweight laboratory rats. Female raptors are particularly prone to this after the breeding season, when large amounts of cholesterol are mobilised for yolk production. Hypercholesterolaemia is hereditary as well as dietary in raptors, but it can be reduced by regular exercising and feeding of lean, low-fat prey. Saturated animal fats provide a supply of cholesterol in excessive amounts for seed and fruit eaters, causing atherosclerosis in older parrots fed on meat and fatty foods.

Preen gland impactions have many causes but may be associated with a deficiency in EFAs and vitamins A and E (see Figure 12.3)

Carbohydrates

Carbohydrates are mainly used for rapid energy production. This is particularly important in birds, because they are in constant demand of rapid supplies of energy for their often-hyperactive and high-metabolism lives. Birds that are debilitated in some way will particularly benefit from the supply of high carbohydrate foods.

Fibre

Dietary fibre does not seem to be important for cage and aviary birds, as the presence of excessive volumes of digestive contents does not make good survival sense when trying to evade predators. As raptors are carnivorous, they

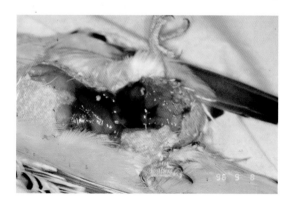

Figure 12.2 Obesity may cause many problems, such as lipoma formation in this budgerigar.

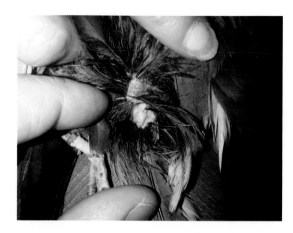

Figure 12.3 Preen gland impaction has been associated with a deficiency in essential fatty acids and vitamins A and E.

do not have a dietary fibre requirement either. Only a few wild birds, such as the ratites (ostriches, emus, rheas and cassowaries) and grouse have large fermenting caeca. The red grouse, e.g. lives predominantly on heather shoots for certain times of the year.

Apart from these general dietary requirements, birds, like all animals, require a variety of vitamins and minerals for a healthy diet.

Vitamins

Vitamins are obviously an essential part of the bird's nutritional requirement.

These compounds are grouped together, although they are widely differing in nature, and all animals have a requirement for various numbers of these. They are categorised into:

- Fat-soluble vitamins A, D, E and K
- Water-soluble vitamins such as the B vitamin complex and vitamin C.

Fat-soluble vitamins

Vitamin A: In cage birds and waterfowl the diet frequently contains only the vitamin A precursors, which are present as carotenoid plant pigments. In birds, the most important version of these, in terms of how much vitamin A can be produced from it, is beta-carotene (Harper & Skinner, 1998). Vitamin A is needed for a number of functions, the best known of which is maintenance of the light sensitive pigment in the retina of the eye. It is also important in the process of epithelial cell turnover and keratinisation, which is why a deficiency in vitamin A has been linked with mite infestations, such as 'scaly face'.

Hypovitaminosis A is a commonly seen problem in companion birds, particularly parrots. This is mainly due to the very low levels of beta-carotenes present in seeds, especially in the much loved sunflower seeds, millet and peanuts. An example of the requirement for vitamin A is quoted as 40 IU per budgerigar, up to a safe maximum of 2500 IU (Harper & Skinner, 1998). The lower levels may be met by as little as 0.4 g of carrot per day, but would require 200 g of millet seed to provide the same amount – i.e. five times a budgerigar's average weight!

If a relative deficiency in vitamin A occurs then mucus membranes become thickened. Oral and respiratory secretions dry up because of blockage of salivary and mucus glands with cellular debris. This leads to poor functioning of the ciliary mechanisms in the airways that have a role in removing foreign particles. This, combined with vitamin A's role in immune system function, leads to respiratory and digestive tract infections (Figure 12.4). One of the most frequently seen infections, particularly in parrots fed an all-seed diet, is the fungal respiratory disease aspergillosis. Sterile pustules and cornified plaques inside the mouth are also commonly seen, with enlargement of the sublingual salivary glands.

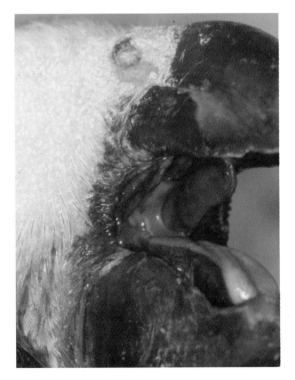

Figure 12.4 Hypovitaminosis A may lead to increased thickening of airway mucus secretions and increased risk of respiratory disease, as in this African grey parrot.

Vitamin A is required for bone growth, for the normal function of secretary glands such as the adrenals and for normal reproductive function. On another level, coloured plumage, particularly the red and yellow, is derived from beta-carotene pigments. Therefore, birds such as the red-factor canaries will become paler in colour if they are fed a diet deficient in this vitamin precursor.

Because it is fat soluble, vitamin A can be stored in the body, primarily in the liver. The recommended minimum dietary levels are 8000–11 000 IU/kg of food offered for both Passeriformes and Psittaciformes (Scott, 1996; Kollias & Kollias, 2000).

Vitamin D: This vitamin is primarily concerned with calcium metabolism, and vitamin D_3 compound is the most active in calcium homeostasis. Plants are not effective as suppliers of this compound.

Cholecalciferol is manufactured in the bird's skin in a process enhanced by ultraviolet light. Indoor-kept birds produce much less of this compound and this can lead to deficiencies. Exposure to just 11–45 minutes of unfiltered sunshine (glass filters out the important ultraviolet light) has been shown to prevent rickets in growing chickens (Heuser & Norris, 1929). Cholecalciferol must then be activated, first in the liver and then by the kidneys, before it becomes functional. It works with parathyroid hormone to increase reabsorption of calcium at the expense of phosphorus from the kidneys. It also increases absorption of calcium from the intestines and mobilises calcium from the bone, increasing the blood's calcium levels.

Hypovitaminosis D_3 affects with calcium metabolism and causes rickets. This is exacerbated by diets low in calcium. Typical sufferers are Psittaciformes, indoor-kept birds fed all-seed diets and raptors fed all-meat diets with no calcium supplementation. This produces well-muscled, heavy birds which have poorly mineralised bones. Radiographical evidence shows flaring of the epiphyseal plates at the ends of the long bones. The end result is bowing of the limbs, especially the tibiotarsal bones. The recommended minimum levels are 500 IU/kg of food offered for Psittaciformes and 1000 IU/kg for Passeriformes (Kollias & Kollias, 2000).

Hypervitaminosis D_3 is caused by over supplementation with D_3 and calcium, and leads to calcification of soft tissues, such as the medial walls of the arteries, and the kidneys. This leads to hypertension and organ failure. The recommended maximum levels are 2000 IU/kg of food offered for Psittaciformes and 2500 IU/kg for Passeriformes (Kollias & Kollias, 2000).

Vitamin E: Vitamin compound is found in several active forms in plants. The most active is alpha-tocopherol. It has an important role in immune system function, particularly lymphocyte cell activity. Vitamin E is combined with selenium into the metalloenzyme glutathione peroxidase. This mops up the free radicals that are produced in the metabolism of dietary polyunsaturated fats, which would otherwise cause cellular damage.

Hypovitaminosis E produces a condition known as 'white muscle disease' in which damage occurs to the muscle bundles and their myoglobin content, leading to pale-coloured muscles and muscle weakness. In addition, birds deficient in vitamin E, such as cockatiels may be more susceptible to the protozoal gut parasite *Giardia* spp. and may pass undigested whole seeds in their droppings.

Hypovitaminosis E may occur due to a reduction in fat metabolism or absorption, as can occur with small intestinal, pancreatic or biliary diseases. It may also occur because of a lack of green plant material in the diet, as this is the main source of vitamin E. Vitamin E deficiency may also occur in birds fed on diets high in polyunsaturated fatty acids, such as fish-eating raptors fed oily fish like tuna. These diets rapidly deplete vitamin E reserves in metabolising the polyunsaturated fats.

Hypervitaminosis E is extremely rare. The recommended minimum level is 50 ppm for both Passeriformes and Psittaciformes (Kollias & Kollias, 2000).

Vitamin K: Because vitamin K is produced by bacteria normally present in the gut, it is very difficult to get a true deficiency, although absorption will be reduced when fat digestion/absorption is reduced as in, e.g. biliary or pancreatic disease.

The consumption of warfarin- and coumarin-derived compounds (such as those found in plants like sweet clovers) can increase the demand for clotting factors. It can also be a problem for raptors that have eaten prey that has been killed by these rodenticides. The deficiency produced causes internal and external haemorrhage, but vitamin K also functions in calcium/phosphorous metabolism in the bones and this may also be affected. The recommended minimum level for raptors, Passeriformes and Psittaciformes is 1 ppm (Wallach & Cooper, 1982).

Water-soluble vitamins

Vitamin B_1 (thiamine): Thiamine is found widely in plant and animal tissues alike. It is concerned with a number of cellular functions, one of which involves the integrity of the central nervous system.

Hypovitaminosis B_1 is uncommon. The most likely cause is the presence of enzymes called thiaminases in the diet, which destroy thiamine. A source of thiaminases is raw saltwater fish, which may be fed to some raptors, such as sea-eagles and ospreys. However, there are thiamine antagonists present in foods such as blackberries, beetroot, coffee, chocolate and tea. When a deficiency occurs, neurological signs such as opisthotonus, weakness and head tremors appear. In addition, the fungal infection aspergillosis is a common sequel to B_1 deficiency. The recommended minimum levels for raptors, Psittaciformes and Passeriformes are 4 ppm (Kollias & Kollias, 2000) or 5 g of usable vitamin B_1 per day for raptors (Wallach & Cooper, 1982).

Vitamin B_2 (riboflavin): Vitamin B_2 is present in particularly small amounts in seeds, and so deficiency is primarily seen in seed-eating birds. Hypovitaminosis B_2 causes growth retardation and curled toe paralysis in chicks. This is due to its function in cartilage, collagenous and nerve cell tissue growth. Birds can be supplemented using commercial powder supplements or simple brewer's yeast. The recommended minimum levels for Psittaciformes and Passeriformes are 6 ppm (Kollias & Kollias, 2000), for game birds 3.6 mg/kg and waterfowl (Austic & Cole, 1971) 4 mg/kg of feed offered (Scott & Norris, 1965).

Niacin: Niacin is found widely in many foods, but the form that occurs in plants has a low availability to the bird. It is used in many cellular metabolic processes.

Birds fed a high proportion of one type of seed, such as waterfowl overfed on sweetcorn, can become deficient. This results in retarded growth, poor feather quality and scaly dermatitis on the legs and feet. Intertarsal joint deformities can occur in the larger waterfowl. The recommended minimum requirements are 50 ppm for Passeriformes and Psittaciformes (Kollias & Kollias, 2000) or 55–70 mg/kg of feed in general (Wallach & Cooper, 1982).

Vitamin B_6 (pyridoxine): Any deficiency of pyridoxine will result in retarded growth, hyperexcitability, convulsions, twisted neck and polyneuritis, although a deficiency is rarely seen. Recommended minimum levels are 6 ppm in Passeriformes and Psittaciformes (Kollias & Kollias, 2000) or 2.6–3 mg/kg of feed for game birds (Scott & Norris, 1965).

Pantothenic acid: Pantothenic acid is found widely in plants and animals and so deficiency rarely occurs. When it does occur in birds, signs include crusting of the feet, eyelids and commissures of the beak, poor feather growth and general epidermal desquamation. The recommended minimum levels are 20 ppm for Passeriformes and Psittaciformes (Kollias & Kollias, 2000) or 35.2 mg/kg of feed in ducks (Scott & Norris, 1965).

Biotin: True deficiencies are rare due to gut bacterial production. Deficiencies produce a range of signs, including exfoliative dermatitis and gangrenous toes. The recommended minimum requirements are 0.25 ppm for Passeriformes and Psittaciformes (Kollias & Kollias, 2000) or 0.09–0.15 mg/kg of feed in waterfowl (Wallach & Cooper, 1982).

Folic acid: Folic acid deficiency leads to severely impaired cell division. This can lead to a number of problems, such as failure of hen birds' reproductive tract development, a macrocytic anaemia due to failure of red blood cell maturation and immune system cellular dysfunction.

Folic acid is needed to form uric acid, the waste product of protein metabolism in birds. Therefore, a relative deficiency of folic acid may occur in some individuals fed a very high protein diet. In addition, some foods, such as cabbage and other brassicas, as well as oranges beans and peas, contain folic acid inhibitors. The use of trimethoprim sulphonamide drugs may also reduce gut bacterial folic acid production. The recommended minimum requirements are 1.5 ppm for Passeriformes and Psittaciformes (Kollias & Kollias, 2000) or 1.25 mg/kg of feed (Scott & Norris, 1965).

Vitamin B_{12}: Vitamin B_{12} is produced by intestinal bacteria so deficiency is uncommon, although it may occur after prolonged antibiotic medication. Vitamin B_{12} is required for many metabolic pathways and neurological function and a deficiency may cause a knock-on deficiency in folic acid. It will cause slow growth, muscular dystrophy in the legs, poor hatching rates and high mortality rates in young birds, as well as hatching deformities. The recommended minimum requirements are for 0.01 ppm in Passeriformes and Psittaciformes (Kollias & Kollias, 2000) or 0.009–0.25 mg/kg of feed offered (Wallach & Cooper, 1982).

Choline: Choline may be synthesised in the body, but not in enough quantities for the growing bird. Because of their interactions, the need for choline is dependent on levels of folic acid and vitamin B_{12}. Excess dietary protein increases choline requirements, as does a diet high

in fats. Deficiencies cause retarded growth, disrupted fat metabolism, fatty liver damage and perosis (slipping of the Achilles tendon off the intertarsal joint groove). The recommended minimum requirements are 1500 ppm for Passeriformes and Psittaciformes (Kollias & Kollias, 2000) or 1300–1900 mg/kg of feed offered (Wallach & Cooper, 1982).

Vitamin C: There are only a few wild birds that have a direct need for vitamin C. These include the red-vented bulbul (*Pycnonotus cafer*) and the willow ptarmigan/red grouse (*Lagopus lagopus*) as well as the crimson sunconure, a form of parrot. Birds in general do not need vitamin C in their diets as it can be produced from glucose in the liver. If a bird is suffering from liver disease, therefore, it may require a dietary source of vitamin C.

Vitamin C is needed for the formation of elastic fibres and connective tissues and is an excellent anti-oxidant similar to vitamin E. Deficiency leads to scurvy in which there is poor wound healing, increased bleeding due to capillary wall fragility and bone weakness.

Vitamin C also increases gut absorption of some minerals, such as iron. This may be important for chronically anaemic patients, but can be a danger for softbills, such as the mynah and toucan families, as these birds are prone to liver damage from excessive dietary uptake of iron.

Minerals

There are two main groups of minerals:

- Macro-minerals
- Micro-minerals

Macro-minerals (such as calcium and phosphorus) are present in large amounts in the body. Micro-minerals or trace elements (such as manganese, iron and cobalt) are all necessary for normal bodily function, but are needed in far lower quantities.

Macro-minerals

Calcium: The active form of calcium in the body is the ionic, double-charged molecule Ca^{2+}. Lowered levels of this form lead to hyperexcitability, fitting and death. This can occur even though the overall body reserves of calcium are normal.

Calcium levels in the body are controlled by vitamin D_3, parathyroid hormone and calcitonin working in opposition to each other. The ratio of calcium to phosphorus is particularly important – as one increases, the other decreases and vice versa. A ratio of 2:1 calcium to phosphorus is desirable in food for growing birds and

1.5:1 for adults. In periods of high egg laying though, to keep pace with the output of calcium into the shells, a ratio of 10:1 may be needed (Brue, 1994). A known deficiency problem occurs in many birds fed an all-seed diet due to the lack of calcium in such a diet and the presence of phytates (phosphorus containing compounds) which bind calcium in the gut and prevent absorption. This is particularly a problem in African Grey Parrots (*Psittacus erithacus*), which may present with collapse or seizures due to low blood calcium levels. Excessive calcium in the diet (>1%), however, reduces the use of proteins, fats, phosphorus, manganese, zinc, iron and iodine and combined with a high level of vitamin D_3 may lead to calcification of soft tissue structures.

Phosphorus: Phosphorus, like calcium, is used in bones. It is also used in the storage of energy as adenosine triphosphate (ATP), and as a part of the structure of cell membranes. Levels of phosphorus are controlled in the body as for calcium, the two being in equal and opposite equilibrium with each other. Nutritional secondary hyperparathyroidism may occur when dietary phosphorus exceeds calcium, and this can lead to progressive bone demineralisation and renal damage due to high circulating levels of parathyroid hormone.

High dietary phosphorus, particularly as phytates, will reduce the amount of calcium which can be absorbed from the gut, as it forms complexes with the calcium present there. This can be a big problem in cage birds which are predominantly seed eaters, as cereals are high in phosphorus and low in calcium. It may also be a problem for raptors fed pure meat with no calcium/bone supplement.

Magnesium: Most of the magnesium in the body is found in the bone matrix. However, it is also essential for phosphorus transfer in the formation of ATP, and cell membranes in soft tissues such as the liver. Most magnesium is absorbed in the small intestine, and is affected by large amounts of calcium in the diet, which will reduce magnesium absorption. The recommended minimum levels are 600 ppm (Kollias & Kollias, 2000) or 475–550 mg/kg of feed (Wallach & Cooper, 1982).

Sodium: Sodium is the main extracellular, positively charged ion and regulates the body's acid–base balance and osmotic potential. Along with potassium, it is responsible for nerve signals and impulses.

A true dietary deficiency (hyponatraemia) is rare, but may occur due to chronic diarrhoea or renal disease. These disrupt the osmotic potential gradient in the

kidneys leading to further water loss and dehydration. Excessive levels of sodium in the diet (greater than ten times recommended levels) lead to poor feathering, polyuria, hypertension, oedema and death. Minimum levels are quoted as 5–10 mg/kg of feed offered (Wallach & Cooper, 1982) or around 0.12% of the diet offered (Kollias & Kollias, 2000).

Potassium: As with mammals, potassium is the major intracellular positive ion. It is essential in maintaining membrane potentials and it is the principal intracellular cation affecting acid–base reactions and osmotic pressure. Rarely is there a dietary deficiency, but, severe stress may cause potassium deficiency, hypokalaemia. This is caused by an increased kidney excretion of potassium due to an elevation in plasma proteins which is often seen at times of stress. This can lead to cardiac dysrhythmias, muscle spasticity and neurological dysfunction.

Potassium is present in high amounts in certain fruits such as bananas. It is controlled in the body in equilibrium with sodium under the influence of the adrenal hormone aldosterone, which promotes sodium retention and potassium excretion. The recommended minimal level is 0.4–1.1 mg/kg (Scott & Norris, 1965).

Chlorine: This mineral is the major extracellular negative ion. It is responsible for maintaining acid–base balances in conjunction with sodium and potassium. Deficiencies are rare due to its combination with sodium in the diet as salt.

Micro-minerals (trace elements)

Iron: Iron is required for the formation of the oxygen-binding centre of the haemoglobin molecule. Absorption from the gut is normally relatively poor as the body is very good at recycling its iron levels from old red blood cells.

Certain species have a greater ability to absorb iron from the small intestine. The mynah and toucan/toucanet families are examples. This ability may become a problem when diets rich in iron are presented to these species. For example, rodents and day-old chicks may be fed to toucans, and so occasionally are various brands of dog or monkey biscuits. In addition, vitamin C increases iron absorption by converting the iron into the more easily absorbed ferrous (Fe^{2+}) state. This can lead to a condition known as haemochromatosis, where the liver becomes fatally overloaded with absorbed iron. The recommended minimum requirement for Passeriformes and Psittaciformes is 80 ppm, but for toucans and mynahs a maximum of 60 ppm, or less than 160 mg/kg of feed, is recommended (Worrell, 1991). Dietary deficiencies rarely occur. However, ground foraging species reared on impervious surfaces such as wire or concrete have suffered iron deficiency. This is because soil consumption, which occurs during ground feeding, is another source of iron.

Copper: Copper is used for haemoglobin synthesis, collagen synthesis and the maintenance of the nervous system.

Deficiencies occur, as with iron, in some ground feeding species like pheasants and other game birds, reared on surfaces such as concrete where soil consumption during the foraging process does not occur. Signs include chronic anaemia with general weakness, limb deformities and hyperexcitability. The recommended minimum requirements are 8 ppm for Passeriformes and Psittaciformes, and 4 ppm for Galliformes (Wallach & Cooper, 1982).

Zinc: This is a vital trace element for wound healing and tissue formation, forming part of a number of enzymes.

Deficiencies can occur in young, rapidly growing birds fed on plant material high in phytates such as cabbage, wheat bran and beans. This is because, as with calcium, the phytates bind zinc and prevent its absorption from the gut. In addition, high dietary calcium itself decreases zinc uptake. Deficiencies cause retarded growth, poor feathering, enlarged intertarsal joints and slipped Achilles tendon (perosis). The minimum recommended requirement is 50 ppm for Passeriformes and Psittaciformes (Kollias & Kollias, 2000).

Manganese: Manganese is primarily found in plant materials but is often present in unavailable forms. Efficient bile salt production is required for its absorption, so birds with hepatic and biliary dysfunction are most at risk of a deficiency.

Manganese is necessary for normal bone structure; hence deficiencies are most commonly manifested by the swelling and flattening of the lateral condyles of the intertarsal joint, allowing the Achilles tendon to slip out of the groove created for it (a condition known as perosis). In addition, the tibiotarsus and tarsometatarsus may exhibit lateral rotation. Young may be born with retracted beaks and shortened long bones. The recommended minimum requirement is 55–60 mg/kg of feed (Wallach & Cooper, 1982).

Iodine: The sole function of iodine is in thyroid hormone synthesis. Deficiencies cause goitre, and produce effects such as reduced growth, stunting and neurological problems. It is a relatively common finding in budgerigars fed on an all-seed diet without additional supplementation. They adopt a classic, hunched posture on the perch because the enlarged thyroid gland constricts the tracheal lumen. They may also be seen to regurgitate seed from the crop. Goitre is one of the differential diagnoses in a vomiting budgerigar. Levels of 4 mg per budgerigar per week prevent goitre from developing (Blackmore, 1963).

Selenium: Its functions are similar to vitamin E, as it is found in the enzyme glutathione peroxidase. If there is a general deficiency in both selenium and vitamin E, a condition known as exudative diathesis will occur. This is when the smaller, subcutaneous blood vessels become damaged and leakier. Fluid then moves rapidly out into the subcutaneous spaces and oedema forms over the neck, wings and breast. This is often followed by stunted growth, limb weakness and death.

The selenium content of plants is dependent on where they were grown and the levels of selenium in the soil. The recommended minimum requirement is 0.1 ppm for Passeriformes and Psittaciformes (Kollias & Kollias, 2000).

Examples of food types for Psittaciformes and Passeriformes

As a rough example of food types suitable for commonly kept cage and aviary birds, please examine the list given below.

Seeds

Rape seed, millet, canary seed, hemp and linseed are useful for smaller species such as finches, canaries, budgerigars and cockatiels.

Safflower, sunflower and pumpkin seeds are useful for larger parrots but beware of addiction to sunflower seeds!

Nuts

Almonds, walnuts, Brazil nuts and hazel nuts are useful for larger parrots, but be careful of addiction to peanuts and *Aspergillus* spp. toxin poisoning. Peanuts and pine nuts may also be fed. Nuts are high in calories.

Fruits

A wide variety of fruits are useful foods. Examples include apple, pear, melon, mango, papaya, pomegranate, guava, apricot, peach, nectarine, oranges and bananas. Grapes and kiwi fruit should be fed sparingly due to their high sugar content, which can cause diarrhoea. Oranges should also only be fed in small amounts, since excess can cause gastric upset, and they should not be fed to toucans and mynah birds due to their high vitamin C content and iron absorption facilitation.

Vegetables

Broccoli, watercress and wild rocket are good sources of vitamin A and calcium. Other good vegetables include Swiss chard, kale, sweet pepper, carrot, beetroot, boiled potato, peas, mung beans (particularly sprouted ones), cauliflower, tomato and sweetcorn.

Do not feed avocados as these cause severe fatty liver damage in birds. Lories, lorikeets and hummingbirds are all nectar feeders and so require a specialised artificial syrup food. Many are commercially produced. They may also take very ripe fruits, and enjoy eating the pollen from flowers.

Specific nutritional requirements

Nutritional requirements for growth

Embryonic growth

The egg is a perfect capsule of nutrients providing all that is needed for the developing embryo. The hen must be fed a balanced diet to ensure that she has the nutrients available to instil into the egg. If she is fed a poor or deficient diet then the egg may not be fertile. It could also undergo:

- Early embryonic death (EED). This is often signalled by a blood ring left in the yolk, which suggests a vitamin A deficiency.
- Retarded embryonic development (RED). This is often associated with vitamin B deficiencies.
- Embryonic deformities, which may be seen with manganese, zinc or other trace element deficiencies.

Post-hatch growth

Hatching occurs after the developing chick has absorbed the external yolk sac, and the chick must then be supplied within 3–4 days with high levels of energy and protein for the growth phase. The remaining internal yolk sac supply will last that long.

When feathers are produced, a huge demand for protein occurs, as feathers are made of keratin, a protein, and will eventually make up one-tenth of the bird's weight. In addition, there will be several feather changes during the first 2 years of life, as juvenile down plumage is replaced by adult plumage. Young birds also have a much larger requirement for calcium and vitamin D_3 for developing bones. On average, sexual maturity for the larger parrots, such as African grey parrots, macaws and cockatoos, is not reached until 2–4 years of age, so this growth phase may be prolonged.

If, during this growth phase, disease or low environmental temperatures are introduced, energy is diverted to immune system function and heat supply. This results in less energy for growth and in slowing of the growth rate. This may be reversed in later periods of growth, assuming no permanent damage has been caused. The obvious side-effect of this, though, is that adult weights are achieved at a later age. If a retarded bird is supplied with excess nutritional levels after this period of leanness, a compensatory growth spurt may occur and the chick appears to grow more rapidly than other birds of that age group.

For all of this growth to occur, it has been estimated that minimum energy requirements for small Psittaciformes and Passeriformes are five times that of adults. Young chicks nearly double their weights over 48 hours, and require a protein level of 15–20%, as opposed to an adult's protein need of 10–14% (Harper & Skinner, 1998). Commercial and home-prepared diets for chicks are usually preformulated mashes with this level of protein, eggs and dairy products which have a good broad spectrum of amino acids supplementation and 20% protein levels.

Excessive protein supplementation may be equally damaging. Levels greater than 25% of diet have been shown to lead to behavioural problems, and claw, beak and skeletal deformities, particularly if combined with a lack of calcium. Levels of 0.6–1.2% of the diet as calcium have been quoted for chick growth (Brue, 1994) with a calcium:phosphorus ratio of 2:1 maintained.

Nutritional requirements for breeding

These requirements include those needed for egg production as well as for courtship behaviour. The requirements for egg production are high, with large volumes needed of fats for the yolk, calcium for the shell and proteins for the albumen (egg white). As egg production commences, the hen bird will increase the volume of food consumed, so removing the need to increase the energy concentration of the diet being offered. It is, however, essential that the diet offered is a balanced one, with increased protein content, particularly from methionine and cystine (the sulphur containing amino acids) and lysine.

In addition, a moderate increase in the amount of calcium and vitamin D_3 offered (an increase of 0.35% of the adult maintenance requirement for calcium) is needed, so that levels approach 1% of diet (Harper & Skinner, 1998). This not only helps to ensure proper calcification of eggshells and the developing embryo, but also to prevent egg-binding in the hen. This is when poor calcium reserves lead to low calcium blood levels, weakness, uterine muscular paresis, egg retention, shock and death.

Other compounds which, if supplied above the minimum daily requirements mentioned earlier, help with egg production, include vitamins A, B_{12}, riboflavin and the mineral zinc. In addition, it is useful for improved hatching rate, to increase the levels of the B vitamins biotin, folic acid, pantothenic acid, riboflavin (B_2) and pyridoxine (B_6), as well as vitamin E, iron, copper, zinc and manganese to above the minimum daily requirements.

Nutritional requirements for the older birds

As with cats and dogs, the aim is to provide a diet of high digestibility whilst reducing slightly the protein, sodium and phosphorus levels. This preserves renal function and prevents hypertension.

In addition, lowering cholesterol and unsaturated fat levels is important, as atherosclerosis is common in older birds. The levels of vitamins A, E, thiamine (B_1), B_{12}, and pyridoxine (B_6), the mineral zinc, amino acid lysine and fatty acid linoleic acid should also be slightly increased to ensure that any decrease in digestive function and age-related cellular damage is contained.

Special nutritional requirements for debilitated birds

Extra nutritional support for debilitated and diseased birds is vital and plays an essential role in ensuring recovery of the avian patient after disease or debility. Enteral nutrition is currently the most usual method of supporting the debilitated patient, with parenteral (intravenous) nutrition still being in its infancy in avian therapeutics.

First, fluid requirements should be assessed, as any animal will succumb to dehydration long before starvation. The reader is referred to chapter 14 for a more detailed discussion of this topic.

Second, energy requirements should be estimated. These can be calculated roughly from the MER by multiplication as follows:

Starvation $= 0.5 \times$ MER

Trauma $= 1.5 \times$ MER

Sepsis $= 2.5 \times$ MER

Burns $= 3–4 \times$ MER

From these crude estimations, a rough idea of the levels of nutrition demanded and the energy concentration of the diet can be derived.

Third, protein requirements should be evaluated, as debilitation will increase amino acid and protein turnover. This may be through the increased use of proteins in the immune system response, or for repair of damaged tissue or simply after using tissue proteins as an energy source.

Birds with liver disease

Birds affected by hepatic dysfunction should be fed a diet which reduces liver use by decreasing its need to convert body tissues into blood glucose, and decreasing its need to break down the waste products of excess protein metabolism. Therefore birds should be fed a diet high in digestible carbohydrates, such as boiled rice, pasta or potatoes, for energy and sugars. Protein sources should be of a high biological value (high in essential amino acids) such as those found in whole eggs. This is in an attempt to keep to a minimum the overall amount of protein fed, particularly purine-producing proteins such as are found in fish, meat, etc. These protein sources lead to the greater build-up of waste products of protein digestion, which the liver then has to detoxify and eliminate via the kidneys. The feeding of frequent, small meals is also advisable for liver disease patients, as is the addition of vitamin B supplements to the diet.

Birds with renal disease

Like the liver, the kidney is responsible for eliminating the waste products of protein metabolism (Figure 12.5). It is therefore important in renal disease to reduce protein levels, and ensure that the protein sources provided have a high biological value.

In addition, restricting phosphorus in the diet is helpful, as excess may lead to demineralisation of the bone, increased levels of parathyroid hormone and further renal damage.

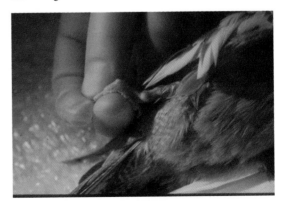

Figure 12.5 Gout crystals may form in joints (articular gout) as in this cockatiel (*Nymphicus hollandicus*) with renal disease.

Finally, restricting sodium is important to reduce fluid retention and decrease hypertension. Vitamin B supplementation can help as an appetite stimulant. It is advisable to supplement it in any case as being a water-soluble vitamin, it can be flushed out of the body where polyuria occurs, leading to deficiency.

Birds with heart disease

Heart disease is commonly seen in older parrots and some raptors, particularly females. It is also seen as a sequel to iron storage disease (haemochromatosis) in toucans and mynahs. Reduction of sodium in the diet to reduce hypertension due to fluid retention is helpful. So too is lowering cholesterol levels by removing saturated fats, such as dairy products and overly fatty prey for raptors. Avoiding meat in general for birds such as parrots is advised. For toucans, mynah birds and related species, the avoidance of high iron-containing diets is essential to prevent haemochromatosis and the cardiac damage which can ensue.

Birds suffering from maldigestion and malabsorption syndromes

Birds suffering from maldigestion and malabsorption syndromes such as pancreatic disease should be fed highly digestible carbohydrate foods such as rice, potatoes and pasta, whilst reducing all fats in the diet such as seeds, meat, etc. The addition of pancreatic enzyme supplementation is to be considered, along with B-vitamin supplementation.

Birds suffering from anaemia

Anaemic patients should have the cause of their anaemia investigated, as common causes include heavy-metal poisoning and chronic disease processes. Other aids to increasing red blood cell production (erythropoiesis) are supplementation with iron and with smaller increases in copper and cobalt levels. Vitamin B_{12}, niacin, and folic acid levels should be six times the normal minimal values to ensure that the extra demands caused by increased red cell production are met.

Other dietary factors and conditions

Other factors which are known to aid the recovery of debilitated birds are given in Table 12.1.

Hypocalcaemic tetany

A specific disease of African grey parrots commonly between the ages of 2 and 4 years is hypocalcaemic tetany.

Table 12.1 Examples of dietary deficiencies in avian species.

Vitamin or mineral	Functions
Vitamin A	Seems to improve the activity of the mononuclear immune system as well as governing cellular turnover of epithelial surfaces
Vitamin B complex	Thiamine especially helps stimulate appetite, and many B vitamins are useful in protein and energy metabolism, making them important during recovery periods
Vitamin C	Also seems to aid immune system function, and may be in short supply if the avian patient is suffering from hepatic disease, since it is the liver which manufactures vitamin C
Vitamin D	Production of this vitamin may also be impaired due to renal or hepatic dysfunction. However, it is worthwhile noting that excess vitamin D_3 can cause soft tissue mineralisation, including in the kidney itself
Vitamin E	Aids immune system function and helps reduce free radical oxidation of tissues
Vitamin K	This may become deficient due to prolonged antibiotic therapy, where intestinal bacteria are depleted or where a raptor has consumed a warfarin poisoned rodent
Zinc	This mineral helps the healing process, particularly in skin diseases, but can also help immunity, particularly with respect to phagocytosis

This is due to a failure to mobilise calcium into the blood stream. The afflicted parrot will become weak, collapse and start fitting which may progress to a coma and death. It appears to be a hereditary condition and birds often grow out of it if carefully managed. Afflicted birds appear to have plenty of calcium in their bones, but seem unable to mobilise it. Management, therefore, consists of providing sufficient dietary calcium so that blood levels remain normal.

Obesity

In overweight or obese birds, particularly where a fatty liver syndrome is suspected, a strict diet management is indicated.

Correcting dietary deficiencies
Attempting to encourage new food consumption

Birds are highly intelligent, particularly members of the Psittaciformes order. This means that the introduction of new foods, in an attempt to correct dietary deficiencies, can be a significant problem. The following techniques may be employed to tempt a cage bird to accept new food items.

Overcoming unfamiliarity

Just because the bird was not interested in the food item today is no reason to suspect that it may not try the food tomorrow. Just like children, birds may view a new or unfamiliar food with suspicion and reject it purely for that. The key is to keep representing the food, preferably on the top of its food bowl, so that the bird has to remove it to get to the usual food underneath. The bird may eventually become used to its sight, smell and taste, and may therefore start to eat it.

Tempting the bird with food

Many birds want to eat what their owners are eating, as obviously it must be better than the rubbish in their own food bowl! This can be used to our advantage, as the owner can sample the food in front of the bird and then offer it to the bird. This can trigger acceptance.

Fooling the bird with food

Covering the food item that you wish the bird to eat in the flavour or colour of a food item it already likes can work well. An example would be honey- or peanut butter-coated broccoli or carrot.

Pelleted commercial diets

Many excellent pelleted avian diets are available for species ranging from flamingos to toucans, parrots to ducks. Their main advantage is homogeneity – the bird cannot pick and choose what it wishes to eat, but is rather forced to eat a balanced, pre-prepared diet.

The disadvantages include the problem of selection. Some of these diets are multi-coloured and birds have good colour vision and may pick out one coloured biscuit to eat only. This is fine if all of the biscuits are of the same composition no matter what the colour, but does lead to wastage. In addition, palatability can be a problem, so getting a bird to eat some of these diets can be difficult.

Fresh water must be available at all times, as these diets are dry pellets and chronic dehydration can occur.

Avian mineral and vitamin supplements

These are very important, particularly for species fed a home-prepared diet. They are produced by many companies and cover all aspects of supplementation. Some are put in the food itself, some in water. The latter may be problematic as the taste may prevent water consumption

or the vitamins may encourage bacterial growth in the water bowl. Multivitamin and mineral preparations may be used as a general supplement to a diet where the individual bird will not take a wide variety of food types; an example is the seed-obsessed parrot. They should be used though, not as an excuse to give up on offering other food types, but more to ensure nutritional balance whilst trying to encourage the bird onto a more stable diet. They may also be used, even when a balanced diet is being fed and eaten, to supplement a bird at certain times of its life when requirements for minerals and vitamins increase, such as during egg-laying, growth, moulting and old age.

Dietary requirements peculiar to specific families

Larger members of the Psittaciformes order

Larger members of the parrot family, such as cockatoos, macaws, Amazons and African grey parrots, have slightly different requirements from the smaller members of the family, such as the conures and parakeets. Many of their larger parrots require slightly more fats in their diets, to increase their calorific density, than their smaller cousins. This is not so surprising considering that the normal wild diets of these parrots involve a moderate amount of oil-based nuts and seeds. It is advisable therefore, that larger nuts, such as hazel nuts, Brazil nuts, cashews, etc. should be included in the diet of these species.

An example of the MER of some of the larger species of parrot include 452 kJ per day for a scarlet macaw (*Ara macao*) as opposed to 200 kJ per day (Nott & Taylor, 1993) required by the lesser sulphur-crested cockatoo (*Cacatua sulphurea*). Therefore, to maintain calorific intake, a scarlet macaw will have to eat far more of a seed such as the sunflower seed, which has an energy content of approximately 24 kJ per gram of dry matter (18 g dry matter or nearly 22.5 g fresh), as opposed to the cashew nut which has an energy content of 32 kJ per gram of dry matter (14 g dry matter or nearly 17 g fresh).

However, many of the larger parrots, especially the Amazons and African grey parrots, are also prone to atherosclerosis, or hardening of the major arteries, due to cholesterol deposition in their walls. This happens if their diets are persistently high in saturated fats, such as meat and dairy products, but may also occur with chronic over-consumption of high fat nuts and seeds. Hepatic lipidosis, or the obliteration of the liver cells with fat, is also a common sequel to over-supplementation of the diet with high fat nuts and seeds in parrots. So it is important to get the balance right.

In formulating these diets it is also important that attention is paid to calcium and mineral levels, as seeds and nuts are extremely poor suppliers of these. Nuts may also be a potential source of fungal growths of *Aspergillus* spp. These can not only produce spores which may cause respiratory disease, but can also produce highly poisonous toxins, known as aflatoxins and gliatoxins, which may cause sudden death, neurological damage or chronic hepatic damage, depending on the dose consumed.

The most commonly seen deficiencies in the larger psittacines occur with vitamin A, vitamin D_3 and the mineral calcium. This is particularly the case with African grey parrots because of hypocalcaemic tetany – an inherited condition of 2- to-4-year-old birds, where blood calcium levels cannot be maintained. This can lead to hypocalcaemic fits. In addition, African grey parrots fed an all-seed diet, are very prone to respiratory infections, especially aspergillosis (the air sac and lung infestation with the fungus Aspergillus fumigatus). This is often associated with hypovitaminosis A.

However, as with so many nutrients, too much is as bad as too little. Excessive levels of vitamin D_3 commonly cause toxicosis in African grey parrots and macaws, leading to soft tissue calcification and renal damage. Excessive vitamin A can also cause problems in the large parrots and in hand-reared chicks, causing liver damage, kidney damage and haemorrhage.

Raptors

Raptors are carnivorous. They therefore require regular fresh rodent or avian prey. If fed whole, these usually provide a balanced diet. To determine the amounts of prey to be fed, a rough rule of thumb is that the larger the raptor, the smaller the food consumption is, as a percentage of that bird's weight. A golden eagle, e.g. may consume 5–7% of its body weight per day, whereas a sparrowhawk would perhaps consume 25% body weight per day.

For raptors in training, the main aim is to keep the birds lean and slightly hungry to make it easier to hand-train them. If underfed, however, the consequence is starvation; if overfed the bird will become obese, and atherosclerosis is a major problem in overfed raptors. To try to prevent under- or overfeeding a useful technique is to weigh the raptor on a daily basis to ensure constant weight levels. This is not always possible, however; e.g. when breeding the raptors they must not be handled, and so at certain times of the year it may be difficult to assess their condition. During this period, however, it is useful, as with any animal to increase the levels of nutrition to

ensure healthy egg production. Care should be taken with egg-laying female raptors though, to ensure they are not fed obese prey items, as the presence of cholesterol and lipids for yolk production in their blood stream makes them very prone to atherosclerosis at this time.

Water consumption

Water consumption is of course vital. Dehydration may occur due to the feeding of previously frozen and then thawed prey, only because the freezing process causes dehydration of the carcass. Therefore, when defrosting the rodent or avian prey item, it is advisable to soak it in water.

Food composition

Protein levels are as expected for a carnivorous family, relatively high, at 15–20% (Cooper, 1991) and this is desirable for full fitness. However, excessive levels of protein (greater than 30%) should be avoided, as this can lead to an excess of protein degradation products in the bloodstream, such as purines. These are converted into uric acid for renal excretion, but if the levels are excessive, the uric acid concentration will exceed that which can be dissolved in the blood. This will lead to the precipitation of uric acid causing gout.

Optimum fat levels in prey offered for raptors have been estimated at 20–25% (Cooper, 1991). Prey such as some laboratory rats and mice, as mentioned, can cause hypercholesterolaemia and atherosclerosis in underworked raptors.

Mineral supplementation may be necessary. This is especially so in chicks which are often fed small pieces of meat, rather than whole prey. This can result in calcium deficiencies, as muscle tissue is low in calcium and high in phosphorus. A ratio of calcium to phosphorus of 2:1 or at least 1.5:1 should be maintained.

Prey

The feeding of certain types of prey should be done with care. For example, pigeons fed to larger birds of prey can be a source of *Trichomonas gallinae* infestation. This is a protozoal parasite which invades the crop and digestive system, causing regurgitation, vomiting and weight loss in the affected raptor. Therefore, it is recommended that if pigeon is to be fed, it be deep frozen and then thoroughly defrosted to kill any *Trichomonas* spp. organisms present in the carcass.

Other parasites such as the worm *Capillaria* spp. can also be transmitted from prey bird to raptor. In other avian and mammalian prey, the presence of lead shot is again a potential hazard and a cause of lead poisoning in raptors.

Other problems due to poisoning from prey offered are pesticides and herbicides, particularly the organochlorines and organophosphates. These concentrate in animal fats and so pass up through the food chain, producing highest concentrations in top predators such as raptors.

In addition, there are compounds such as the polychlorinated biphenyls (PCBs). These are used for a number of purposes, including insulation and electrical circuitry, and may enter the food chain through small rodents. These also concentrate in animal fats, so concentrating their levels in the tissues of animals, as one moves up the food chain. They cause problems similar to those caused by the pesticides: reproductive problems, chick mortalities and neurological tremors which can lead to death.

Food management for racing pigeons

The day-to-day feeding of racing pigeons includes the provision once or twice a day of a grain-and-pulse-based diet. For racing pigeons, one trend is the feeding of carbohydrate-based foods, such as grains, early on in the course of a week, and then increasing the protein levels with supplements and pulses as the racing day, often a Saturday, approaches. Many companies now produce homogenous pelleted feeds for racing pigeons, containing differing levels of protein depending on whether they are actively training or rearing young. Grit can be given freely. It is insoluble and aids in the grinding of grain in the gizzard. This is important in species such as pigeons, which do not de-husk seed before swallowing it. Water is offered, as with game birds, from communal feeders, and pigeon owners will often add multivitamins, minerals and medicants to these fountain feeders.

Waterfowl

Nutrition of waterfowl receives less attention, as many geese and ducks are kept in outdoor smallholding settings and so live predominantly on grass and other herbage. Geese in particular need ample grass for grazing. It is essential to ensure that access to poisonous plants or trees, such as laburnum and foxgloves, is restricted, as these birds will eat almost anything. In poor weather, or with limited grass production, commercial pelleted food should be given. There are now commercial duck and geese pellets available. Alternatively the use of poultry 'layer' pellets can be tried.

Commercial pellets come in four main categories:

- Pellets designed for the brooding, egg-laying female, which are higher in calcium and protein
- Pellets for the very young waterfowl chick up to 2–3 weeks of age (known as 'starter pellets' or 'crumbs')
- Pellets for the juvenile growing waterfowl (up to 4–6 months)
- Adult non-breeding maintenance pellets.

The differences lie in the provision of proteins and calcium, with the highest being in the starter pellets (at around 20% protein) through to the lower end as adult pellets (14% protein). There are now companies which also produce special diets for other ornamental waterfowl such as sea duck and flamingos. (Flamingos require more protein and a selection of salts to encourage plumage colouration.)

Duck and geese enclosures need to be routinely examined for evidence of foreign objects, such as lead shot, barbed wire fragments and so on. This is because of these birds' desire to consume any and every loose potential food item they can find when foraging.

References

Austic, R.E. and Cole, R.K. (1971) Impaired uric acid excretion in chickens selected for uricemia and articular gout. *Proceedings of the 1971 Cornell Nutritional Conference*, November 2–3, Buffalo, Colorado.

Blackmore, D.K. (1963) The incidence and aetiology of thyroid dysplasia in budgerigars (*Melopsittacus undulatus*). *Veterinary Record*, **75**, 1068–1072.

Brue, R.N. (1994) Nutrition. *Avian Medicine: Principles and Application* (eds B. Ritchie, G. Harrison & L. Harrison), pp. 63–95. WB Saunders, Philadelphia, PA.

Cooper, J.E. (1991) Nutritional diseases including poisons. *Veterinary Aspects of Captive Birds of Prey*, pp. 124–142. Standfast Press, Glos.

Harper, E.J. and Skinner, N.D. (1998) Clinical nutrition of small psittacines and passerines. *Seminars in Avian and Exotic Pet Medicine*, **7**(3), 116–127.

Heuser, G.F. and Norris, L.C. (1929) Rickets in chicks III: The effectiveness of mid-summer sunshine and irradiation from a quartz mercury vapour arc in preventing rickets in chickens. *Poultry Science*, **8**, 89–98.

Kollias, G.V. and Kollias, H.W. (2000) Feeding passerine and psittacine birds. *Small Animal Clinical Nutrition* (eds M.S. Hand, C.D. Thatcher, R.L. Remillard & P. Roudebush), 4th edn, pp. 979–991. Mark Mervis Institute, Marceline, Missouri.

Nott, H.M.R. and Taylor, F.J. (1993) The energy requirements of pet birds. *Proceedings of the Association of Avian Veterinarians*, pp. 233–239.

Scott, M.L. and Norris, L.C. (1965) Vitamins and vitamin deficiencies. *Diseases of Poultry* (eds H.E. Biester & L.H. Schwarte), 5th edn. Iowa State University Press, Ames, Iowa.

Scott, P.W. (1996) Nutrition. *Manual of Psittacine Birds* (eds P.H. Beynon, N.A. Forbes & M.P.C. Lawton), pp. 17–26. BSAVA, Cheltenham, Gloucester.

Wallach, J.D. and Cooper, J.E. (1982) Nutritional diseases of wild birds. *Non-infectious Diseases of Wildlife* (eds G.L. Hoff & J.W. Davis), pp. 113–126. Iowa State University Press, Ames, Iowa.

Worrell, A. (1991) Serum iron levels in rhamphastids. *Proceedings of the Association of Avian Veterinarians*, pp. 120–130.

Further reading

Stahl, S. and Kronfield, D. (1998) Veterinary nutrition of large Psittacines. *Seminars in Avian and Exotic Pet Medicine*, 7(3), 128–134.

Chapter 13

Common Avian Diseases

Skin and feather disease

Feather plucking

Feather plucking can be one of the most complicated conditions in avian medicine to accurately diagnose and treat. The causes of feather plucking can vary tremendously. For examples, see below (Figure 13.1).

1. Ectoparasites
2. Endoparasites
3. Skin infections (bacterial, viral and fungal)
4. Iatrogenic (e.g. poor wing clip)
5. Behavioural
6. Organopathy
7. Heavy metal poisoning (lead, zinc)
8. Psittacosis
9. Salmonellosis
10. Hormonal
11. Environmental contaminant (e.g. nicotine-tainted feathers).
12. Viral diseases affecting other organs (e.g. bornavirus) (the causal agent of proventricular dilatation disease)
13. Pain
14. Hepatitis/hepatomegaly (e.g. hepatic lipidosis)
15. Atopy/allergic skin disease

Diagnosis requires a full, detailed history to be taken as well as a full health examination. A diagnosis of a behavioural condition can only be made accurate by extensive history taking and elimination of medical conditions from the picture.

Behavioural feather plucking

The most basic classification is to divide feather pluckers into two types. The first is the true feather plucker which removes the whole feather. The second is the feather chewer which just mutilates the feather but leaves it embedded in the skin. In addition, some species of Psittaciform bird such as the cockatoos may also exhibit self-mutilation of the body as well as feather plucking.

The condition is mainly seen in members of the Psittaciformes, although some of the hawk family such as Harris' Hawk are also susceptible.

Behavioural feather plucking may be diagnosed often only after the ruling out of infectious/pain causes.

Ectoparasites

Ectoparasites are not as commonly seen in cage birds as might be expected. There are, however, many important skin and feather parasites of raptors, game birds and waterfowl kept in captivity.

Mites

Knemidocoptes: They are seen mainly in the budgerigar and canary. These eat cell debris and cause the conditions known as 'scaly beak' and 'tassle foot'. The presenting signs are crusting and enlargement of the cere at the base of the beak, and thickening and proliferation of the skin of the legs. Another mite peculiar to pigeons is the depluming mite (*Knemidocoptes laevis*). This mite causes disintegration of the feather quill, causing it to break off close to the skin and producing bald areas.

Sarcoptes: Scabies mites (*Sarcoptes* spp.) are uncommonly seen, but have been reported in macaws. The symptoms are feather loss and widespread self-trauma.

Dermanyssus: The red feather mite (*Dermanyssus gallinae*) has been reported in raptor flights, pigeon lofts and in some cases, cage and aviary birds such as parrots, particularly those in outside flights. This mite does not live on the bird permanently. It hides in the cracks and crevices of the cage or shelter during the day and crawls out to attack the bird when it is roosting at night. It is a blood sucking mite and can cause anaemia and weakness in heavily parasitised birds.

Ornithonyssus: Another blood sucking mite is the northern fowl mite (*Ornithonyssus sylviarum*). This mite inhabits the host continuously, so it is easier to detect and to treat.

Veterinary Nursing of Exotic Pets, Second Edition. Edited by Simon J. Girling. © 2013 John Wiley & Sons, Ltd. Published 2013 by John Wiley & Sons, Ltd.

PART II: AVIAN SPECIES

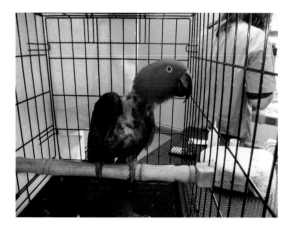

Figure 13.1 Feather plucking may have many causes.

Other mites such as the skin mites, *Backericheyla* spp. and *Neocheyletiella media* in passerine birds, and *Epidermoptes bilobatus* and *Michrolichus avus* may also cause pruritus. Quill mites such as *Dermatoglyphus* spp. and *Syringophylus* spp. may also cause pruritus, feather picking and loss.

Lice

All avian lice belong to the order Mallophaga, and so cause their damage by chewing the feathers. They are generally elongated, squeezing in between the barbs of the feathers. They are more commonly seen in outdoor-housed birds and the main route for infestation is from wild birds.

The waterfowl mite is *Holomenopon* spp. It has been associated with damage of feathers, leading to a lack of normal structure and loss of waterproofing. This causes the feathers to look bedraggled and soggy so-called 'wet feather' disease.

In pigeons, two main types of louse are seen. The body louse (*Menapon latum*) and the slender louse (*Columbicula columbae*) are seen on the wings. They cause damage to the structure of the feather, damaging the interlocking of the barbs which keep the feather's shape intact, and so give the pigeon a somewhat ragged appearance.

Raptors are prone to lice and a wide variety of species-specific lice are found. The mites destroy feather integrity and this leads to poor flight.

Flies

The blow fly family, such as the blue, black and green bottles, may be drawn to birds with diarrhoea or with wounds. The maggots of these species then eat their way into the bird with devastating results, and allow the colonisation of the wounds by smaller species of fly maggot.

The Hippoposcidae genus contains such species as the sheep and horse keds, which are however capable of infesting aviary birds, particularly raptors. The juvenile form of the fly is flightless and so spends large amounts of time living on its host. These species will often create infection and anaemia. They can also transmit blood-borne parasites, e.g. avian malaria, *Haemoproteus* spp. and *Leucocytozoan* spp., which may cause anaemia and immunosuppression. The pigeon louse fly (*Pseudolynchia canariensis*) has been associated with transmission of *Haemoproteus* spp., but also pigeon adenovirus 1 and possibly pigeon pox virus.

Mosquitoes

They have been shown to cause irritation and to act as a vector for avian malaria in penguins, as well as causing the spread of other blood parasites and viruses, such as West Nile fever eastern and western encephalitis viruses.

Gnats

Gnats can transmit blood-borne parasites such as *Leucocytozoan* spp.

Ticks

These can rapidly be fatal to birds, possibly due to the presence of a toxin in the saliva of the tick. They are seen relatively uncommon, but can occur in raptors being used for hunting, as ticks are ground dwellers. They are also common in aviary-kept birds which are overhung by surrounding trees. The ticks may be carried on wild birds and so drop-off roosts and nests into an aviary beneath. Again, they may transmit many bacteria, such as members of the Rickettsia family, as well as blood-borne parasites and viruses.

Endoparasites

The parasite *Giardia* spp. can infest cockatiels leading to internal irritation, which causes the affected bird to pluck the feathers over its flanks and ventrum. In addition, severe ascarid nematode infections have been associated with feather plucking in psittacine birds.

Viral diseases affecting the skin

Psittacine beak and feather disease

Psittacine beak and feather disease (PBFD) is caused by a member of the circovirus family. There is evidence of the presence of different strains of the virus in different species. As its name suggests, it is mainly seen in Psittaciformes, although many other orders of birds have been found to be affected. Some species may recover from infection, such as many lorikeets and lories. In many species, circoviral disease is a terminal infection. Grey parrots (*Psittacus erithacus*) are an example where two main forms of the disease are commonly seen: An acute form which is seen in juvenile birds that present with clinical anaemia and immunosuppression (and frequently aspergillosis); and a chronic form which causes increasing feather, nail and beak dystrophia, death finally occurring due to dysphagia and inanition (see Figure 13.2). In many birds, the first feathers to be affected are the powder feathers – this is more obvious in cockatoos which normally have a very dusty beak – those infected with circovirus have a shiny beak free of dust.

In Eclectus parrots and Lovebirds, early circoviral disease can present with self-mutilation making circoviral infection a differential in feather plucking. In Budgerigars, the disease is known as 'French moult', with birds from 4–5 weeks becoming depressed then showing necrosis of developing feathers. Some may die after 1–2 weeks with diarrhoea and crop stasis. Transmission of circovirus in psittacine birds is by feather dander, oral and faecal routes. In Columbiformes, a typical disease pattern occurs in young squabs between 2 months and 1 year of age. Incubation periods are 2 weeks. Clinical signs include anorexia, diarrhoea, weight loss, respiratory disease and lethargy. Death commonly occurs within 3–5 days. The disease produces immunosuppression and therefore concurrent infections are common-most, typically *Chlamydophila psittaci* or *Aspergillus* spp. infections.

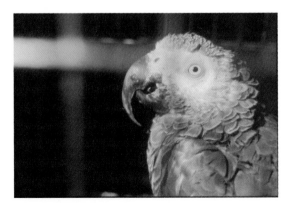

Figure 13.2 PBFD in an African grey parrot – note the overlong beak, which is splitting, and some poor feather quality.

Diagnosis is based on polymerase chain reaction (PCR) demonstration of the viral antigen in blood or feather pulp – it is advised that both are submitted as frequently one can be negative depending on the stage of the disease. Others have suggested liver biopsy in Grey parrots as this appears to be the target organ (Grund *et al.*, 2005). Alternatively, histopathology of skin biopsies can demonstrate viral inclusions and at postmortem in young birds, depletion of B lymphocytes from the Bursa of Fabricius with viral inclusions in the bursa, thymus and in the bone marrow. There is no treatment for the virus although avian gamma interferon therapy has been tried with varying degrees of success. Vaccination has been attempted, but if the bird is already infected, then vaccination has been shown to actually deteriorate the bird's condition.

Polyomavirus

Avian polyomavirus (APV) infection is common and causes systemic disease in various species of psittacine, gallinaceous, passerine and raptor birds. In budgerigars (*Melopsittacus undulatus*), it is the cause of budgerigar fledgling disease/feather duster disease. In this condition, neonates in infected flocks may die suddenly at around 10–15 days. Others may develop abdominal distension, reduced feathering and haemorrhages under the skin. Some may show neurological signs such as ataxia and tremors of the head. If infected after 15 days of age, they will often survive but develop feather abnormalities preventing flying. In juvenile finches (primarily Gouldian finches), clinical signs include weight loss, fluffed appearance, diarrhoea and dehydration. A polyomavirus has also been identified in canaries (*Serinus canaria*) with similar signs plus loss of feathers and some neurological signs. Many of these had secondary infections.

Diagnosis is based on clinical signs and PCR testing of cloacal swabs or tissues at postmortem. Testing indicates that the canary and finch strain are different (Shivaprasad *et al.*, 2009). Clinical gross postmortem and basophilic intranuclear inclusion bodies on histopathology are suggestive.

There is no treatment for this condition, although there is now a vaccine in the United States (Biomune II Psittimune®). Detecting virus DNA particles from a cloacal swab or faecal sample is the standard test.

Avipox viruses

These can occur in all avian species, although none have so far been recorded in Strigiformes. Signs include pox-like lesions, occurring predominantly on the face, eyelids, feet and cere. These become secondarily infected, and may lead to more extensive lesions. Respiratory tract disease is also seen and may cause sloughing of the lining of the trachea and smaller airways, causing asphyxiation. Transmission may occur directly from bird to bird, and by flying insect vectors. The pox virus affecting canaries is particularly virulent and may cause serious mortality in canary flocks and has been associated with lung neoplasia.

Diagnosis is based on demonstrating the classical Bollinger bodies, seen due to virus particles inside infected cells, as well as the clinical signs described.

Papillomavirus

This may lead to proliferative skin masses on the feet and legs of passerine birds and they are considered enzootic in some populations of waterfowl, Gruiformes and Ciconiiformes and may mimic mite infestations. Rarely in psittacine birds, proliferative lesions on the face and around the beak may be seen. Papillomas of the digestive tract are now thought not to be caused by a papillomavirus but rather by a herpesvirus. Diagnosis is by histopathological demonstration of intranuclear inclusion bodies. There is no treatment at present.

Bacterial disease affecting the skin

Examples include *Salmonella typhimurium* var. copenhagen joint infection of pigeons, which may then erupt as a boil visible on wing joints such as the elbow; and *Staphylococcal* spp. and *E. coli* infections of the feet of many species, which cause bumblefoot.

Bumblefoot

In raptors, it is more frequently seen in falcons. Persistent pressure on the same parts of the sole of the foot when perching restricts the blood flow to these areas. This will ultimately lead to hypoxia and death of tissues, followed by open sores and deep pedal infections. Bacteria most commonly seen such as *E. coli* and *Staphylococci* spp., but yeasts such as *Candida* spp. may also be seen in cases that have been on antibiotics for prolonged periods of time. Many categorisations for the differing stages of bumblefoot have been described, the most basic being proposed by Cooper (1985):

- Type I: This is when the injuries are restricted to smoothing of the normally papillated underside of the foot. There may or may not be the presence of a corn and sometimes a mild scab.

- Type II: This is the next stage, wherein the mild scabs become deeply infected. This condition may also be caused by the raptor puncturing its own foot with one of its claws. The bacteria involved include *Staphylococcus aureus*, *E. coli*, *Pseudomonas* spp. and occasionally yeasts.
- Type III: This is the worst lesion, with deeper structures such as bones within the toes, ligaments etc., all becoming infected. These birds are often not possible to treat. The feet are very swollen and painful and hot to the touch.

More recently, bumblefoot has been further refined in classification into five categories from the mildest at I, with early devitalisation of the plantar aspect of the foot, to severe osteomyelitis of the phalangeal bones at V (Oaks, 1993; Remple, 1993).

Fungal diseases affecting the skin

These tend to be secondary to other injuries, or skin mutilation. *Candida albicans* has been reported in lorikeets and associated with hypovitaminosis A. It has also been seen in lovebirds with feather loss around the eyes, beak and neck with scaling.

Malessezia spp. have been associated with pruritus in galahs, eclectus parrots, mynah birds and cockatiels (Reavill *et al.*, 1990).

Dermatophytosis has been recorded in Galliformes where it is known as favus, and is generally seen most commonly around the wattles and comb.

Allergic skin conditions

There is some evidence that allergic skin disease is a problem in Psittaciformes. Serological tests do not seem to be reliable in birds, but intradermal skin testing has been shown to be useful in determining allergens and has been shown to give significantly different results in feather plucking and normal birds (MacWhirter *et al.*, 1999). Codeine phosphate is used as the positive control as it gives more consistent results than histamine (Colombini *et al.*, 2001). The intradermal skin test is carried out using the skin either side of the keel over the pectoral muscles which limits the amount of allergens which can be tested for in one go and also due to the thin nature of the avian skin requires the bird to be anaesthetised with isoflurane. However, the results indicate that some feather plucking parrots do have an allergic response to allergens, such as sunflower seeds, house dust mites and *Aspergillus* spp. Hypovaccination has not been tried on any major scale but this author has had some effects with hypovaccines.

Miscellaneous diseases affecting the skin

Split keel

Split keel is commonly seen in young, overweight, hand-reared birds, particularly those which have been carelessly wing clipped. It occurs when the bird attempts to fly off a high perch, and, either due to poor wing muscling or lack of flight feathers, drops like a stone and hits the ground with force. This often splits the thin skin covering the prominent keel area and this split may become secondarily infected. This delays healing, and may necessitate the use of antimicrobials or even surgery to achieve wound healing.

Ulcerative skin disease

Ulcerative skin disease can be due to bacterial infections, for example, *Staphylococcus* spp., or may be due to fungal infections such as infection by *Aspergillus* spp. Birds most commonly affected are species such as lovebirds, cockatoos and cockatiels.

The bird traumatises the skin underneath each wing, leading to a weeping ulcerative dermatitis. The infections may be primary or secondary. Little is known about the true initial causes of this condition, although some suggestions recently have included allergic skin conditions similar to those seen in dogs.

Psittacosis/chlamydophilosis

Systemic infection with *Chlamydophila psittaci* has been implicated in some parrots with feather plucking and generally poor feather quality (Figure 13.3).

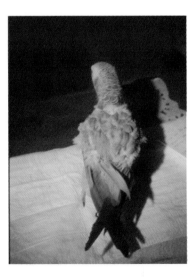

Figure 13.3 Infection with *Chlamydophila psittaci* may cause many conditions, one of which may be feather plucking as seen here.

Changes in feather colouration and structure

This may occur due to a lack of one nutrient, such as the paler colour seen in some canary breeds, for example, red factors, when deprived of vitamin A. Vitamin A in particular is required for the production of the yellow and red colouration of feathers. Other colour changes which can be seen include the following:

- Vasa parrots will develop white feathers rather than their normal grey, when they are infected with PBFD virus.
- Red colouration of the grey feathers in African grey parrots may also be seen with hepatic disease and with PBFD virus.
- Black feathers appearing in green-coloured birds such as Amazons can suggest liver disease.

Fret marks

Fret marks are another common feather abnormality seen in birds with a history of illness. These are breaks in the integrity of the feathers due to poor production of the interlocking barbs. This produces a noticeable band on all of those feathers which were growing at this time. The presence of fret marks suggests some systemic disease or malnutrition at the time the feathers were being produced, and can be a useful external indicator of a bird's recent past health, although they say nothing about its current health status.

Hormonal skin disease

Hypothyroidism has been recorded in chickens and African grey parrots. Clinical signs include slow growth and poorly coloured feathers, which often lack the interlocking barbules and so appear ragged. Diagnosis is based on the thyroid stimulating hormone (TSH) test where 1 IU/kg of TSH is administered intramuscularly after measurement of basal T4 levels. T4 levels are then measured 24 hours later, over which time a 2.5 times increase in T4 should have occurred. Failure to do so suggests hypothyrodism. It has been suggested that an underlying cause of hypothyroidism may be a dietary deficiency of iodine.

Tumours and feather cysts

The more common skin tumours include subcutaneous lipomas, and the so-called xanthoma seen particularly along the distal wings of birds (e.g. budgerigars). This is more an accumulation of fat deposits within the cells, producing a thickening of the area, and a characteristic yellow colouring of the skin.

Feather cysts are seen commonly in budgerigars and canaries (Figure 13.4). The condition occurs when a new growing feather fails to find its way through the skin surface, and so continues to grow while trapped under

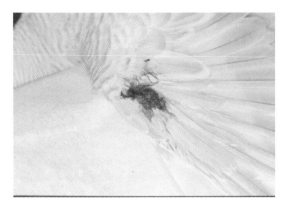

Figure 13.4 A bleeding feather cyst on the wing of a budgerigar.

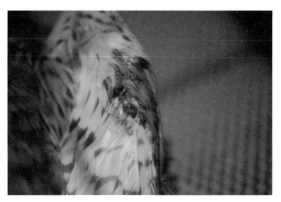

Figure 13.5 Wing tip oedema in a kestrel (*Falco tinnunculus*).

the skin. The feather cyst becomes an enlarging caseous nodule, which can ulcerate and become secondarily infected. It is thought that the condition is hereditary and the affected birds should be removed from breeding stock.

Oil spills

Sea birds and shore birds alike become coated with crude oil, making them flightless and removing their waterproofing. Many also succumb to the toxic and irritant effects of the oil itself.

Treatment is based on a number of principles which include stabilisation of the often dehydrated and malnourished bird, followed by prevention of further irritation and absorption of oil across mucous membranes, and finally removal of the oil from the pelage (feathers and skin) (Chapter 6).

Heavy metal toxicosis

Acute heavy metal (principally lead and zinc) toxicosis has been associated with neurological and renal disease in birds. However, chronic lead toxicosis in particular is also implicated in feather plucking. Older houses often have wooden surfaces that have decades of lead based paints, which parrots are adept at chewing off! Kitchen units use lead in the 'leading' of glass doors. Solder and many pewter items contain lead. Diagnosis is via blood testing – the cutoff level for lead is >0.2 ppm (20 ug/dL or 1.25 umol/dL) measured in lithium heparin whole blood. Levels >0.5 ppm (50 ug/dL or 2.6 umol/dL) are diagnostic. Some argue that as lead is not required for any bodily system function and therefore the presence of any lead is significant.

Wing tip oedema

This, as its name suggests, is seen clinically as swelling and oedema of the wing tips (carpus distally) and is most commonly associated with frostbite in raptors. It will often lead to avascular necrosis of the wing tips once the oedema has subsided if not treated quickly (see Figure 13.5).

Digestive disease

Crop

Ingluvitis

Ingluvitis is inflammation of the crop. It can be caused by an overgrowth of the yeast *Candida albicans* or bacteria such as E. coli and other Gram-negatives. *Candida albicans* infection tends to be confined to the crop and gastrointestinal tract. It is often a sequel to prolonged antibiotic therapy such as tetracycline treatment of chlamydophilosis or in neonate psittacine birds. Clinical signs usually involve regurgitation and delayed crop emptying. Diagnosis is by visualising the thickened crop lining, which has been likened to a towel surface and by demonstration of typical peanut-shaped budding yeasts. Presence of pseudohyphae indicates deeper tissue involvement and worsens the prognosis.

Ingluvitis can also be due to parasites such as *Trichomonas* spp., which are a common cause of regurgitation of seed in budgerigars and cockatiels. In pigeons and raptors, *Trichomonas* spp. cause a condition, known as 'canker' or 'frounce', which results in caseous yellow nodules at the corners of the oropharynx and the proximal oesophagus. It can however spread throughout the body and result in high levels of mortality, particularly in raptors. The feeding of wild-caught pigeons to raptors is a prime means of transmitting this particular pathogen. If a raptor owner is to feed wild-caught pigeon, then it should first be frozen for 3–4 weeks and then thoroughly defrosted before being fed, so as to kill off any *Trichomonas* spp. present. Diagnosis of the causal agent is by crop wash. The volume of crop wash saline used varies from 0.5 ml in a budgerigar up to 10 ml in a large macaw. The sample should then be examined using both Gram's stain and Diff-Quik® style dichrome stains. *Trichomonas* spp. may be difficult to pick up using this method, as it is often in the lining of the crop. Treatment has to be given on the assumption that this disease exists, once all of the other possibilities have been ruled out. Willette *et al.* (2009) describe trichomoniasis as the most clinically significant parasitic disease in birds of prey. Certain species however seem more; for example, resilient-peregrine falcons, which naturally feed on wild Columbiformes, are less likely to suffer from trichomoniasis. Conversely, Northern Goshawks (*Accipter gentilis*), gyrfalcons (*Falco rusticolus*) and barn owls (*Tyto alba*) are much more susceptible. In addition, young birds seem more susceptible.

Bacterial infections causing ingluvitis due to *E. coli*, *Pseudomonas* spp. and *Aeromonas* spp. are also not uncommon, particularly in juvenile birds and neonates.

Sour crop

Sour crop in Psittaciformes is associated with juvenile birds. It occurs when the contents of the crop ferment, producing a foul-smelling acidic environment. This condition may be life-threatening. In raptors, it may be associated with overconsumption of food. The crop has a neutral pH and so if food is present for too long a period of time it can ferment and go off leading to sour crop.

Crop impaction

Crop impaction occurs in juvenile birds that may overeat. Some may occur due to poor motility associated with neurological conditions such as lead poisoning or proventricular dilatation disease. Alternatively, they may eat the floor covering, and, if this is composed of shavings or sawdust, impaction may occur (this is particularly common in pheasants and other young game birds).

Capillariasis

Capillariasis is the name given to the infestation of the crop lining with the nematode *Capillaria* spp. This is mainly a problem for pigeons and raptors, but is also seen in Passeriformes (e.g. finches and canaries), as well as species of Galliformes (e.g. pheasants and grouse). It is much rarer in Psittaciformes.

Clinically, raptors flick their head from side to side when eating, and will regurgitate. In pigeons, acute infections are associated with high mortality because of intense vomiting. In cases of capillariasis, characteristic bipolar eggs may be seen in the faeces. The life cycle is often indirect and may involve earthworms.

The parasite *Streptocara* spp. have been associated with oesophageal damage in waterfowl similar to that caused by *Capillaria* spp. in other birds.

Crop burns

These are frequently seen in hand-reared Psittaciformes. They occur when the owner has fed the juvenile bird a rearing formula porridge that has been microwaved and not thoroughly stirred and allowed to stand resulting in 'hot spots' within the mixture, which will cause local burns. These can be full thickness, causing the skin to slough after 7–10 days.

Foreign bodies

Many larger Psittaciformes may consume foreign objects, which become lodged in the crop and may cause irritation, retching, and may lacerate the thin crop lining. Retrieval of the object via endoscopic examination under anaesthesia is advised, with repair of any lacerations.

Associated crop disorders

The lack of iodine in an all seed diet will cause thyroid gland enlargement (goitre). This enlarged gland will press on the crop and proximal oesophagus, so limiting its ability to empty and fill. Often seen in budgerigars, they will adopt a horizontal posture lying across the perch with the head slightly raised. There is frequent intermittent regurgitation of seed.

Proventriculus

Proventriculitis

Inflammation of the true stomach (proventriculus) can be caused by the yeasts *Candida* spp. and *Macrorhabdus ornithogaster* (formerly known as 'Megabacteria'). Signs can include the vomiting of food, the passing of undigested seed in the faeces, and in the case of Psittaciformes, anorexia, diarrhoea and weight loss.

In budgerigars, the incidence of *Macrorhabdus ornithogaster* infection is relatively high. Many birds are carriers with no clinical signs, but a percentage of a flock will show a 'going light' syndrome. They will eat voraciously, but lose weight, often passing undigested seed in their faeces. Diagnosis is by finding the typical bacillus-like Gram-positive chains of the yeast in faeces.

'Megabacteriosis' is seen in a wide host of other species including finches, canaries, parrotlets, cockatiels, lovebirds, ostriches and domestic poultry (ducks, chickens, turkeys and geese).

Proventricular dilatation disease

Proventricular dilatation disease (PDD) has been reported in over 50 species of psittacine and nonpsittacine birds. It was first reported in Macaws (aka 'Macaw wasting disease') and its current name is derived from the lymphoplasmacytic ganglioneuritis, which damages the nerves supplying the proventriculus resulting in progressive muscular flaccidity leading to a maldigestion syndrome, starvation and eventually death (see Figures 13.6 and 13.7). The disease appears to be able to affect the central nervous system as well as the myenteric and so

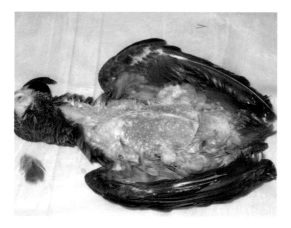

Figure 13.6 Severe emaciation and death is the clinical outcome of proventricular dilatation syndrome (breast feathers have been manually removed to show extent of weight loss).

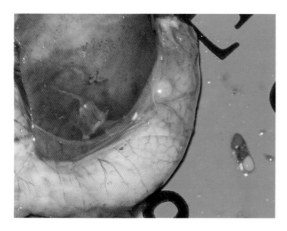

Figure 13.7 An enlarged proventriculus (cream structure curving around the darker liver) is seen on examination.

affected birds may show signs of ataxia, nervous tremors, central blindness, fitting and torticollis (Steinmetz *et al.*, 2008). The median age of onset appears to be 3–4 years but has been reported as early as 5 weeks of age and as old as 17 years (Phalen, 2006a; Smith, 2009).

The virus is an avian Bornavirus (Gancz *et al.*, 2009; Gray *et al.*, 2009; Shivaprasad *et al.*, 2009) with Koch's postulates being fulfilled in the cockatiel (*Nymphicus hollandicus)* (Hoppes *et al.*, 2010) and Patagonian Conures (Gray *et al.*, 2010). They cause most of the clinical signs by stimulating the body's own immune system. Multi-bird households have a significantly higher incidence of infection with avian Bornavirus than single bird households (71.4% versus 51.3%). Infection may be associated with higher incidences of feather plucking (76% of positive cases showed plucking behaviour) (Zantop, 2010). Transmission is suspected to be faeco-oral but respiratory transmission is also suspected (Perpinan *et al.*, 2007). Incubation period may be rapid as witnessed by the young age of some cases, but may also take up to 7 years to manifest itself.

Definitive diagnosis is difficult. Clinically, the disease has been diagnosed based on histopathology of a proventricular or crop biopsy. Diagnosis by crop biopsy is less accurate ([66–76%] Doolen, 1994; Gregory *et al.*, 1996); although trying to ensure a blood vessel is incorporated to increase the likelihood of sectioning a nerve increases the chances of success. Proventricular biopsy although more accurate is more challenging due to the risk of postoperative coelomitis. Other supportive diagnostic tests include positive contrast radiography demonstrating a dilated proventriculus and displacement of the ventriculus to the right side with prolonged emptying times. These signs may be mimicked by other disease such as neoplasia, foreign bodies and heavy metal poisoning. PCR serology and crop biopsy have so far showed a poor correlation between the three (Clubb & De Kloet, 2010). Villaneuva *et al.* (2010) have shown that western-blotting techniques to test for antibodies to avian Bornavirus was effective; however, of the 117 psittacine birds detected as positive, only 30 could be confirmed on histopathology suggesting that subclinical carriers of avian Bornavirus are common. The same study also showed that many seronegative birds also were positive on detected antigen in faeces by PCR again showing further discrepancies.

Proventricular/ventricular impaction

If insoluble grit is fed, the grit builds up can block the gizzard. Other causes of impaction are seen in juvenile cockatoos (*Cacatua* spp.) and African grey parrots

(*Psittacus erithacus*), which often compulsively ingest items in their environment such as fragments of wood, plastic etc. These birds present as vaguely unwell, losing condition, rarely with vomiting although recurrent bacterial enteritis has been reported (Speer, 1998).

Endoparasites

Helminths

Ascaridia *spp:* Ascarids are commonly seen in cage and aviary birds, particularly those that have a deep litter or earth floor to their aviary, as this allows maturation of any worm eggs that are passed in the faeces. Species seen include *Ascaridia platycerci* (psittacine birds), *A. hermaphrodita* (in a Hyacinth macaw), *A. columbae* (found in psittacine birds and Columbiformes), *A. columbae* (Columbiformes) and *A. galli* (found in Galliformes and psittacine birds).

Infected individuals may show no external signs, but if parasitised heavily enough they may lose weight, have diarrhoea or, in severe cases, may experience intestinal blockage and death. Ascarids have a direct life cycle. This means that the eggs passed in the faeces of an infected bird, after a few days, can be directly infectious to another bird without having to be taken up by an intermediate host. Diagnosis is made by finding the thick-walled eggs in the faeces of the affected bird.

Capillaria *spp:* In pigeons, *Capillaria obsignata* burrows into the lining of the intestine where it can cause severe diarrhoea and regurgitation, often with fatal consequences. Diagnosis is by demonstrating the presence of the bioperculate eggs in the faeces or regurgitated material produced by the infected bird. Its life cycle is direct, as with the ascarid family.

Other digestive system worms seen in birds

Other species of worm found in the digestive system are largely nematodes and include *Ornithostrongylus quadriradiatus* which is found in the intestine of pigeons. It is a blood-sucking worm, similar to the hookworms. Its eggs are thin walled and more spherical than the *Capillaria* spp. eggs.

Waterfowl: There are many different species of nematode worms. *Echinuria* spp. cause a high mortality rate in young ducks and swans. It is transmitted via the intermediate host *Daphnia* spp., the water flea. It can produce tumour-like lumps in the lining of the proventriculus and gizzard, which may lead to partial blockage of these organs.

Epomidostomum and *Amidostomum* spp. which infest the gizzard of geese, cause bleeding into the lumen, diarrhoea, enteritis and weight loss. In young birds, it causes growth retardation and even death.

Game birds: Heterakis isolonche is a significant cause of mortality in young pheasants, causing severe damage to the caecal lining. In many Galliformes, such as turkeys and chickens, this worm carries another pathogen with it – *Histomonas meleagriditis,* a single-celled protozoan parasite that can cause significant focal liver necrosis, giving the disease its name of black spot.

Corvids and thrushes: Porrocaecum spp. have been associated with weight loss and intestinal/stomach granulomas.

Non-helminth digestive system parasites

Motile protozoan parasites: Giardia psittaci are commonly found in cockatiels and budgerigars. Signs of the disease vary, and in the case of the cockatiel, it has been associated with a deficiency in vitamin E, producing feather plucking.

Diagnosis is by finding the parasites on faecal smears. The sample is suspended in saline and examined using the x400 microscope lens. The sample must be fresh, as the parasite disintegrates rapidly once the faeces dry. When fresh, movement of the organism which has eight flagellae can be observed.

Hexamita spp. are commonly found in pigeons. It produces weight loss and diarrhoea. It is seen in young birds towards the end of the breeding season when environmental contamination is high. Diagnosis is by finding large numbers of the motile, eight-flagellae-bearing, elongated protozoa using the x400 microscope lens on a slide of fresh faeces suspended in saline.

Trichomonas spp. may affect the intestines as well as the crop.

Cochlosoma spp. are a flagellate single-celled protozoal parasite, which has been associated with widespread mortalities in Australian finches. It causes diarrhoea, dehydration and moulting abnormalities particularly in birds between 10 days and 6 weeks of age.

Coccidiosis: Eimeria spp. infest many species, from pigeons and cage birds to Galliformes and waterfowl. They contribute to the 'going light' syndrome where the bird loses condition. In pigeons, heavy burdens of *E. columbarum* and *E. labbeana* may affect racing performance. Clinical signs may appear before oocysts are detected in the faeces. In canaries, *Isospora canaria* affects canaries of

2 months of age and older producing diarrhoea and emaciation, primarily damaging the duodenum which may be oedematous at postmortem. In hill mynah birds, *Eimeria* spp. have been associated with haemorrhagic enteritis.

Caryospora spp. cause crop and intestinal damage. There is often high mortality in young birds, with adults exhibiting abdominal discomfort. There are over seven species of *Caryospora* known to affect birds of prey, the two most commonly seen in captivity being *C. falconis* and *C. neofalconis* (Forbes and Simpson, 1997; Heidenreich, 1997). Transmission is by direct means although there is evidence that rodent prey can act as a heteroxenous host. Clinical signs include general debility, diarrhoea, weight loss and anorexia and are most commonly seen in young raptors between 3 and 6 months of age. The parasite sexually reproduces in the gut, but encysted forms can be found in the muscle and central nervous system, and result in an encephalitis with neurological signs such as torticollis. Merlins (*Falco columbarius*) appear particularly susceptible with sudden death occurring. Diagnosis can be made on clinical signs and the presence of huge numbers of oocysts in the faeces with a typical single sporocyst with eight sporozoites within it.

In canaries and other Passeriformes, *Atoxoplasma* spp. may be found. It spreads from the gut into the mononuclear white blood cells and is carried through the bloodstream affecting organs such as the liver, resulting in hepatomegaly known as 'black spot' because it is visible through the thin skin of the canary's abdomen. Diarrhoea or death may be seen, but the disease may be asymptomatic.

Diagnosis of coccidiosis is by finding the oval to round oocysts in the bird's faeces using sugar flotation methods, or by direct smear of the liver.

Cryptosporidium *spp:* This coccidian organism appears to be able to infect any epithelial surface and so has been reported in the gastrointestinal, respiratory and urinary tracts. It has a direct life cycle and the transmission route is faeco-oral, in food (other avian prey) or by respiratory aerosol. In psittacine birds, the proventricular form is the most commonly observed, with birds co-infected with *Macrorhabdus ornithigaster* being most likely to die (Messenger & Garner, 2010).

Bacterial gastrointestinal disease

Bacteria such as *E. coli*, *Campylobacter* spp., *Clostridium* spp., *Pseudomonas* spp., *Salmonella* spp., *Yersinia* spp. and *Chlamydophila psittaci* may all cause diarrhoea and even toxaemia, septicaemia and death. *Salmonella* spp. may be particularly difficult to treat as the bacteria become entrenched in the lining of the intestines. The main salmonellae seen in birds are *Salmonella typhimurium* and *S. arizonae*. Clinical signs resemble those seen in yersiniosis but are generally more chronic. However, significant mortality can occur, particularly in finches and other small passerine birds. In pigeons, *S. typhimurium* var. *Copenhagen* typically produces swollen joints, especially on the wings referred to as 'boils' by pigeon racers and fanciers. In addition, weakness, lethargy, green urates, diarrhoea and death of young hatchlings may all point to a salmonella problem. In pigeons, after paramyxovirus 1, salmonellosis is the next most common cause of neurological signs and may also mimic mycobacterial disease when infecting bones. Culture and sensitivity testing using specific *Salmonella* spp. culture medium should always be performed on avian faecal samples in cases of diarrhoea and weight loss. *Escherichia coli* are generally absent from the intestines of passerine and psittacine birds (Dorrestein, 2009), but are typically found in 97% of all pigeon intestinal tracts (Harlin & Wade, 2009). Clinical signs of *E. coli* infection include diarrhoea and sudden death, and may be associated with epizootic mortalities in imported finches. *Clostridium* spp. have been associated with gastrointestinal disease and death of a wide range of birds. They may be found in the gastrointestinal tract of many species notably raptors. *Clostridium perfringens* is considered a normal part of the flora of a raptors digestive system. However, as with clostridial bacteria in rabbits, overgrowth may occur in poor conditioned birds resulting in enterotoxaemia. In addition, food spoiled by clostridial toxins will result in rapid death of the raptor.

In addition, the mycobacterium *Mycobacterium avium*, the cause of avian tuberculosis, is often seen in waterfowl and raptors. It inhabits the gut and associated organs and is thus spread via the faecal–oral route. It is often implicated in chronic wasting diseases, and produces classical caseous nodules throughout the gut. Diagnosis is made on Ziehl–Neilsen stains demonstrating the acid-fast bacteria, and bacterial culture of the faeces. It is not treatable and, as it is a zoonotic disease, affected birds should be euthanased.

Viral gastrointestinal disease
Duck plague virus
The duck plague virus is a member of the alpha herpesvirus family. It affects both ducks and geese. It is spread in the faeces and oral secretions and may be carried latently with

no clinical disease, or can cause death with no premonitory signs. Alternatively, it may cause violent diarrhoea, anorexia and neurological tremors. It can be associated with mass outbreaks in ducks. Death usually occurs within 3–12 days of infection, and 1–10 days after developing clinical signs. Diagnosis is made on the clinical signs and isolation of the virus from faeces, or on demonstration of intranuclear inclusion bodies in the gut wall on postmortem.

Avian papillomatosis

This condition is thought to be due to a herpesvirus. It occurs in members of the Psittaciformes family causing papillomas throughout the digestive system frequently in the cloaca. In the cloaca, it often leads to irritation and eversion or even prolapse due to repeated straining. Other clinical signs include regurgitation, recurrent bouts of enteritis, passage of blood in the faeces and infertility. Papillomatosis is also linked with a high incidence of liver and pancreatic cancer in affected birds.

Diagnosis is made in the live bird by visualising the papillomas aided by applying 5% acetic acid to the lesion, which will cause the papillomas to turn white while normal mucosal folds will remain pink.

Liver disease
Haemochromatosis

Haemochromatosis is where excessive amounts of iron are deposited in the liver. Birds affected are commonly members of the toucan, toucanette, mynah and starling families. In the wild, these species often live in iron poor soil areas, and their digestive systems are therefore adapted to absorb as much iron as possible. When presented with an iron-rich diet, high levels of vitamin C (which encourages iron absorption from the gut), too much iron is absorbed. This iron is then deposited in the liver, leading to damage and failure.

Clinical signs include ascites, dullness, dyspnoea (due to the ascites pressing on the air sacs), abdominal swelling and sudden death. Diagnosis is based on species, clinical signs, and liver biopsy to assess iron levels. This can be a dangerous procedure, particularly if the bird has ascites. There is then a real danger of rupturing air sacs and drowning the bird.

Avian tuberculosis (*Mycobacterium avium* infection)

Avian tuberculosis may produce liver disease, causing classical caseous nodules throughout the structure, and is also associated with intestinal disease.

Other liver bacterial diseases

Any bacteria, such as *Salmonella* spp., *E. coli* and *Pseudomonas* spp., which breaches the gut wall may affect the liver directly via the enterohepatic circulation. In addition, the pansystemic infection of *Chlamydophila psittaci* will cause hepatitis manifested, as with so many hepatic disorders, by green-to-yellow coloured urates. Diagnosis is based on clinical signs, biochemistry and isolation of the bacteria from the gastrointestinal tract and, if possible, from hepatic swabs.

Viral liver diseases

Psittacid herpesvirus isolates 1, 2 and 3 have been recorded, all of which can cause 'Pacheco's disease' in psittacine birds. Old World psittacine birds appear more resistant to infection than New World ones with Amazon parrots and conures being considered the most susceptible. Clinical signs may be sudden death for New World birds, or a more prolonged course of depression, anorexia, regurgitation and green diarrhoea before death in more resistant species. Occasionally, haemorrhagic diarrhoea may be seen. Some cockatoos have been reported as surviving infection (although probably remain persistently infected). Transmission appears to be in oropharyngeal secretions and faeces. At postmortem, the liver is often bronze in colour and enlarged. The kidneys may also be enlarged and the intestines and brain congested. Intranuclear inclusion bodies (Cowdry type A) with hepatocellular necrosis are suggestive. Diagnosis can also be made using PCR technology on cloacal or oropharyngeal swabs. A vaccine is available in the United States.

Raptor herpesviruses: Currently have three distinct isolates: Falconid herpesvirus 1 (FHV1); strigid herpesvirus 1 (SHV1) and accipitrid herpesvirus 1 (AHV1). All cause hepatitis and splenitis with typical herpesvirus inclusion bodies. Wernery and Kinne (2004) suggest that transmission is via the ocular/intranasal route in falcons.

Falconid herpes virus: This virus affects Falconidae and occurs mainly in Europe and the Middle East. It is usually fatal, particularly in gyrfalcons and causes liver and spleen swelling and necrosis, bone marrow necrosis and gut inflammation with haemorrhage. It is transmitted directly from bird to bird and via prey items.

Strigid (Owl) herpes virus: This virus causes liver, spleen and bone marrow necrosis and is specific to the owl family. It is invariably fatal within 3–9 days. Yellow nodules may be found in the gut and the pharyngeal mucosa. It is spread in urine and faeces, as well as respiratory secretions. Some birds that survive will remain latently infected. There is no treatment or vaccine available.

Pigeon herpesvirus: This can cause a mild pharyngitis/oesophagitis with cellular necrosis in young birds. Older birds are frequently immune but remain persistent carriers. Anorexia, regurgitation and sometimes neurological signs in conjunction with green urates are suggestive. Inclusion body hepatitis can be seen on biopsy of affected livers.

Duck viral hepatitis: Duck viral hepatitis affects chiefly young ducklings under 3 weeks of age and is caused by a member of the Picornaviridae. It is rapidly fatal and produces severe liver damage and haemorrhage from the liver surface.

Avian reovirus: Not all are pathogenic but some can cause significant disease particularly in budgerigars and Grey parrots. High mortalities have been reported in the United Kingdom in budgerigar flocks (Manvell *et al.*, 2004; Pennycott, 2004). Clinical signs include anorexia, fluffed up appearance, dyspnoea, nasal discharge, diarrhoea and sudden death. Postmortem reveals hepatitis, nephritis, serositis with ascites, pneumonia and splenitis with subcutaneous haemorrhages. There is often lymphoplasmacytic infiltrates of various organs, haemosiderosis, haemorrhage and fibrin deposition. Infections are commonly associated with other pathogens such as *C. psittaci*, adenovirus and *M. ornithogaster* infections.

Avian leukosis/sarcoma virus: This family group of viruses is known to induce a tissue borne leukaemia in Psittaciformes, Galliformes and Passeriformes (such as the canary). It destroys the liver and kidneys, which become infiltrated by rapidly dividing lymphocytes. Hen birds seem more susceptible than cock birds, and it is shed in the faeces, oral/respiratory secretions and semen. It is also passed in genetic material from mother to young in the egg. Clinical signs include hepato- and renalomegaly, ascites, respiratory distress, weight loss, green coloured urates, polydipsia and polyuria. There is no treatment.

Hepatic lipidosis

Hepatic lipidosis is usually diet related. High fat diets (such as the all-seed diets so beloved of Psittaciformes) and lack of exercise lead to obesity and fat deposition in the liver cells or hepatocytes. Liver function suffers as a consequence. This condition may also be seen in raptors

that are not working, but are still being well fed. Affected birds are often sleek, plump birds, which then become dull and lethargic, and may exhibit signs varying from ascites, to respiratory distress and clotting defects.

Toxic liver conditions

Toxins from a number of sources may cause hepatic damage in the avian patient. These include the heavy metal toxicoses such as lead and zinc poisoning. It may also include other metals such as copper, chromium and mercury.

Lead poisoning: Lead poisoning is frequently seen in waterfowl, which have inadvertently eaten lead shot from hunting or fishing. Psittaciformes may also be affected, as they will consume or destroy many household items that contain lead. These include

- Lead window effects on kitchen units
- Lead weights in curtains or blind drawer cords
- Lead in the foil used for wine bottles
- Metallic cloths used for sanding/polishing metals
- Lead paints in older houses
  Clinical signs include
- Weakness (S-shaped neck of the swan)
- Lethargy, vomiting, passage of blood in the faeces (very common in Psittaciformes)
- Passage of lime green faeces (very common in raptors)
- Chronic non-regenerative anaemia
- Seizures
- Kidney and liver damage
- Death
  Diagnosis is by finding blood lead levels in excess of 0.2 ppm (12.5 mmol/L). Those in excess of 0.4–0.6 ppm (25–37.5 mmol/L) are diagnostic. In addition, radiography will often show lead particles as radiodense areas in the proventriculus and ventriculus.

Zinc poisoning: It is mainly seen in Psittaciformes shortly after they have been moved into a new cage ('new wire cage disease'). Occasionally, the finish of these cages is of a poor quality and a fine powder of zinc oxide forms the surface of the wires. The parrot manoeuvres itself around the cage with feet and beak, and takes in small volumes of this powder on a daily basis. After 4–6 weeks, liver and kidney damage will occur, and the bird may present weak, lethargic, having seizures and with anaemia. Other sources of zinc include some forms of coin, some plastics and other alloys. Diagnosis is made on clinical signs, history and finding zinc blood levels above 2 ppm (2000 mg/L).

Other poisons affecting the liver: Aflatoxins released by *Aspergillus* spp., are known to be hepatotoxic and carcinogenic, as are the organic poisons found in rapeseed, ragwort and the castor bean. Treatment is rarely possible.

Pancreatic disease

Diabetes mellitus is a common condition in budgerigars and cockatiels. It may be hereditary, although pancreatitis can result in the development of this disease.

Clinical signs include polydipsia and polyuria, often with dramatic weight loss despite a healthy appetite.

Diagnosis is made on the clinical signs in conjunction with persistently raised blood glucose (often above 25 mmol/L up to 44 mmol/L). Some glucose may be found in the urine normally, but high levels (>1%) are strongly suggestive of disease.

Pancreatitis can be seen in birds. It has been linked with infections due to Paramyxovirus III (e.g. cockatiels). The passage of partially digested seed or pasty tan coloured faeces may be seen combined with weight loss.

Respiratory disease
Upper respiratory tract
Nostrils

Clinically often feathers are stained just above the nares, and there may be sneezing and head flicking due to the discharge.

Rhinoliths, concretions of dried secretions that form a ball of solid material blocking the entrance to the nasal passages, may be caused by dietary insufficiencies such as hypovitaminosis A, and/or may involve local or deeper infections due to bacteria such as *Mycoplasma* spp. (e.g., pigeons), or *Chlamydophila psittaci* (e.g. Psittaciformes).

Fungi, such as *Aspergillus* spp., or viruses, such as the avipox virus group, are also the causes. The mite *Knemidocoptes* spp. may also contribute to the blockage of the nostrils (e.g. Psittaciformes and raptors).

Some species of parrot, such as Amazons, are susceptible to nasal irritation in dry environments, and in the presence of feather dander, produced by African grey parrots and cockatoos.

A congenital defect is the absence of a patent internal choanal slit. This prevents the normal nasal secretions from draining ventrally into the oropharynx. The secretions then present as a clear nasal discharge.

Theromyzon tessulatum is the duck nasal leech and is a common parasite. It may lead to secondary infections of the nasal passages.

Pigeon herpesvirus (PHV) affects young (<6 months) pigeons. It causes a nasal discharge, sneezing and necrotic plaques to form inside the mouth and upper airways. It may also cause the cere to become discoloured and crusty. In severe cases death may occur. There is no specific treatment or vaccine available, although many will survive.

Sinusitis may be seen in conjunction with rhinoliths and nasal discharges. It may be visible as a swelling on the face, often ventral to the eye in the area of the infraorbital sinus.

Lower respiratory tract
Trachea

Gape worm infection: *Syngamus trachea* is found in Galliformes, pigeons and raptors (e.g. buzzards). This parasite uses the earthworm as its intermediate host before finally maturing in the windpipe of the afflicted bird. There it causes irritation and secondary infection, and may be present in sufficient numbers to suffocate the bird. Diagnosis is made by finding the characteristic Y-shaped worms (the male and female worms are permanently joined in copulation!) in the mucus of the mouth and trachea.

Avipox virus: In Amazon parrots, a severe form of avipox virus may cause the sloughing of the lining of the windpipe, resulting in dyspnoea, pneumonia and even death from secondary infection. All avipox viruses cause pox lesions on the face, particularly around the eyes and mouth, the pharynx and trachea, but may also produce lesions on the feet. Secondary infections are common. In pigeons there are vaccines available. Diagnosis is confirmed by finding the characteristic Bollinger bodies that are the reproductive centres of virus replication within the host cells.

Aspergillosis: The fungus *Aspergillus* spp., can produce a growth that blocks the windpipe in a matter of days (see Figure 13.8). This condition is particularly common in raptors and many Psittaciformes such as African grey parrots. Diagnosis is discussed below.

Air sac mites: Air sac mites, *Sternostoma tracheacolum*, are common in Passeriformes such as canaries, Lady Gouldian finches and goldfinches where they prefer the trachea and bronchi, and cause dyspnoea. The mites may be seen if the feathers of the neck region are wetted and a bright, cold light is shone from behind the bird. The mites are silhouetted as dark pinheads within the trachea. Another form of air sac mite, known as *Cytodites nudus*, is seen in waterfowl, and produces dyspnoea often with a cough.

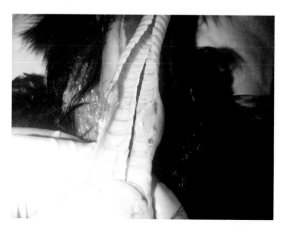

Figure 13.8 An aspergilloma growing in the trachea of this raptor resulted in asphyxiation and its death.

Avian cholera: This is a disease of waterfowl caused by the bacterium *Pasteurella multocida*. It causes a thick mucoid discharge from the mouth and trachea, dyspnoea and often death in young birds. A related bacterium, *Reimerella (Pasteurella) anatipestifer,* will cause tracheal and upper airway discharge in ducklings and a condition known as duck septicaemia. It is a common cause of mortality.

Lungs and air sacs

The absence of a diaphragm in avian species means that any disease causing fluid retention or production, such as liver damage, has the potential to affect breathing. This is particularly so when a thin-walled air sac ruptures and allows fluid to access the respiratory system. The bird may then become suddenly severely dyspnoeic.

Chlamydophila psittaci infection: This bacterium produces the condition chlamydophilosis, also known as ornithosis and psittacosis.

Psittacosis refers to the condition in Psittaciformes, ornithosis to the condition in other avian species and chlamydophilosis may be applied to both. The bacterium is of great significance first because of its widespread presence, particularly in the smaller species such as cockatiels and budgerigars, and secondly because birds may act as carriers of the bacteria for months to years without necessarily showing any signs of disease. They may shed the bacterium into their faeces and oral secretions intermittently, which can make detection of carriers difficult.

The disease is spread via faecal, oral and respiratory secretions and feather dander, and different strains of the bacteria affect different species of bird. Not all strains are as potent, either to the bird or to human.

Pigeons are commonly affected by chlamydophilosis showing persistent conjunctivitis and sneezing. Conversely, in species such as the macaw family, the first sign of psittacosis may be death! The strain of *C. psittaci* seen in Psittaciformes is more virulent and more zoonotic than the strains seen in pigeons, waterfowl and other species.

C. psittaci can infect almost every internal organ, including the spleen, the liver and the kidneys. It has also been reported as a cause of otitis media, meningoencephalitis and bursitis. It would be more accurate therefore, in species such as the Psittaciformes, to consider chlamydophilosis as a systemic disease with respiratory symptoms.

Diagnosis of chlamydophilosis

Because of the intermittent shedding of the bacteria into the environment that frequently occurs in carrier status individuals no one diagnostic technique is 100% accurate. Radiography and white blood cell counts are useful, as infected Psittaciformes often have marked enlarged spleens on radiography and white blood cell counts in excess of 30×10^9/L, if infected.

The standard test is the PCR used to detect the bacteria in droppings, or, on postmortem, from internal organs. Due to intermittent shedding, faecal testing may not pick up all cases but collecting droppings over 3–5 days helps to minimise false negatives.

The Immunocomb® test (Biogal Labs) detects antibodies (Ig$_Y$) produced by the bird's immune system, and so is beneficial in testing birds which may be carriers of the disease and not shedding it into the environment. The disadvantage of the test is that the bird may not be currently infected, and yet still have antibodies against the disease if it was infected in the past.

Chlamydophilosis is a zoonosis: All humans are susceptible, but those most at risk include
- The very young
- The very old
- Those on immunosuppressive medication (e.g. corticosteroids, chemotherapy)
- Those with immunosuppressive diseases (e.g. diabetes mellitus, AIDS).

If the owner falls into one of these categories, then serious thought should be given to rehoming or even euthanasing the bird.

In a pet shop situation, where the public are at risk, the affected livestock must be removed from public areas into a specific quarantine area. All handlers of birds during the treatment period should wear face masks and protective clothing when in the same air space as the birds. Faeces should be incinerated.

The owner should also be informed of the symptoms of chlamydophilosis in humans, and advised to contact his or her doctor immediately to receive testing or medication if any of these occur.

The symptoms of chlamydophilosis in humans include all or some of the following:

- A dry, non-productive cough
- 'Flu-like muscle pains and fever
- Migraines
- Kidney and liver damage
- Dyspnoea
- Heart damage
- Occasionally death

Despite all of these problems, chlamydophilosis is not a notifiable disease unless it is diagnosed in domestic poultry. This does not, however, diminish the veterinary surgeon's responsibility under Health and Safety guidelines to ensure that all staff, as well as owners, are aware of the risks and health hazards, and that all precautions are taken to ensure adequate protection of staff dealing with the infected birds.

Veterinary nurses and technicians are equally obliged to follow practice protocols and health and safety procedures, when dealing with positive cases.

Aspergillosis: This is the fungal condition caused by *Aspergillus* spp., frequently *Aspergillus fumigatus*. This is an environmental contaminant and so any bird may be affected. It is not infectious from one bird to another. Certain environments will contain more airborne microscopic spores of this fungus. These include areas near rotting vegetation, which includes the bottom of a parrot cage which has not been cleaned out recently!

Certain species are very susceptible, including most raptors (e.g. gyrfalcons, golden eagles, Northern Goshawk and snowy owls), penguins (e.g. Gentoo and King) are extremely susceptible. In Psittaciformes, all species can suffer from this condition, but African grey parrots are more likely.

Younger birds are more commonly affected than adults. Aspergillosis may also be seen in birds that are immunosuppressed due to concurrent illness, or immunosuppressive medication (e.g. corticosteroids).

The fungal spores settle out on the surface of the respiratory tract, particularly in the region of the syrinx, the abdominal air sacs and the lung structure itself. This can lead to blockage of the airway in the case of the syrinx, or it can lead to the production of large balls of fungus, known as 'fungal granulomas', within the air sacs.

The fungus progressively blocks airways leading to dyspnoea and death through asphyxiation, or it invades the bloodstream and is transported to other organs, such as the liver, kidneys and central nervous system.

Aspergillus spp. can also produce a toxin known as aflatoxin. This is highly toxic to birds and rapidly causes liver damage, failure and death. In addition, a gliatoxin may also be released causing central nervous system damage with paresis, fitting and other neurological signs being observed.

There is some evidence to suggest that due to its important role in cellular turnover of the airway linings and local immunity, hypovitaminosis A may play a part in the disease.

Diagnosis of aspergillosis

Full blood cell counts are useful as the condition will often cause a markedly elevated white blood cell count ($>30 \times 10^9$/L). Radiographs are useful to show thickening of the air sacs, and any fungal granulomas within them.

Rigid endoscopy is frequently essential to examine the syrinx and the internal air sacs allowing sampling for culture.

Tracheal and lung washes may be performed with sterile saline (0.5–1 mL/kg of bird) flushed into the trachea of the anaesthetised bird, and then immediately aspirated.

Recent work has confirmed the difficulty in diagnosing aspergillosis: Antibody results can be positive in birds not currently infected with aspergillosis and negative due to anergic responses; *Aspergillus* galactomannan tests used in humans for invasive aspergillosis can also produce positive results in noninfected birds although confirmed cases had 2.6 times the levels than presumptive healthy birds; derangements in the plasma protein electrophoresis trace however were 2.4 times more likely in positive cases than healthy ones with specific elevations of beta and gamma globulins (Cray *et al.*, 2009, 2010). Girling (2002) describes typical plasma protein electrophoresis responses to aspergillosis in a number of psittacine species. Variations in response are dependent on species and sexual maturity includes the following: *Ara* spp. produced a significantly higher alpha-1 globulin level when infected compared with other psittacines, whereas *Psittacus* spp. and *Amazona* spp. produced a higher alpha-2 globulin response; elevations in beta globulins were significant in cases of aspergillosis and across the species elevations above 3.5 times normal were considered significant indicator of aspergillosis.

Paramyxovirus/Newcastle disease: This is a condition seen primarily in pigeons, and is important, as Newcastle disease and paramyxovirus-1 (PMV-1) are notifiable due to their ability to cause mortality and debility in commercial poultry.

Symptoms of paramyxovirus disease may include:

- Dyspnoea
- Tachypnoea
- Periocular oedema
- Listlessness and neurological signs, e.g. wing drooping
- Head tilt and circling (torticollis)
- Sudden death

The virus is thought to be transmitted via droppings. Diagnosis is based on the symptoms and confirmation is made using viral haemagglutination inhibition tests.

Other paramyxoviruses have been recorded with serotype 5 being seen in the 1970s in budgerigars manifested by depression, diarrhoea and high mortality. Paramyxovirus serotype 3 has been reported in small psittacines more recently causing torticollis and circling (Jung *et al.*, 2009).

Influenza virus disease: Avian influenza viruses are all of type A, enveloped single stranded RNA viruses belonging to the orthomyxoviridae family and have high genetic variability. They are classified according to the properties of the envelope haemagglutinin (HA) and neuraminidase (NA) glycoproteins. They are also classified according to their pathogenicity (high [HPAI] and low [LPAI] pathogenic). All known HPAI are of the H5 or H7 subtype (although not all H5 and H7 strains are HPAI). Clinical signs of influenza A virus infection vary between different influenza A strains and different avian species. In HPAI virus infection (e.g. H5N1), widespread mortality in domestic poultry with peracute deaths is reported. However, it is possible for certain breeds of birds, such as waterfowl, to carry the virus asymptomatically and so introduce the virus to new areas. In pigeons, gross pathological findings were mild and confined to the nervous system with lymphohistiocytic meningoencephalitis (Klopfleisch *et al.*, 2006).

If certain strains are isolated (H5 and H7) then compulsory culling will be enforced of captive birds. In the face of an outbreak, it is possible in England and Wales to vaccinate valuable and genetically rare avian species to prevent infection (under EU Decision 2006/474) –

requests must be made to the Government Agency AH-VLA. This is not currently possible in Scotland.

Prevention of infection should revolve around the use of virucidal footbaths, careful storage of feed to prevent spoiling by wildlife and avoiding wearing the same clothing outside the aviary system. Commercial quarantine aviaries should have completely separate airspaces for separate consignments. Negative pressure ventilation systems are also advised. New arrivals should be quarantined for a minimum of 30 days before being introduced to the rest of the collection.

Bacterial pneumonias and air sacculitis: Psittacosis has already been mentioned and may result in bacterial pneumonia and air sacculitis.

Mycoplasmosis: Mycoplasma spp. have been isolated from most species of bird. In many pigeons, small passerine and psittacine bird's clinical signs include conjunctivitis and upper respiratory disease. *M. gallisepticum* has been implicated in many of these outbreaks.

Others are due to secondary bacterial infections such as those occurring in raptors after infestation by the raptor air-sac mite *Serratospiculum spp.*

Diagnosis is made upon clinical signs, full blood cell counts and full body radiographs.

Pasteurellosis: Pasteurella multocida is the cause of avian cholera. *P. multocida* serotypes 1 and 3 are seen most commonly. In passerine birds, the disease is usually spread via aerosol or contaminated equipment. In raptors, it often gains access to the body via infected prey, causing an oesophagitis, pharyngitis and can lead to septicaemia. For falconry birds, vaccination has been recommended using commercial polyvalent killed pasteurella vaccines (Willette *et al.*, 2009).

Other bacteria: Aeromonas spp. and *Pseudomonas* spp. bacteria have been reported in cases of upper respiratory tract and gastrointestinal disease (the former may present as a septicaemic syndrome as well). *Bordatella avium* can cause an upper respiratory tract infection and has been associated with the lockjaw syndrome in cockatiels. *Klebsiella pneumoniae, K. ozaenae* and *K. oxytoca* have all been associated with contaminated water whether for drinking or in incubators. It tends to colonise the gut first and then spread via the bloodstream to the respiratory tract.

Enterococcus faecalis has been linked to chronic tracheitis, air sacculitis and pneumonia in canaries.

Diagnosis is made on clinical signs, full blood cell counts and full body radiographs.

Toxins: Teflon® and smoke-inhalation toxicity: Birds are extremely sensitive to the odourless fumes given off by overheated Teflon® coated pans. The consequence can be a reaction causing pulmonary oedema with severe dyspnoea and often death before treatment can be initiated. A similar situation is seen with poisoning due to the toxic fumes from smoke, or cooking fat inhalation.

Cardiovascular disease
Congenital heart defects
With the success of breeding programmes to produce colour variants, the incidence of congenital heart defects has increased.

Atherosclerosis
It is often because of lack of exercise and inappropriate, high fat diets. The major arteries become thickened with cholesterol deposits, their lumen diameter decreases and they become less elastic, so blood pressure increases (Figure 13.9). Calcification of the plaques often occurs, particularly if excessive amounts of vitamin D_3 and calcium are consumed.

Arterial calcification
Over-supplementation of calcium and vitamin D_3 may lead to loss of elasticity and increased blood pressure, heart failure and organ damage.

Vegetative endocarditis and myocarditis
Chlamydophilosis can lead to myocardial damage, as can a number of septicaemic and bacteraemic conditions. It can also lead to vegetative endocarditis.

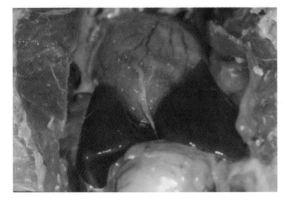

Figure 13.9 An enlarged heart in an African grey parrot (*Psittacus erithacus*) due to atherosclerosis. Note also the white granular gout crystals covering the pericardium due to secondary renal failure.

Streptococcus gallolyticus (formerly known as *S. bovis*) has resulted in acute/peracute death of pigeons. Initial clinical signs include inability to fly and drooping wings followed by anorexia, polyuria/polydipsia, green urates and ascites. Peracute cases have evidence of septicaemia with pericarditis.

Many Gram-negative bacteria such as *E. coli, Klebsiella* spp. and *Pseudomonas* spp. can also lead to syndromes such as vegetative endocarditis.

Mycobacterial disease has also been associated with myocarditis and pericarditis.

Parasites such as those causing toxoplasmosis and sarcocystosis have both been reported in birds as a cause of myocarditis heart failure and death.

Cardiomyopathy
Dilated cardiomyopathy has been reported in birds and associated with rapid growth, hypoxia, high altitude, furazolidone, monensin and sodium toxicities, vitamin E and selenium deficiencies, rancid fat in the diet and inbreeding (Strunk & Wilson, 2005). The mechanism by which the disease develops appears to be the same as for mammals.

Haematological disease
Anaemia may be due to heavy metal, such as lead or zinc, poisoning, debilitation or haemoparasites. *Leucocytozoan* spp. inhabit red and white blood cells and causes intravascular haemolysis leading to anaemia, and spleen and liver damage where the parasite multiplies. It is transmitted by black flies and is known to cause serious problems in young Galliformes, raptors and Anseriformes.

Other significant blood parasites include malarial parasites, *Plasmodium* spp., which can cause severe anaemia, lethargy, vomiting, seizures and death, particularly in penguin species, snowy owls and gyr falcons and their hybrids. *Plasmodium* spp. are transmitted by mosquitoes of the *Anopheles* spp. or by direct blood to blood transfer during fighting. Clinical signs include mucous membrane pallor, lethargy, haemoglobinuria and death. A common haemoparasite, *Haemoproteus* spp., which inhabit the avian red blood cell, generally does not cause disease. It is transmitted via biting flies (Hippoboscids).

Atoxoplasmosis caused by *Isospora (Atoxoplasma) serini* in canaries can multiply in the liver resulting in massive liver enlargement ('black spot disease' due to the projection of the liver beyond the caudal sternum ventrally). It tends to occur in juvenile canaries from 2–9 months with clinical signs of general debilitation, diarrhoea and in around one-fifth cases of neurological signs. It has been implicated in the 'going-light' syndrome of Greenfinches (Cooper *et al.*, 1989). Mortality can be significant around the 80% marker. Impression smears of the cut surface of the liver and spleen will show the intracellular coccidian in the cytoplasm of monocytes indenting the monocyte nucleus into a crescent shape. Faecal examination is often unrewarding due to the low number of oocysts shed after the initial acute phase of the disease.

Blood-borne leukaemia is uncommon in birds. Much more commonly seen are the tissue associated lymphomas. Avian type C retrovirus group (avian leucosis-related viruses) includes avian leucosis and sarcoma virus (ALSV). Transmission is both horizontal (faeces and saliva) and vertical via gonadal cells. Female birds are more susceptible than males and the incubation period can be many months. It may result in immunosuppression and has been associated with discrete renal tumours in budgerigars resulting in unilateral leg paralysis.

A type C retrovirus unrelated to SLV is the cause of lymphoma in turkeys. Marek's disease is a gamma herpesvirus affecting Galliformes, inducing lymphomatous changes in peripheral nerves, bursa, thymus and visceral organs.

Urinary tract
Acute renal disease
Aetiology

This is often due to bacterial causes. It may also be caused by poisons such as zinc antifreeze and chocolate or due to nonsteroidal ant-inflammatory drugs (e.g. diclofenic acid that causes the precipitous decline of white-backed vultures in India). Viruses such as APV in Psittaciformes and infectious bronchitis virus in Galliformes have also been implicated. Another cause in geese is the coccidial parasite *Eimeria truncata*, producing lethargy, rapid weight loss and diarrhoea with high mortality rates. An acute syndrome in adult Merlins (*Falco columbarius*) exists where the kidneys become damaged by fatty degeneration, the bird often dying in good body condition. Its exact aetiology is unknown. Acute renal failure may also be due to shock – cardiogenic or more commonly hypovolaemic.

Diagnosis

PCR tests are available for many viral diseases such as polyomavirus and bacteria such as chlamydophila.

Otherwise, it is based on clinical signs such as anuria or oliguria, and extreme depression, with a history of exposure to the relevant poison. Blood tests may show a massively elevated uric acid level (>1500 umol/L) and sometimes potassium levels (>5 mmol/L). It should be noted that a moderate rise in uric acid levels will occur, particularly in raptors, for several hours after a meal. Urea levels may also be measured and compared with uric acid levels to ascertain if pre-renal azotaemia or renal disease is present as pre-renal azotaemia will cause a predominant rise in urea. The problem is the ratios need to be worked out for each species – the ratio is calculated by multiplying the plasma urea level (in mmol/L) by 1000 and then comparing it with plasma uric acid level (in umol/L). In peregrine falcons, the ratio is >6.5 (Lumeij, 2000). Birds are often anuric with acute renal failure and so urinanalysis is not possible.

Chronic renal disease
Aetiology

As with acute nephritis, this has a number of causes. The causes could be

1. Toxicity/poisonings (e.g. lead)
2. Chronic infection
   a. Bacterial (e.g. *Pseudomonas* spp.)
   b. Viral (e.g. infectious bronchitis)
   c. Fungal (e.g. aspergillosis)
   d. Parasitic (e.g. microsporidia such as *Encephalitozoon hellum*)
3. Excessive levels of calcium and vitamin D_3 in the diet
4. Long-term excessive levels of protein in the diets of Psittaciformes.
5. Neoplasia (e.g. ALSV in budgerigars)
6. Chronic dehydration (e.g. in hen's incubating eggs)
7. Renal lipidosis (e.g. Galliform chicks, adult Merlins correlated with a high-fat/low-protein diet, starvation, biotin deficiency and chronic liver disease)
8. Amyloidosis (e.g., aged waterfowl).

Bacteria may get into the kidneys either via the reflux or via the ureters from the cloaca, or via the bloodstream directly from the intestinal tract due to the renal portal system that exists in birds.

Excessive supplementation of calcium and vitamin D_3 can lead to calcification of soft tissue structures, leading to renal calcinosis and failure.

In laying hens, renal urolithiasis, which can lead to post renal failure due to blockage of the renal tubules, occurs due to the high circulating calcium levels present during egg laying, some of which overspill into the urine. This may be exacerbated if the bird becomes egg-bound due to pressure on the kidneys, so restricting renal blood flow and creating ischaemia.

ALSV infection in budgerigars results in renal tumours in birds of 3–6 years old. Clinically, this may present as unilateral limb paresis/paralysis due to pressure on the ischiatic nerve that passes through the kidney, or with coelomic distension and no other clinical signs. Other suspected ALSV infections have been reported in psittacine birds, Galliformes, Columbiformes and passerine birds resulting in lymphoid neoplasia often in the liver, spleen or kidneys.

Diagnosis

Diagnosis of chronic renal disease in birds is based on a number of tests:

1. Uric acid measurement exceeding 500 umol/L. This should be performed in a fasting bird, as (particularly in the meat-eating raptors) a recent meal can elevate the levels falsely.
2. Excessively high levels of calcium (>3 mmol/L) suggesting over-supplementation, providing the bird is not an inlay hen, when blood levels may rise high normally due to calcium mobilisation for shell production.
3. Radiography may show kidney enlargement in the case of nephritis and tumours. It will also show increased radiodensity in cases of calcinosis. Normally, the avian kidney is difficult to see as it is located in the roof of the synsacrum, but with renalomegaly, it often projects cranially in front of the ilium on a lateral view. Urography may be used to assess renal excretion. The ulna vein is used and iodine-based contrast is injected at 2 mL/kg with the first view being taken after 30 seconds. The dye should have reached the ureters by 1 minute post injection.
4. Ultrasound examination is difficult owing to the presence of air sacs. However, it may be of use in some species where the probe can be placed on the lateral body wall without coming up against the ribcage (e.g. Galliformes and Columbiformes) and where large neoplasias are present.
5. Urinanalysis: Green urates indicate bilverdinuria and liver disease. Normal specific gravity levels tend to be 1.005–1.020 g/mL. The pH is variable but is between 6 and 8 depending on species and diet fed (more acidic in laying hens and more alkaline in bacterial nephritis cases). Ketones may be found in cases of beta oxidation of fats , which can occur

in disease but also during migration stress. An examination for protein or fat casts should be made. Small numbers of red cells and bacteria (from faecal contamination) and uric acid crystals are normal. Large amounts of blood may indicate heavy metal toxicosis or neoplasia. Protein levels up to 2 g/L are normal. Glucose levels should be low. High levels of GLDH indicate severe kidney cell damage. The presence of coccidia or cryptosporidia is of course also significant. Rosskopf et al. (1986) describes the change of casts from granular/cellular to haemoglobin casts as resolution of an inflammatory process. Finally, early work on measurement of N-acetyl-gamma-D-glucosaminidase (NAG) in the urine of birds has shown its level's increase when tubular damage occurs, but normal values are not currently available for birds.

6. Blood pressure monitoring may show hypertension (see Chapter 16) with chronic renal failure.

Renal biopsy can be used to ascertain definitive diagnoses of the condition. This can be performed through a left or right flank approach using rigid endoscopy.

Renal failure will lead to a buildup of uric acid, which rapidly reaches its saturation point. After this, the crystals of uric acid form in the bloodstream and adhere to vital structures. This causes encasement of these structures in the hard, white crystalline uric acid, further damaging them.

Sites initially and preferentially found with uric acid deposits in them include the kidneys themselves (see Figure 13.10), the heart, pericardial sac, liver and of course the joints.

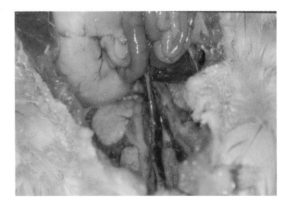

Figure 13.10 Chronic renal failure in an African grey parrot (*Psittacus erithacus*). Note the pale colour of the kidneys and the multiple small white dots of gout crystals or tophi.

Renal urolithiasis

Renal urolithiasis is common in laying hens. It can lead to renal failure due to blockage of the renal tubules. It happens because of the high levels of calcium that circulate during egg laying, some of which spills over into the urine. The situation may be exacerbated if the bird becomes egg-bound, pressing on the kidneys, restricting renal blood flow and creating renal ischaemia.

Renal tumours

Renal tumours are common (e.g. budgerigars) due to ALSV as described earlier.

Reproductive tract disease

Egg binding

This is the most common complaint of the avian reproductive system. There is a history of compulsive egg laying and poor diet, high in seeds and low in calcium. The hen bird becomes lethargic, dull and sits on the floor of its cage. Egg abnormalities or uterine rupture may also contribute (too cold).

Diagnosis of egg binding

Clinical signs plus palpation of the egg if it is situated in the lower reproductive tract, just caudal to the sternum. Radiography is useful for more cranially situated eggs.

Salpingitis

Salpingitis is also known by the name of vent gleet because of the discharge from the cloaca which accompanies it. It is due to infection of the uterus, or, more correctly, the portion of the uterus corresponding to the salpinx. Signs may vary from nonspecific malaise, with a bird becoming intermittently dull and lethargic, to an obvious purulent discharge.

Prolapsed oviduct

This may be a sequel to egg binding and often involves prolapse of the cloaca. Tissues become rapidly desiccated and infected if outside of the body.

Egg yolk coelomitis

This is a life-threatening situation where internal laying of yolks occurs. If the yolk membrane ruptures, the lipids it contains cause an intense inflammatory reaction and coelomitis (see Figure 13.11). This may then become secondarily infected. In any case, it generates an inflammatory response including a raised white cell count (often $>30 \times 10^9$/L) There is often a history of regular egg laying followed by a cessation and then lethargy and collapse. It is more regularly seen in cockatiels, budgerigars, macaws

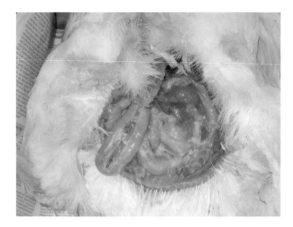

Figure 13.11 Egg yolk coelomitis in a chicken. Note the yellow fibrin tags, the increased coelomic fluid and the congested nature of the coelomic organs.

and Galliformes. Diagnosis can be confirmed with ultrasound and needle aspiration, although care should be taken to avoid puncture of air sacs.

Neoplasia

Ovarian tumours are the most commonly seen female reproductive tract tumour. They can enlarge dramatically and so cause dyspnoea. Adenocarcinomas, adenomas and granulosa cell tumours are the most commonly reported. They may be associated with leg paresis in the same way as of kidney neoplasia. A similar problem is seen in males as testicular neoplasia, involving one or both testes, is also commonly seen in budgerigars. These tumours metastasise to the liver. Most are inoperable due to their size and vascularity.

Musculoskeletal disease

Fractures

The assessment of injuries is essential to triage patients. Fractures occur commonly in many cage and aviary birds. The fractures which occur are often open fractures due to the brittle nature of the bones, which produce very sharp fragments. Any bird that has injuries so bad that a leg needs to be amputated should be euthanased as no bird manages well on one leg, particularly if over 150 g. Wing amputations will mean no release of wild birds and no breeding potential for males as they cannot mount the female successfully.

Carpometacarpal luxation

This condition is often known by its colloquial name of angel wing and is seen commonly in budgerigars, macaws, geese and other waterfowl. It is when the carpometacarpal joints in either wing rotate and subluxate so that the distal primary feathers point dorsally giving a fanlike appearance. It is thought that the condition may have a connection with calcium/vitamin D_3 deficiency (rickets) and excess dietary protein levels, as it is a growth deformity.

Nutritional osteodystrophy/metabolic bone disease

Nutritional osteodystrophy is due to a deficiency in vitamin D_3 and calcium. Several syndromes are seen. The most common is bowing of the tibiotarsal and tarsometatarsal bones. This is because the weight of the growing bird cannot be properly supported by poorly mineralised bones. Often the diets of the birds have high levels of protein as well as low calcium and vitamin D_3, promoting rapid growth and further exacerbating the situation.

Pinwheel

Pinwheel is a developmental deformity of the stifle joint of young pigeons. It occurs around 2–4 weeks of age. The squab cannot flex its stifle, and since only one leg is usually affected, it leads to the circling or pinwheeling, which gives the condition its name. It seems to occur in well-fed chicks reared in flat-bottomed nests with little nesting material. Prevention is the key to success. Treatment is usually ineffective.

Articular gout

Articular gout is seen commonly in older cage and aviary birds and has been discussed under chronic renal disease.

Neurological disease

Fitting

This condition has many aetiologies, including
- Trauma (flying into glass windows etc.)
- Nutrition (hypoglycaemia, hypocalcaemia, hypovitaminosis B_1)
- Heavy metal poisoning (lead and zinc primarily)
- Plant and pesticide poisons
- Meningoencephalitis (bacterial, viral or protozoal)
- Organopathy (particularly hepatic disease)
- Idiopathic epilepsy (reported in red-lored Amazons)
- Vestibular disease
- Cardiovascular disease (fat emboli during egg production, atherosclerosis)
- Cancer
- Congenital CNS disease (cerebellar hypoplasia seen in lutino colour birds).

The breed of bird may suggest a condition, for example, a fitting African grey parrot between the ages of 2 and 4 years may well have hypocalcaemia syndrome, and waterfowl is prone to lead poisoning from lead shot and fishing tackle weights.

Heavy metal toxicosis

Heavy metal toxicosis is common in Psittaciformes, waterfowl and raptors. In raptors, it is often due to feeding wild lead-shot prey. In waterfowl, it is often lead fishing weights or again spent lead shot. In Psittaciformes, it may be due to lead paints on woodwork of old buildings, lead strips on windows/kitchen units, pewter ware/wine tops etc. Zinc poisoning is generally a disease of Psittaciformes and may be associated with housing in zinc-galvanised cages. The Psittaciform manoeuvres itself around the cage using beak and feet and so will take in small amounts of zinc oxide; after 4–6 weeks enough may have been consumed to cause toxicity.

In all cases of heavy metal poisoning, a range of clinical signs can be seen that include weakness, paresis (raptors often rock back onto their intertarsal joints with one foot holding the other, waterfowl have serpentine necks and are unable to fly), liver problems (diarrhoea and biliverdinuria), regurgitation/ileus, kidney failure (polydipsia/polyuria), anaemia and fitting. Diagnosis is made on clinical signs and confirmed by radiography to demonstrate metal particles in the gizzard and blood levels of lead >0.2 ppm or zinc >2 ppm.

Other causes of neurological disease

Hypocalcaemic syndrome of African grey parrots

This is seen in African grey parrots between the ages of 2 and 4 years. It occurs where, although bone calcium quality is adequate, the parrot is unable to mobilise calcium reserves to maintain blood calcium levels. This is often compounded by low calcium, that is all seed, diet. This leads to hypocalcaemia, muscular weakness, tremors, collapse, fits and death. Blood ionized calcium levels should be between 0.96 and 1.22 mmol/L in healthy African grey parrots.

Hypoglycaemia seizure/collapse

In the case of small raptors, such as kestrels, sparrow hawks etc., which have a high metabolic rate, the condition of hypoglycaemia is seen in malnourished or highly stressed birds. There is often a history of being flown in poor weather and failure to monitor body weight regularly during the flying season.

Hyperglycaemia

One or two species of raptor, such as the Northern Goshawk, are prone to hyperglycaemia. This species is prone to hyperglycaemia when retraining at the start of the season occurs and the bird is possibly overweight. Blood glucose levels often exceed 30 mmol/L (normal range is 12–17 mmol/L).

Kidney tumours

Unilateral leg paralysis is a common peripheral neuropathy in budgerigars. It is often due to tumours of the kidneys induced by ALSV infection (see above).

Kidney disease

Any form of kidney disease which results in swelling of the renal parenchyma can theoretically place pressure on the leg nerves and so produce varying signs of paresis and paralysis.

Egg binding

Egg binding is a common cause of bilateral hind limb paresis and paralysis in hen birds. The egg becomes stuck in the pelvic inlet, placing pressure on the nerves in the roof of the pelvis that innerve the legs. Radiography will aid in diagnosing this condition.

Wing paralysis

Wing paralysis is common after flying injuries or fracture of the humerus. This fracture results in rotation laterally of the distal fragment, often lacerating the radial nerve.

Spinal abscesses and fungal infection

Spinal abscesses and fungal infection can occur in birds. Spinal abscesses may occur from bacteria, which have spread there via the bloodstream, particularly after spinal trauma, such as bruising after a flying injury. Fungal granulomas are common in cases of aspergillosis, and may invade the spinal cord as many vertebrae are pneumonised and so connected to the air sac system.

Paramyxoviruses/Newcastle disease

Paramyxovirus is frequently isolated from pigeons. The condition is preventable by vaccination, which is compulsory in pigeons presented at races and shows under the Disease of Poultry Order 1994 (SI 1994/3141). In addition to respiratory problems, the virus can also cause neurological diseases. Signs of this include wing drooping, circling, torticollis and opisthotonus.

An overview of avian biochemistry

Biochemical parameters may be measured using heparinised blood or clotted blood samples. As mentioned in the section on anatomy and physiology, haematological parameters are best measured in potassium edetate collected blood samples, but in some species of bird, potassium EDTA causes lysis of erythrocytes (e.g. many penguins and corvids).

Liver biochemical parameters

The most reliable test for liver function in avian species is that for bile acids. Normal ranges vary from species to species, but commonly range from 20–80 mmol/L.

Other useful tests include aspartamine transaminase (AST) rather than the mammalian AST. Alkaline phosphatase (ALKP) is too nonspecific for birds to be of great use. AST activity is also found in muscle tissue, so often the two other biochemical tests of lactate dehydrogenase (LDH) and creatinine phosphokinase (CPK) are performed. This allows some differentiation between liver and muscle damage, as CPK is only found in muscles. LDH is released in the early stages of liver disease, but also has some skeletal and cardiac muscle distribution. The enzyme glutamate dehydrogenase (GLDH) is released when liver and kidney cells die or are disrupted. As the renal source of this enzyme goes into the urine directly, and not the bloodstream, blood levels of GLDH reflect any hepatocyte damage. Levels greater than 2 IU/L are considered elevated in psittacines (Hochleithner, 1994).

Kidney biochemical parameters

The only reliable test for renal function is uric acid. Neither urea nor creatinine is useful in avian species. However, uric acid is not a sensitive test, and is only elevated once the majority (>75%) of the renal mass ceases to function. Levels may be falsely elevated in raptors immediately after feeding, so samples should be taken in the fasted bird. Levels greater than 420 mmol/L in psittacines, 550 mmol/L in fasted raptors and 750 mmol/L in racing pigeons are suggestive of renal problems. Blood tests in chronic renal failure may show a massively elevated uric acid level (>1500 umol/L) and sometimes potassium levels (>5 mmol/L). Urea levels may also be measured and compared with uric acid levels to ascertain if pre-renal azotaemia or renal disease is present as pre-renal azotaemia will cause a predominant rise in urea. The problem is the ratios need to be worked out for each species – the ratio is calculated by multiplying the plasma urea level (in mmol/L) by 1000 and then comparing it with plasma uric acid level (in umol/L). In peregrine falcons, the ratio is >6.5 (Lumeij, 2000).

Calcium and phosphorus

Levels of calcium and phosphorus depend on nutritional levels and renal function as well as on the presence of vitamin D_3 and functional parathyroid glands. Normal values quoted for total calcium are 2–2.8 mmol/L in most psittacines and 1.9–2.6 mmol/L in pigeons, or 0.96–1.22 mmol/L ionized calcium in African grey parrots. Excessively high levels of calcium (>3 mmol/L) may suggest over-supplementation, providing the bird is not an inlay hen, when blood levels may raise this high normally due to calcium mobilisation for shell production. For phosphorus, 0.9–5 mmol/L in psittacines and 0.57–1.33 mmol/L in pigeons are considered normal. Elevated phosphorus and calcium may suggest renal dysfunction. Low calcium and high or normal phosphorus suggest nutritional deficiency or the hypocalcaemic syndrome seen in African grey parrots.

Plasma proteins

These are very useful in birds to allow an assessment of nutrition and hepatic function. To gain accurate values for albumin and globulins though, it is necessary to perform protein electrophoresis. The laboratory practice, dry chemistry systems, used for mammals are not accurate enough for this. Plasma protein electrophoresis is a useful technique to assess whether the bird is mounting an immune response, when the values of some acute phase proteins may rise, and the pattern of this can be suggestive of some types of disease. An example would be in cases of aspergillosis where elevations in beta globulins are commonly seen (Girling, 2002).

Blood glucose

Blood glucose measurement is useful in raptors, where the values should range between 17–22 mmol/L. If levels fall below 15 mmol/L, hypoglycaemic fitting and coma may develop in small species of raptor. If levels exceed 27 mmol/L, hyperglycaemic fitting can occur. Diabetes mellitus is seen in Psittaciformes such as budgerigars. Here values greater than 30 mmol/L may be observed. It is worth noting though that small elevations in blood glucose commonly occur in stressed birds and should not necessarily be taken to suggest clinical disease.

References

Clubb, S. and De Kloet, S. (2010) Comparison of crop biopsy, serology and PCR for diagnosis of subclinical proventricular dilatation disease. *Proceedings of the Annual Conference of the Association of Avian Veterinarians*, San Diego, California, pp. 3–9.

Colombini, S., Foil, C.S., Hosgood, G. and Tully, T.N. (2001) Intradermal skin testing in Hispaniolan parrots (*Amazona ventralis*). *Veterinary Dermatology*, **11**, 271–276.

Cooper, J.E. (1985) Foot conditions. *Veterinary Aspects of Captive Birds of Prey*, 2nd edn, pp. 97–111. Standfast Press, UK.

Cooper, J.E., Gschmeissner, S. and Greenwood, A. (1989) Atoxoplasma in greenfinches (*Carduelis chloris*) as a possible cause of 'going light'. *Veterinary Record*, **124**, 343–344.

Cray, C., Reavill, D., Romagnano, A., *et al.* (2009) Galactomannan assay and plasma protein electrophoresis findings in psittacine birds with aspergillosis. *Journal of Avian Medicine and Surgery*, **23**, 125–135.

Cray, C., Watson, T., Rodriguez, M. and Arheart, K. (2010) Serodiagnostic testing options for avian aspergillosis. *Proceedings of the Annual Conference of the Association of Avian Veterinarians*, pp. 371–372.

Doolen, M. (1994) A low risk diagnosis for neuropathic gastric dilatation. *Proceedings of the Annual Conference of the Association of Avian Veterinarians Lake Worth*, Florida, pp. 193–196.

Dorrestein, G.M. (2009) Bacterial and parasitic diseases of passerines. *Veterinary Clinics of North America: Exotic Animal Practice*, **12** (3), 433–451.

Forbes, N.A. and Simpson, G.N. (1997) *Caryospora neofalconis*: An emerging threat to captive-bred raptors in the United Kingdom. *Journal of Avian Medicine and Surgery*, **11**, 110–114.

Gancz, A.Y., Kistler, A.L., Greninger, A., *et al.* (2009) Avian Bornaviruses and proventricular dilatation disease. *Proceedings of the Annual Conference of the Association of Avian Veterinarians*, pp. 5.

Girling, S.J. (2002) Plasma protein electrophoresis: Variations in health and disease in the family Psittaciformes *Dissertation as Part-fulfillment for the RCVS Diploma in Zoological Medicine*, RCVS Library.

Gray, P., Hoppes, S., Suchodolski, P., *et al.* (2010) Use of avian Bornavirus isolates to induce proventricular dilatation disease in conures. *Emerging Infectious Diseases*, **16**, 473–479.

Gray, P., Villaneuva, I., Mirhosseini, N., Hoppes, S., Payne, S. and Tizard, I. (2009) Experimental infection of birds with avian Bornavirus. *Proceedings of the Annual Conference of the Association of Avian Veterinarians*, pp. 7.

Gregory, C.R., Latimer, K.S., Campagnoli, R.P. and Ritchie, B. (1996) Evaluation of crop biopsy for the diagnosis of proventricular dilatation syndrome in psittacine birds. *Journal of Veterinary Diagnostic Investigation*, **8**, 76–80.

Grund, C.H., Kohler, B. and Korbel, R.T. (2005) Evaluation of various tissues for diagnosis of psittacine beak and feather disease (PBFD). *Proceedings for the 8th European AAV Conference – 6th Scientific ECAMS Meeting*, Arles, France, 24–30 April, 2005.

Harlin, R. and Wade, L. (2009) Bacterial and parasitic diseases of Columbiformes. *Veterinary Clinics of North America: Exotic Animal Practice*, **12** (3), 453–473.

Heidenreich, M. (1997) Parasites. *Birds of Prey: Medicine and Management*, pp. 133. Blackwell Science, Oxford.

Hochleithner, M. (1994) Biochemistries. *Avian Medicine: Principles and Applications* (eds B. Ritchie, G. Harrison & L. Harrison), pp. 223–245. W.B. Saunders, Philadelphia, PA.

Hoppes, S., Gray, P.L., Payne, S. and Shivaprasad, H.L. (2010) The isolation, pathogenesis, diagnosis, transmission and control of avian Bornavirus and proventricular dilatation disease. *Veterinary Clinics of North America: Exotic Animal Practice*, **13**, 495–508.

Jung, A., Grund, C., Muller, I. and Rautenschlein, S. (2009) Avian paramyxovirus serotype 3 infection in *Neopsephotus*, *Cyanoramphus* and *Neophema* species. *Journal of Avian Medicine and Surgery*, **23**, 205–208.

Klopfleisch, R. Werner, O., Mundt, E., Harder, T. and Teifke, J.P. (2006) Neurotropism of highly pathogenic avian influenza virus A/Chicken/Indonesia/2003 (H5N1) in experimentally infected pigeons (*Columba livia f. domestica*). *Veterinary Pathology*, **43**, 463–470.

Lumeij, J.T. (2000) Pathophysiology, diagnosis and treatment of renal disorders in birds of prey. *Raptor Biomedicine 3* (eds J.T. Lumeij, J.D. Remple, P.T. Redig, *et al.*), pp. 169–178. Zoological Education Network, Lake Worth, FL.

MacWhirter, P., Mueller, R. and Gill, J. (1999) Ongoing research report: Allergen testing as part of diagnostic protocol in self-mutilating Psittaciformes. *Proceedings of the Annual Conference of the Association of Avian Veterinarians*, pp. 125.

Manvell, R., Gough, D., Major, N. and Fouchier, R.A. (2004) Mortality in budgerigars associated with a reovirus-like agent. *Veterinary Record*, **154**, 539–540.

Messenger, G.A. and Garner, M.M. (2010) Proventricular cryptosporidiosis in small psittacines. *Proceedings of the Annual Conference of the Association of Avian Veterinarians*, pp. 55–58.

Oaks, J.L. (1993) Immune and inflammatory responses in falcon staphylococcal pododermatitis. *Raptor Biomedicine* (eds P.T. Redig, J.E. Cooper, J.D. Remple & D.B. Hunter), pp. 72–87. University of Minnesota Press, Minneapolis, MN.

Pennycott, T. (2004) Mortality in budgerigars in Scotland: Pathological findings. *Veterinary Record*, **154**, 538–539.

Perpinan, D., Fernandez-Bellon, H., Lopez, C. and Ramis, A. (2007) Lymphoplasmacytic myenteric, subepicardial and pulmonary ganglioneuritis in four nonpsittacine birds. *Journal of Avian Medicine and Surgery*, **21**, 210–214.

Phalen, D. (2006a) Implications of viruses in clinical disorders. *Clinical Avian Medicine* (eds G. Harrison & T. Lightfoot), pp. 721–760. Spix Publishing Inc., Palm Beach, FL.

Reavill, D.R., Schmidt, R.E. and Fudge, A.M. (1990) Avian skin and feather disorders: a retrospective study. *Proceedings of the Annual Conference of the Association of Avian Veterinarians*. Phoenix, AZ, pp. 248–254.

Remple, J.D. (1993) Raptor bumblefoot: A new treatment technique. *Raptor Biomedicine* (eds P.T. Redig, J.E. Cooper, J.D. Remple & D.B. Hunter), pp. 154–160. University of Minnesota Press, Minneapolis, MN.

Rosskopf, W.J., Woerpel, R.W. and Lane, R.A. (1986) The practical use and limitations of the urinalysis in diagnostic pet avian medicine: With emphasis on the differential diagnosis of polyuria, the importance of cast formation in the avian urinalysis and case reports. *Proceedings of the Annual Conference of the Association of Avian Veterinarians*, Miami, Florida, pp. 61–73.

Shivaprasad, H.L., Franca, M., Honkavuori, K., Briese, T. and Lipkin, W.I. (2009) Proventricular dilatation disease associated with bornavirus in psittacines. *Proceedings of the Annual Conference of the Association of Avian Veterinarians*, pp. 3–4.

Smith, J. (2009) Unusual outbreak of PDD in a psittacine nursery. *Proceedings of the Annual Conference of the Association of Avian Veterinarians*, pp. 9–13.

Speer, B.L. (1998) Chronic partial proventricular obstruction caused by multiple gastrointestinal foreign bodies in a juvenile umbrella cockatoo (*Cacatua alba*). *Journal of Avian Medicine And Surgery*, **12** (4), 271–275.

Steinmetz, A., Pees, M., Schmidt, V., Weber, M., Krautwald-Junghanns, M.E. and Oechtering, G. (2008) Blindness as a sign of proventricular dilatation disease in a grey parrot (*Psittacus erithacus erithacus*). *Journal of Small Animal Practice*, **49**, 660–662.

Strunk, A. and Wilson, G.H. (2005) Avian cardiology. *Veterinary Clinics: Exotic Animal Practice* (ed A. Rupley), pp. 221–240. Elsevier Saunders, Philadelphia, PA.

Villaneuva, I., Gray, P., Mirhosseini, N., *et al.* (2010) The diagnosis of proventricular dilatation disease: use of a Western blot assay to detect antibodies against avian bornavirus. *Veterinary Microbiology*, **143**, 196–201.

Wernery, U. and Kinne, J. (2004) How do falcons contract a herpesvirus infection? Preliminary findings. *Falco*, **23**, 16–17.

Willette, M., Ponder, J., Cruz-Martinez, L., *et al.* (2009) Management of select bacterial and parasitic conditions of raptors. *Veterinary Clinics of North America: Exotic Animal Practice*, **12** (3), 491–517.

Zantop, D.W. (2010) Bornavirus: Background levels in 'well' birds and links to non-PDD illness. *Proceedings of the Annual Conference of the Association of Avian Veterinarians*, pp. 305–310.

Further reading

Chitty, J. and Harcourt-Brown, N. (eds) (2005) *BSAVA Manual of Psittacine Birds*, 2nd edn. BSAVA, Quedgeley, UK.

Chitty, J. and Lierz, M. (2008) *BSAVA Manual of Raptors, Pigeons and Passerine Birds*. BSAVA, Quedgeley, UK.

Cray, C. (1997) Application of aspergillus antigen assay in the diagnosis of aspergillosis. *Proceedings of the Annual Conference of the Association of Avian Veterinarians*, pp. 219–220.

Harrison, G. and Lightfoot, T. (2006) *Clinical Avian Medicine*. Spix Publishing Inc., Palm Beach, FL.

Payne, L.N. and Purchase, H.G. (1991) Leukosis/sarcoma group. *Diseases of Poultry* (eds B.W. Calnek), 9th edn, pp. 388–439. Iowa State Press, Ames, IA.

Redig, P.T., Brown, P.A. and Talbot, B. (1997) The ELISA as a management guide for aspergillosis in raptors. *Proceedings of the 4th Conference of the European Committee of the Association of Avian Veterinarians*, pp. 223–226.

Ritchie, B. (1995) *Avian Viruses Function and Control (ed).* Wingers Publishing Inc., Lake Worth, FL.

Ritchie, B., Harrison, G. and Harrison, L. (1994) *Avian Medicine: Principles and Applications*. W.B. Saunders, Philadelphia, PA.

Samour, J. (ed) (2008) *Avian Medicine*, 2nd edn. Mosby Elsevier, Edinburgh, IN.

Chapter 14

An Overview of Avian Therapeutics

FLUID THERAPY

Maintenance requirements

In birds there is almost no water lost as sweat as they have no proper skin sweat glands. However, there are greater losses compared with cats and dogs, due to their increased metabolic rates and because of their high body surface and lung area to body weight ratio. This means that proportionately large amounts of fluids are lost through respiration.

To compensate, birds can conserve water more efficiently than mammals. Unlike urea, their waste protein excretory product, uric acid, requires very little water to be excreted. However, the losses and gains equal out, so that maintenance levels in companion birds have been estimated as 50 mL/kg/day, which is the same as for cats and dogs.

The effect of disease on fluid requirements

With any disease the need for fluids increases, even if no obvious fluid loss has occurred. The disease process may affect the kidneys causing increases in the glomerular filtration rate or reduction in water reabsorption by the collecting ducts, leading to increased urine output, or there may be a loss of absorption of water from the small or large intestine. For example, the endotoxins produced in cases of *E. coli* septicaemia or enteritis cause a reduction in the response of the renal collecting ducts to arginine vasotocin (AVT) (the avian equivalent of antidiuretic hormone (ADH) released from the pituitary). This will lead to less concentration of the urine, more fluid loss and dehydration.

Respiratory disease is common in avian patients, especially in cases of chlamydophilosis, hypovitaminosis A and aspergillosis, all of which may lead to fluid loss.

Individuals suffering from diarrhoea will experience fluid loss and often metabolic acidosis due to prolonged loss of bicarbonate. There may also be chronic losses of potassium.

Most avian patients have the potential to regurgitate. Fluid loss by this route is therefore not uncommon. The secretions of the crop are mainly neutral to alkali, and so losses are more likely to give straightforward neutral water loss. However, more severe true vomiting will occur in birds with proventricular disease, such as PDD or 'megabacteriosis', and metabolic alkalosis due to loss of hydrogen ions will ensue.

Another route of fluid and electrolyte loss is through skin disease. Lovebirds and cockatiels in particular are prone to ulcerating skin conditions, particularly under the wings. These produce lesions which resemble chemical or thermal burns, and leave large areas of weeping, exudative skin which allow fluid and electrolyte loss.

Post-surgical fluid requirements

Surgical procedures bring their own requirements for fluid therapy. There is the possibility of intrasurgical haemorrhaging, necessitating vascular support with an aqueous electrolyte solution or, in more serious blood losses (>10%), colloidal fluids or even blood transfusions (Figure 14.1).

Even if surgery is relatively bloodless, there are inevitable losses via the respiratory route because of the drying nature of the gases used to deliver the anaesthetics commonly used in avian surgery. Smaller birds have larger surface areas in relation to volume, and this applies to the lung fields as well as the skin. Avian patients also have an air sac system, which increases the surface area for fluid loss even further.

Many patients are not able to drink immediately after surgery. The period without food or water intake may stretch to a few hours, enough time for any avian to start to dehydrate. Finally, some forms of surgery, such as prosthetic beak repair procedures, will lead to inappetence for a period.

Veterinary Nursing of Exotic Pets, Second Edition. Edited by Simon J. Girling. © 2013 John Wiley & Sons, Ltd. Published 2013 by John Wiley & Sons, Ltd.

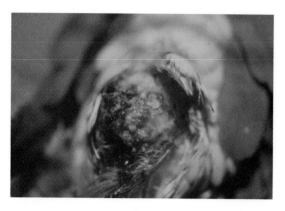

Figure 14.1 Removal of tumours, such as this uropygial gland tumour from an African grey parrot, will result in blood loss and require fluid replacement therapy.

Electrolyte replacement

In cases of chronic fluid loss, electrolytes as well as fluids will often need replacing. Chronic diarrhoea, such as in megabacteriosis or *Giardia* infestations, will cause loss of food, water and electrolytes to waste. The main electrolyte losses involve bicarbonates and potassium.

Because they have a crop between the mouth and the true stomach, birds may well regurgitate rather than vomit. The crop contents are alkaline to neutral, and so metabolic alkalosis is unlikely to occur with regurgitation or crop problems, indeed metabolic acidosis is more likely. However, in serious proventriculus disease, such as the viral condition 'macaw wasting syndrome', stomach megabacteriosis or ulcers, loss of hydrogen ions will occur and metabolic alkalosis can ensue.

Fluids used in avian practice

Lactated Ringer's/Hartmann's

This is useful for rehydration and to supply maintenance needs. It is useful for avian patients suffering from metabolic acidosis, e.g. those with chronic gastrointestinal disease and bicarbonate loss, but it can also be used for fluid therapy after routine surgical procedures. The quantity of potassium present in lactated Ringer's solution is unlikely to cause a problem in birds with hyperkalaemia (such as those suffering from rapid weight loss or with serious skin or tissue trauma). The use of calcium gluconate (5 mg/kg) or the addition of a glucose-containing fluid will help drive the potassium ions into the cells and so reduce the hyperkalaemic threat.

In hypokalaemic birds (such as those suffering from chronic diarrhoea, vomiting, burns or on long-term

glucose/saline fluids), the addition of potassium to the fluids at rates of 0.1–0.3 mEq/kg body weight may help stimulate appetite and reduce the risk of cardiac arrhythmias.

In cases of metabolic acidosis, an assessment of bicarbonate ion loss can be made from a blood sample. However, in many cases it is not possible in practice to measure it. Therefore, if persistent vomiting or chronic weight loss or trauma occurs and metabolic acidosis is suspected, a rough approximation may be made. Give a sodium bicarbonate supplement at 1 mEq/kg at 15–30-minute intervals until a maximum of 4 mEq/kg has been reached. (This supplement must not be given with the lactated Ringer's solution as it will precipitate out.)

Hypertonic saline

This may be used in birds with acute hypovolaemia. It works by rapidly drawing fluid from the cellular and pericellular space into the circulation to support central venous pressure. See chapter 16, Avian Emergency and Critical Care Medicine, for further details of its use. It must be administered intravenously or intraosseously.

Glucose/saline combinations

Glucose/saline solutions are useful for small avian patients. These may well have been through periods of anorexia prior to treatment and therefore may be borderline hypoglycaemic. The concentration to start with when dehydration is present is 5% glucose, 0.9% saline. Once dehydration has been reversed, the avian patient may be moved on to the 4% glucose, 0.18% saline concentration for maintenance purposes.

Protein amino acid/B vitamin supplements

Protein and vitamin supplements can be very useful for nutritional support. Products such as Duphalyte® (Fort Dodge) may be given at the rate of 1 mL/kg/day. They are particularly useful to replace nutrients in cases where the patient is malnourished or has been suffering from a protein-losing enteropathy or nephropathy. They are also good supplements for patients with hepatic disease or severe exudative skin disease such as thermal burns.

Colloidal fluids

Colloidal fluids have been used in avian practice only by the intravenous route, but they can be used via the intraosseous route. They are used in the same way as with cats and dogs:

- When a serious loss of blood occurs
- Where severe hypoproteinaemia is seen
- In order to support central blood pressure

This is due to their ability to stay in the bloodstream for several hours after administration whereas crystalloids remain in circulation for just 15–30 minutes on average. Colloids may be used as a temporary measure whilst a blood donor is selected, or, if a donor is not available, the only means of attempting to support such a patient. Bolus treatment with gelatin colloids such as Gelofusine® (Millpledge) and Haemaccel® (Hoechst) may be given at 10–15 mL/kg intravenously four times over a 24-hour period to aid in the treatment of hypoproteinaemia. Use of Hetastarch® which has a larger colloid particle size and so stays in the circulation for up to 24 hours is preferred where this is available. See section Chapter 16 for Shock fluid therapy.

Blood transfusions

Blood transfusion should be considered if the PCV (packed cell volume) drops below 15%. Birds are more tolerant of blood loss than mammals as the oxygenation of their blood is more efficient. However, transfusions are sometimes required. Donors should be from the same species, e.g. African grey parrot to African grey parrot, or budgerigar to budgerigar. Blood can be collected from the donor into a container or syringe with acid citrate dextrose anticoagulant or, in an emergency, a heparinised syringe may be used. Ideally, a blood filter should be used before blood is transfused into the recipient bird, but frequently this is not possible in general practice, and so collection and administration should be done with care, to reduce haemolysis and clumping.

It is useful to remember that one drop of blood is roughly equal to 0.05 mL and that the estimated blood volume of an avian patient is 10% of its body weight in grams. Volumes that can be transfused range from 0.25 mL in a budgerigar to 5 mL in an African grey parrot.

Oral fluids and electrolytes

Oral fluids may be used in avian practice for those patients experiencing mild dehydration, and for 'home' administration. Many products are available for cats and dogs, and may be used for birds. One electrolyte in particular may be useful and that is Avipro® by VetArk. This is a probiotic, but used at the correct concentration may also be used as an oral electrolyte solution. The lyophilised bacteria are useful to aid digestion, which is also often upset during periods of dehydration.

Calculation of fluid requirements

A critically ill avian patient is assumed to be at least 5–10% dehydrated. As with cats and dogs, you should assume that 1% dehydration is equal to the need to supply 10 mL/kg body weight of fluid in addition to maintenance requirements. Assumptions then have to be made on the degree of dehydration of the bird concerned. Roughly,

- 3–5% dehydrated – increased thirst, slight lethargy, tacky mucous membranes, increased heart rate
- 7–10% dehydrated – increased thirst, anorexia, dullness, tenting of the skin and slower return to normal over eyelid or foot, dry mucous membranes, dull corneas, red or wrinkled skin in chicks
- 12–18% dehydrated – dull to comatose, skin remains tented after pinching, desiccating mucous membranes, sunken eyes

These deficits may be large and the volume required for replacement will be difficult to administer rapidly. Indeed, it may be dangerous to overload the patient's system with these fluid levels all in one go. To spread the deficit evenly, it is advised that the following protocol be used:

- Day 1: Maintenance fluid levels +50% of calculated dehydration factor
- Day 2: Maintenance fluid levels +50% of calculated dehydration factor
- Day 3: Maintenance fluid levels.

If the dehydration levels are so severe that volumes are still too large to be given at any one time, it may be necessary to take 72 hours rather than 48 hours to replace the calculated deficit.

To add to the problem, debilitated avian patients may also be anaemic, and therefore PCVs may appear misleadingly normal, so total protein levels are an additional parameter to look at when assessing dehydration. Uric acid levels may also be measured, as these will often increase in cases of moderate to severe dehydration. Other useful parameters include weight measurement and of course fluid intake and urine output. Table 14.1 gives some normal PCV and total protein values.

Equipment for fluid administration

The equipment required to administer fluids to birds is often very small in size. For example, the blood vessels available for intravenous medication are often 30–50% smaller than their cat or dog counterparts and tend to be highly mobile and much more fragile and prone to rupture.

Table 14.1 Normal packed cell volumes (PCV) and total blood proteins for selected avian species.

Species	PCV l/l	Total protein (g/L)
Budgerigar	0.45–0.57	20–30
Amazon parrot	0.41–0.53	33–53
African grey parrot	0.42–0.52	26–49
Macaw	0.43–0.54	25–44
Cockatoo	0.42–0.54	28–43
Cockatiel	0.43–0.57	31–44
Mallard duck	0.42–0.56	32–45
Canada goose	0.35–0.49	37–56
Mute swan	0.32–0.5	36–55
Chicken	0.24–0.43	33–55
Pheasant	0.28–0.42	42–72
Pigeon	0.36–0.48	21–35
Peregrine falcon	0.37–0.53	25–40
Barn owl	0.42–0.51	29–48
Tawny owl	0.36–0.47	27–46

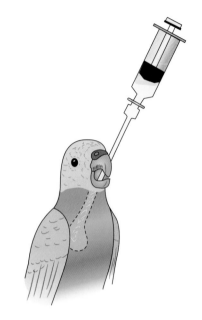

Figure 14.2 Method of inserting a crop tube. Approach from left side of beak and aim towards the lower right neck region.

Crop tubes

They are useful as a route for fluid and nutrition administration. Crop tubes come either as straight or curved metal tubes, both with blunt ends. To insert a crop tube, extend the bird's head. Starting from the left side of the inside of the lower beak, pass the tube down the proximal oesophagus into the crop at the right side of the thoracic inlet. Maximal volumes which may be given vary from 0.5 mL in a budgerigar to 15 mL in a large macaw (Figure 14.2).

Catheters

Because they have a length of tubing attached to the needle, butterfly catheters are extremely useful for the small and fragile avian vessels. If the syringe or drip set is connected to this piece of flexible tubing rather than directly to the catheter, there is less chance of the catheter becoming dislodged; should the bird draw back after the catheter is inserted. Also, the piece of clear tubing on the catheter allows you to see when venous access has been achieved, as blood will flow back into this area without having to draw back on the syringe (which would collapse the fragile veins anyway).

It is advised to flush any catheter with heparinised saline prior to use to prevent clots forming. Twenty-five to twenty-seven gauge sizes are recommended and will cope with venous access for budgerigars through to small conures. Twenty-three to twenty-five gauge sizes will suffice for larger parrots and some of the bigger waterfowl and raptors.

Ordinary over-the-needle catheters may also be used for catheterisation of jugular veins. The latex catheter is useful for long-term maintenance of venous access, as butterfly catheters tend to rupture the vessels if left in for long periods. It is better to use an over-the-needle catheter which has plastic flanges so that it can be sutured to the skin at the site of insertion to prevent removal.

Hypodermic or spinal needles

Spinal needles have a central stylet to prevent clogging of the lumen of the needle with bone fragments after insertion and are therefore useful for intraosseous catheterisation. Twenty-one to twenty-five gauge spinal needles are usually sufficient for most cage birds. Straightforward hypodermic needles may also be used for the same purpose, although the risks of blockage are higher. Hypodermic needles may also be used, of course, for the administration of subcutaneous fluids. Generally, 21–25 gauge hypodermic needles are sufficient for cage birds.

Syringe drivers

For continuous fluid administration, such as is required for intravenous and intraosseous fluid administration during anaesthesia, syringe drivers are becoming more widely used. They are less useful in the conscious bird due to poor tolerance of drip tubing; hence bolus fluid therapy is more commonly used in avian practice.

Collars

It may be necessary to place some of the psittacine family into an Elizabethan-style collar as they are the world's greatest chewers! There is also a selection of lightweight Perspex neck braces which may be better tolerated. However, these are not so useful when jugular vein catheters are used.

Routes of fluid administration

There are four main routes available for administration of fluids to birds. They are

- Oral
- Subcutaneous
- Intravenous
- Intraosseous

The advantages and disadvantages of the four routes are given in Table 14.2. The intraperitoneal route used in mammals is not available for use in birds, due to the lack of a diaphragm and the presence of air sacs. This means that any injection into the body cavity (or coelom) may inadvertently enter an air sac and thence on to the bird's airways, resulting in drowning.

Oral

Lactated Ringer's solution, probiotic or electrolyte solutions such as VetArk's Avipro® and Critical Care Formula® or 5% dextrose solutions may be used. The maximum volumes which may be administered via crop tube are given below.

- Budgerigar: 0.5–1 mL
- Cockatiel: 2.5–5 mL
- Conure: 5–7 mL
- Cockatoo: 10 mL
- African grey: 8–10 mL
- Macaw: 10–15 mL

Subcutaneous

Table 14.2 gives the advantages and disadvantages of subcutaneous fluid therapy. The sites for subcutaneous fluid administration are located in the inguinal web of skin which attaches the leg to the body cranially, the axillary region immediately under each wing, and the dorsal interscapular area.

Table 14.2 Advantages and disadvantages of various avian fluid therapy routes.

Route	Advantages	Disadvantages
Oral	Reduced stress (if competent handler) Physiological route Less trauma Home therapy possible	Increased stress (if inexperienced) Not useful in cases of digestive tract dysfunction or disease Risk of aspiration pneumonia if regurgitates Slow rate of rehydration (not good for serious hypovolaemia) Inaccurate method of dosing (unless crop tubing)
Subcutaneous	Faster uptake of fluids than oral route Volumes given may be large, reducing dosing frequency	Reduced uptake in severe dehydration or peripheral vasoconstriction May be painful in smaller species Only hypotonic or isotonic fluids may be used
Intravenous	Rapid rehydration and support of the central venous pressure Use of hypertonic and colloidal fluids possible Good for waterfowl where medial metatarsal veins can take indwelling catheters or multiple venipuncture	Venous access may be difficult in some species Veins may be fragile Some species will not tolerate permanent indwelling intravenous catheters
Intraosseous	Rapid rehydration and support of the central venous pressure Useful in smaller species where venous access is difficult May be better tolerated for indwelling catheters than intravenous routes Use of hypertonic and colloidal fluids possible	Potentially painful procedure requiring analgesia and, local or general anaesthetic Risk of bone fracture or osteomyelitis Bolus of fluids takes longer to administer due to rigid confines of bone cortices Avoid use of pneumonised bones (e.g., humerus and femur) as will cause drowning.

Intravenous

Table 14.2 gives the advantages and disadvantages of intravenous fluid therapy in avian species.

Blood vessels used for intravenous therapy

Veins which may be used for intravenous therapy include the basilic and ulnar veins, which run on the underside of the wing in larger species. The right jugular vein may be used for bolus injections in all species down to the size of a canary. In raptors, a jugular vein catheter is very well tolerated for repeated bolus injections (see Figure 14.3). In waterfowl, such as swans and ducks, raptors and some larger parrots, the medial metatarsal vein, which runs along the medial aspect of the lower leg, can be used. Avian species will tolerate catheterisation of this vessel extremely well for several days.

Volumes of fluid which may be administered intravenously

Isotonic solutions may be given at 10–15 mL/kg per bolus, although volumes up to 30 mL/kg rarely cause problems. Maximum intravenous bolus volumes are given below:

- Finch: 0.5 mL
- Budgerigar: 1 mL
- Cockatiels: 2 mL
- Conure: 6 mL
- Amazon parrot: 8 mL
- Owl: 10 mL
- Cockatoo: 14 mL

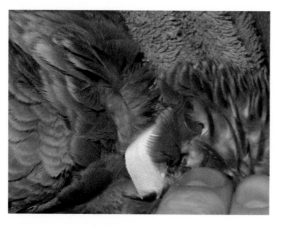

Figure 14.3 A jugular catheter placed in the right jugular of a parrot. Note the silk tape which is then sutured to the bird's skin to hold the catheter in place. Note also the bung as intravenous fluids in birds are generally given as boluses rather than continuous rate infusion due to the intolerance of drip sets etc.

- Buzzard: 12–14 mL
- Macaw: 14 mL
- Swan: 25–30 mL

Placement of intravenous catheters

Right jugular vein catheterisation

1. Sedate or lightly anaesthetise the avian patient, preferably with isoflurane, to ensure no trauma occurs and to minimise stress.
2. The feathers overlying the area should be wetted and parted. An area of no feather growth (known as apterylae) lies over the immediate area of the right jugular vein.
3. Raise the vein at the base of the neck with a thumb and swab the area lightly with surgical spirit.
4. Use a 23–25 gauge over-the-needle catheter, pre-flushed with heparinised saline. Insert it in a caudal direction, as these are often better tolerated than cranially pointing ones, particularly when administering fluids.
5. Once in place, suture the catheter securely to the skin on either side with fine nylon and re-flush to ensure it is properly in the vein. Then attach the intravenous drip tubing or catheter bung to the end of the catheter.
6. Sometimes a light bandage may be necessary to protect the catheter. In severe cases, an Elizabethan bird collar may be used (although the latter may catch on the catheter). Many avian patients will tolerate a catheter unprotected at this site for 24–48 hours.

Medial metatarsal catheterisation for waterfowl: This procedure may be used for larger Psittaciformes and raptors. It may also be performed with the bird conscious, particularly in waterfowl, as the blood vessel is less mobile and likely to rupture.

1. Wipe the inside of the lower leg with surgical spirit or povidone-iodine just above the intertarsal joint.
2. The vessel runs from the anterior aspect distally to a more medial aspect proximally, and is obvious without digital pressure.
3. Use a 23–25 gauge over-the-needle catheter inserted in a proximal direction (i.e., in the direction of blood flow up the leg).
4. Tape the catheter in place using zinc oxide tape and apply a catheter bung after flushing with more heparin saline.

Intraosseous

Table 14.2 gives the advantages and disadvantages of intraosseous fluid therapy in avians.

Bones used for intraosseous fluid therapy

The two bones most commonly used for intraosseous fluid therapy are the ulna and the tibiotarsus. The ulna may be accessed from a distal or proximal aspect, and the tibiotarsus is accessed from a cranial proximal aspect through the crest just distal to the stifle joint.

Placement of intraosseous catheters

Proximal tibiotarsus: This is the procedure for placing a tibiotarsal intraosseous catheter.

1. Sedation or anaesthesia is needed for conscious animals. In all cases good analgesia must be administered.
2. Pluck the area overlying the cranial aspect of the tibial crest and surgically prepare this with dilute povidone-iodine.
3. Insert a 21–25-gauge needle through the tibial crest (depending on the size of the patient), screwing it into the bone in the direction of the long axis of the tibiotarsus distally.
4. Flush the needle with heparinised saline. The advantage of using a spinal needle is that it has a central stylet, which helps prevent it from becoming plugged with bone fragments.
5. Tape the needle securely in place and apply an antibiotic cream around the site. Radiographing the area to ensure correct intramedullary placement of the needle is advised.
6. Once correct placement has been assured, attach the needle to intravenous tubing and a syringe driver and bandage this securely in by wrapping bandage material around the limb. If the catheter has merely been placed for use later, insert a catheter bung and bandage in place.
7. Finally, fit an Elizabethan collar or avian neck brace if the patient shows signs of trying to remove the catheter.

Distal ulna in all species (Figures 14.4 and 14.5): Sedation or isoflurane anaesthesia is often required.

1. Pluck the feathers over the distal aspect of the carpal joint of the wing to be used.
2. Surgically prepare the site with povidone-iodine or surgical spirit and flex the distal tip of the wing caudally. This flexure exposes the distal aspect of the radius and ulna bones within the carpal joint. The ulna is the larger of the two bones, unlike in mammals, but as with mammals it lies caudal to the radius.
3. Palpate the end of the ulna with the carpal joint maximally flexed, and using a 23–25-gauge hypodermic or

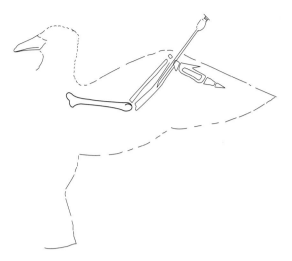

Figure 14.4 Method of inserting an intraosseous catheter into the distal ulna. Note the flexed carpal joint and that the ulna runs caudal to the radius.

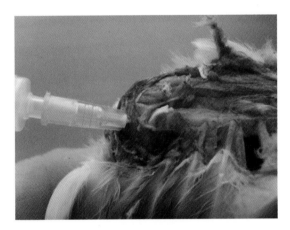

Figure 14.5 Simple method of giving a bolus of fluids via the distal ulna in a cadaver using a hypodermic needle and syringe.

spinal needle, screw into the medullary cavity of the bone along the long axis of the ulna from a distal to proximal direction.
4. Flush the catheter with heparinised saline and place a catheter bung over the end. Radiographs may be taken to ensure accurate placement, and antibiotic cream can be used at the site of insertion.
5. Bandage the wing to the side of the bird to immobilise it. Encircle the thorax and pass both cranial and caudal to the opposite wing's attachment at the chest wall, otherwise the bird may flap wildly and loosen the catheter or traumatise itself.

PART II: AVIAN SPECIES

6. The catheter may then be used for either intermittent slow bolus injections or for attachment to a syringe driver for continuous perfusion.

TREATMENT OF AVIAN DISEASES

As this text is aimed at the veterinary technical nurse, it is not intended to give exhaustive lists of treatments or drug dosages, rather to give an idea of the treatments possible and the techniques useful to aid recovery. For drug dosages, the reader is referred to one of the many excellent texts listed in the additional reading list at the end of this chapter.

Avian dermatological disease therapy

Table 14.3 highlights some of the treatments and therapies commonly used for the management of avian skin diseases. In addition, the management of the bacterial pododermatitis problem known as 'bumblefoot' as well as behavioural feather plucking is also discussed.

Treatment and prevention of bumblefoot

This condition is seen in almost any species, and prevention is better than cure. Some methods to prevent bumblefoot from developing include the following:

- Provide a variety of different diameter natural wood perches for cage and aviary birds. These will allow the feet of the bird to expand and contract as they grip the differing perches allowing blood to be pumped through the foot, preventing devitalisation, and also applies pressure to different areas, preventing corns.
- For falcons and raptors, perches should be covered in padding such as Astroturf®, particularly if they are tethered for days at a time. This cushions the foot and prevents excessive pressure that causes ischaemia.
- A good quality diet is vital. Vitamin A is particularly important for skin integrity and local immunity, as well as the vitamin B complex and minerals such as calcium. Preventing obesity is also important as this will lead to increased pressure on the feet.

In the case of existing pododermatitis:

- For type I–II lesions (Cooper, 1985; Oaks, 1993, padding the perches is a simple solution. In the case of raptors, increasing the time spent flying helps, and the use of antibiotics has been recommended where inflammation is present.
- If a scab exists, it should be debrided under sedation with antiseptic such as povidone-iodine, followed by padding of the foot. The padding is formed from a non-adherent dressing such as Coflex®/Vetband®, which is wound in small strips around the base of each digit. This lifts the plantar aspect of the foot off the perch, thus allowing increased circulation.
- For type III–IV lesions (Oaks, 1993), it is recommended that a culture of the lesion is taken in order

Table 14.3 Treatment of avian skin diseases.

Diagnosis	Treatment
Ectoparasites	**Mites** (e.g. *Knemidocoptes* spp.): Ivermectin at 0.2 mg/kg once, orally, topically or by injection. Repeat after 10–14 days.
	Lice: Commercial louse powders are available containing cis-permethrin or piperonyl butoxide. Fipronil sprayed onto a cloth and wiped over feathers or pyrethrin based powders. *Dermanyssus gallinae* will require treatment of cage/aviary environment as they only live on the host at night. Pyrethrins are available.
Avipoxvirus	No specific treatment. Antibiosis and topical treatment with dilute povidone-iodine are useful.
Psittacine circovirus (PBFD)	Avian gamma interferon (not commercially available) has been used with success at 1×10^6 IU injected once daily for 90 days (Stanford, 2004).
	Prevention is possible by live vaccine (produced in Australia), but this must not be given to already infected birds as it accelerates the course of the disease.
Psittacine polyomavirus	No treatment is available. Prevention may be attempted using a commercial vaccine from the USA (Biomune II Psittimmune®)
Pigeon poxvirus	Vaccine available for prevention. Columbovac PMV/Pox® (Pfizer Animal Health) given subcutaneously over the dorsal neck.
Neoplasia and feather cysts	Surgical excision in the case of neoplasia. For cysts excision or marsupialisation (opening the cyst and sewing the capsule to the skin surface).
Ulcerative dermatitis	Appropriate antibacterial and antifungal medication. Behavioural aspects, e.g. environmental enrichment or exposure to UV light, need to be considered. Possibility of allergic skin disease

to choose the correct antibiotic. The wounds should be repeatedly debrided with dilute povidone-iodine and the toes bandaged. In more severe cases, the application of a ball bandage (where a wad of padding is placed in the grip of the foot and the foot bandaged to this ball) may be necessary (see Figure 14.6). Alternatively, casting materials may be used to create a large but lightweight 'corn plaster', which removes pressure from the affected area of the foot. It is usually necessary to do this to both feet to avoid putting pressure on the non-affected foot.

- For type V–VI lesions (Oaks, 1993), the process is the same as for type III–IV. If bone is involved, the outlook is poor but antibiotic-impregnated polymethylmethacrylate (AIPMMA) beads have been shown to improve healing and recovery rates. These beads are implanted and sewn into the wounds where they release antibiotic slowly at the site of the infection over a period of weeks. Alternatively, drains may be placed in the affected foot, exiting proximally on the caudal aspect of the tarsometatarsus. This allows the wounds to be flushed with antibiotics for a number of days. The foot should be placed into a ball bandage dressing, which should be changed after each flush.

Treatment of behavioural feather plucking

This can be extremely difficult and it cannot be stressed enough that a full work-up to rule out infectious, nutritional or pain causes of feather plucking/mutilation should be carried out. For example, subclinical PDD,

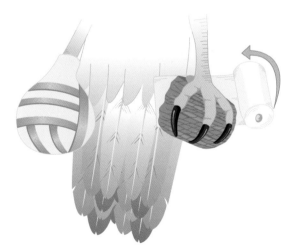

Figure 14.6 Application of a ball bandage to the feet of a raptor with bumblefoot. Note gauze packing to support the foot before using elasticated bandage material.

chlamydophilal or circoviral disease can mimic self-mutilation.

If the cause is sexual frustration due to the keeping of a single parrot, these cases may improve by the pairing with a suitable mate. Alternatively, the reproductive hormone axis may be blocked temporarily by reducing daylight to less than 10 hours to mimic the nonbreeding season. Or, more permanently, by using GnRH agonists such as leuprolide acetate (100 ug/kg IM which lasts for 3–4 weeks) or deslorelin (4.7 mg implant lasts 6–10 months). The latter is more readily available in a long-acting implant form in the United Kingdom and is implanted subcutaneously over the back of the head where it cannot be removed by the parrot. Remember that this drug works by initially stimulating the sex hormonal axis; therefore, the condition may initially worsen until the axis is shutdown.

Many larger parrots develop feather plucking disorders due to lack of socialisation as they have been hand-reared, would normally spend many years with their parents and so have not developed any avian social interactive skills. These can be more difficult to manage, but training these individuals to accept basic commands and to learn their place in the household. The owner and all other household members should be dominant to the parrot. Top birds are always higher up than the subdominant; therefore, the parrot's cage should never be placed so that the bird perches higher up than its owner's shoulder. Never let parrots perch on your shoulder as this also allows them to feel dominant. Training parrots to simple commands such as 'up' to step up onto a hand or proffered perch, 'down' to step back onto its own perch, 'no' when an undesirable action has occurred and vocal praise plus a treat when the parrot does what you want are good places to start this.

Environmental enrichment is essential to take the bird's mind off self-mutilation and to give its beak something else to work on! Food puzzles, toys and regular changing of these to reduce boredom are important. Background noise such as a low level of radio sound is also important as very quiet environments are stressful to prey species as this often indicates the presence of a predator. Access out of the cage is important, but they should have free access back into it as the cage should be seen as a safe zone.

Physical prevention of self-mutilation may be necessary in the form of Elizabethan collars or neck braces. These have a role to play, but they should not be used on their own without correction of the underlying psychological problem.

Psychotropic drugs similarly should not be used without attempting to alter the underlying cause. Diazepam has been used at 0.5 mg/kg for short-term control of self-mutilation in cockatoos with anxiety and hysteria. Haloperidol has been used in those where skin mutilation has occurred and appears to be the most successful in the more extreme self-mutilation cases at 0.1 mg/kg orally q12 hours. Clomipramine (0.5–1 mg/kg q12–24 hours) has also been used but seems less successful if behavioural modification therapy is not included and has been associated with deaths (possibly due to its arrhythmogenic effects).

Avian digestive tract disease therapy

Table 14.4 highlights some of the treatments and therapies commonly used for the management of avian digestive tract diseases.

Avian respiratory tract disease therapy

Table 14.5 highlights some of the treatments and therapies commonly used for the management of avian respiratory tract diseases. Avian nasal sinus flushing is described, which is useful in the treatment of upper respiratory tract disease. Air sac tube placement may be necessary during surgery or treatment of tracheal/syringeal disease, or when a tracheal/syringeal obstruction occurs.

Performing a sinus flush

Apply the hub of a syringe (minus its hypodermic needle!) to one external nostril. To make a snug fit between syringe and nostril it is often helpful to remove the rubber stopper of a 2 mL syringe, pierce a hole through its centre and attach this to the hub of the syringe containing the medication.

Table 14.4 Treatment of avian diseases of the digestive system.

Diagnosis	Treatment
Nematodes (e.g. *Capillaria* spp.)	Fenbendazole 15–20 mg/kg orally daily for 3–5 days for *Capillaria* spp. – care during moult can damage growing feathers. Radiomimetic effects reported and suppression of white blood cell counts have been seen. For ascarids, once dosing with 20 mg/kg and then repeating in 2 weeks for heavier burdens may be sufficient. Flubendazole available as an in-feed wormer for poultry and game birds (Flubenvet® Janssen). Ivermectin 0.2 mg/kg orally or by injection once. May repeat 10–14 days later.
Protozoa (e.g. *Trichomonas* spp., *Hexamita* spp., *Giardia* spp.)	Metronidazole 10–30 mg/kg orally twice daily for 3–5 days. May need 50 mg/kg orally for *Hexamita* in pigeons for 7 days. Watch for toxicity. Carnidazole (e.g. Spartrix® – Harkers) for pigeons with *Trichomonas* infections but can be used in other birds as well at 20–25 mg/kg orally once. Ronidazole (e.g. Harkanker® – Harkers) for pigeons with *Trichomonas* infections – 1 × 400 mg sachet in 4L as drinking water for 5 days. Same dose for cochlosomiasis. Doses of 0.1–0.2 g/L for canaries.
Coccidiosis	*Caryospora* spp. – clazuril 5–10 mg/kg orally every other day for 3 doses or 5–10 mg/kg daily for 2 doses. *Eimeria* and *Isospora* intestinal phase sulfadimethoxine (e.g. Coxi-plus® Dechra Veterinary Products) in water for 5 days – beware use in birds with renal disease or during the laying period. Products containing lasalocid have been used in feed for game birds (e.g. Avatec® Pfizer Animal Health), but these can be toxic to some cage birds. Toltrazuril (Baycox 2.5% oral solution® Bayer Animal Health) has also been used but must be diluted at 1 mL/L drinking water for 2 days as it is highly alkaline in nature.
Bacterial/fungal infections	Based on culture and sensitivity results. *Macrorhabdus ornithogaster* – amphotericin B for 3–5 days (e.g. in water 2% preparation Megabac-S® 5 g/L for 5 days). Cider vinegar added to drinking water at 60–120 mL/L to acidify water and reduce spread in the flock. *Candida albicans* – nystatin 300,000 units/kg orally twice daily. Alternatively 10 mg/kg itraconazole orally twice daily (warning has toxicity issues in grey parrots). Associated with a lack of vitamin A
Sour crop	Food should leave crop after 3–4 hours. If not crop, wash and remove manually. May need antimicrobials plus sodium bicarbonate (antacid) plus metoclopramide.
Crop impaction	Crop wash under anaesthetic with warm water. Milk the contents out. Make sure the bird is intubated with a snug fitting tube or lightly inflate the cuff to avoid inhalational pneumonia
Crop burns	Leave until full extent of skin slough develops (often 5–7 days) and treat with covering antimicrobials and pain relief +/– fluid therapy. Surgically debride the necrotic skin and underlying tissues and close in separate layers using monofilament dissolving suture material. Large deficits may require flaps or grafts.
Duck plague	No treatments. A vaccine is available for prevention (Nobilis Duck Plague® MSD Animal Health)

Diagnosis	Treatment
Haemochromatosis	Iron chelation agent, e.g. deferoxamine, 100 mg/kg once daily. Phlebotomy (bleeding 1–2 mL blood/kg once weekly). Diet should contain <60 ppm iron levels for susceptible species and low vitamin C, which facilitates iron uptake.
Cloacal papillomas	Surgical removal using caustic silver nitrate under anaesthesia
Hepatic lipidosis	Reduce fats and proteins in diet but maintain biological value of proteins. Vitamin B and K supplements are advisable. Use of hepatic supporting drugs such as inisotol and L-carnitine, or *Spirulina* as dietary supplements. Lactulose syrup (0.3 mL/kg) orally once daily.
Lead/zinc poisoning	Heavy metal chelation agent, e.g. sodium calcium edetate, 20–50 mg/kg twice daily by injection for 5 days minimum. D-penicillamine at 50–55 mg/kg orally twice daily may also be used. Beware of renal toxicity so fluid therapy is essential. Flushing out proventriculus/ventriculus to remove all metal particles is also advisable.
Diabetes mellitus	Protamine zinc insulin 0.1–1 unit/kg. Dilute in saline to allow accurate dosing. Rarely however controls blood glucose. Aim is rather to stop weight loss. Twice daily dosing often required.
Proventricular dilatation disease	No treatment. Has been managed with dietary changes (switch to rearing formulas) plus use of NSAIDs such as celecoxib (10 mg/kg orally once daily) and meloxicam (0.2 mg/kg orally once daily).
Pacheco's disease and other herpesvirus infections	Limited success if caught early in the course of the disease with the use of acyclovir at 80 mg/kg orally every 8–12 hours.

Table 14.5 Treatment of avian respiratory system disease.

Diagnosis	Treatment
Upper respiratory tract disease	Antimicrobial therapy based on culture/sensitivity. Swab from the choanal slit. Surgical removal of rhinoliths, sinus flushes (see below), parenteral antimicrobials.
Respiratory parasites (e.g. *Syngamus trachea* and air-sac mites	Ivermectin 0.2 mg/kg once. May be repeated in 10–14 days to catch the recently hatched eggs.
Ornithosis/psittacosis/ infection with *Chlamydophila psittaci*	Use of doxycycline advised. In water preparation licensed in United Kingdom (Ornicure® Dechra Veterinary Products) for pigeons and cage birds. Many larger parrots will not take in water medications so injections of 75–100 mg/kg human intravenous doxycycline hycylate (Vibravenos® Pfizer) once weekly may be used. Periods of 42 days plus are advised (the life span of the alveolar macrophage in which the organism often resides). Candida overgrowth of the gut is a common sequel.
Aspergillosis	Treatment is difficult and prolonged. Surgical debridement of granulomas, possible air sac tube placement (see below). Nebulisation with amphotericin B/diluted F10® 3–4 times daily particularly for the first 1–2 weeks is useful. Intravenous amphotericin B at 1.5 mg/kg for 3–5 days has been described but it is nephrotoxic, so care should be used. Oral itraconazole 10 mg/kg twice daily is effective but this drug is toxic in African grey parrots. Voriconazole has been used in raptors. Terbinafine may be used at 10–15 mg/kg orally twice daily instead. Treatment periods are often 3–12 months.
Bacterial lower respiratory tract disease	This depends on bacterial culture and sensitivity testing. However, mycoplasmosis tends to respond to fluoroquinolones (e.g. Baytril® Bayer Animal Health) and tetracyclines (e.g. Ornicure® Dechra Animal Health), and pasteurellosis will respond to fluoroquinolones and sometimes pencillins.
Paramyxovirus	No treatment. Prevention is via vaccination in pigeons (e.g. Colombovac PMV® (Pfizer Animal Health) and Nobilis Paramyxo P201® (MSD Animal Health). Essential for racing pigeons in United Kingdom by law (Disease of Poultry Order 1994 (SI 1994/3141)).
Smoke inhalation toxicity	Supportive therapy. Furosemide 1–4 mg/kg intravenously/intramuscularly (beware of nephrotoxicity). Oxygen-enriched atmosphere is advised, and in severe cases methylprednisolone at 10–20 mg/kg or prednisolone at 6 mg/kg for lung oedema may be given. Beware of corticosteroids immunosuppressive drugs, side effects as aspergillosis and bacterial infections may appear.

The bird is held inverted and the contents of the syringe (0.5 mL for a budgerigar, up to 5–7 mL for a large macaw or raptor) are expelled into the nostril. The mixture should exit through the infraorbital sinus and out through the eye, and through the internal choanal slit and out of the mouth. Holding the bird upside down minimises aspiration of this mixture.

Repeat the procedure for the other nostril.

Air-sac tube placement

In many cases of syringeal aspergillosis or when performing tracheal washes in a dyspnoeic bird, the placement of an air-sac tube may be vital to keep a patent airway. This is further discussed in chapter 16.

Nebulisation

A nebulisation circuit may be used to administer oxygen or drugs in aerosol form to avians with respiratory disease (Figure 14.7). Antibiotics such as gentamicin that are effective against Gram-negative bacteria, but which if given intravenously can be nephro- and ototoxic, may be administered by nebulisation as they will not cross the air–blood barrier.

Avian reproductive tract disease therapy

Egg binding

The supplementation of 100 mg/kg calcium given intravenously, slowly or intramuscularly is the first step where there is suspicion of hypocalcaemic flaccidity.

The hen should then be placed in a warm environment and kept in a quiet situation. Fluid therapy is also advisable, as the reproductive tract frequently becomes dry and friable due to the pressure of the retained egg.

Historically, the hen was often administered 0.1–1 unit/kg of oxytocin by intramuscular injection, once. However in birds, oxytocin is not produced (they produce vasotocin) and in reality it results in cardiovascular effects and very painful but often ineffective smooth muscle contractions.

Prostaglandin E2 gel, dinoprost at 0.02–0.1 mg/kg topically on the entrance of the reproductive tract to the cloaca, to allow dilation of the vaginal sphincter has also been used. It may be necessary to lubricate the exit of the reproductive tract with a sterile gel.

If none of these methods work, then collapse the egg within the bird in order to reduce the pressure which causes the ischaemia of the intestines and kidneys. This may be done either by passing a hypodermic needle of 23 gauge attached to a 2 mL syringe or through the cloaca and into the end of the egg that is visible. The contents are aspirated. This collapses the egg. It is not necessary to go in after the shell fragments, as these will usually be passed over the next 24 hours.

If the egg is not visible via the cloaca, then the needle may be passed through the body wall in midline ventrally. Again the contents of the egg are then aspirated and the egg gently collapsed.

Covering antibiotics and analgesia should also be considered, particularly if collapse of the egg has been carried out.

Prevention

Firstly, it is important to provide a well-balanced diet, which is correctly supplemented in calcium.

Secondly, if the hen has started to lay eggs, or has a history of problems, a few environmental changes may be performed to reduce further stimulus to lay. The first of these is to reduce daylight length to a maximum of 10 hours/day. This tries to mimic the conditions found in mid-winter, and should help to discourage reproductive activity in the hen.

It is also useful to remove nest boxes from the cage to reduce the visual stimulus to nest and reproduce.

The use of plastic commercial egg replacers to fool the hen in thinking she has produced a full clutch of eggs is useful with indeterminate egg layers such as cockatiels which will keep laying eggs until they reach a certain clutch size. If egg replacers are not available then do not remove the eggs. With budgerigars, it doesn't matter as they are determinate egg layers, i.e., they will lay a set number of eggs irrespective of whether they are removed or not.

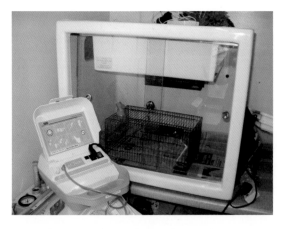

Figure 14.7 A nebulisation circuit that may be attached to an oxygen supply or preferably a nebulisation unit to administer drugs in aerosol form to avian patients with respiratory disease.

If egg laying persists, then hormonal therapy may be tried to suppress the reproductive cycle. Progesterone injections had been the mainstay of hormonal modulation such as medroxyprogesterone acetate. The down side to this medication is the damaging effect the progesterone has on liver function, as well as the risk of iatrogenic diabetes mellitus. Human chorionic gonadotrophin hormone has been used at 500–1000 IU/kg on days 1, 3 and 5. This has fewer side effects and can stop egg laying for up to 6 weeks. More recently, gonadotropin releasing hormone (GnRH) agonists have been used – specifically deslorelin implants that can last for many months. These work by making the GnRH – pituitary – ovary axis to become refractory to stimulation and so they shut down.

The last resort is spaying of the bird. This is a risky operation, and involves the removal of just the uterus. The ovary is left, due to its multiple arterial blood supply making removal dangerous.

Table 14.6 highlights some of the other treatments and therapies commonly used for the management of avian reproductive tract diseases.

Avian urinary tract disease therapy

Table 14.7 highlights some of the treatments and therapies for avian urinary tract diseases.

Avian musculoskeletal system disease therapy

Table 14.8 highlights some of the treatments and therapies commonly used for the management of avian musculoskeletal system diseases. The process for splinting a fractured wing is also described.

Temporary wing splinting

Splinting of wing fractures may be performed with bandage material. It should be noted, though, that when a bird's joint is kept immobilised for a few days it starts to stiffen. This can be disastrous for raptors and wild birds. Bandaging techniques are therefore more suitable for cage and aviary birds, and also for emergency support dressings, or where it is possible to maintain joint movement.

The technique for humeral/radial/ulna fractures is described below:

- Flex the wing using coflex/vet wrap.
- Starting from the point of the elbow, take the bandage over the dorsal aspect of the wing to a point just distal to the point of the carpus.
- Place the bandage over the ventral aspect of the wing, heading back to the point of the elbow.
- Cover the dorsal aspect of the wing to a point just proximal to the carpus.
- Put the bandage onto the ventral aspect of the wing towards the digits.
- Roll it over the leading edge of the wing and the dorsal aspect once more and back to the elbow.

This 'figure of eight' technique bunches the primary feathers together and so uses them as a splint.

Avian neurological system disease therapy

Table 14.9 highlights some of the treatments and therapies commonly used for the management of avian neurological system diseases.

Table 14.6 Treatment of reproductive system diseases.

Diagnosis	Treatment
Prolapsed oviduct	May be a sequel to egg binding and often involves prolapse of the cloaca. Uterus is the most commonly prolapsed part of the oviduct. Tissues become rapidly desiccated and infected, if outside of the body. If the tissues are not too devitalised, they may be pushed back with a moistened cotton bud under anaesthetic. Two simple interrupted sutures may be placed, one either side of the vent, to try and reduce the aperture and prevent recurrence. If the oviduct is devitalised, then removal may be necessary. The cloaca may need to be sutured in place if it repeatedly prolapses also.
Salpingitis	This is by first identifying the bacteria involved by bacterial culture and sensitivity from a swab of the reproductive tract. However, even when the correct antibiotic is chosen for the bacteria isolated, the infection may not be fully cleared. This may be due to the area affected which walls off the infection from the body and results in the need to consider spaying the bird.
Egg yolk coelomitis	Abdominocentesis may be necessary to relieve pressure from the air sacs but should be performed cautiously via midline ventrally under anaesthesia. Antibiotics are also required effective against Gram-negative bacteria (particularly coliforms) and supportive therapy for shock. Short-term shutdown of the reproductive tract with GnRH agonist implants should be considered, but long-term treatment may require laparotomy and debridement of granulation tissue, lipid and surgical spay. The prognosis is guarded.

Table **14.7** Treatment of avian urinary tract disease

Disease	Treatment
Acute renal disease	This is aimed towards encouraging urine production using fluid therapy (see chapter 16) and diuretics, particularly if shock is present. The diuretic used is principally furosemide at 1–4 mg/kg intravenously or intramuscularly. Specific therapy for heavy metal poisoning is based on the chelating agent, e.g. sodium calcium edetate, at 10–30 mg/kg twice daily, intramuscularly for 5 days. For renal coccidiosis, the use of clazuril at 5–10 mg/kg orally every third day on three occasions, or sulphadimidine at 25 mg/kg orally, twice daily for 3 days, resting for 2 days and repeating for 3 days. For chlamydophilosis, doxycycline is the antibiotic of choice (see respiratory tract section), but for Gram-negative bacteria, fluoroquinolones or third-generation cephalosporins are advised.
Chronic renal disease	Even once the causative agent is removed/treated, management of chronic renal failure is challenging. Fluid therapy is required in the early stages of treatment (chapter 16). Supplementation of water-soluble vitamins (B vitamins) and the use of anabolic steroids (to reverse catabolism and bone marrow suppression) have also been advocated. The use of allopurinol at 10–15 mg/kg orally q12 hours is advised when uric acid levels are high, but in some species (e.g. red-tailed hawk) this has been associated with an increase in uric acid levels (Lumeij & Redig, 1992). Colchicine is used in humans to reduce uric acid and can be used in birds at 0.02–0.04 mg/kg orally q12–24 hours. Many birds are too ill to stabilise and euthanasia should be considered where uric acid levels remain >1000 umol/L. Surgery may be performed to remove gout crystals, in joints and alleviate some of the pain and discomfort. However, the underlying renal disease needs to be rectified. Diet of a high bioavailable but lower protein source is sensible. Omega-3 fatty acids have been suggested as useful (Pollock, 2006).

Table **14.8** Treatment of avian musculoskeletal system diseases.

Diagnosis	Treatment
Fracture management	In all cases it is important, particularly for wild birds, to obtain as near a 100% successful repair otherwise there could be a welfare issue releasing such a bird into the wild. *Coracoid, furcula* These usually recover with rest alone – occasionally, they may require an intramedullary pin. *Humerus* This is the most common fracture in raptors (especially hawks). The bone is pneumonised and mid-shaft fractures often traumatise radial nerve. A tie-in external fixator is often required. *Elbow dislocation* Poor prognosis as transarticular fixation is needed so a return to full flight is unlikely. *Ulna and radius* If only the ulna is fractured and there is no displacement – cage rest generally effective with restricted wing movement for 2–3 weeks. If the radius is fractured then intramedullary pin fixation is required. NB: Watch for synostosis between ulna and radius. *Femur* This is uncommon but may be seen in heavier birds. The bone is pneumonised in raptors but often not in Psittaciformes. A tie-in external fixator will be required. *Tibiotarsus and tarsometatarsus* Often associated with trapping or jess injuries in raptors. If a crushing injury occurs then there is a poor prognosis. If it is a clean break but still viable then good prognosis. An external fixator with a tie-in is needed unless it involves small species in which case an 'Altman splint' may be used with two pieces of zinc oxide tape applied on either side of a reduced fracture (see Figure 14.8). *Digit injuries* These may be dressed with a ball bandage (see Figure 14.4) or if amputation is necessary, a light padded elasticated support (see Figure 14.9).
Carpometacarpal luxation	Bandage wings to the body wall for 4–6 weeks if early on in the condition. Once rotation has occurred, the only option is surgical. Poor prognosis for wild release.
Nutritional osteodystrophy	Once bones are deformed and mineralised the only options are surgical. Prevention is geared to adequate diet, calcium supplementation, etc., and not providing excess proteins which generate too rapid growth rates.

Table 14.9 Treatment of avian nervous system diseases.

Diagnosis	Treatment
Hypocalcaemic syndrome of African grey parrots	Acute collapse: Slow intravenous/ intramuscular injection of 100 mg/kg calcium gluconate. Diazepam (0.2 mg/kg) or diazepam (2 mg/kg) intramuscularly to control fitting. Prevention requires adequate dietary calcium and vitamin D_3. This can be achieved through nutritional supplements, ultraviolet light provision (strip lamps if indoors or obviously access to unfiltered natural sunshine) and access to vegetables and some dairy products (e.g,. bioyoghurts and cottage cheese). Most birds grow out of the condition by 5–6 years of age.
Seizuring	Treatment is based on diagnosis of the cause. For heavy metal toxicity see Digestive System Diseases. For hypocalcaemic syndrome, see above; also seen in young raptors. Symptomatic treatment – dimmed lighting, reduced noise levels, careful handling. Use of diazepam/midazolam 0.3–1 mg/kg intravenously/intramuscularly. If the condition occurs in a small raptor, it may be hypoglycaemia. Administer 40% glucose/dextrose w/v intravenously and slowly at 0.25–1 mL/bird depending on the size. Northern goshawks are also prone to hyperglycaemia at the start of the training season. Diagnosis is blood glucose >30 mmol/L. To treat use protamine zinc insulin 0.1 unit and repeat until glucose levels fall below 15 mmol/L (Forbes, 1996b). Lories and lorikeets fed on home prepared nectar formulations may experience hypovitaminosis B1 and seizure. Injections of 3 mg/kg once followed by dietary supplementation at 35 mg/kg food are successful if the bird is treated quickly.
Newcastle disease/PMV-1	Treatment is not possible but vaccination for PMV-1 pigeon paramyxovirus is compulsory in racing pigeons in the United Kingdom. Vaccines include Colombovac® (Pfizer Animal Health) and Nobilis Paramyxo P201® (MSD Animal Health). Pigeon paramyxovirus is notifiable in the United Kingdom and so should be reported to the local Animal Health and Veterinary Laboratories Agency (AHVLA) office.
Proventricular dilatation disease	This may result in central nervous system disease such as torticollis, circling, central blindness and fitting. See Digestive System Diseases for management of proventricular atony. See Seizuring above for control of fitting. Prognosis is poor with CNS signs.
Spinal disease	Fractures of lumbar spine are common sequels to window/car strike incidents. Surgery to stabilise can be attempted with postoperative use of anti-inflammatories such as meloxicam 0.2 mg/kg once daily and physiotherapy of the pelvic limbs. Prognosis is frequently poor. Aspergillomas may also invade the spinal canal from the underlying lung or air sacs. Treatment is as for aspergillosis in Respiratory System Diseases. Prognosis is again poor.

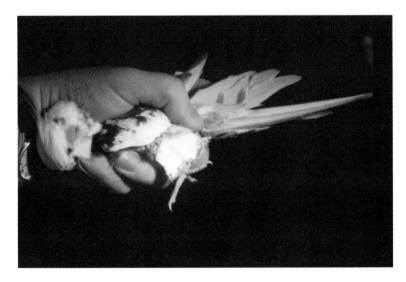

Figure 14.8 An Altman splint applied to the tibiotarsus of this cockatiel (*Nymphicus hollandicus*) for a simple closed fracture. Two pieces of heavy zinc oxide tape are used to sandwich the proximal and distal fragments together.

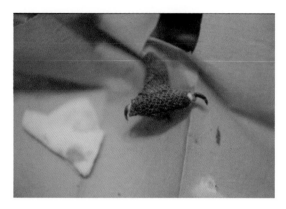

Figure 14.9 A light padding and elasticated bandage support for a toe amputation.

Miscellaneous conditions

Oil spills

Stabilisation

This involves fluid therapy to correct dehydration, due to diarrhoea. Birds are often hypothermic due to plumage damage. Gentle warming in warm air, such as that from a hair dryer, can be used to bring body temperature to near normal. Heated cages with dimmed lighting to reduce further stress are also advisable. As these birds may have been unable to feed for days, readily digestible liquid food should be provided – if necessary by crop tube.

Initial treatment

Oral administration of adsorbents, such as activated charcoal, prevents further absorption of oil. Covering antibiotics and further fluid and nutritional support may also be necessary. Due to the extreme stress of the situation, many birds succumb to systemic fungal diseases such as aspergillosis and this may necessitate additional treatment.

Cleaning

The best cleaning agent for removal of oil is washing-up liquid, which should be diluted 1 part to 50 parts water. This should be lathered into the oil and sprayed off using a shower head attachment. The water supply should be kept at around the bird's own body temperature (between 40 and 45°C) to reduce further loss of body heat. This is important as it may take up to an hour to clean some birds. Attention must be paid to thoroughly cleaning all of the feathers, so a cleaning pattern or routine should be used. Washing can stop when the water starts to form small, bead-like droplets on the feathers.

Once the oil has all been removed, the feathers should be dried initially using a hair dryer, and then by placing the bird in a heated cage. After cleaning and ensuring that the birds are feeding properly and maintaining condition, it is often necessary to retain waterfowl in captivity for a few days to ensure that they are regularly preening to waterproof their feathers.

Lead poisoning

It is often caused by the bird consuming lead shot from shotgun discharges or old lead weights from coarse fishing (which are now banned but can still be found in the environment). Commercial mining may also occasionally contribute to discharges of lead and other heavy metal discharges, such as zinc and tin.

Diagnosis should be made by radiographing the bird to demonstrate radiodense particles in the gizzard or ventriculus. However, many affected birds no longer have lead particles in their digestive system but are still suffering from lead poisoning. Therefore, a blood sample to demonstrate elevated levels of lead is required. Normal levels are below 0.4 ppm, while levels over 0.5 ppm, and particularly over 2 ppm, are diagnostic for lead poisoning.

Treatment with sodium calcium edetate at 20–50 mg/kg twice daily intramuscularly is recommended as a chelating agent – fluid therapy should also be administered as both the heavy metal and the drug are nephrotoxic. Treatment should continue until a return to 'normal' blood levels of lead (<0.2 ppm) or zinc (<2 ppm) are seen assuming all radiodense material has been removed from the gut. The latter may be facilitated by a proventriculus wash with warmed saline under anaesthetic. A tube may be passed with care through the oesophagus and past the crop and into the proventriculus. This is then flushed out by tilting the bird head down. It is essential that an endotracheal tube is used in this process, and that it is snug fitting or has a light amount of air inserted into the cuff. If the particulate matter has moved on, the use of peanut butter on bread for Psittaciformes or waterfowl has been suggested as a means of 'sticking' heavy metal particles and allowing passage out of the ventriculus and gut.

References

Cooper, J.E. (1985) Foot conditions. *Veterinary Aspects of Captive Birds of Prey*, 2nd edn, pp. 97–111. Standfast Press, Gloucestershire.

Forbes, N.A. (1996b) Fits and incoordination. *Manual of Raptors, Pigeons and Waterfowl* (eds P.H. Beynon, N.A. Forbes & N.H. Harcourt-Brown), pp. 197–207. BSAVA, Cheltenham, UK.

Lumeij, J. and Redig, P. (1992) Hyperuricaemia and visceral gout induced by allopurinol in red-tailed hawks (*Buteo jamaicensis*). *Proceedings Tagung der Fachgruppe Gefluegelkrankheiten*, Giessen, Germany.

Oaks, J.L. (1993) Immune and inflammatory responses in falcon staphylococcal pododermatitis. *Raptor Biomedicine* (eds P.T. Redig, J.E. Cooper, J.D. Remple & D.B. Hunter), pp. 72–87. University of Minnesota Press, Minneapolis.

Pollock, C. (2006) Diagnosis and treatment of avian renal disease. *Veterinary Clinics of North America, Exotic Animal Practice*, **9**, 107–128.

Stanford, M. (2004) Interferon treatment of circovirus infection in grey parrots (*Psittacus e. erithacus*). *Veterinary Record*, **154**, 435–436.

Further reading

Chitty, J. and Harcourt-Brown, N. (eds) (2005) *BSAVA Manual of Psittacine Birds*, 2nd edn. BSAVA, Quedgeley, UK.

Chitty, J. and Lierz, M. (2008) *BSAVA Manual of Raptors, Pigeons and Passerine Birds*. BSAVA, Quedgeley, UK.

Forbes, N.A. (1996a) Respiratory problems. *Manual of Raptors, Pigeons and Waterfowl* (eds P.H. Beynon, N.A. Forbes & N.H. Harcourt-Brown), pp. 147–157. BSAVA, Cheltenham, UK.

Harrison, G. and Lightfoot, T. (2006) *Clinical Avian Medicine*. Spix Publishing Inc., Palm Beach, FL.

Lightfoot, T.L. (1998) Approach to avian obstetrics. *Proceedings of the North American Veterinary Congress*, pp. 757–778.

Ritchie, B. (ed) (1995) *Avian Viruses Function and Control*. Wingers Publishing Inc., Lake Worth, FL.

Samour, J. (ed.) (2008) *Avian Medicine*, 2nd edn. Mosby Elsevier, Edinburgh.

Chapter 15 Avian Diagnostic Imaging

Physical restraint

Purpose built perspex restraint boards may be purchased. The basic design is a flat sheet of perspex with at one end a neck vice which constrains the head. A couple of attached fine ropes can be applied to the legs, and a strap will restrain the wings in a dorsal extended position.

This author prefers to use chemical restraint when radiographing avian species to minimise stress.

The only occasions where this is not possible is in the use of positive contrast digestive system studies, where transit times are important and anaesthesia will of course alter these. Also in the case of horizontal beam radiography, which may be used to determine fluid lines in an ascitic patient, the avian patient needs to be conscious and perching!

Chemical restraint

In general, the method of chemical restraint preferred by this author is isoflurane gaseous anaesthetic in 100% oxygen to both induce the patient (at 3–4%) and to maintain (at 1.5–2%) preferably after intubation. Sevoflurane may also be used (induction of 4–6% in 100% oxygen; maintenance at 2–3% in 100% oxygen).

Ketamine may be used at doses of 20–50 mg/kg (Beynon *et al.*, 1996b) for psittacines or as 15 mg/kg in combination with 150–350 mg/kg of medetomidine for raptors (Beynon *et al.*, 1996a). However, recovery time is less predictable and longer, and the results less satisfactory.

Avian patient radiography

As with other species, the traditional two views are required. In avian patients though the wings have a habit of getting in the way, and therefore to maximise the potential of this medium, the wings must be fully abducted and placed extended over the dorsum of the bird when taking lateral views. In addition, the legs should be pulled caudally to avoid excessive overlying of the caudal coelom (see Figures 15.1 and 15.2).

Positive contrast techniques

Barium

This is routinely used to highlight foreign bodies in the gastrointestinal tract, and to differentiate opacities in the caudal coelom, such as retained eggs, from the rest of the coelomic contents. Usually, it is only performed in stabilised patients as it requires 3–4 hours fasting to empty the gut out, and it requires that the patient be conscious for serial radiographs, which is stressful (although it may be performed using horizontal beam radiography with the bird on a perch). For the smaller birds such as cockatiels and budgerigars, 3–5 mL of a 25–30% barium mixture should be crop tubed. For larger birds such as African grey parrots and Amazons, 12–15 mL may be used, and for the larger macaws, 20–30 mL. Serial radiographs are taken at 30 minutes and then hourly until 2 hours post administration, then at 4, 8 and 24 hours post administration.

Transit times vary with species, an African grey parrot's proventriculus will empty around 10–30 minutes post administration of barium sulphate into the crop, reaching the small intestines around 30–60 minutes, the large intestine at 60–120 minutes and the cloaca at 120–130 minutes (see Figure 15.3). Many hawks on the other hand will show proventriculus emptying times around 5–15 minutes post crop tubing, reaching the small intestine around 15–30 minutes, the large intestine around 30–90 minutes and the cloaca around 90–360 minutes (McMillan, 1994).

Barium will also highlight dilations of the crop, and proventriculus as can occur in some neuropathies, or parasitic diseases, as well as swellings, growths, ulcers, etc.

Iodine

Iodine, aqueous-based techniques may be used for intravenous excretory urography examinations when examining the kidney structures for the presence of abnormalities, or for angiography (although fluoroscopic techniques rather than traditional film cassette-based radiography is required for this) techniques.

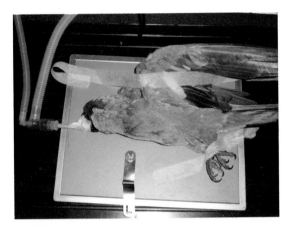

Figure 15.1 Positioning for a right lateral view radiograph in a bird.

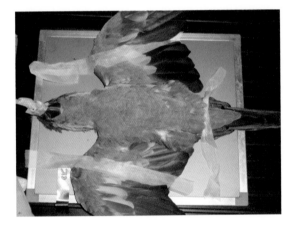

Figure 15.2 Positioning for a standard ventrodorsal view radiograph in a bird.

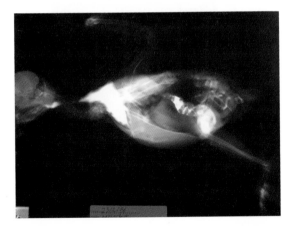

Figure 15.3 Lateral barium digestive tract study in a normal African grey parrot.

In addition, conditions such as choanal atresia, which is a common cause of a permanent clear sinus discharge, may be elucidated by iodine-based contrast techniques injected into the nasal sinuses.

Normal radiographic findings

The avian skeleton is significantly different from its mammalian cousin. Many bones have become fused, e.g. no tarsal bones survive; the proximal row having fused to the distal end of the tibia, forming the tibiotarsus; and the distal row fusing with the proximal metatarsals forming the tarsometatarsus. Birds possess a prominent keel in many species, particularly Psittaciformes, formed from the fusion and extension of the sternal vertebrae (see Figures 15.4 and 15.5). However, some species such as the ratite family and many waterfowl have a flattened, more boat-shaped sternum without the prominent midline crest. Many bones are pneumonised (i.e. connected to the air sac system and therefore have an air-filled medullary cavity rather than bone marrow); common examples include the femur and the humerus, although individual species vary. The pelvis is not fused having two separate slender pubic bones projecting caudal to the femur. The dorsal aspect of the pelvis forms a protective dome fusing with the sacral bones forming the synsacrum. The thoracic vertebrae and sacral vertebrae are both largely fused and immobile. In contrast the cervical vertebrae are highly mobile.

The body cavity, as with reptiles, is not divided into a thorax and abdomen as there is again no diaphragm. In addition, the avian lungs are a rigid structure, paired and closely adherent to the dorsal body wall in the cranial coelom and appear homogenously mottled on lateral radiographs. The air sacs which fill the coelom appear as marked

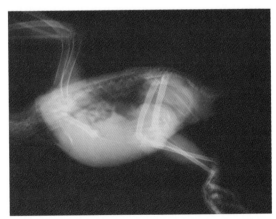

Figure 15.4 Right lateral view of a normal African grey parrot.

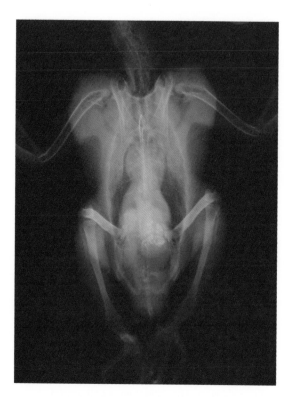

Figure 15.5 Ventrodorsal view of a normal African grey parrot.

radiolucent areas, and allow clear definition of many internal organs. The trachea is mobile and elongated, and may have many coils in certain species of waterfowl such as the trumpeter swans. In many ducks, such as the common mallard, the trachea may have a swelling at its base formed by a bulla, which is a perfectly normal finding.

On lateral radiographs, the heart may be clearly seen with the major arterial and venous trunks leaving and entering it. The caudal border of the heart merges with the liver shadow. Dorsal to the liver lies the spleen, which is spherical in many cage birds, and enlarges markedly during infectious diseases such as chlamydophilosis. In addition, in this region lies the 'true' acid secreting stomach or proventriculus, and immediately caudal to this lies the often grit filled in granivorous species, ventriculus, gizzard or second stomach. Caudal to this lie the intestinal mass. The kidneys lie on the dorsal body wall within the shadow of the pelvis and may be seen to project cranially when enlarged due to inflammatory disease or tumours.

The ventrodorsal view is useful to compare the thoracic and abdominal air sacs, which are prime sites for fungal granuloma formation in diseases such as aspergillosis. The heart shadow is clearly outlined on the ventrodorsal

view, and forms the upper part of an hour glass shape, with the lower chamber being produced by the shadow of the liver. Some species such as the larger cockatoos may have a small heart shadow and/or a small liver shadow which may be a normal radiographic finding. The gizzard or ventriculus is often clearly seen in grit consuming birds, lying to the left of midline in the caudal coelomic region.

Abnormal radiographic findings
Skeletal

Evidence of fractures may be obvious as with most long bone fractures, or slightly less blatant, as with femoral head fractures.

Metabolic bone disease is common in juvenile birds that are fed inappropriate diets, and the bones most commonly affected are the long bones, especially the tibiotarsus, which may bend into a complete right angle (see Figure 15.6).

Other skeletal deformities include polyostotic hyperostosis which is often associated with cystic ovarian disease and persistent hyperoestrogenaemia, leading to a mottled appearance to the long bones.

Soft tissue

Enlargement or reduction in size may be noted in any of the internal organs if affected by disease.

An enlarged liver often present as a reduction in the 'waist' of the hourglass shape created by the heart and liver shadows on the ventrodorsal view, an increase in the width of the liver area and narrowing of the caudal air

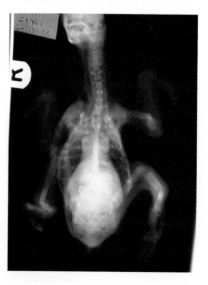

Figure 15.6 Ventrodorsal view of an eclectus parrot chick with metabolic bone disease. Note the deformed long bones and rib cages, the growth plates and the poor bone quality.

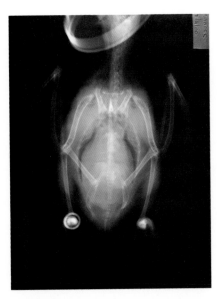

Figure 15.7 Ventrodorsal view of an Amazon parrot with hepatomegaly. Note the reduced caudal air-sac space, the reduction in the 'waist' of the hourglass shape of the major body organs and the increase in width of the liver shadow.

sacs (see Figure 15.7). A reduction in the size of the liver may be seen as a visible gap between the caudal border of the heart and the cranial border of the liver.

An enlarged proventriculus may be seen in gastric dilatation syndrome, and is shown by a fluid-filled organ dorsal to the heart and liver shadow on a lateral radiograph (see Figure 15.8). On a ventrodorsal view, the enlarged proventriculus which lies on the left hand side can be mistaken for an enlarged liver shadow which overlies it (see Figure 15.9).

An enlarged spleen as mentioned may be clearly seen on lateral radiographs dorsal to the liver shadow, around the mid-femur level in infectious disease states, particularly chlamydophilosis/psittacosis (see Figure 15.10).

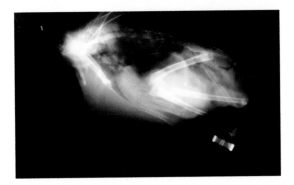

Figure 15.8 Lateral view of an African grey parrot with an enlarged proventriculus seen as a gas-filled viscus above the liver and heart.

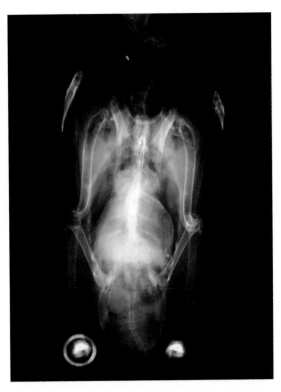

Figure 15.9 Ventrodorsal view of the parrot in Figure 15.8 showing an enlarged proventriculus on the bird's left hand side (our right), which may be mistaken for an enlarged liver.

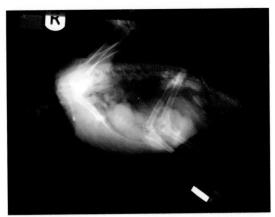

Figure 15.10 Lateral view of a macaw with psittacosis/chlamydophilosis showing an enlarged spleen (the spherical organ mid coelom, at the level of the mid femur).

Enlarged or damaged kidneys may appear more radiodense, or they may project cranially out from the boundaries of the pelvis, or may move dorsocaudally to obliterate a section of the abdominal air sac which normally lies over the dorsal aspect of the caudal kidney area.

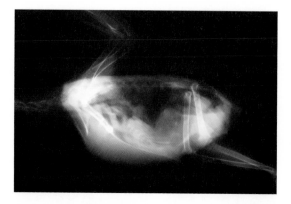

Figure 15.11 Lateral view of an African grey parrot with thickening and increased radiodensity of the major vessels exiting the heart, typical of atherosclerosis.

The great vessels exiting the heart may become dilated, or more radiodense with either atherosclerosis or metastatic mineralisation (see Figure 15.11). The heart itself may also become enlarged with progressive failure in older or diseased birds.

Foreign bodies may also be seen using radiography, particularly metallic elements, which may result in heavy metal (e.g. lead and zinc) poisoning. They will often lodge in the ventriculus (gizzard) in psittacine birds (see Figure 15.12).

Infections of the air sacs are common in psittacine birds and raptors. The most frequently seen disease is perhaps aspergillosis – a fungal infection of the lungs and air sacs. This may produce subtle changes initially but may go on to produce significant radiographic changes in advanced chronic disease (see Figure 15.13).

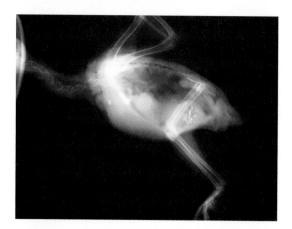

Figure 15.12 Lateral view of an African grey parrot with lead poisoning. Note the radiodense metallic particles present in the ventriculus (gizzard).

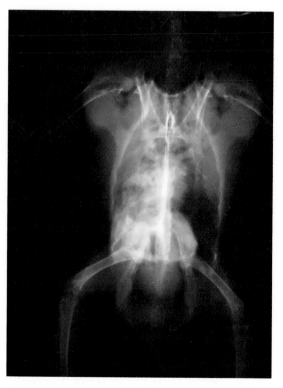

Figure 15.13 Ventrodorsal view of an Amazon parrot with advanced chronic aspergillosis. The bird's right side (our left) is completely obliterated with fungal growth obscuring the air sacs and anatomical structures.

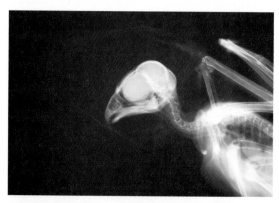

Figure 15.14 Lateral view of a Kestrel's skull showing the prominent hooked beak and large eye sockets and scleral ossicles – the small bones that support the structure of the eye around the scleral junction.

Species variations

There are considerable species variations. Raptors have notable adaptations of the head (see Figure 15.14) and feet (see Figure 15.15) amongst others. Many passerine birds and other nonpsittacine birds have a more elongated body

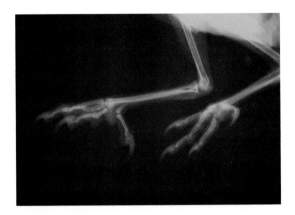

Figure 15.15 Lateral view of a Kestrel's feet showing the anisodactyl limb (as opposed to the zygodactyl limb of psittacine birds) and prominent claws.

form and do not have the hourglass shape comprised of heart and liver but rather a more rectilinear shape.

Ultrasonography

Positioning

The transducer is usually applied to the skin caudal to the keel, ventrally, or in Galliformes and other species where the ribs do not extend as far caudally, access may be gained from the lateral body wall just in front of the leg. Therefore, restraint in lateral or dorsal recumbency, with the head elevated to allow the organs to fall towards the transducer is preferable. It may be possible to image raptors, e.g. on their perches if they are hooded.

Normal ultrasound findings

For most imaging of birds above 150–200 g, it is possible to use a 7.5 MHz sector probe. A 10 MHz probe or a standoff may be required for such a small species as a budgerigar though. Adequate amounts of coupling gel should be applied and allowed to soak into the skin before imaging. It may be necessary to pluck a few feathers as well, although careful wetting and parting of the feathers, particularly immediately caudal to the sternum on the ventrum, will allow access to the skin without this.

The main problem with ultrasound examination of birds is the presence of the air sacs which of course completely block the passage of ultrasound waves. It is possible to use organs as 'windows' to view other organs, and this is usually the case with the liver which is easily accessible from the caudal sternum position and may be used to image the heart. Where ascitic/coelomic fluid is present, of course this modality becomes much more useful.

Liver: The liver as mentioned is easily imaged from a ventral approach immediately caudal to the sternum. As with mammals, the normal liver is homogenous in density (see Figure 15.16). Blood vessels may be seen readily within the parenchyma as hypoechoic areas. Most of the commonly seen species in general practice do not possess a gallbladder.

Heart: The heart can be seen as a four-chambered structure, although there is a disproportionate difference between the size of the larger left ventricle and the smaller right ventricle (see Figure 15.17). It is generally difficult to see all four chambers in one section as the right and left atria are in a slightly different plane from the ventricles. The left ventricle also has a thinner wall than the right ventricle. The right ventricle ends before reaching the cardiac apex.

The valves of the heart may also be distinguished. The right atrioventricular (AV) valve is normally thickened, muscular and is singular. The left AV valves are similar

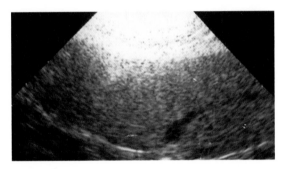

Figure 15.16 Liver structure should be homogenous. Note the blood vessel creating a hypoechoic line arcing across the lower right of the structure.

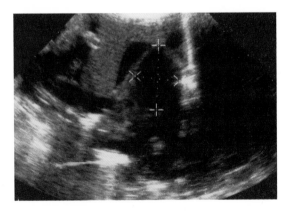

Figure 15.17 Image of the heart. Note the liver at the top of the picture, which is used as the acoustic window to visualise the heart.

to that seen in the cat and dog. The aortic valves are also easily seen and are paired.

Normal values for the heart parameters have been published for African grey and Amazon parrots by Pees *et al.*, 2004.

Other organs: It is not normally possible to image many of the healthy organs of birds due to the presence of the air sacs, these include: Kidneys, spleen and reproductive organs. Shelled eggs in the oviduct appear obviously hyperechoic, but laminated eggs, i.e. those without a shell yet formed around the yolk and albumen, may also be seen in the oviduct. The yolk tends to be more hyperechoic, and the albumen hypoechoic in structure (see Figure 15.18).

Abnormal ultrasound findings

Liver: Liver enlargement is difficult to assess using ultrasound as the full extent of the liver cannot be determined in one view. However, the protrusion of the liver beyond the caudal sternum/xiphoid is usually taken as an indication of hepatomegaly.

Where the liver is markedly enlarged, it may be possible to see dilated vessels within the parenchyma and increased echogenicity of their walls. Hepatic lipidosis (fatty liver degeneration) is seen as increased echogenicity and liver size. Hepatic tumours, whether primary or secondary, may of course be identified with ultrasound techniques as areas of increased and decreased echogenicity, although these may be difficult to separate from granulomas and areas of hepatic necrosis unless a discrete capsule to the neoplasm is seen. Hepatic enlargement and necrosis seen as large hypoechoic areas is a common finding in liver diseases such as haemochromatosis (iron storage disease).

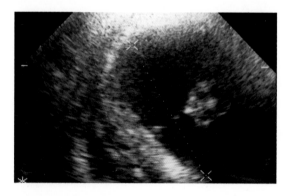

Figure 15.18 Egg in the coelomic cavity. The outer albumin is hypoechoic and the central yolk is hyperechoic.

Heart: The presence of a pericardial effusion, as with mammals is considered abnormal in birds. Overall cardiac enlarged, as associated with cardiomyopathies is also easily diagnosed. Valvular defects have been reported in birds and ultrasound may be used to diagnose these (Rosenthal & Stamoulis, 1993).

Kidneys: Renal tumours, such as those commonly seen in budgerigars, may be diagnosed, as they often enlarge rapidly from the cranial pole of a kidney and may be cystic in nature.

Reproductive system: Coelomic deposition of eggs (so-called 'internal laying') may occur with some cage birds and may result in egg yolk peritonitis. Such eggs may be seen either as hypoechoic or multilaminate structures.

Other organs: Where ascitic/coelomic fluid is present, most of the organs may be imaged easily. In cases of cystic ovarian disease, the classical hypoechoic 'bunches of grapes' may be seen as the ovary becomes enlarged enough to push ventrally. Egg yolk peritonitis will present with a marked coelomic effusion which has a turbid appearance, and so has areas of increased echogenicity whereas a true ascitic effusion tends to be hypoechoic in nature.

Dilatation of the proventriculus may also be imaged, due to its distended size, and a thinning of its wall may further enhance a diagnosis. Splenomegaly, particularly in cases of chlamydophilosis, may also be diagnosed by ultrasound, as the spleen pushes ventrally towards the body wall caudal to the proventriculus. The spleen in most Psittaciformes is rounded, and will have increased echogenicity in comparison to the liver, but is normally homogenous in character. Splenic tumours are rare, but may also present as with mammals with hypoechoic areas within the parenchyma.

MRI and CT scanning

Both these modalities have been reported in avian patients. CT scanning of the head to examine fractures of jaw bones such as the quadrate bone which is easily damaged when birds fly into windows is far easier than trying to make the same diagnosis using radiography. MRI scanning of the heart and liver is useful as these are difficult sometimes to visualise on radiographs and ultrasound examinations owing to their encasement within the ribcage.

Endoscopy

Rigid endoscopes are extremely useful to enable visualisation and guided sampling of lesions. They can be used to look down the trachea for syringeal aspergillomas, into the crop and on into the proventriculus for upper GI tract examination, into the cloaca to look for papillomas etc. In addition, the presence of air sacs within the bird makes it an ideal candidate for laparoscopic endoscopy.

Access to coelom

The point of access is the lateral body wall. The boundaries of the entrance point are taken as the cranial edge of the iliotibial muscles (with the bird in lateral recumbency and the legs pulled caudally) and the caudal edge of the pectoral muscles. This site is between the last two ribs for a psittacine bird (may be just caudal to the last rib in a passerine or raptor) (see Figure 15.19). The skin is incised with scissors and the body wall muscles are bluntly dissected using a pair of mosquito haemostats.

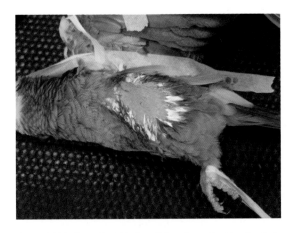

Figure 15.19 Site and positioning of the avian patient for standard rigid endoscopic examination of the coelomic cavity.

The left flank is used when wishing to examine the gonads for sexing, as well as being useful for examining the spleen, gizzard, pancreas left kidney and left lung. The right flank is preferable for examining the right testis, right kidney and right lung. For views of the liver, the bird should be in dorsal recumbency and the access point is immediately caudal to the sternum and midline.

References

Beynon, P.H., Forbes, N.A. and Harcourt-Brown, N. (1996a) Formulary. *Manual of Raptors, Pigeons and Waterfowl*. BSAVA, Cheltenham, UK.

Beynon, P.H., Forbes, N.A. and Lawton, M.P.C. (1996b) Formulary. *Manual of Psittacine Birds*. BSAVA, Cheltenham, UK.

McMillan, M.C. (1994) Imaging techniques. *Avian Medicine: Principles and Applications* (eds B.W. Ritchie, G.J. Harrison and L.R. Harrison), pp. 246–326. Wingers, Fort Worth, FL.

Pees, M., Straub, J. and Krautwald-Junghens, M.E. (2004) Echocardiographic examinations of 60 African grey parrots and 30 other psittacine birds. *Veterinary Record*, **155**, 73–76.

Rosenthal, K. and Stamoulis, M. (1993) Diagnosis of congestive heart failure in an Indian hill mynah (*Gracula religiosa*). *Journal of Association of Avian Veterinarians*, **7** (1), 27–30.

Further reading

Chitty, J. and Harcourt-Brown, N. (eds) (2005) *BSAVA Manual of Psittacine Birds*, 2nd edn. BSAVA, Quedgeley, UK.

Chitty, J. and Lierz, M. (2008) *BSAVA Manual of Raptors, Pigeons and Passerine Birds*. BSAVA, Quedgeley, UK.

Harrison, G. and Lightfoot, T. (2006) *Clinical Avian Medicine*. Spix Publishing Inc., Palm Beach, FL.

Krautwald, M.E., Tellhelm, B., Hummel, G., Kostka, V. and Kaleta, E.F. (1991) *Atlas of Radiographic Anatomy and Diagnosis of Cage Birds*. Paul Parey, Berlin.

Ritchie, B. (ed) (1995) *Avian Viruses Function and Control*. Wingers Publishing Inc., Lake Worth, FL.

Samour, J. (ed) (2008) *Avian Medicine*, 2nd edn. Mosby Elsevier, Edinburgh.

PART II: AVIAN SPECIES

Chapter 16 | Avian Emergency and Critical Care Medicine

Triage

Any bird presented unconscious, fitting, with evidence of head trauma or respiratory distress should be attended to immediately. Birds that are off colour and dull should be moved into a quiet, warm (29–30°C), dimly lit area with supplemental oxygen, if there is any evidence of tachy/hyperpnoea and should be examined as soon as possible.

Cardiopulmonary-cerebral resuscitation in birds

The ABC may be followed for birds as for mammals – although there is now some feeling that the correct order should be CAB as the circulation contains enough oxygen to maintain life, providing it can keep moving around the body even with temporary loss of breathing.

A for airway and B for breathing

During anaesthesia with isoflurane or sevoflurane, cardiac arrest is usually preceded by respiratory arrest when it occurs. The prognosis, providing the bird is intubated and the anaesthetist vigilant and the process is spotted before cardiac arrest, is good. The anaesthetic should be stopped immediately and mechanical ventilation initiated. If intubation is not possible, a tight-fitting face mask may be used; but it is preferable to consider placing an air-sac tube (see below). Doxapram may be used to stimulate respiration centrally by applying a drop to the oral mucosa or injecting intramuscularly 1–2 mg/kg (roughly 0.1 mL for birds 200 g).

Where the trachea may be blocked as with a foreign body or an aspergilloma, it may be necessary to place an air-sac tube. This is where a tube is inserted through the body wall into an air sac due to the fact that birds can extract oxygen from the air on both inspiration and expiration, it does not matter which way the air enters the respiratory tract. A typical air-sac tube is placed as follows:
1. Place the bird in the right lateral recumbency position. The bird may first be anaesthetised, or in emergencies this may be performed in the conscious bird.
2. Elevate the uppermost wing (left). Another operator pulls the uppermost leg caudally.
3. Make a small skin incision just caudal to the last rib, and just ventral to the pelvis at its conjunction with the spine (see Figure 16.1).
4. Pass either a specifically designed air-sac tube (see Figure 16.2) through the body wall or a short length of 2–3.5 gauge endotracheal tubing is grasped with a pair of haemostats and pushed through the body wall. The cuff on the endotracheal tube or air-sac tube may be inflated and the tube sutured to the body wall.
5. The outlet of the anaesthetic circuit may then be attached to the free end of the tube to administer anaesthetic or oxygen. Alternatively, in the conscious bird the air-sac tube is cut short and may be left in place for normal breathing for 3–4 days whilst the bird's condition is treated.

C for cardiovascular system

Bradycardia often precedes cardiac arrest and is due to heart blocks developing (similar to those in small mammals). If this is detected quickly, administration of atropine (0.01–0.02 mg/kg IM/IV) or glycopyrrolate (0.01 mg/kg IM/IV) may be enough to reverse this.

If cardiac arrest has occurred, then the prognosis in birds is poor. This is owing to the fact that the heart is protected behind the keel/sternum and ribs and so external massage is less effective than in mammals. In addition, there is no diaphragm and so clinicians cannot use the thoracic pump mechanism to increase overall negative thoracic pressure. Adrenaline may be administered, preferably intratracheally, at 0.01–0.02 mg/kg with atropine 0.02–0.04 mg/kg. Application of regular compressions on the caudal sternum can be attempted to start cardiac massage. The patient is best placed in dorsal recumbency to allow better compression of the heart with the sternum, but be aware that positive pressure ventilation is more difficult in this position owing to the pressure of the viscera on the lungs and heart.

Veterinary Nursing of Exotic Pets, Second Edition. Edited by Simon J. Girling. © 2013 John Wiley & Sons, Ltd. Published 2013 by John Wiley & Sons, Ltd.

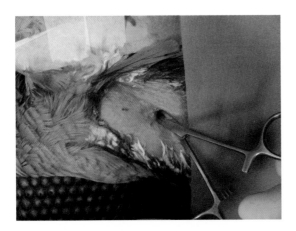

Figure 16.1 A stoma in the caudal body wall being made using blunt dissection with a pair of haemostats to allow the insertion of an air-sac tube.

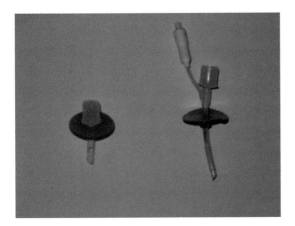

Figure 16.2 Commercially available (Cook Veterinary Products®) air-sac tubes.

D for drugs

See Table 16.1 for tabulated information on emergency drugs in birds. In cases of respiratory arrest, administration of 0.5 mg/kg doxapram, *per os* or intravenously, is advised followed by intubation and manual or machine-assisted IPPV. If cardiac arrest occurs, then intubation and intratracheal administration of adrenaline (0.05 mL for a budgie and up to 0.5 mL for a grey parrot) followed by compression of the cranial chest wall between finger and thumb five times in a row, followed by five breaths via an ET tube, and then five compressions of the chest wall etc. may allow revival. Intubation should be attempted wherever possible. However, if it is not possible, then a face mask with 100% oxygen is used and the resuscitator places the bird in lateral recumbency and grasps the uppermost wing at the carpal joint and rhythmically pumps the wing up and down. This has the effect of raising and depressing the chest wall, thus simulating inspiration and expiration.

Other drugs used before a diagnosis can be accurately made include broad spectrum antibiosis. Often combinations of a fluoroquinolone (e.g., enrofloxacin (Baytril2.5%® Bayer Animal Health) at 10 mg/kg b.i.d. or marbofloxacin (Marbocyl Small Animal Injection® Virbac) at 10 mg/kg s.i.d.) and a potentiated penicillin (e.g., amoxicillin/clavulanate at 150 mg/kg b.i.d.) are advised as these will cover most of the bacterial pathogens seen in avian medicine. If aspergillosis is suspected, then nebulisation of drugs such as Amphotericin B (Fungizone® Squibb) and F10® (Health and Hygiene Pty) may be of some help, as is an intravenous bolus of Amphotericin B (at 1.5 mg/kg IV) or oral itraconazole (Itrafungol® Janssen) (at 5–10 mg/kg b.i.d.) or oral terbinafine (at 10–15 mg/kg b.i.d.).

In the case of birds such as grey parrots or in laying hens/birds on poor quality diets where a possible calcium deficiency may be a cause for collapse of the patient, the use of calcium gluconate is advised. Doses of 50–100 mg/kg IM have been quoted. Doses of 0.2–0.5 mg/kg diazepam may be needed to control seizure initially in some of these cases.

Where heavy metal poisoning (mainly lead or zinc) is suspected, the chelating agent sodium calcium edetate should be used at 20–50 mg/kg IM b.i.d. Fluid therapy should always be used as heavy metals and possibly this drug itself may be nephrotoxic.

Where egg binding has occurred, it is vital to keep the patient warm, quiet and well hydrated. Use of prostaglandin E2 gel applied directly to the oviduct sphincter inside the cloaca is necessary to help release the sphincter and encourage contraction of the uterine muscle. In some circumstances, collapsing the egg inside the bird either by puncturing it through the cloaca with a needle or via a midline ventral abdomen insertion of a needle attached to a syringe may be necessary to relieve pressure from the abdomen, which can cause ischaemic necrosis of the vital organs due to the relatively large size of bird eggs.

E for ECG

ECG traces may be taken from birds, although it is preferable to anaesthetise the bird to perform them. It is also helpful to blunt the alligator teeth on the clamps as these can traumatise the skin very easily. The bird is placed in dorsal recumbency and the clips attached to the skin of the thighs and the skin of the propatagium (the bit of

Table **16.1** Commonly used emergency and recovery medications for birds.

Drug	Dosage	Notes
Adrenaline	0.05–0.5 mL depending on patient size	Use intratracheally after intubation and IPPV with 100% oxygen
Amoxicillin/clavulanate	150 mg/kg b.i.d.	Useful where anaerobes may be present (e.g.. cat bites etc.)
Amphotericin B (Fungizone® Squibb)	1.5 mg/kg IV	Aspergillosis. Always use aggressive fluid therapy as nephrotoxic
Calcium EDTA	20–50 mg/kg b.i.d. IM	Chelating agent for lead or zinc poisoning. Always use aggressive fluid therapy to avoid renal damage
Calcium gluconate	50–100 mg/kg IM	Hypocalcaemic fits, particularly African grey parrots
Diazepam	0.2–0.5 mg/kg IM/IV	Muscle necrosis if given IM
Doxapram	0.5 mg/kg PO/IV	Intubate and use IPPV
Doxycycline (Vibravenosa® Pfizer)	75–100 mg/kg IM every 5–7 days for 42 days	Treatment for psittacosis. Human drug and requires VMD authorisation for import to United Kingdom. Causes muscle necrosis.
Doxycycline (Ornicure® Dechra Animal Health)	In water medication	Works if patient drinks water. NB is licensed for treatment of psittacosis in cage birds and pigeons in the United Kingdom.
Enrofloxacin (Baytril 2.5%® Bayer Animal Health)	10 mg/kg b.i.d.	Licensed antibiotic for birds. Useful against Gram-negative bacteria but not against anaerobes. Can cause muscle necrosis.
Furosemide	0.1–2 mg/kg	Diuretic. Lories (type of nectar eating parrot) are very sensitive
Itraconazole (Itrafungol® Janssen)	5–10 mg/kg b.i.d.	Aspergillosis – do not use in African grey parrots
Midazolam	0.2–0.5 mg/kg IM/IV	Less likely to cause muscle necrosis than diazepam
Meloxicam	0.2 mg/kg IM/PO s.i.d.	Beware use if already has renal damage
Prostaglandin E2 gel	Apply 0.1 mL/100 g bird	Apply direct to oviduct sphincter inside vent to relax sphincter, increase uterine tone and aid egg passage.

PART II: AVIAN SPECIES

skin between the shoulder and carpus of the wing on the wings' leading edge). Alternatively, place hypodermic needles through the skin of the wings and thighs, and attach the clamps to these.

In most avian species, the lead II trace appears as a mammalian one, except the QRS complex appears inverted. This is not the case, but rather it occurs because the S wave is the dominant deflection and the Q wave hardly records at all. For this reason, bird's QRS waves are often referred to as 'rS' waves. P and T waves are as for mammals (see Figure 16.3). Occasionally in some species (pigeons, some parrots), there is a small depression wave known as a Ta wave immediately after the P wave and this is normal (it represents atrial repolarisation) see Figure 16.4. In addition, the P on T phenomena (where the P wave is superimposed onto the following T wave) is a normal finding in some African grey and Amazon parrots.

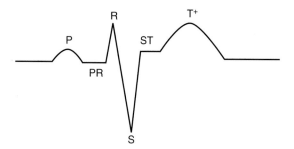

Figure 16.3 Normal lead II annotated ECG trace for a bird.

Values for ECGs in birds have been published but vary between species and exceed the scope of this text. Many birds have heart rates too fast to record on even 50 mm/ second traces. It is more important to look for arrhythmias such as severe bradycardia (a common abnormality before cardiac arrest in anaesthetised birds) instead.

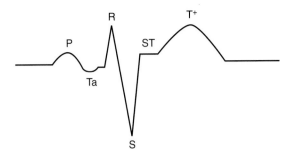

Figure 16.4 Normal lead II annotated trace for pigeons and some psittacine birds showing the Ta wave associated with atrial repolarisation.

Monitoring of CPCR responses

Assessment of cardiac output by using end-tidal CO_2 level has been suggested (Lichtenberger, 2007). A steady increase in end-tidal CO_2 during CPCR should occur and if it has not exceeded 10 mm Hg after resuscitation has been ongoing for 15–20 minutes, the prognosis is poor.

Venous blood is preferable for assessment of blood gases and pH as this more closely represents the body organ's status than arterial blood does.

Mucous membrane colour should be assessed where possible – the lining of the cloaca or the mouth are the two best sites in birds. Cloacal temperature may also give an indication of peripheral perfusion and should be 40–42°C.

Blood pressure may be monitored as described below under monitoring of acute hypovolaemia.

Initial clinical assessment of the avian patient

Do not be too quick to physically restrain the sick avian patient, particularly if it is a small species and/or in respiratory distress. Severe respiratory distress is obvious, with respiratory stertor, wheezes and whistles, but subtle changes such as an increase in respiratory rate, tail bobbing and nasal discharge/blocked nares may all indicate relatively serious respiratory pathology. Birds have no diaphragm and therefore rely on the outward movement of the ribcage and downward movement of the keel to allow inspiration. Any restriction of this (coupled with a stress response increase in oxygen demand) will lead to hypoxia, possible cardiac ischaemia and arrest.

Examine in cage first, use dimmed/blue/red lighting. If in doubt, admit to place the patient in an oxygen-enriched atmosphere +/− nebulisation with saline first. Then see if you can physically restrain the patient for examination. It

may be anaesthetising the patient in 100% oxygen with isoflurane is the preferred method.

Initial assessment should look at the following points:
1. Feather condition – chewed feathers, fret lines, discolouration, feather loss etc.
2. Are the feathers fluffed up?
3. Are the eyes closed?
4. Are the corneas bright?
5. Is there respiratory noise?
6. Is there tail bobbing when breathing indicating dyspnoea/hyperpnoea?
7. Are the nares clear or is there a serous or purulent discharge?
8. Is there any faecal clumping to the feathers around the vent?
9. What is the recent faecal output like?
10. Are the urates green/mustard yellow? (may indicate liver disease)
11. Is there any blood in the faeces (may indicate haematuria such as is seen in heavy metal poisoning)?
12. Is there undigested seed in the faeces? (may indicate proventricular dilatation disease or pancreatitis)
13. What is the bird's weight, and what is the muscle condition of the pectoral area like? (body scores of 0–5 may be given as with other animals)
14. What is the stance of the bird like? (upright on the perch, on the floor, leg weakness, respiratory distress etc.)
15. Is there evidence of vomitus/regurgita on the feathers around the head?

All of these assessments can be made relatively quickly and often without actually handling the patient.

Detailed examination of the avian patient

Once it is assumed safe to handle the patient, a more detailed examination may be made.

See Table 16.2 for some normal biological parameters of selected birds.

Examination

A detailed examination should include the following:
1. An intraoral examination using a mouth gag or a pen/pencil to encourage the bird to open its beak. This should allow a close examination of the tongue, the internal nostril or choanal slit (the communication between the nasal passages and the mouth), and the palate. The glottis may also be visualised. Abnormalities such as a discharge from the choanal slit, loss of

Table 16.2 Biological parameters for selected bird species.

Species	Order	Heart rate at rest (bpm)	Respiration rate at rest (bpm)	Average weight	Diet
Canary	Passeriformes (perching birds)	275	60–80	25–30 g	Seeds, grasses
Zebra finches	Passeriformes (perching birds)	300	90–110	15–20 g	Seeds, grasses
Budgerigar	Psittaciformes (parrot)	250	60–75	25–45 g	Seeds, vegetables and fruits
Cockatiel	Psittaciformes (parrot)	200	40–50	50–60 g	Seeds, vegetables and fruits
African grey parrot	Psittaciformes (parrot)	150	15–45	400–500 g	Seeds, nuts, pulses, vegetables and fruits
Blue-fronted Amazon	Psittaciformes (parrot)	150	15–45	400–550 g	Seeds, nuts, pulses, vegetables and fruits
Blue and gold macaw	Psittaciformes (parrot)	100	20–25	650–850 g	Seeds, nuts, pulses, vegetables and fruits
Ringed-neck parakeet	Psittaciformes (parrot)	175	30–45	80–100 g	Seeds, vegetables and fruits
Tawny owl	Strigiformes (owl)	150	15–40	400–550 g	Chicks, rodents
Barn owl	Strigiformes (owl)	150	15–40	400–500 g	Chicks, rodents
Harris hawk	Falconiformes (bird of prey)	100	20–40	0.75–1.5 kg	Chicks, rodents
Peregrine falcon	Falconiformes (bird of prey)	125	30–45	0.65–1 kg	Chicks, rodents
Golden eagle	Falconiformes (bird of prey)	90	10–20	3–6 kg	Chicks, rodents, rabbits

NB: All birds body temperature is higher than mammals, and all are broadly similar at around 41–42°C. Birds do not seem to show significant physiological pyrexia in the presence of infection.

papillae on the palate, an abnormal or foul odour and evidence of white or yellow plaques on the mucosa should all be noted, and if possible, sampled with a swab dampened with sterile water.

2. A detailed examination of the nares and the eyes. This will allow an assessment of any upper respiratory tract disease. Clinical signs of this include: abnormal shaped nare(s); loss of the rostral concha(e) (operculum); sinking of the globe of the eye; swelling below the globe of the eye (the region of the infraorbital sinus); discharge from the eye itself; swelling of the conjunctiva; and corneal blemishes.

3. A detailed examination of the feathers themselves. This is particularly useful regarding the blood or newly emerged 'pin' feathers. These may be plucked from the body area and the sheath carefully slit to reveal the pulp, which may then be made into a smear and stained. This can give evidence for skin/feather pulp infections. Examination of the shaft and vane of the feather may also reveal evidence of lice and mites.

4. A detailed auscultation of the lungs and air sacs. The lungs are best auscultated from the dorsum between the wings as they are closely attached to the ventral aspect of the thoracic area. The air sacs are dispersed throughout the body. The most easily auscultated, and thankfully those with often the most pathology are the abdominal and caudal thoracic air sacs that may be auscultated on the ventral aspect of the body caudally, just behind the keel bone. The heart may be auscultated from the lateral body wall just underneath the wings.

5. A detailed examination of the wings may be made. When anaesthetised, an idea of wing integrity and the elasticity of the propatagium (wing web) may be made by placing the bird on its sternum and extending both wings laterally to an equal distance and then letting them go. They should both recoil equally. Any asymmetry should be noted and may indicate joint or propatagial injury.

6. A detailed examination of the vent and caudal abdomen should also be made. The caudal abdomen, unprotected by the keel bone, should be naturally concave. Any

convexity may indicate a space-occupying mass in the coelomic cavity of the bird, such as hepatomegaly, or the presence of ascites. In smaller birds (<300 gm) slightly wetting the feathers over the ventrum in this region will allow the clinician to see through the thin skin of the body wall, and if hepatomegaly is present, the dark black-brown shadow of the liver will be seen. Normally, the liver does not extend caudal to the keel bone.

Monitoring and vital sign assessment

Pulse assessment

Assessing a pulse can be very difficult in birds owing to their rapid heart rates and thin-walled vessels which can be easily occluded. In most cases, assessments of pulse are made using Doppler ultrasound probes that can be attached to the following blood vessels:

1. Basilic vein (runs over the ventral aspect of the elbow joint of the wing)
2. Medial metatarsal vein (runs over the medial aspect of the lower unfeathered leg and may be clearly seen in waterfowl)

Capillary refill times should be less than 2 seconds as with mammals. They may be assessed on mucous membranes around the mouth and face or vent.

Cardiac and respiratory auscultation

To auscultate the lungs of a bird, the stethoscope diaphragm must be placed over the dorsum of the bird as the lungs are closely adherent to the underside of the dorsal thoracic wall. Air sounds may be heard over the flanks and ventrum, but these are due to referred sounds and the sounds of air moving through the air sacs (balloon-like structures inside the bird). The lungs being rigid, and there being no diaphragm, the bird inspires by moving its keel bone ventrally and ribcage laterally, which creates a negative pressure inside the single body cavity (coelom). This allows air to be drawn in through the trachea, down to the lungs (which do not inflate or deflate significantly being semirigid in nature) where gaseous exchange occurs. As the lungs do not inflate, air already in the lungs moves into the air sacs caudally. On expiration, the process is reversed, and means that air in the caudal air sacs is pushed back through the lungs, allowing extraction of oxygen on both inspiration and expiration. It then goes into the cranial air sacs. In fact, the whole process, from the moment any one air molecule enters the trachea to its final expulsion, occurs over two cycles of inspiration and expiration.

The heart may be auscultated over the pectoral area. Heart rates are usually very fast even in the larger parrots and so hearing murmurs is difficult. Arrhythmias, however, may be detected.

Neurological assessment

Fitting or collapsed birds may be affected by heavy metal poisoning (particularly lead, but also zinc); hypocalcaemia (particularly in a hen bird that is egg laying and on an unsupplemented diet or a young African grey parrot as the latter species has a particular hypocalcaemia syndrome); hypoglycaemia (particularly common in birds of prey that are underweight and being flown regularly); or a CNS infection whether it be due to parasites (usually protozoa) or bacteria.

Assess whether the bird can perch using both legs. If held in the hand, see if the bird can grasp a finger/towel with both feet. Unilateral leg paresis through to full paralysis is common, particularly in small psittacine birds such as the budgerigar where they are often associated with a renal or gonad tumour (the gonads are of course internal in birds in both males and females). This is due to the mass pressing against the sciatic nerve (referred to as the ischiatic nerve in birds), which passes through the kidneys before entering the leg. The same syndrome may be seen in toxicities such as heavy metal (lead or zinc) poisoning or organic toxins such as those associated with aspergillosis infection of the airways.

Birds of prey that are suffering from lead poisoning, having consumed lead shot in the prey that they have been fed, will often sit on the floor, rocked back onto their 'hocks' with drooped wings and a slightly drunk appearance.

Assess whether the bird is holding both wings normally. One wing drooping is most likely to be associated with a muscular/skeletal injury. Both wings drooping is more likely to be lead or permethrin/organophosphate poisoning.

Birds will not demonstrate eye nystagmus as they are relatively large in comparison to the skull. Instead, birds with central nervous system disease affecting the vestibular section of the brain will often demonstrate a whole head nystagmus. In addition, head tilts are common with peripheral and central vestibular disease.

Pupillary reflexes do not work well in birds as they have a significant amount of skeletal muscle in their irises which is under conscious control. Also the eyes are so big and the bone separating them from each other in midline is often so thin, that light shone into one eye frequently passes through the bony septum and into the opposite eye as well!

Pulse oximetry

Pulse oximeter probes may be attached to distal legs over the medial metatarsal area or over the basilic (brachial) vein on the ventral aspect of the elbow. However, it should be noted that avian haemoglobin is different from mammalian and therefore the accuracy of pulse oximeter readings is questionable. It is still useful to use the probe to assess *changes* in the SpO$_2$, but actual values (providing the readings stay above 90%) are not reliable.

Blood biochemistry

There are so many species of birds that any meaningfully accurate table would be too large to include here. Instead, Table 16.3 below gives broad ranges of common biochemical parameters for birds routinely seen in practice. It should be noted that, as with reptiles, uric acid is the only useful indicator of renal function, although usually less than one quarter of the kidneys need to be left functioning before uric acid levels become elevated. Urea and creatinine levels do not provide information on renal function in birds and reptiles.

Haematology

As with biochemistry, values vary between species. Some indication of PCVs across avian species has been given in chapters 9 and 14. In general, white cell counts are in the range of 10–18 $\times$ 10^9/L. In parrots, three main conditions will push the white cell count over 30 $\times$ 10^9/L and these are

1. Psittacosis (infection with *Chlamydophila psittaci*)
2. Egg yolk coelomitis (equivalent to peritonitis but where the yolk ruptures internally instead of being shed into the oviduct)
3. Mycobacteriosis (rare)

Occasionally, infections such as aspergillosis (a fungal infection usually of the airways) may stimulate a similar response, although more commonly the patient has a low white cell count when severely affected.

The avian equivalent of the neutrophil is the heterophil so named because of its part basophilic part eosinophilic staining with Romanowsky stains. It has a bi-trilobed nucleus and brick red cigar-shaped granules in its cytoplasm. Evidence on a blood smear of degranulation of these and rupture of the cells (toxicity) is a strong indicator of active and severe infection.

Erythrocytes and platelets in birds are nucleated. The erythrocytes are rugby ball shaped with a similar shaped nucleus. The platelets are oval and smaller. Other cells are similar to those seen in mammals.

Urinalysis

This is less useful than for mammals owing to the faecal contamination that occurs with avian urine. However, it is important to look at the urates (white portion of the dropping) to see if there is any blood, or if the

Table 16.3 Average plasma biochemistry values for birds.

Parameter	Value	Notes
Total protein g/L	30–50	
Albumin g/L	16–32	
AST IU/L	100–350	Not liver specific, also found in muscle
CK IU/L	50–300	Only found in muscle
LDH IU/L	150–450	Not liver specific, also found in muscle including cardiac
Calcium mmol/L	2–3.25	May be elevated in hen birds around egg production. Total calcium levels may appear within normal range whilst bird is still showing signs of hypocalcaemia (especially African grey parrots) as ionised calcium is the biologically active fraction (African grey parrot ionised calcium results around 0.96–1.22 mmol/L)
Phosphorus mmol/L	1–1.85	
Glucose mmol/L	10–20	Note: Budgerigars may be seen with glucagon-associated diabetes mellitus; birds of prey may be seen with hypoglycaemia associated with exercise when malnourished-glucose levels usually 30 mmol/L
Uric acid μmol/L	150–350	Gout (precipitation of uric acid) occurs when levels exceed 1500. May be transiently elevated in birds of prey immediately after a meal.

urates have turned mustard yellow or lime green. If the latter has occurred, this is evidence of biliverdinuria, which in birds is an indicator of liver inflammation/damage (common with psittacosis in parrots and lead poisoning in birds of prey). Biliverdin is the main excretory product of the liver as opposed to bilirubin in mammals.

Volumes of water/true urine should be small in a healthy bird's dropping. If they are very watery, as opposed to diarrhoea, then this may indicate polyuria.

Blood in the urates is often associated with heavy metal, particularly lead poisoning.

Monitoring and treatment of acute hypovolaemia

Systolic blood pressure monitoring can be performed by placing a cuff on the distal humerus or femur and the Doppler probe on the medial surface of the proximal ulna (proximal ulnar artery) or tibiotarsus (medial metatarsal artery). Cuff widths should be 40% of the circumference of the humerus or distal femur, which means that for small avian patients, the available commercial cuffs are really too large. Systolic blood pressure monitoring using the indirect method correlate better with directly measured blood pressure in birds than is the case in mammals (Lichtenberger & Ko, 2007). Central venous pressure monitoring in birds has not been quantified and is technically difficult.

Anything below 90 mm Hg is considered hypovolaemic for birds (and anything above 200 mm Hg is hypervolaemic). Bolus administration of fluids should be attempted intravenously or intraosseously (see below for access sites) until correction of blood pressure. Crystalloids are administered at a rate of 10 mL/kg and colloids such as Hetastarch or Oxyglobin® can be administered at 5 mL/kg – usually one or two boluses are required. In larger species 5 mL/kg of 7.5% hypertonic saline may be used once to increase systolic blood pressure.

Calculation of fluid therapy requirements in birds

Please refer to Chapter 14 for standard fluid requirements and administration in birds.

Nebulisation

This can be a good method to deliver medications for the respiratory system and also to deliver moisture aiding in rehydration, particularly in small species. For further information, see Chapter 14.

Supportive therapy
Ongoing medication
Details of antibiotics useful in birds have been given in Table 16.1. Chelation therapy for heavy metal poisoning is also listed. Prokinetics are not necessary.

Ongoing nutritional supplementation with calcium/vitamin D_3 replacers is useful in cases of African grey parrot hypocalcaemia and examples include Nutrobal® and Zolcal-D® produced by Vetark Professional Ltd.

Other mineral and vitamin supplements are often required if the diet is poor or restricted to seeds in the case of parrots (as well as trying to introduce fruit and vegetables), particularly vitamin A.

Critical care nutrition including calculation of energy requirements
Calculation of energy requirements can be made using the formula

$$BMR = k \times (weight\ (kg))^{0.75}$$

where k the constant is 78 for parrots and 129 for other birds. Remember that MER (metabolic energy requirement) is generally 1.5–2× the basal metabolic requirement (BMR) and if disease is present, then this further amplifies the required calories (sepsis and burns for example may increase MER by 2–3×).

Assisted feeding techniques and foods
The majority of cage birds are granivorous/herbivorous/frugivorous. Members of the parrot family should not be fed meat or dairy products as these can result in renal, hepatic, and cardiovascular diseases. Many cage birds can feed themselves; however, emergency nutrition may need to be used such as Vetark Professional Ltd's Critical Care Formula, or even vegetable-based baby foods (avoid lactose in these products) and these may need to be crop tubed. This process preferably involves the use of a purpose designed, steel blunt-ended crop tube that can be attached to a syringe containing the food formula. The beak is opened and a gag inserted whilst the tube is advanced from the bird's left side, dorsally over the base of the tongue and glottis and down to the base of the neck slightly to the right of midline. See section headed 'Crop Tubing' for maximum values that may be crop tubed at one time.

Raptors are of course by nature carnivores and should preferably be fed whole prey such as rodents or day-old chicks. However, in the practice environment, this may not be possible and therefore 'crop tubing'/gavaging is necessary. This can be performed by making use of products such as Hills a/d®, Virbac's Reanimyl or other related cat/dog high-protein/calorie diets. Care should be taken initially to ensure that the patient is correctly hydrated before loading large amounts of protein into it. It may be better in a severely weakened bird to start off with simple sugar/amino acid products such as Vetark's Critical Care Formula® before moving on to high-protein/fat diets.

Crop tubing

Once rehydrated, crop tubing with critical care support formulas (such as 'Critical Care Formula®' Vetark) may be crop tubed (see Figures 16.5 and 16.6). An idea of maximum volumes that may be safely crop tubed into an avian patient at any one time are given in Table 16.4.

Nursing of wounds

Avian wounds generally gape as their skin is not very elastic. However, the skin is often very thin and has a low bacterial burden, so traumatic wounds if relatively clean may be cleaned briefly with dilute povidone–iodine or chlorhexidine, and then either staple or glue it closed. An Elizabethan collar should be applied to the bird, making sure it is reversed to point caudally as parrots cannot move around their cage or eat with the collar projecting cranially (see Figure 16.7).

For deeper wounds associated with bites etc., particularly if they occur over the legs distally, debridement of the wound under anaesthetic is essential to prevent infections of the avascular tendons or worse, osteomyelitis. Once cleaned, the wounds may be dressed with

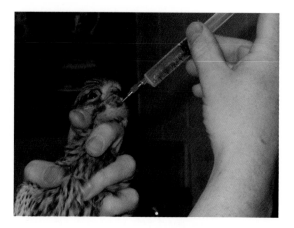

Figure 16.6 Crop tubing a Kestrel with support formula.

Table 16.4 Maximum volumes that may be safely administered via crop tube.

Species	Maximum volumes
Budgerigar	0.5–1 mL
Cockatiel	2.5–5 mL
Conures	5–7 mL
Cockatoos	10 mL
African grey	8–10 mL
Macaws	10–15 mL

GranuFLEX® (Convatec UK Ltd.) to aid granulation, or covered with Veterinary Biosist® (Cook Products Ltd.) that may be sutured over the deficit. Secondary and tertiary bandage material may be applied over the top to protect the wound further. A collar should always be used in parrots, although many birds of prey will leave dressings alone, particularly if they are hooded (falcons).

For fracture stabilisation, a figure-of-eight bandage may be used on wing fractures for a short period (<48 hrs) to contract the wing and bind it to the lateral body wall. Any longer immobilisation leads to fibrosis of the joints and will result in severe impairment in wing function.

Leg fractures in small cage birds such as canaries, may be stabilised using the so-called 'Altman' splint. This is simply two pieces of heavy zinc tape applied laterally and medially to the fractured leg, sandwiching the leg between them. These can be left on or replaced as the bird chews them off for the duration of the healing process.

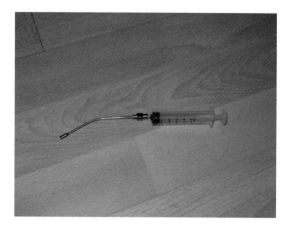

Figure 16.5 A curved, stainless steel crop tube attached to a disposable syringe.

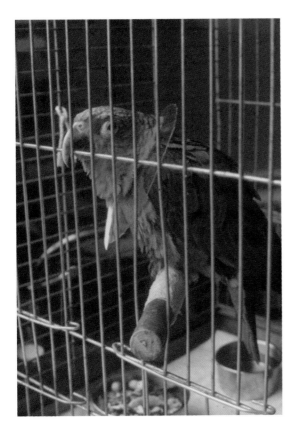

Figure 16.7 When applying an Elizabethan collar to birds, make sure it is positioned to face backwards otherwise the bird cannot eat or limb around its cage.

Finger splints or tongue depressors may be used in larger birds for temporary stabilisation, but these will generally require a surgical fixation.

Placement of tubes

Feeding tubes are generally not used in birds owing to the fragile nature of their skin and the presence of air sacs throughout the body.

Air-sac tubes are mentioned above.

References

Lichtenberger, M. (2007) Shock and CPCR in small mammals and birds. *Veterinary Clinics of North America: Exotic Animal Practice*, **10**, 275–291.

Lichtenberger, M. and Ko, J. (2007) Critical care monitoring. *Veterinary Clinics of North America: Exotic Animal Practice*, **10**, 317–344.

Further reading

Chitty, J. and Harcourt-Brown, N. (eds) (2005) *BSAVA Manual of Psittacine Birds*, 2nd edn. BSAVA, Quedgeley, Glos.

Chitty, J. and Lierz, M. (2008) *BSAVA Manual of Raptors, Pigeons and Passerine Birds*. BSAVA, Quedgeley, Glos.

Harrison, G. and Lightfoot, T. (2006) *Clinical Avian Medicine*. Spix Publishing Inc., Palm Beach, FL.

Rosenthal, K. and Stamoulis, M. (1993) Diagnosis of congestive heart failure in an Indian hill mynah (*Gracula religiosa*). *Journal of Association of Avian Veterinarians*, **7** (1), 27–30.

Samour, J. (ed) (2008) *Avian Medicine*, 2nd edn. Mosby Elsevier, Edinburgh.

PART II: AVIAN SPECIES

Part III Reptiles and Amphibians

Classification

Reptiles are classified into many different family groups, according to a number of physical, anatomical, and evolutionary factors. It is useful to know to which group a reptile belongs, as this gives an indication of the other reptiles to which it is related. This is of some help when faced with a species that you have not seen before.

Table 17.1 contains some of the more commonly encountered family groups of reptiles seen in general and reptile orientated practices.

SNAKES

Like the bird, the snake has no diaphragm, so no separate thorax and abdomen. Instead it has a coelomic, or common, body cavity.

Musculoskeletal system

All true snakes have no limbs. This distinguishes them from species such as the slow worm, which is actually a lizard with vestigial limbs. There are some remnants of limbs in one or two of the older evolutionary species of snake such as the boid family (pythons and boa constrictors). These can possess vestigial pelvic remnants, having claw-like spurs either side of the vent representing the hind limbs.

The snake skull possesses a small cranial cavity containing the brain and a large nasal cavity. The maxilla has 4 rows of teeth, two on either side. The mandible has the more normal two rows of teeth (Figure 17.1). The teeth vary somewhat between the genera. The more commonly seen non-poisonous species such as the colubrid family (containing the kingsnakes and rat snakes) and the boid family, have simple, caudally curved, peg-like teeth. Some of the more poisonous species have specialist adaptations. Rattlesnakes, for example, have hinged, rostrally situated fangs which swing forward as they strike. All teeth are replaced as they are lost, including fang teeth in poisonous species. It is worth mentioning that owners (other than zoos) of poisonous species of snake, such as pit vipers

and rattlesnakes, must be licensed and registered in the United Kingdom under the conditions of the Dangerous Wild Animals Act of 1976.

The anatomy of the snake's head has a number of adaptations that allow it to swallow large prey. In all snakes, the two halves of lower jaw are loosely held together rostrally and the mandibular symphysis can separate. In addition, the snake has no temporomandibular joint. Instead it possesses a quadrate bone, which articulates between a mandible and the skull and allows the mandibles to be moved rostrally and laterally, 'dislocating'. The maxilla also hinges only loosely with the rostral aspect of the cranium, so allowing the nose of the snake to be raised, increasing the oral aperture.

The skull articulates with the atlas vertebra via a simple joint containing only one occipital condyle, rather than the mammalian two. The coccygeal vertebrae (those caudal to the vent) are the only vertebrae with no ribs attached. Instead they have paired, ventral, haemal processes between which the coccygeal artery and vein run. This vein can be used for venipuncture both for sampling and for intravenous injections. The site for this is one third the distance from the vent to the tail tip on the ventral aspect.

The ventral scales, known as scutes or gastropeges, overlie the muscular casing of the snake's torso. This muscle is segmental and supplied by intervertebral nerves. It is by alternately contracting and relaxing these segmental muscles that the snake can propel itself across the ground, the caudal edge of each ventral scute providing friction.

A very few species of snake, such as the glass snake, exhibit autotomy. That is, they will shed their tail if roughly handled or caught by a predator. They will regrow their tail later.

Respiratory system (Figure 17.2)
Upper respiratory system

The nostrils are paired and open into the roof of the mouth. Snakes, like all reptiles other than crocodilians, do not have a hard palate. When the mouth is closed,

Veterinary Nursing of Exotic Pets, Second Edition. Edited by Simon J. Girling. © 2013 John Wiley & Sons, Ltd. Published 2013 by John Wiley & Sons, Ltd.

Table 17.1 Basic classification of reptiles.

Superorder	Description
Chelonia	Contains all shelled reptiles, e.g., the order Testudines which itself contains most turtles and tortoises such as the true 'tortoises' (Family Testudinidae - e.g., *Testudo* spp. Mediterranean tortoises)

Lepidosauria	Classically this superorder contains the order Squamata which contains the:
	    Suborder Serpentes (i.e., the snakes) suborder Lacertilia (i.e., the lizards) suborder
	      Amphisbaenia (the worm-lizards)
	More recently the order Squamata has been divided into the:
	Suborder Iguania (containing the Agamids, Iguanids, Chameleons and New world lizards)
	Suborder Scleroglossa which itself is then split into the following infraorders
	    Anguimorpha (Monitor lizards, Heloderma lizards, slow worms etc.)
	    Amphisbaenia (worm lizards)
	    Gekkota (the geckos)
	    Scincomorpha (skinks, whiptail lizards and European Lacertid lizards)
	    Serpentes (the snakes)

Crocodylomorpha	Contains the order Crocodylia which contains the following families
	    Gavialidae (the gharial)
	    Alligatoridae (the alligators and caimans)
	    Crocodylidae (the crocodiles)

the internal nostrils are positioned directly above the entrance to the trachea. This is guarded by the glottis. An epiglottis may be present in vestigial form, but there is often fusion of the cartilages here to form a glottal tube. This tube is rigid enough to withstand the pressures placed upon it when the snake is swallowing whole prey. At rest the glottis is held closed, only opening when the snake breathes. The glottis then opens into the trachea which, in the snake family, is supported by C-shaped cartilages similar to those of the cat and dog.

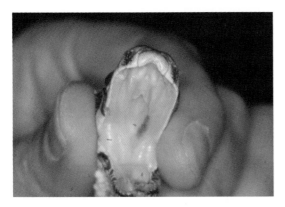

Figure 17.1 Intraoral view of a young Burmese python showing the four upper and two lower rows of teeth, as well as the glottal tube and tracheal entrance, rostral to which is the tongue sheath.

Lower respiratory system

In the majority of colubrid species, such as rat snakes and kingsnakes and some Viperidae, the right lung is the major lung, the left having regressed to a vestigial structure. The vestigial left lung is often replaced by a vascularised air sac and so can take part in gaseous exchange. In the evolutionarily older species such as the Boidae there are two lungs.

The trachea bifurcates at the level of the heart. The lungs occupy the first half of the middle third of the body of the snake. As there is no diaphragm, inspiration is purely due to the outward movement of the ribs and intercostal muscles. This is aided by elastic tissue present within the lung structure, which allows the lungs to expand and recoil. Expiration is facilitated by contraction of abdominal and intercostal muscles, and the elastic recoil of the lungs themselves. A 'tracheal lung' is often present as an outpouching of the lining of the trachea from the open part of the C-shaped cartilages. This is thought to aid respiration when main lungs are being compressed during the swallowing of large prey items.

The stimulus for respiration is a lowered partial pressure of oxygen, rather than an increase in the partial pressure of carbon dioxide, as is the case in mammals.

Digestive system
Oral cavity

The tongue sits in a basal sheath at the rostral end of the oral cavity just in front of the glottis and can be pushed out through the lips even when the mouth is closed through

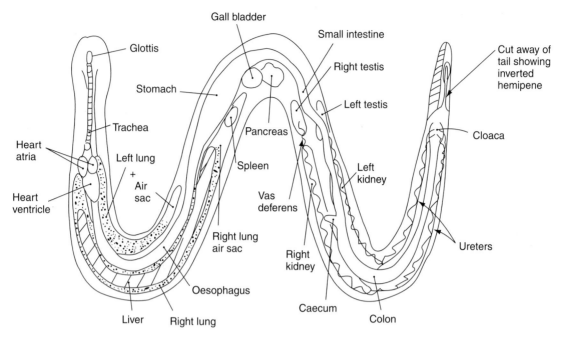

Figure 17.2 Diagram of a male snake (ventral aspect).

the labial notch. The tongue is bifid (split into a forked end) and is used to catch odours on its moist surface. These are then pushed into the roof of the mouth into the vomeronasal organ. The vomeronasal organ is connected to the olfactory region of the brain and is a primitive but effective pheromone and scent detector. The oral cavity contains salivary glands which are stimulated to release saliva during mastication. The mouth is normally free of saliva at other times.

The oropharynx passes on into the oesophagus, which is an extremely distensible muscular tube travelling ventral to the lungs and entering the stomach in the second half of the middle third of the snake's body.

Stomach, associated organs and intestine

The stomach is a tubular organ, populated with compound glands secreting both hydrochloric acid and pepsin (mammals having two separate cells) and separate mucus secreting glands. There is no well-defined cardiac sphincter. The majority of the digestive process occurs in the stomach and is continued by the small intestine. The only substance which cannot be digested is the hair of the prey, known as the 'felt', which is passed out in the stool.

The stomach empties into the duodenum, which is poorly defined from the jejunum and ileum. The spleen,

pancreas and gall bladder are found at the point where the pylorus empties into the small intestine. Some snakes have a fused splenopancreas. The gall bladder is found at the most caudal point of the liver, which is an elongated structure extending from the mid-point of the lungs to the caudal stomach.

The small intestine empties into the large intestine, which is distinguished from it by its thinner wall and larger diameter. In the Boidae there may be a caecum at this junction.

The large intestine empties into the coprodeum portion of the cloaca, which, as with birds, is the common emptying chamber for the digestive, urinary and reproductive systems.

Urinary system

There are paired elongated kidneys (Figure 17.3), situated in the distal half of the caudal third of the snake's body, attached to the dorsal body wall. The right kidney is cranial to the left and both has a single ureter each which travels across their ventral surface to empty into the urodeum of the cloaca, caudal to the proctodeum. There is no urinary bladder in snakes. The caudal portions of the kidneys in male snakes are the 'sexual segments', enlarging during the breeding season as they provide seminal fluid.

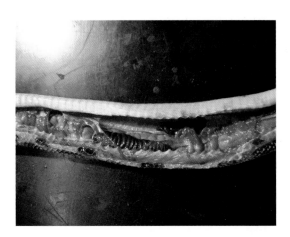

Figure 17.3 Postmortem showing the elongated lobular right and left kidneys of a rainbow boa constrictor (*Epicrates cenchria*).

Renal physiology

As with the majority of reptiles, snakes are uricotelic, that is, like birds their primary nitrogenous waste product is not urea but uric acid. This compound is relatively insoluble allowing conservation of water. This is particularly important for reptiles, as they have no loops of Henle in their kidneys; therefore, they cannot create hypertonic urine as mammals can. To further conserve water, urine in the urodeum portion of the cloaca can be refluxed back into the terminal portion of the gut where more water reabsorption can occur. If the reptile becomes dehydrated, or renal blockage or infection occurs, then excretion of uric acid is reduced and can lead to gout as is seen in birds.

Cardiovascular system

Heart

The heart is three-chambered, with two atria and a common ventricle situated within the pericardial sac, but it despite this functions as a four chambered organ. The heart lies in the caudal half of the proximal third of the snake's body, and is mobile, to allow the passage of large food items through the oesophagus above it. There are two cranial venae cavae and one caudal vena cava entering via the sinus venosus (a narrow tube leading to the right atrium from which it is separated by the sino-atrial valve).

Blood vessels

The snake family has paired aortas. They exit one from each of the two sides of the single ventricle of the heart and then fuse into a single abdominal aorta. The pulmonary artery that leads to the lung(s) also arises here.

As with birds, snakes have a renal portal system. The blood supply from the caudal portion of the snake in the coccygeal artery splits into two and can enter the renal circulation or may bypass it via a series of valves. This is important when administering drugs which are nephrotoxic, or which may be excreted by the kidneys, as it means they might be concentrated there. They should therefore be administered in the cranial part of the snake.

There is also a hepatic portal system from the intestine to the liver. A ventral abdominal vein lies in the midline, just beneath the ventral abdominal musculature, and must be avoided when performing surgery.

Two external jugular veins run just medial to the ventral cervical ribs, and may be reached to place catheters for intravenous fluid administration via a surgical cutdown procedure. The ventral tail vein has already been mentioned and is useful for venipuncture for blood collection.

Lymphatic system

There are no specific separate lymph nodes as seen in mammals, a situation similar to birds. Instead, as with birds, there are discrete accumulations of lymph tissue within most of the major organs, particularly the liver and intestines. There is also a spleen, as mentioned above, which has loosely arranged red and white pulp. Lymphatic vessels are found throughout the body. A lymphatic sinus, for example, runs the length of the snake just ventrolateral to the epaxial musculature immediately below the skin surface on either side of the body. This may be used for small volumes of fluid administration. In the walls of many of the lymphatic vessels there are muscular swellings known as 'lymph hearts' which aid in the return of the straw-coloured lymphatic fluid back to the true heart.

Reproductive system

Male (Figure 17.2)

The paired testes lie intracoloemically (within the coelom or common body cavity, as snakes, like most reptiles, have no diaphragm and so no separate thorax and abdomen; rather they have only a common coelomic cavity). They are situated cranial to each kidney, and caudal to the pancreatic tissue, with the right testis slightly cranial to the left, and are oval in shape. The testes enlarge during the breeding season, often reaching two to three times their quiescent state. Close to the testes lie the adrenal glands. Each testis has a solitary vas deferens leading down to the urodeum portion of the cloaca, where seminal fluids from the reproductive sexual segment of the kidneys are added.

The male snake also has paired penises, known as hemipenes, in its tail. At rest they are like two inverted sacs either side of the midline and lie ventral to two other small invaginations in the tail which form the anal glands. When a hemipene's lining becomes engorged with blood, it everts, forming a finger-like protrusion through the vent. As with the domestic cat, the hemipenes are often covered in spines and barbs, and they each have a dorsal groove into which the sperm drops from the cloaca, and so is guided into the female's cloaca. The hemipenes therefore do not play any part in urination.

Female

The female has paired ovaries, cranial to the respective kidneys, with the right ovary cranial to the left. There are two coiled oviducts starting with the fimbriae opposite each ovary, and moving through the tubular portion of the infundibulum and on into the magnum. From here the tract merges into the isthmus and then the shell gland or uterus before opening into the muscular vagina. This organ ensures that the eggs are laid only when the timing is correct. The vagina empties into the urodeum section of the cloaca. The vascular supply is from the dorsally suspended oviduct mesentery, rather than the caudocranial route employed in mammals.

Most females are stimulated to reproduce in the spring, when the weather warms and the daylight length increases. The tropical boas (such as the boa constrictor) and the Burmese python (*Python molurus*), however, start breeding when the temperature drops slightly during the cooler portion of the year.

Some species of snake are oviparous (i.e., they lay eggs), others are viviparous (i.e., they bear live young). The latter are, for example, the garter snakes (*Thamnophis sirtalis*) and the boid family, which have a vestigial egg structure more closely resembling a placenta. Other species make nests, and some species of python will incubate eggs by contracting and relaxing skeletal muscles, so creating warmth.

Sex determination and identification

Snakes are chromosomally dependent for sex determination, as with most mammals. This is in contrast with the Chelonia, Crocodylia and some lizards, in which sex may be temperature dependent.

Sex identification is best made by surgical probing. A fine, sterile, blunt-ended probe is inserted through the vent and advanced just to one side of the midline in a caudal direction. If the snake is a male, then the probe will pass into one of the inverted hemipenes to a depth of 8–16 subcaudal scales. In the female, there are anal glands in this region, and so the probe may be inserted only to a depth of 2–6 subcaudal scales. In some species, such as the boid family, the males possess a paracloacal spur. This is the remnant of the pelvic limb and may be found on either side of body, ventrally, at the level of the cloaca. In very young snakes it may be possible carefully to evert the hemipenes manually, a technique known as 'popping'.

Skin

The outer epidermal layer in snakes is thrown into a series of folds forming scales, which cover the whole surface of the snake. There are different sizes of scale over the body, with smaller, less raised ones covering the head and larger and more raised scales over the main portion of the body. Some species have scales with ridges on their surface to add greater grip; other species have smooth scales. In some snakes, such as the sea snakes, the skin is very loose fitting, and apparently has few elastic fibres. Other snakes have elastic skin which relatively quickly returns to its normal shape. The reptile skin has little or no skin glands. Its outer layer, or stratum corneum, is heavily keratinised, and composed of three layers of dead cells filled with keratin. These cells become progressively more flattened as they approach the surface. On the ventral surface of the snake there is a single row of scales which span the width of the snake, and are known as the ventral scutes or gastropeges. The caudal edge of each overlaps the cranial edge of the following scale (Figure 17.4).

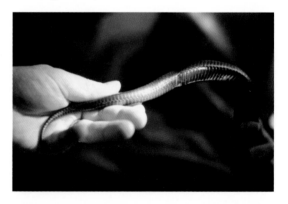

Figure 17.4 The vent of a rat snake showing the division of the ventral scales from single scutes cranial to the vent to paired scales caudally.

Ecdysis

Ecdysis is the regular shedding of the entire skin. Other reptiles also shed their skin, but the Chelonia and Crocodylia shed individual scutes, and the lizards shed in patches. Only the snakes shed all of their skin (including the clear, fused eyelids, or spectacle) in one go. The stimulus can be dependent on time of year, health status and age of the snake and the process is partly controlled by the thyroid gland.

First, the new layer of skin is formed deep to the old one. Once it is complete, the snake secretes a proteinaceous lymph fluid between the new layer of skin and the old one. At this time the snake will become dull in colour, and often exhibits blueing of the eyes. The fluid forces the outer layer of old skin to separate away from the new, and often contains enzymes to help in this process. Once separation has been achieved the fluid is reabsorbed and the snake's eyes may be seen returning to normal. A few days later the snake will shed the old skin. It starts the process by rubbing the corners of its mouth on some abrasive surface. The shedding proceeds with the head skin first and the snake then rolls the old skin back until the tail is the last to emerge.

In a healthy snake all of the skin should come away at once. If the skin does not shed the condition is known as dysecdysis. There can be many reasons for this. Disease, dehydration (which causes too little fluid to be produced), scars on the skin surface or lack of an abrasive surface upon which to remove the skin can all be factors. Regular bathing and soft but abrasive damp surfaces may be needed to aid shedding, and any underlying disease should be attended to.

Special cutaneous adaptations in snakes

There are one or two special structures associated with the skin of snakes. These include the lateral spurs of the Boidae, which have been mentioned earlier. The male possesses larger spurs than the female.

Snakes do not have mobile eyelids. Instead, the eyelids have become fused together and transparent, forming the so-called 'spectacle'.

Many snakes also have special sense organs on the head. The older snake families such as the Boidae have labial pits – a series of depressions running along the dorsal border of the upper jaw. These function as rudimentary heat sensors. In the more evolutionarily advanced species, such as the pit vipers, the heat sensing organs can actually focus on their prey, and are composed of bilateral, forward-facing pits midway between the nares and the eyes. They are supplied by branches of the trigeminal nerves, and, in the case of pit vipers, may be sensitive enough to detect changes of heat as small as 0.002°C!

Snakes do not possess an external eardrum or middle ear. They can, however, hear airborne sounds and can of course detect ground tremors.

LIZARDS
Musculoskeletal system

Lizards have a musculoskeletal system more familiar to those used to dealing with mammalian forms. They possess, in the majority, four limbs, an axial skeleton and much of the anatomical layout of small mammals. There are some exceptions, one being the slow worm, a native of mainland Britain and northern Europe which resembles a snake, having no obvious external limbs. It is actually, however, a highly evolved lizard with rudimentary limbs.

The skull is more rigid than its snake counterpart, having less mobile jaws. There are four rows of teeth, one to each jaw. These are peg-like in shape and are continually replaced in lizards except for the Agamidae and Chamaeleonidae. There are no fang teeth in lizards, but the beaded lizard (*Heloderma horribilis*) and the Gila monster (*Heloderma suspectum*) have hollow teeth which allow the venom from sublingual venom glands to ooze through them into the prey when they bite them. These two species are therefore currently classified as dangerous wild animals under the Dangerous Wild Animals Act 1976 (as amended), in the United Kingdom requiring a special licence to keep them in captivity outside of a zoological collection.

The skull articulates with the atlantal cervical vertebra via a single occipital condyle. The thoracic vertebrae and lumbar vertebrae generally have paired ribs on either side. The coccygeal vertebrae possess ventral haemal arches, between which it is possible to access the ventral tail vein for venipuncture.

In many lizards, the tail possesses fracture planes which allow the tail to break off during escape from a predator. These fracture planes occur in the mid to caudal portions of the tail, but not proximally, where vital structures such as the male reproductive organs and fat pads are stored. Only certain species exhibit this tail autotomy. This includes most of the Iguanidae, but does not include the Agamidae, monitor lizards and true chameleons. When the tail is regrown in these species, the coccygeal vertebrae are not replaced, instead a cartilaginous rod of tissue forms the rigid structure. In addition the rows of scales over the new tail surface are often haphazardly arranged and do not match the size and shape of the rest of the tail (Figure 17.5).

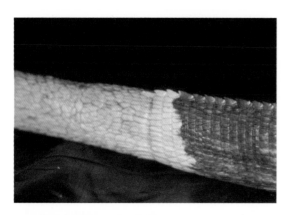

Figure 17.5 Regrowth of the tail is possible in many species of lizard, but the scales which regrow are arranged haphazardly, and the vertebrae lost are replaced by a rod of cartilage.

Respiratory system (Figure 17.6)
Upper respiratory system
Lizards have paired nostrils situated rostrally on the maxilla. To the side, or just inside the nares, particularly in iguanids, there is often situated a pair (one on each side) of salt-secreting glands. These are responsible for excreting excess sodium as sodium chloride so helping

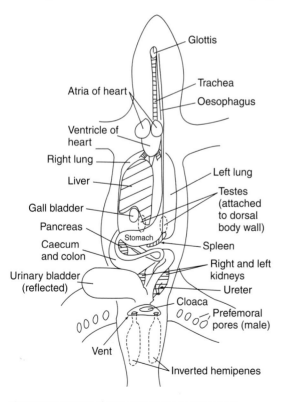

Figure 17.6 Diagram of male green iguana (ventral aspect).

to conserve water. The sodium chloride may be seen as a white crystalline deposit around the nostrils which is often sneezed out by the lizard. The nostrils enter into the rostral part of the oral cavity, there being no hard palate.

The entrance to the trachea is guarded by a rudimentary larynx which often lacks an epiglottis and vocal folds. Some species, such as the Geckonidae, do possess vocal folds and are capable of producing a variety of sounds. In most species, the trachea is supported by incomplete cartilaginous C-shaped rings similar to those of the cat and dog.

Lower respiratory system
The trachea bifurcates into two main bronchi in the cranial thorax to supply two lungs. In more primitive lizards, the lungs are sac-like structures with large bulla-like divisions and alveoli. In the more advanced lizard species, the lungs are more like the mammalian sponge-like system, with finer divisions and more structured alveolar systems. Lizards will often overinflate their lungs in an attempt to make themselves look bigger, when threatened.

There is no diaphragm in any lizard species, so there is no clear distinction between the thorax and abdomen, rather there is a common body cavity, known as the coelom, as in snakes and birds.

Respiration is thought to be stimulated by falling partial pressures of oxygen in the blood stream. The act of inspiration is due to the mechanical contraction of the intercostal muscles causing an upwards and outwards movement of the rib cage. This is aided by the elastic tissues that are present within the lung structures themselves. Expiration is by contraction of the abdominal and intercostal muscles, and by the elastic recoil of the lung tissue.

Digestive system
Oral cavity
The majority of lizards have a large, fleshy tongue which is frequently mobile. In some species however, such as the chameleons, the tongue has become specialised. It lies coiled in the lower jaw and can be projected out at a flying insect or other potential prey item. The green iguana has a more traditional fleshy tongue, which has a much darker tip. This is not to be confused with pathological changes. A vomeronasal organ is present.

Stomach, associated organs and intestine
The stomach is a simple sac-like structure in most species. The glands are combined hydrochloric-acid- and

pepsin-secreting glands lining the walls. There are also separate mucus-secreting glands for lubrication.

The small intestine is better developed in more carnivorous species such as the monitor lizards and the insectivorous water dragons. In herbivorous species it is relatively short. It is poorly divided into jejunum and ileal structures. In a few, mainly herbivorous, species, at the junction between the small and large intestines lies the caecum. The liver is roughly bilobed in structure and is situated ventral to the stomach and lungs. There is usually a gall bladder, with the primary bile pigment being biliverdin, as with birds, rather than the bilirubin of mammals.

The large intestine is more highly developed in herbivorous species than in carnivorous or omnivorous species. Examples include the green iguana and the chuckwalla. These have a large intestine which is often sacculated and divided into many chambers by leaf-like membranes. These increase the intestinal surface area so that microbes, upon which these species depend for vegetation digestion, may colonise it.

The large intestine then empties into the coprodeum portion of the cloaca. The cloaca itself is then continued, as with birds and snakes by the other two segments, the urodeum which receives the urogenital openings, and the proctodeum which is the last chamber before waste exits the cloaca through the vent.

Urinary system

The kidneys are paired and often bean-shaped organs. Their position is variable depending on the species. In some, such as the green iguana, they are both situated in the pelvis, attached to the dorsal body wall (see Figure 17.6). Other species, such as chameleons, have longer kidney structures which extend cranially into the coelomic cavity. As with snakes, the males of some species have a specially developed caudal portion of the kidneys known as the 'sexual segment', which enlarges during the breeding season and contributes to the production of seminal fluid. The kidneys empty into the ureters which empty into the urodeum portion of the cloaca.

Many lizards have a bladder. This is not, however, like the sterile bladder of mammals, as it is not connected directly to the ureters. Instead, it is joined to the cloaca, and so urine has to enter the cloaca, before entering the bladder. There is some evidence that the bladder is able to absorb some fluid from its contents, or it may function as a fluid storage chamber, flushing its contents back into the caudal large intestine for further fluid absorption.

Renal physiology

The renal physiology is similar to that already described for snakes. The main differences lie in the variable presence of the urinary bladder, which may have some water reabsorption capabilities.

Cardiovascular system
Heart

The lizard heart is very similar to the snake model, with paired atria and a single common ventricle which nevertheless functions as two. The majority of the deoxygenated blood is channelled to the pulmonary arteries and the oxygenated blood enters the paired aortas.

Blood vessels

The two aortas fuse dorsally, after giving off paired carotid trunks, to form the abdominal aorta. Lizards also possess a hepatoportal venous supply and a renal portal system, hence, as with birds and snakes, intravenous injection into the caudal half of the lizard of medications which are excreted through the renal tubules, could result in their failure to reach the rest of the lizard's body. It could also increase the toxicity of substances known to be renally toxic if given by this route.

Lizards, like snakes, also possess a large ventral abdominal vein, which returns blood from the tail area and passes just beneath the body wall, ventrally and in the midline. This must be avoided when performing abdominal surgery. This vessel can be used, carefully, for venipuncture for blood sampling in lizards, although the preferred vessel is the ventral tail vein. For intravenous use, the cephalic vein may be accessed on the cranial aspect of the antebrachium, via a cut-down procedure, in the larger species.

Lymphatic system

The lymphatic system is similar to that of snakes, with no discrete lymph nodes.

Reproductive system
Male

The paired testes are situated cranial to the respective kidneys in those species which have abdominally positioned kidneys (Figure 17.6). In those where the kidneys are more pelvic in position, the testes are located just caudal to the end of the lungs and liver, in the middle part of the coelomic cavity. They are supplied by several arteries each and drained by several veins. Both are very tightly adhered to their vascular supply, the left testicle being separated from the left renal vein (into which the left testicular veins drain) by the left adrenal gland. The right testicle is tightly attached to its right renal vein, which separates it from the right adrenal gland. This positioning, so close to such vital structures, makes castrating aggressive lizards a difficult operation. The testes enlarge during the breeding season and regress out of it. Each testis drains into a vas deferens which has a tightly coiled course over the ventral surface of the respective kidney before emptying into the urodeum portion of the cloaca. Some species, such as the Chameleonidae, have a pronounced epididymis extending caudally from each testicle.

The male lizard has paired penises, as with the snake, known as hemipenes. These lie in the base of the tail structure, either side of midline, and function as with the snake family. At rest they are inverted sacs in the tail base. During copulation, one will engorge with blood and evert itself, creating a groove along its dorsal surface. Into this groove sperm and spermatic fluid will drop from the cloaca, and the hemipene will guide this into the female lizard's cloaca.

Female
The female lizard has much the same anatomy as that described for the snake.

Egg-producing physiology
Reproductive physiology in the female lizard is broadly similar to that of the avian patient. Some species, such as some of the Chameleonidae, are ovoviviparous. That is, they produce live young instead of laying eggs, although the eggs are produced internally. Some species are viviparous, in which a form of placenta or thin-walled egg structure allows the foetus to develop and live young are produced. Many other species are oviparous: that is, they lay eggs. One or two species are parthenogenic: that is, the females produce entire females with no need for a male lizard – some species of Lacerta and Hemidactylus (geckos) are capable of this.

Reptile eggs are generally soft shelled and more leathery than those of their avian cousins. Sexual maturity varies according to the species, green iguanas, for example, reaching it at 2–3 years.

Sex determination and identification
Sex determination is largely dependent on chromosomes. However, geckos as a family are temperature dependent, with 99% of eggs incubated between 26.7–29.4°C

being female whereas if the temperature was greater than 32.2°C, 90% of the offspring would be male.

Sex may be identified by surgical probing as mentioned above. This is often the only method available for some species such as the beaded lizard, some monitors and the Gila monster. However, in most other species there are external physical differences. These include the prominent pre-femoral pores of males that are seen on the caudoventral aspect of the thigh of iguanids (see Figure 17.6). Some male lizards have a series of pre-anal pores just cranial to the vent. Males have wider tail bases than the females to house the large hemipenes (Figure 17.7). Some males have greater ornamentation (Figure 17.8). Male green iguanas and plumed basilisks have larger crests, male Jackson's chameleons have horns, male water dragons have larger crest spines and many male geckos have a wider vent size and hemipenal bulge.

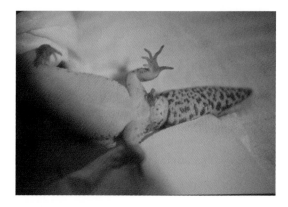

Figure 17.7 Eversion of a hemipene in a male leopard gecko to remove a hemipenal plug (accumulation of dried secretion).

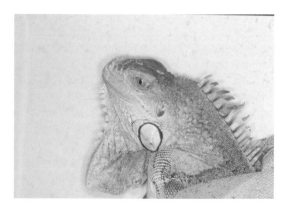

Figure 17.8 Greater ornamentation: more spines and larger dewlaps as well as brighter colouration distinguish the male green iguana.

Skin

Lizard skin is much the same as that of snakes. The scales in most cases are much smaller than the snake equivalent.

Special cutaneous adaptations in lizards

There are some specialised skin glands and structures in lizards. The males of certain species, such as the green iguana, have secretory glands or pores. The green iguana's are on the ventrocaudal aspect of the femoral area. Some geckos have precloacal pores.

Many lizards have large numbers of chromatophores in their skins. These are connected to neural networks, allowing them to alter the colour they produce according to external stimuli and mood. This ability is seen in the chameleons, and, to a lesser extent, in green iguanas and many other species.

Unlike snakes, lizards have a tympanum, located ventrocaudal to the eye, and a middle ear.

Many males will have large amounts of ornamentation on their body surface for display purposes. Examples include the male green iguana, which often has large coloured scales on the head and a bluish sheen to the head and neck colouring. Others, such as male anoles, have extendable chin flaps which are often brightly coloured and can be 'flashed' in display. Some males, such as the male plumed basilisks, have larger nuchal crests than the female.

Many lizards, such as the green iguana have a parietal eye. This is a special adaptation on the very top of the skull midway between the eyes. It is connected directly, via neural pathways, to the pineal gland in the brain and it is responsible for informing the lizard about light intensity and daytime lengths. These in turn influence feeding and reproductive behaviour. In the tuatara, which is found in New Zealand, a primaeval lizard in its own class of the reptile family, this parietal eye actually has a vestigial lens within it.

CHELONIA (TORTOISES, TURTLES AND TERRAPINS)
Musculoskeletal system

Chelonia have a rigid upper and lower jaw structure similar to that of the lizard family, but unlike lizards they have no teeth. Instead, the maxillae and mandibles are edged with tough keratin to form a horny beak, similar to that seen in birds. The skull articulates with the atlantal cervical vertebra via a single occipital condyle, similar to birds and other reptiles. There are two strong muscles attached to the back of the chelonian skull, connecting it to the point of fusion of the cervical vertebrae with the shell. These are responsible for the retraction of the head in Cryptodira, those species which can pull their heads back into the shell. There are some turtles (the side necked or Pleurodira turtles) which, as their name suggests, fold their head sideways into the shell, rather than fully retracting it in a craniocaudal manner. The thoracic vertebrae are fused with the dorsal shell, becoming flattened and elongated. The same is true of the lumbar and sacral vertebrae. The coccygeal vertebrae emerge distally to form the mobile tail.

Chelonia are distinguished from other animals by the presence of their shell. This structure is composed of fused living dermal bone covered by keratinised epidermis. It therefore can feel sensations and pain and so should never be used to tether tortoises to ropes or chains. The shell is composed of an upper section, known as the carapace (Figure 17.9), and a lower, flatter ventral section, known as the plastron (Figure 17.10). These two sections of the shell are connected either side between the fore- and hind limbs by the pillars of the shell. The carapace is a fusion of dermal bone, ribs, thoracic and lumbar vertebrae. The scutes (the individual segments of the shell epidermis) are given specific names. They do not overlie directly the bone sections of the shell, there is some overlap. Some tortoises, such as the box turtle (*Terrapene carolina*), possess a hinge to the plastron allowing them to close themselves into their shells even further.

Some of the Mediterranean species of tortoise such as the spur-thighed tortoise (*Testudo graeca*) can have caudal plastral hinges. This can be particularly useful in females, when they can increase the caudal exit space of the shell for egg laying.

Another unusual feature of Chelonia is that the scapulae are to be found on the inside of the shell: that is, inside the ribcage, due to the shell structure. This is unique in the animal world. In addition, the elbow joint is effectively rotated through nearly 180° to cause the twisted forelimb so characteristic of tortoises.

The fore- and hind limbs are supplied with extensive muscles making them extremely strong for their size. The Horsfield's tortoise (*Testudo horsfieldii*) differs from most Mediterranean species in that it is generally smaller than most but it has the unique four toed/clawed forelimbs whereas the rest have five.

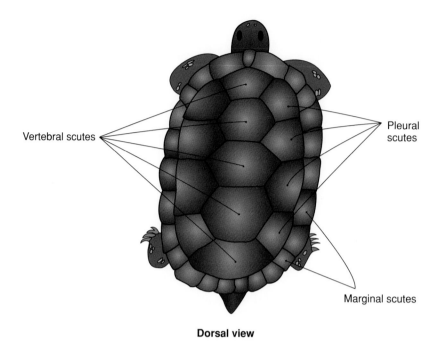

Dorsal view

Figure 17.9 Dorsal view of carapace.

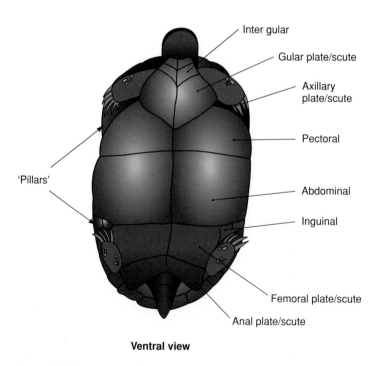

Ventral view

Figure 17.10 Ventral view of plastron.

Respiratory system (Figure 17.11)

Upper respiratory system

Chelonia have paired nostrils leading to the rostral portion of the oral cavity. As with other reptiles (excepting the crocodylians) there is no hard palate. The entrance to the trachea is guarded by the glottis, which, as with lizards and snakes, is closed at rest. It opens into the trachea, which has complete cartilaginous rings, and bifurcates relatively far cranially, often in the neck area, allowing the chelonian to breathe easily even when the neck is withdrawn deep into the shell.

Lower respiratory system

The two bronchi supply two lungs. These structures are situated in the dorsal aspect of the coelomic cavity against the inside of the carapace, and above the liver and digestive system. Between the lungs and the rest of the body organs, there is a membrane but no true diaphragm. The lungs are sponge-like in structure and contain smooth-muscle and elastic fibres, forming essentially a non-collapsible structure. In some aquatic species the lungs have air sacs that act to increase buoyancy.

Respiration is aided by movement of the limbs and neck, which act to pump the air into and out of the confined lungs. In addition, there are muscles attached to the membrane that separates the lungs from the rest of the viscera. In breathing, these contract and relax. Many chelonians can survive without breathing for several hours if necessary. The stimulus for respiration is, as with other reptiles, a fall in blood partial pressure of oxygen.

Digestive system

Oral cavity

The tongue is relatively tightly attached, but is fleshy in structure with the glottis at its base. Salivary glands secrete mucus only when eating to lubricate food. The pharynx is wide and passes into a distensible smooth-muscle covered oesophagus. Many of the aquatic turtles have caudally curved spines present in the caudal pharynx and oesophagus, which are thought to aid in swallowing slippery prey such as fish.

Stomach, associated organs and intestine

The stomach sits on the left side ventrally in the mid-coelomic cavity. It has a strong cardiac sphincter, making vomiting in the healthy chelonian rare. The stomach leads to the duodenum and a short but highly coiled small intestine. At the junction of the small and large intestine

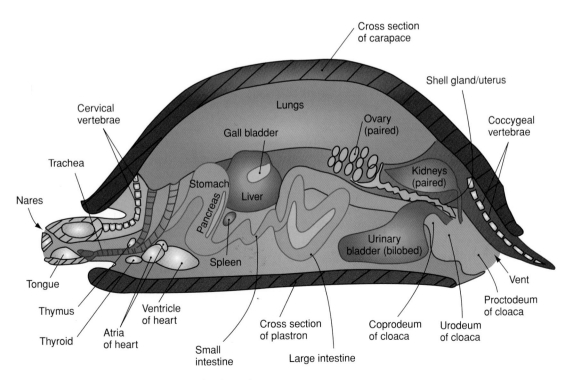

Figure 17.11 Section through the midline of a female tortoise.

lies the caecum, which is often a rounded bag-like object. The large intestine itself has a large diameter and, for herbivorous chelonia such as tortoises, is the principal site of fermentation. It then narrows to form the rectum. Next come the coprodeum and the urodeum, then the proctodeum of the cloaca, and finally the vent.

The liver is a bilobed structure situated transversely across the mid-section of the coelomic cavity, dorsal to the digestive system, and ventral to the lungs. There is a gall bladder to the right of the midline.

Urinary system

The paired kidneys are situated caudally within the shell, tightly adhered to the ventral surface of the inside of the carapace and caudal to the acetabulae of the pelvis. There is a difference in the marine species where the kidneys are situated cranial to the acetabulae. Two ureters empty into a urogenital sinus, a common chamber for the opening of the urinary and reproductive systems, which also connects with the urinary bladder. The latter organ is a large, bilobed, thin-walled structure which has some ability to reabsorb water. The urogenital sinus empties into the urodeum portion of the cloaca.

Cardiovascular system

Heart

As with lizards and snakes, the chelonian heart is a three-chambered organ situated within the pericardial sac. The two cranial vena cavae and one caudal vena cava merge to form the sinus venosus, which enters the right atrium.

Blood vessels

Paired aortas give rise to the carotid arteries that supply the head and neck. They then curve dorsally to fuse into the abdominal aorta. Just before fusing, the left aortic arch gives rise to arteries supplying the digestive tract, and the right aortic arch produces the brachiocephalic trunk that supplies the head and forelimbs. The abdominal aorta then courses down the ventral aspect of the vertebrae, supplying the shell and dorsal structures via intercostal arteries. The shell itself has a blood supply arising from cranially placed subclavian and caudally placed iliac arteries which anastomose widely.

The venous return of blood follows a similar pattern to lizards and snakes. Another bypass system exists whereby blood from the caudal vessels may cross from one side of the body to the other via transverse pelvic veins. From these, the blood may enter the paired abdominal veins which run along the floor of the coelomic cavity. It is

these latter vessels which must be carefully negotiated when performing abdominal surgery in chelonians.

Lymphatic system

The lymphatic system is essentially the same as in the snake and the lizard. The spleen is situated close to the caecum.

Reproductive system

Male

The testes are internal and often yellow cream coloured oval organs cranial to the kidneys. As with the liver, there may also be some dark pigmentation to the testes. The testes empty into the associated epididymal organs that overlie their surface. The sperm then enter the vas deferens, which courses over the ventral surface of the kidneys, and enters the urogenital sinus adjacent to the urodeum portion of the cloaca.

The phallus is a large fleshy organ, and, unlike in snakes and lizards, there is only one of them. It lies on the ventral aspect of the cloaca at rest. When engorged, the free caudal end of the phallus is projected through the vent and curves cranially. In so doing, a dorsal shallow seminal groove is formed to guide sperm into the female's vent (see Figure 17.12).

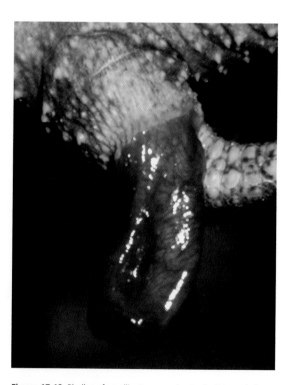

Figure 17.12 Phallus of an alligator snapping turtle (*Macrochelys temminckii*).

Female

Paired ovaries are suspended from the mid-dorsal aspect of the coelomic cavity. They shed their ova into the infundibulum portion of the oviduct. This is connected to similar structures as in the snake and lizard families, including a magnum and a uterus. This finally connects to the smooth-muscle lined vagina which is responsible for keeping the oviduct closed to the outside world until egg laying occurs. The oviducts empty into the urogenital sinus and then into the urodeum portion of the cloaca.

Reproductive physiology

Folliculogenesis is stimulated by the time of year. In those chelonians such as the Mediterranean species of tortoise, hibernation is an important factor. This period is necessary for the pre-programming of the thyroid gland and the reproductive cycle. Two bouts of egg production can occur per year. On average, 10–30 eggs are laid each year depending on the species. Most Mediterranean tortoise species do not become sexually mature until they are 7–10 years of age.

The female tortoise will start to form fertile eggs after a successful mating. These are carried in her reproductive system for a period of time varying anywhere from 4 weeks to 3–4 years which means that it is possible for Mediterranean species to carry eggs through hibernation. The female can also store the sperm from a successful mating for long periods of time, eventually allowing fertilisation to occur many months to years after exposure to the male, a factor which makes identification of the father sometimes rather difficult!

Sex determination and identification

As with many reptiles, tortoise sex determination depends on the temperature at which the eggs were incubated. Spur-thighed tortoises (*Testudo graeca*) will produce males if the eggs are kept at 29.5°C and females if kept at 31.5°C. It seems that this fact can be applied to a large number of other tortoise species, with males being predominantly produced at the lower temperatures, and females at the higher ones. If the temperature range is kept from 28 to 31°C, a mixture of sexes is likely to be achieved.

Male Chelonia have longer tails, the vent being found on the tail caudal to the edge of the carapace, in order to house the single phallus. Males of many Mediterranean species of tortoise and turtles possess a dished plastron, and a narrower angle to the caudal plastron in front of the cloaca than the egg bearing female. Some female Mediterranean species have a hinge to the caudal part of the plastron to allow easier egg laying. The male of the box turtle (*Terrapene carolina*) has red coloured irises whereas the female has yellow/brown ones. The female leopard- (*Stigmochelys pardalis*) and Indian starred tortoises (*Geochelone elegans*) have longer hind limb claws for digging than the males. The male red-eared terrapin (*Trachemys scripta elegans*), has longer forelimb claws than the females. Some males, such as the Horsfield's tortoise (*Testudo horsfieldii*), have a large, hooked scale at the tip of their tails. In some species there is a size difference between the sexes, the female of the Indian starred tortoise and the red-eared terrapin species is larger than the male when full grown, but the reverse is true of the red-footed tortoise (*Chelonoidis carbonaria*).

Skin

The skin covering the head, neck, limbs and tail of the chelonian is much the same as that of snakes and lizards. Many species of tortoise have enlarged scales over their forelimbs, and some have horny spurs on their hind limbs. The skin is particularly tightly adhered to the underlying bony structures over the distal limbs and the head.

Tortoises and most other Chelonia have visible auditory membranes covering the entrance to the middle ear. These lie caudoventral to the eyes at the rear of the skull.

The shell is formed from the fusion of islands of bone produced within the chelonian's dermal layer the skin, rather than from the limbs or ribs. The overlying epidermis is highly keratinised and pigmented. The lines joining individual scutes on the shell are not directly above the corresponding suture lines in the bony part of the shell. There is some considerable overlap which reinforces the structure.

CROCODYLIA (CROCODILES, ALLIGATORS, CAIMANS AND GHARIALS)

Musculoskeletal system

The body plan for the Crocodylia is not dissimilar to that of the lizards. The basic structure is a quadruped reptile, with an elongated tail, but instead of the short- to medium-length head, the crocodylians have elongated jaws. This is particularly accentuated in the long thin jaws of the fish eating gharial family.

The teeth are continually replaced and are held in crude sockets. One of the distinguishing features between the more bad-tempered crocodiles and the alligator family is that the fourth mandibular tooth on either side is visible in the crocodiles. In the alligator subfamily the tooth is hidden in a maxillary pocket.

The articulation point of the upper and lower jaws is located at the rear of the skull, giving more room for teeth and allowing a larger gape. The jaws are powered by strong temporal and pterygoid muscles, allowing immense crushing forces to be applied. Interestingly though, the muscles responsible for opening the jaws are relatively weak; hence once closed and taped shut, a crocodilian cannot easily open its mouth again.

There are eight pairs of ribs arising from the thoracic vertebrae, with additional dermal bones embedded in the ventral body wall known as gastralia or floating ribs. There are also thickened transverse processes of the sacral vertebrae which float freely alongside the respective vertebral bodies and have also been called ribs. The femur is proportionally longer than that of the lizards, leading to a raised appearance to the crocodylian hindquarters.

Respiratory system

Upper respiratory system

The nares of the Crocodylia are frequently protected by lateral skin flaps which can be contracted medially to close them when submerged. The nasal passages have excellent neural endings in the ethmoid/olfactory chamber area allowing an acute sense of smell. The crocodiles have a true hard palate that separates the oral and nasal passages. The internal nostrils open caudally; therefore the glottis guarding the trachea is also situated caudally.

The entrance to the larynx is guarded by the glottis but also by gular and a basihyal fold which originate in, respectively, the floor and roof of the oropharynx and can close access to the glottis from the mouth when a crocodilian is submerged. This allows them to drag prey underwater at the same time preventing any water from entering the caudal aspect of the pharynx. Providing its nostrils are above water, the crocodilian can still draw air in through the nasal passages.

The trachea is composed of complete cartilage rings, similar to Chelonia and birds.

Lower respiratory system

The trachea bifurcates within the 'chest' into two primary bronchi, each supplying a well-formed lung structure. The lungs are basic in design, and do not contain well-defined lobules, as do their mammalian counterparts, although they are very well vascularised. There are air sacs more caudally which can be inflated to provide some buoyancy. More importantly, they can function as a gas reserve, allowing them to remain submerged for up to 1–2 hours before anaerobic respiration takes over. The lungs are also different from those of other reptiles in that there is a muscular, crude diaphragmatic structure separating the dorsally situated lung fields from the ventrally situated heart and digestive system. The diaphragm and the intercostal muscles are important for respiration in crocodylians.

Digestive system

Oral cavity

The crocodylian tongue is large and fleshy, but immobile. Caudally, the floor of the mouth forms a transverse fold, as does the palate above. This shuts the oropharynx off completely from the glottis and nasopharynx.

Stomach, associated organs and intestines

The crocodilian stomach is large and divided into two areas, known as the body and the pars pylorus. The body area is heavily populated by mucus-secreting glands and surrounded by a thick band of smooth muscle. It is in this area that stones swallowed by the crocodilian may be found, and therefore this area seems to be responsible for grinding and massaging food into smaller pieces, similar to the action of the avian gizzard. The pars pylorus has acid- and pepsin-secreting glands and empties into the small intestine through the well-developed pyloric sphincter.

The small intestine meets the large intestine at the ileocaecal sphincter. The large intestine empties into the coprodeum portion of the cloaca, which opens into the urodeum, then the proctodeum before ending at the vent to the outside world.

Urinary system

There are paired kidneys located in the caudal abdomen, and extending into the pelvis. The aquatic crocodile kidney excretes waste protein nitrogen as ammonia rather than as the more usual reptilian uric acid, although the latter can also be produced, particularly when the animal is dehydrated. Osmoregulation, the maintenance of the electrolyte and water balance within the body, is not solely performed by the kidneys, as with many other reptiles. Instead, there are salt-secreting glands in the mouth which aid excretion of excess sodium as sodium chloride. There are no truly marine crocodilians, although the saltwater crocodile and the American crocodile will spend time in brackish water and will venture out into the sea.

The oral salt-secreting glands of the alligator subfamily are not as highly developed, reflecting their more freshwater habitat. The kidneys empty through the ureters which travel into the urodeum portion of the cloaca.

Cardiovascular system
Heart
The crocodilian heart is different from that of other reptiles in that it has four chambers, similar to the mammalian model. There is however a small 'hole in the heart' between the two ventricles, known as the foramen of Panizza, which allows some mixing of oxygenated and deoxygenated blood.

The rate of mixing is dependent on the pressures within the left and right ventricles. While the animal is breathing, the left ventricle has higher pressure and so blood moves from the oxygenated side to the deoxygenated side. More important for the crocodilian is what happens when he is submerged and not breathing. The increased pulmonary resistance so produced forces blood from the right ventricle to the left and out through the abdominal aorta, decreasing the blood flow to the non-functional lungs and sending it back around the body. The left ventricle blood, still returning from the lungs and so still relatively well oxygenated, is diverted through the brachiocephalic trunk to the head and heart muscle which need more oxygen to keep functioning. This allows the crocodilian to function in conditions of reduced oxygen and anaerobic metabolism for up to 6 hours!

Blood vessels
The basic structure of the blood vascular system is similar to the lizard's. There are paired aortas from the right and left ventricles which fuse to form a single abdominal aorta after giving off the brachiocephalic trunk, which supplies the head and forelimbs.

The venous system has many parallels with the lizard's. There is an hepatoportal system supplying the liver directly from the intestines and a renal–portal system wherein the blood returning from the hind limbs and tail enters a venous circle around the kidneys.

There is a large venous sinus caudal to the occiput of the skull on either side of the midline which may be used for venipuncture. Alternatively, the ventral tail vein may be used for blood sampling purposes.

Lymphatic system
The lymphatic system parallels the lizard's system.

Reproductive system
Male
The testes are long, thin organs situated medial to their respective kidneys either side of the caudal vena cava. The vasa deferentia travel to the urodeum portion of the cloaca. The testes enlarge during the reproductive season.

On the ventral aspect of the cloaca lies the phallus. This is a fibrous organ which has little erectile tissue, but once everted it forms a dorsal groove into which the semen is deposited (Figure 17.12). There are two accessory ducts entering this groove which supply seminal fluids from the caudal kidney area.

Female
The paired ovaries are also to be found medial to their respective kidneys. Each ovary is slightly flattened and has a central medullary area which is supplied with nerves and blood vessels. The rest of the reproductive system consists of the fimbria or ostium which catches the ova, and then there is a muscular portion followed by the isthmus and the shell gland or uterus. The paired oviducts open into the urodeum of the cloaca, adjacent to the clitoris.

Reproductive physiology
Follicular activity is triggered by increasing day length in March–May, there being one cycle per year. An average clutch of follicles varies from 20 to 80 per cycle.

Sex determination and identification
This varies with species. In the case of alligators and caimans, the lower incubation temperatures (from 28 to 31°C) produce all females. An intermediate temperature (from 31 to 32°C) produces males and females, and a higher temperature (from 32 to 34°C) produces all males. In the case of crocodiles, temperatures at the lower end of the range (from 28 to 31°C) also produce all females. Intermediate temperatures (from 31 to 33°C) produce some females but predominantly males. For higher temperatures (from 33 to 34°C), predominantly female crocodiles, with some males, are produced.

The best method of sex identification is by manual palpation of the ventral surface of the cloaca for the presence of the phallus. This is an obvious structure if present, as otherwise the cloaca is completely smooth walled. The crocodilian involved must be in dorsal recumbency and adequately restrained in order to perform this!

Skin

The epidermis and dermis of Crocodylia are composed of thickened scales which are joined together like a patchwork quilt by elastic tissue. The skin is tightly attached to underlying bone over the feet and the skull. The skin covering the dorsum has layers of dermal bone present within it, making this area extremely thick and impossible to penetrate for injections. The caimans have areas of bone in the skin covering their ventral surface as well.

Specialised skin areas

Within the majority of the scales of the crocodile subfamily are present integumentary sense organs (ISO). These are absent in the alligator subfamily. Their function is to determine underwater pressure sensations which can be used to locate prey whilst submerged.

Overview of reptilian haematology

The cells found in the reptilian bloodstream broadly mirror those seen in mammals. There are however a few important differences:

- The reptilian (and amphibian) erythrocyte is oval in shape rather than biconcave and has a nucleus even when fully matured.
- The reptile, like the avian patient, has a slightly different version of the mammalian neutrophil, known as the heterophil. This white blood cell has a bilobed nucleus, like the neutrophil, and contains cytoplasmic granules, but these stain a variety of colours with Romanowsky stains, rather than remaining neutral as seen in neutrophils. The heterophil performs similar functions to the neutrophil, being a first line of defence for infection. However, although its numbers may be increased during infections, they may stay the same, in which case the only tell-tale sign of an inflammatory process occurring is vacuolation and degranulation of the cell (the so-called 'toxic' cell). This makes cytological examination more important than cell counts in reptiles.
- An additional mononuclear cell is the azurophil. It stains a blue-red colour and is a large, single nucleated cell with moderate cytoplasm present. It is found normally in small numbers, but if elevated in lizards and Chelonia, it suggests an inflammatory/infectious process. It is particularly associated with chronic granuloma formation.

- Eosinophils and basophils are present in most species, basophils being common in turtles. Basophils generally stain blue, and are small, spherical cells with a non-lobed nucleus. The eosinophil is a larger spherical cell with eosinophilic cytoplasmic granules and a mildly lobed to elongated nucleus. However, in the green iguana they often stain blue!
- Lymphocytes may vary with the season showing a decrease in the 'winter'/colder months in tropical species. Unlike mammals, the B lymphocyte can change into the plasma cell form within the bloodstream during chronic or severe infections of reptiles. Hence, the eccentrically placed nucleus and pale staining 'clock-face' cytoplasm of the plasma cell may be seen in blood smears of reptiles.
- The thrombocytes (platelets) of reptiles, like avian species, are also nucleated.

Most importantly, when collecting blood samples from reptiles, it is better to do so into heparinised containers for haematology, rather than potassium EDTA tubes used in birds and mammals. This is because the blood cells, particularly erythrocytes, of many species (particularly the Chelonia) will rupture in potassium EDTA. An air-dried smear for staining made at the time of sampling is also useful, as heparin interferes with the Romanowsky stains.

AMPHIBIANS
Classification

Amphibians are classified into many different family groups, according to a number of physical, anatomical and evolutionary factors. It is useful to know to which group an amphibian belongs as this gives an indication of the other amphibians to which it is related. This is of some help when faced with a species that you have not seen before.

Table 17.2 contains some of the more commonly encountered family groups of amphibians seen in general and exotic species orientated practices.

Table 17.2 Basic classification of amphibians.

Order	Description
Anura (Salientia)	Includes frogs and toads
Gymnophiona (Apoda)	Includes caecilians (legless amphibians)
Caudata (Urodela)	Includes salamanders and newts

Musculoskeletal system

The body plan of Amphibia in general varies greatly within the family from the classic lizard shape of the salamanders and newts, through to the tailless quadruped form of the anurans (frogs and toads) through to the worm-like caecilians.

In the case of the anurans and the salamanders, the skeletal structure is very basic but similar to the lizard model described above. The main differences lie in the anurans, which have long femurs, tibias and fibulas, and metatarsals which are developed into the well-muscled hind limbs. There is a basic spinal column of cuboid vertebral bodies joining to the primitive pelvis caudally and the single occipital condyle of the skull cranially.

The skull possesses a mandible and maxilla with, in many cases, simple peg-like, open-rooted and continually replaced teeth. The eye sockets are large in anurans, as is the well-developed eardrum that leads to the middle ear. Sight is mainly based on movement rather than sharp focus, but the sense of hearing is very good, although low frequency sounds are transmitted through the bones of the forelimbs, and high frequency ones through the actual eardrum.

The majority of anurans have five digits on the forelimbs and four on the hind limbs (see Figure 17.13). Many salamanders and newts have four digits on their forelimbs and four or five digits on their hind limbs. Many salamanders will show autotomy or tail shedding when roughly handled as with many lizards.

Many amphibians possess vestigial rib structures, and the majority also have a sternum. The pectoral and pelvic girdles are fused to the spine, giving increased rigidity to the body structure.

The caecilians have a much simpler body plan with few if any bones. Their body plan is more worm-like, although they are amphibians rather than insects; but they do possess jaws, a primitive skull and a fibrocartilaginous spinal column. They also have small eyes and nostrils in the head (see Figure 17.14).

Respiratory system

In aquatic amphibians such as the primitive axolotl, gills are still present. Indeed, as an amphibian metamorphoses through from egg to larval or tadpole form it will also have gills, although these may be lost as the adult form is reached.

Terrestrial amphibians, such as many of the anurans, have an internal lung structure. This is often no more than a simple air sac structure. There are no internal alveolar areas to this lung, although it may be folded to increase its surface area. No diaphragm is present, giving a continuous body cavity or coelom; hence respiration for those amphibians possessing lungs occurs due to intercostal muscle and limb movements pulling the chest wall up and outwards.

Many amphibians will use the skin surface for gaseous exchange, whether they possess an internal lung structure or not. Indeed, the skin is often solely used for gas exchange during periods of low oxygen requirement, such as during hibernation. For other skin breathers, such as the plethodontid salamanders, other adaptations, such as increasing the skin's surface area by having folds of skin,

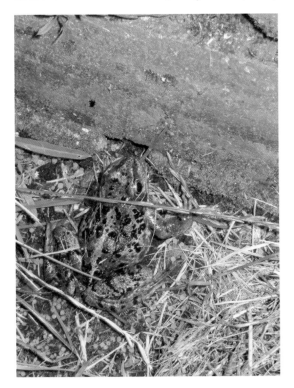

Figure 17.13 The European frog (*Rana temporaria*) like many Anurans has four digits on the hind limbs and five on the forelimbs.

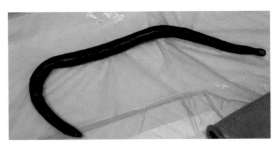

Figure 17.14 The caecilians have a very basic, worm-like body plan.

or by having 'hairs' on their surface (for example, the African hairy frog (*Trichobatrachus robustus*), or reducing oxygen demands/metabolic rates, are necessary.

Digestive system

Most adult amphibians are carnivorous, and their digestive systems are adapted to this diet. The majority possess a tongue which can be projected at high speed towards their prey. It is covered in fine sticky cilia, as in many anurans, enabling it to capture flying prey. The salamanders, newts and most anurans have vestigial peg-like teeth. There are frequently cilia within the oral cavity and oesophagus, which aid in the propelling of food into the stomach. Terrestrial amphibians also have mucus-secreting salivary glands to aid in the swallowing of prey.

The stomach is simple in nature, possesses mucus-secreting glands and, in the majority of cases, combined acid- and pepsinogen-secreting glands. The small intestine is short, and little defines its finish and the start of the rectum which empties into the cloaca.

The liver is frequently dark coloured due to melanin pigmentation for protection from ultraviolet light, necessary due to the thin nature of amphibian skin.

Urinary system

As with the reptile family, amphibians cannot concentrate urine beyond plasma tonicity. The main excretory product of aquatic amphibians such as caecilians and aquatic newts and the axolotl, is ammonia. This is actually excreted, as with fish, through the gills if present, and the skin if not, rather than the kidneys.

In terrestrial amphibians, urea is the main waste product of nitrogen metabolism and this is excreted through a primitive paired kidney structure. The cloaca of these species (chiefly the anuran toad family) may also have a pocket forming a primitive bladder. One or two amphibians can produce uric acid. The kidneys empty into ureters which travel to the urodeum portion of the cloaca, before either refluxing into the bladder (if present) or emptying through the vent.

Cardiovascular system
Heart

The circulatory system changes dramatically during the metamorphosis of the amphibian. At the larval stage the circulatory system is more fish-like, with a two chambered heart possessing only one atrium and one ventricle. When the adult form is achieved, the heart has divided itself into three chambers by producing an intra-atrial septum, and has also rerouted its circulation away from the gill arches of the larvae to the adult respiration organ (the skin, lungs or again gill arches).

Blood vessels

As far as the more peripheral vascular system is concerned, the amphibians differ from the reptiles in that the caudal body drainage goes through the hepatic portal system rather than the renal portal system. This is important for the administration of hepatically metabolised drugs or hepatotoxic drugs in the caudal half of an amphibian.

Lymphatic system

There is a large lymphatic drainage system, with paired dorsal lymph sacs in anurans lying cranial to the hind limbs laterodorsally. These help propel lymph fluid as well as draining it via lymph hearts back to the true heart. They may also play a role in electrolyte balance through the skin overlying them.

Reproductive system

There are paired internal testes or ovaries depending on the sex. There is some variation in the size of the gonads during the reproductive season and basic hormones resembling the activity of follicle stimulating hormone (FSH) and luteinising hormone (LH) are produced.

In the female, there are paired oviducts which are responsible for producing the jelly-like material that coats the ova. Most amphibians fertilise their eggs outside the body, but one or two species of anuran, and the caecilians, do have a form of phallus for internal fertilisation. Indeed some caecilians are viviparous and actually secrete a uterine milk to nourish the foetuses within the oviduct.

When hatched, the amphibian then metamorphoses through a series of changes, often known as instars, one of which we all know as the 'tadpole' of the anurans which has external gills and a tail and no legs initially. The stimuli for the metamorphosis seem to come from various external sources, such as environmental iodine levels, as well as internal hormonal influences from the thyroid gland.

Skin

The terrestrial amphibian has a thin stratum corneum which provides extra cutaneous protection above that seen in aquatic species. It also reduces water loss from the skin. The skin is shed regularly, similarly to a snake, and is frequently then eaten by the amphibian. The skin contains many glands which secrete oils and mucus in to further protect against water loss, but amphibians always have to have access to damp conditions or free water to survive.

Many of the toad family have poison glands located in their parotid glands which are used as a form of protection. A similar ploy is used in the poison arrow tree frogs which secrete neurotoxins onto the surface of their skin.

Some anurans, such as the midwife toad *Xenopus laevis*, have claws, but most have very fragile skin, which, as mentioned above, may have capabilities for gas exchange as well as water and electrolyte exchange.

Some male amphibians can be identified by skin colour or ornamentation. The male great crested newt has a larger crest than the female, for example, and many male frogs and toads have a swelling in the 'thumb' area of the hand which contains scent glands. Male caecilians often have a phallus in the cloaca.

Chapter 18

Reptile and Amphibian Housing, Husbandry and Rearing

There are many good books available on the husbandry of reptiles and amphibians, and some are listed at the end of this chapter. This chapter will therefore provide only a brief overview of the main points in housing and caring for reptiles and amphibians. It is essential when treating a reptile patient for the first time that a thorough history is taken. This is particularly important as many problems can arise through improper care as with any captive animal.

Vivarium requirements

Dimensions and construction

Vivarium designs vary, as does their construction material. The main aim though is to ensure that they are durable, easily cleaned for hygiene reasons and that they provide enough space for the captive reptile to demonstrate normal behaviour. Strict cage dimensions are therefore difficult to quantify, as each situation should be judged on its own merits. However, some general principles apply (Figure 18.1). Size of the vivarium/terrarium will depend on the species, number of individuals housed and sexual maturity. It is important that the vivarium is large enough to allow a temperature gradient to be created.

For species which are more arboreal (tree climbing) in nature, for example, the green iguana and many snakes (e.g. the boa constrictor and Burmese python), the emphasis in cage design should be more on vertical height rather than horizontal space. For tortoises, however, the provision of too much vertical space is pointless. Barnard (1996) provided some minimum dimensions in Table 18.1.

Cage materials commonly used include perspex, reinforced glass, sealed wood and fibreglass (Figure 18.2). Wood should be avoided unless it is sealed to prevent moisture damage and rotting. Glass and clear perspex are useful when showing off a collection, but care should be taken as many reptiles cannot see the tank sides, and so may continually rub their snouts along the inside of the vivarium, causing severe abrasions which can become infected. Often the provision of a tape strip on the outside

of the glass at reptile level allows them to appreciate that a barrier exists and prevents this problem.

Heating

Reptiles are ectothermic by nature, i.e. they rely on the environment to provide sufficient heat to warm them to their preferred body temperature (PBT). Their PBT is the body temperature at which their organs and biochemical processes function optimally. To maintain their PBT, the reptile must be provided with a preferred optimum temperature zone (POTZ) within which it may position itself. This necessitates the provision of some form of artificial heating within the tank/vivarium to create a temperature gradient within which the reptile can place itself to either cool down or warm up.

Two main forms of heating are advised. A background, continuous heat source is important to raise the vivarium temperature above the background room temperature. This is often provided in the form of a radiant heat mat, a mat which emits heat continuously, and is placed on the outside wall of the vivarium (Figure 18.1). It then radiates heat through the tank wall. Placing it on the outside of the tank avoids the possibility of the reptile chewing, urinating or defaecating on it, so increasing hygiene and safety. The size of available mats varies, but a rough rule is that one-third to one-half of the longest side of the tank should be covered with the mat. Some form of insulation on the outside of the mat, increasing reflection of heat into the vivarium, is also useful.

In addition, the vivarium requires a focal hot spot, which may be provided in the form of a ceramic, infrared heat or combination heat/UV bulb. This should be suspended from the ceiling of the vivarium, and should be protected from the reptile to avoid the risk of burns. The bulb should be attached to a thermostat, which will allow maximum and minimum tank temperatures to be set. A form of heated, plastic molded rock has been used to provide a basking point for reptiles. These should be avoided

Veterinary Nursing of Exotic Pets, Second Edition. Edited by Simon J. Girling. © 2013 John Wiley & Sons, Ltd. Published 2013 by John Wiley & Sons, Ltd.

Table 18.1 Some minimum vivarium sizes.

Type of reptile	Minimum vivarium sizes
Arboreal lizards	Height should be 2–3 × reptile's length Floor dimensions should be minimum of 2 × reptile's length by 3 × reptile's length
Terrestrial lizards	Height should be sufficient to prevent escape Floor dimensions should be minimum of 2 × reptile's length by 3 × reptile's length
Arboreal snakes	Height should be minimum 1 × reptile's length Floor dimensions should be minimum of 3/4 × reptile's length by 1/3 × reptile's length
Terrestrial snakes	Height should be minimum 1/2 × reptile's length Floor dimensions should be minimum of 3/4 × reptile's length by 1/3 × reptile's length
Terrestrial chelonians	Floor dimensions should be minimum of 5 × reptile's length by 5 × reptile's length
Aquatic chelonians	Height should be enough to prevent escape Floor dimensions should be minimum of 5 × reptile's length by 3 × reptile's length Water depth should be 1/2 × length of reptile

Source: Data from Barnard (1996).

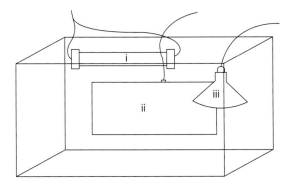

Figure 18.1 Basic diagrammatic representation of a vivarium: (i) Ultraviolet light source (on inside of tank as glass filters out UV light); (ii) radiant heat mat, usually placed on outside of tank for hygiene reasons; (iii) focal heat source such as a heat lamp to provide a temperature gradient.

as should the thermostat break within such a device it can overheat and the reptile will injure itself.

The importance of a focal heat source is that it provides a temperature gradient, allowing the reptile to bask underneath the heat source or to escape to a cooler end of the tank when overheated. The reptile can then maintain

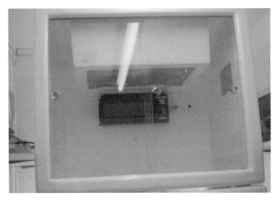

Figure 18.2 Vivarium made of moulded fibreglass.

its PBT by positioning itself at different points in the tank during the course of the day.

The temperatures required for different species of reptile will naturally differ. A list of some species and their temperature requirements is given in Table 18.2.

Humidity

Humidity is also important. Many species of reptile come from dry desert regions, but equally many originate in tropical rain forests. Therefore, their tolerance of water moisture in their environment will vary. A water dragon, basilisk or garter snake, all used to living near or in water, will require a 75–90% humidity level. This may be difficult to maintain in a heated environment; as the hotter the air, the more water droplets the air can hold, and so the relative humidity levels drop. Thus, spraying the enclosures frequently, using a hand-held plant mister, with previously boiled and then cooled water is useful. Alternatively, the provision of water baths or damp substrate within the tank

Table 18.2 Preferred optimum temperature zones and relative humidity for selected species of reptile.

Species	Temperature range (°C)	Relative humidity
Mediterranean tortoises	20–28	30–50%
Green iguana	25–35	75–100%
Leopard gecko	25–34	30–40%
Water dragon	24–30	80–90%
Bearded dragon	25–35	30–40%
Corn snake	23–30	30–70%
Burmese python	25–30	50–80%

can be used to increase humidity. Care should be taken over hygiene levels though, as a too damp and soiled substrate can lead to skin infections such as blister disease, a common problem in garter snakes. In the case of reptiles from more arid climates, a relative humidity between 25 and 50% is often adequate (see Table 18.2). This is around the normal level of the average centrally heated home. However, at certain times even these species require increased levels of humidity. One such example is during the shedding cycle when the old skin layer is sloughed. At this time an increase in humidity is essential to prevent the old skin drying out before it has a chance to peel off and so resulting in constrictions around extremities such as the digits. This is a very common problem in leopard geckos and many adults have lost the ends of their toes through avascular necrosis. To prevent this, it is useful to provide a hide that has an increased humidity level in addition to a normal hide. This can be achieved by placing a shallow dish of water with some cotton wool in it within the hide.

Ultraviolet lighting

Lighting is particularly important for the growing juveniles of many species. In the wild, many of these reptiles live in parts of the world where the intensity of the sun's ultraviolet rays is high. These ultraviolet rays stimulate a number of functions in the reptile; often encouraging mating at certain times of year, and may act as a general appetite stimulus. This seems to be the role of the A section of the ultraviolet waveband.

The B waveband of the ultraviolet spectrum is important in all species in encouraging the production of vitamin D_3 from precursors in the reptile's skin. Vitamin D_3 is intimately involved in the metabolism of calcium and bone growth within the juvenile reptile. Therefore, a lack of ultraviolet light can be responsible for the presence of metabolic bone disease in several species, particularly the green iguana and the Mediterranean tortoises (see chapter 21). Many terrestrial chelonia are kept in open-topped, plastic or wooden enclosures with suspended heat/ultraviolet lamps.

Artificial ultraviolet lighting is therefore important in these species, and should be provided on the inside of the vivarium. This is because glass and perspex will filter out the UV rays if the light is placed on the outside of the tank. In addition, the light source should be positioned close to the reptile, i.e. within 30–45 cm. This is because the intensity of these artificial lights is relatively low, and the inverse square rule tells us that the intensity of the light diminishes with the square of the distance from its source (e.g. the intensity at 2 m from the source is a quarter of that 1 m from its source).

Some species are not so susceptible to ultraviolet deprivation, including more nocturnal species such as the leopard gecko and many snakes. The theory is that these species gain sufficient preformed vitamin D_3 in their diets to cope. This is important if the owner is not feeding them correctly, as metabolic bone disease may then be seen.

It is also worth noting that the type of UV lighting should be tailored to the species. Some species prefer to bask in full sunlight and so a 'sunbeam' method of providing lighting with a high UVB mercury vapour or metal halide light ideally in combination with an incandescent lamp to produce the equivalent of a sunbeam in the basking zone. This should be big enough to get the whole reptile inside the basking zone. This is most suitable for reptiles noted for basking such as fence lizards (*Sceloporus* spp.), bearded dragons, frilled lizards, etc. Others do not bask and prefer a more dappled shade method where an incandescent lamp is used at one end of the vivarium controlled by a dimming thermostat. This creates a suitable temperature gradient and a focal UVB source which then creates a UV gradient in the tank as well with a high point underneath the heat lamp. Shelter is then provided using vegetation and plenty of hides so that the reptile is not continuously exposed to UV light. This is most suitable for reptiles such as rat snakes, anoles, water/garter snakes. More information can be found in Baines and Brames (2010) and Ferguson *et al.* (2010).

Cage 'furniture' and environmental enrichment

Many reptiles are relatively poorly adapted to captivity, being wild animals in a confined space, and so it is important to ensure that their environment adequately caters for their requirements.

As previously mentioned, many arboreal species enjoy exploring vertical space. They should therefore be provided with branches and ramps up, which they may climb. It is often useful to provide an elevated basking spot which they can lie out on near to the focal heat source.

In the case of ground-dwelling species, the provision of some form of floor furniture is important. Tortoises are best kept singly, except when breeding of course, or in the case of small hatchlings which prefer to be in groups. In these cases, the provision of visual barricades which they can hide behind and so escape from one another is useful.

All reptiles should be provided with a hide. This is important particularly for many snakes which will often refuse to eat their prey in the open, but rather prefer to take it back into the hide area away from view. The size of these areas does not need to be that large, in the case of most species a space 2–2.5 times the size of the reptile housed is sufficient. The number of hides should ideally be equivalent to the number of reptiles housed plus one.

Flooring

The substrate of the vivarium, or floor covering, is important. It is vital that any substrate used is nontoxic to the reptiles housed and is easily cleaned. In many cases the provision of newspaper or unbleached household paper is perfectly sufficient, although possibly not so aesthetically pleasing, as more naturalistic substrates. Care should be taken with smaller reptiles with newspaper, as the ink from the newsprint may prove irritant.

Other substrates used commonly include bark chippings, calcite sand and peat. Bark chippings are a good choice for deep litter situations, particularly when providing enough substrate for a pregnant female to dig a nest in which to lay eggs. However, the chips should not be of cedar as the resins from this can be irritant. It is also more difficult to monitor the cleanliness of bark chippings as faeces and urine may fall into the substrate and so avoid detection.

Sand is useful for desert species such as leopard geckos, collared lizards, sand boas, etc., but care should be taken with any reptile on this substrate. If the diet contains mineral deficiencies or if there is intestinal parasitism present, many species will consume the sand and may suffer intestinal blockages.

Peat can be useful for species requiring damper conditions such as water dragons, red-footed tortoises, etc., but care again should be taken with the hygiene of this substrate, as waste materials may build up unnoticed.

Certain types of substrate are best avoided. Coral is not advised as a substrate for ecological reasons as well as the tendency for reptiles to eat the substrate and suffer gut impactions. Corn cobs should also be avoided as these are often inadvertently eaten, swell and cause intestinal blockages.

Aquatic species and amphibians

Some reptile species, such as the terrapins and turtles, require large areas of free water; some, such as frogs and toads, a small area but damp environmental conditions (Figure 18.3).

In the case of freshwater species, tap water may be used, but it should be dechlorinated. This may be done by standing it in an open container for 24 hours prior to use

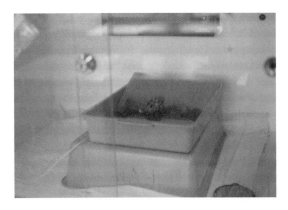

Figure 18.3 Example of hospital tank provision for an amphibian, in this case an Argentinian horned frog.

or by using any commercial dechlorinating tablets available from aquarists. In addition, the tap water should be allowed to come up to room temperature before being introduced to avoid cold shocking the reptile or amphibian.

Where large areas of water are provided, it is important to keep them clean. It is advisable for terrapins and soft-shelled turtles that their habitat provides an area in which they can immerse themselves completely in water, and an area into which they can pull themselves out to bask and dry themselves off, preferably with a focal heat source above it. It is often advisable to remove them from the water and place them in a separate, dry or water-containing feeding tank. This is because they are extremely messy eaters and will quickly contaminate their water with food. The food acts as a substrate for bacteria, and this can increase the risk of shell infections and septicaemia. An alternative would be a powerful water filtration device placed in the tank to cope with the large volumes of organic debris produced. Even if a feeding tank is provided, regular water changes or filtration is required, as they will of course still urinate and defaecate in their water.

Many anurans will appreciate a small amount of free water, but the rest of their vivarium should be well supplied with moisture-retaining substrate such as mosses or peat substitute mulches. These retain moisture and increase the humidity of the tank, ensuring protection of the sensitive amphibian's skin. Other amphibians, such as newts and salamanders, require more access to free fresh water and precautions similar to those mentioned for freshwater turtles and terrapins should be taken. In addition, for all these species, the construction of the vivarium should ensure that it is waterproof!

Egg incubation of reptiles

It is necessary for successful egg incubation to use an incubator. The basic components of a reptile egg incubator are as follows: A plastic, perspex or toughened glass tank with a plastic lid containing aeration holes that can be covered to regulate humidity and temperature; nesting substrate is placed into small open containers within the tank; and the eggs are placed in slight depressions within the substrate – a useful substrate is the loft insulating material vermiculite. Alternatives include damp sand, sphagnum moss or even peat.

When the eggs are retrieved from the nest site particular care should be taken to maintain the same position of the egg in the incubator. The eggs should not be turned during the incubation process as this can cause significant foetal mortality.

The tank requires a source of humidity and heat production. There are two methods for providing these. The containers containing the eggs and substrate may be placed onto a wire mesh which divides the tank into a top and a bottom compartment. The bottom compartment may then be three quarters filled with filtered water, and a thermostatically controlled water heater placed into it. This technique will provide heat and moisture, and is good for the higher-moisture-requiring species (e.g. water dragons) that need an average 80% humidity.

An alternative set-up is to attach a thermostatically controlled radiant heat mat to the outside of the tank. The tank is then completely filled with the substrate, which is kept moist by regular misting with a plant sprayer, and by placing shallow containers of filtered and previously boiled water in amongst the eggs. This provides a drier atmosphere, more suitable for desert dwelling species.

Care should be taken not to allow the humidity to drop below 50%, as reptile eggs are porous and excessively dry conditions will dehydrate the foetus inside and lead to high levels of mortality. Equally, excessive levels of humidity will lead to an increased risk of fungal infection of the shell and contents and again higher mortality rates. It is therefore important to have both a thermometer and a humidity gauge within the incubator, and both should be monitored regularly.

Temperatures for incubation of reptile eggs vary from 26–32°C with an average incubation period in snakes of 45–70 days. Incubation periods vary from 45–70 days in smaller lizards to 90–130 days for iguanas and larger lizards – see Table 18.3 for more information.

Table 18.3 Incubation times and temperature ranges for selected reptiles.

Species	Egg incubation time (days)	Incubation temperature (°C)
Inland bearded dragon	65–115	28–32
Green iguana	60	25–30
Leopard gecko	150–170	28–32
Corn snake	55–70	28–30
Burmese python	58–63	28–32
Spur-thighed tortoise	56–70	29–32
Hermann's tortoise	85–100	30–33
Horsefield's tortoise	60–75	28–32
Leopard tortoise	140–155	28–32

For chelonians, the colder, northerly climes of the United Kingdom mean the incubation of eggs in an outside environment is not possible. It is therefore necessary to artificially incubate them. Once laid the eggs will hatch for most tortoise species in 8–12 weeks depending on the temperature at which they are incubated. In snakes and non-gecko lizards, the sex of the hatchling is determined by genetics. In chelonians, many geckos and crocodylians, the sex is generally determined by the temperature at which the egg was incubated. For example, the Hermann's tortoise egg if incubated below 29.5°C will produce predominantly male hatchlings and those incubated at or above 32°C will produce predominantly female. In leopard geckos, temperatures at or below 29°C will produce predominantly females, intermediate temperatures 30–32°C produce mostly males and temperatures above 34°C will again produce mostly females (although the latter temperatures are not recommended as they are close to the lethal limit for incubation). It is interesting to note that in leopard geckos incubated at cooler temperatures are also more darkly pigmented than those incubated at higher temperatures.

Quarantine

There are an increasing number of viral diseases being discovered in reptiles as well as other known pathogens that can have long incubation periods and may be difficult to detect ante-mortem. For this reason, it is important to consider quarantining any new reptile before adding it to your collection. Periods of quarantine suggested have varied from 6 weeks to 9–12 months.

Veterinary health tests should be carried out where possible during this period. The new reptile should be housed preferably not only in a separate vivarium but in a separate room to avoid sharing the same airspace. Separate utensils should be used and they should be cleaned out and fed last to avoid cross contamination. Disinfection is important to avoid potential spread of disease. Typical disinfectants suitable for reptiles include quaternary ammonium compound based products such as Ark-Klens® (Vetark Professional Ltd.) and F10® (Health and Hygiene Pty).

Hospitalised reptiles

The guidelines given above for ultraviolet light, humidity and temperature should be applied for any hospitalised reptile. However, some important differences may be made with regards to substrate which in most cases can be of newspaper (avoid coloured print which may be irritant) or unbleached paper towelling to ensure good hygiene and facilitate faecal collection. Space provision may also be compromised for short periods of hospitalisation, but periods of more than 2–3 days, every effort to keep the reptile in the minimum dimensions detailed should be made.

It is vitally important that the vivarium is cleansed thoroughly between patients to avoid disease spread. The use of povidone-iodine-based cleansing agents such as Tamodine-E (Vetark Professional Ltd.) or quaternary ammonium compounds such as F10® (Health and Hygiene Pty) should be considered.

References

Baines, F. and Brames, H. (2010) Preventive reptile medicine and reptile lighting. *Proceedings of the 1st International Conference on Reptile and Amphibian Medicine*, Munich, 4–6 March, pp. 3–13.

Barnard, S.M. (1996) *Reptile Keepers Handbook*. Krieger Publishing, Malabar, FL.

Ferguson, G.W., Brinker, A.M., Gehrmann, W.H., Bucklin, S.E., Baines, F.M. and Makin, S.J. (2010) Voluntary exposure of some western-hemisphere snake and lizard species to ultraviolet-B radiation in the field: How much ultraviolet-B should a lizard or snake receive in captivity? *Zoo Biology*, **29**(3), 317–334.

Further reading

Cooper, J.E. and Jackson, O.F. (eds) (1981) *Diseases of the Reptilia, Volumes 1 and 2*. Academic Press, London.

Frye, F. (1991) *Biomedical and Surgical Aspects of Captive Reptile Husbandry, Volume 1 and 2*. Krieger Publishing, Malabar, FL.

Girling, S.J. and Raiti, P. (eds) (2004) *BSAVA Manual of Reptile Medicine and Surgery*, 2nd edn. BSAVA, Quedgeley, UK.

Mader, D.R. (ed) (2006) *Reptile Medicine and Surgery*, 2nd edn. Elsevier, Philadelphia, PA.

Chapter 19

Reptile and Amphibian Handling and Chemical Restraint

Handling the reptilian patient

Is there a need to restrain the reptilian patient?

Reptiles are less easily stressed than their avian cousins, and so restraint may be performed without as much risk in the case of the debilitated animal. However, it is still worthwhile considering factors that may make restraint dangerous to animal and nurse alike.

- Is the patient in respiratory distress where excessive manual manipulation can be dangerous?
- Is the species a fragile one? Day geckos are extremely delicate and prone to shedding their tails when handled. Similarly some species such as green iguanas are prone to conditions such as metabolic bone disease where spontaneous fractures occur.
- Is the species an aggressive one? Some are naturally so, e.g. snapping turtles, tokay geckos and rock pythons.
- Does the reptile patient require medication or physical examination? In which case restraint is essential?

It should be noted that many species of reptile have *Salmonella* spp. present normally in their gut. Personal hygiene is therefore very important when handling these patients to prevent zoonotic diseases.

Techniques and equipments involved in restraining reptile patients

Lizards

Their main danger areas to the handler are their claws and teeth, and in some species, such as iguanas, their tails – which can lash out in a whiplike fashion.

Geckos, other than tokay geckos, are generally docile as are lizards such as bearded dragons. Others, such as green iguanas, may be extremely aggressive, particularly sexually mature males. They may also be more aggressive towards female owners and handlers as they are able to detect pheromones secreted during the menstrual cycle.

They are best restrained by grasping around the shoulders (the pectoral girdle) with one hand, from the dorsal aspect, so controlling one forelimb with forefinger and the thumb and the other between middle and fourth finger. The other hand is used to grasp the pelvic girdle from the dorsal aspect, controlling one limb with the thumb and forefinger, the other again between middle and fourth finger. The handler may then hold the lizard in a vertical manner, with head uppermost, placing the tail underneath his or her arm (Figure 19.1). It is then possible to present the head and feet of the lizard away from the handler to avoid injury. The handler should allow some flexibility as the lizard may struggle and overly rigid restraint could damage the spine.

More aggressive iguanas may need to be pinned down first. The use of a thick towel to control the tail and claws is useful. Gauntlets may be necessary for particularly aggressive large lizards or for those which may have a venomous bite. It is important to ensure that you do not use too much force when restraining the lizard, as those with skeletal problems, such as metabolic bone disease, may be seriously injured. In addition, lizards do not have a diaphragm and so overzealous restraint will lead to increasing pressure on the lungs.

Day geckos and other fragile species are best examined in a clear plastic container. Other geckos have easily damaged skin, so latex-free gloves and soft cloths should be used for examination. When handling small lizards, they may be cupped in the hand and their heads controlled by holding between the index finger and thumb to prevent biting.

It is important that lizards are never restrained by their tails. Many will shed their tails at this time, but not all of them will regrow. Green iguanas, e.g. will only regrow their tails as juveniles (less than 2.5–3 years of age). Once they are older than this, they will be left tailless. However, there are plenty of lizards that do not undergo autotomy, e.g. many agamids, chameleons, etc.

Vagovagal reflex

The vagovagal reflex can be used to place members of the lizard family into a trancelike state. The eyelids are closed and gentle digital pressure is applied to both eyeballs. This

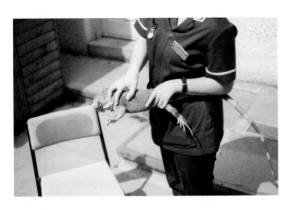

Figure 19.1 The iguana should be approached from above grasping over the pectoral and pelvic areas dorsally and may then be firmly but gently controlled. Tucking the tail underneath the arm prevents eye injuries.

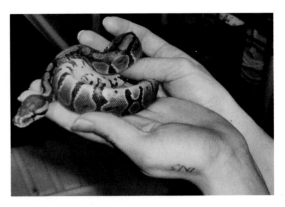

Figure 19.2 Allowing the snake to coil itself around the handler's hand and arms is preferable to over-zealous restraint in non-aggressive species such as this small Royal python (*Python regius*).

stimulates the autonomic parasympathetic nervous system resulting in a reduction in heart rate, blood pressure and respiration rate. Providing there are no loud noises or environmental stimulation, after 1–2 minutes the lizard may be placed on its side, front, back, etc. allowing radiography to be performed without using physical or chemical restraint. A loud noise or physical stimulation will immediately cause the lizard to revert to its normal wakeful state.

Snakes

Snakes are all characterised by their elongated form and absence of limbs. The danger areas for the handler are their teeth (and in the case of the most venomous species such as the viper family, their fang teeth), and, in the case of the constrictor and python family, their ability to asphyxiate their prey by winding themselves around the victim's chest and neck.

With this in mind, the following restraint techniques may be employed. Non-venomous snakes can be restrained by controlling the head initially. This is done by placing the thumb over the occiput and curling the fingers under the chin. Reptiles, like birds, have only one occipital condyle, so it is important to stabilise the occipito-atlantal joint. It is also important to support the rest of the snake's body so that not all of the weight of the snake is suspended from the head. Allow the smaller species to coil around the handler's arm, so the snake is supporting itself (Figure 19.2).

In the larger species (longer than 10 feet) it is necessary to support the body length at regular intervals. This often requires several handlers. Indeed, it is vital to adopt a safe operating practice with the larger, constricting species of snake. A 'buddy system' should be operated wherein any snake longer than 5–6 feet in length should only be handled by two or more people. This ensures that if the snake was to enwrap one handler, the other could disentangle him or her by unwinding from the tail end first. Above all, it is important not to grip the snake too hard as this will cause bruising and the release of myoglobin from muscle cells. This can damage the glomerular filtration membrane in the kidneys.

Venomous snakes or very aggressive species may be restrained initially using snake hooks. These are 1.5–2 feet steel rods with a blunt shepherd's hook on the end. They are used to loop under the body of a snake to move it at arm's length into a container. The hook may also be used to trap the head flat against the floor before grasping it with the hand. Once the head is controlled safely the snake is rendered harmless. Exceptions include the spitting cobra family where handlers should wear plastic goggles, or a plastic face visor as they can spit poison into the prey or assailant's eyes and mucous membranes causing blindness and paralysis.

Chelonia

The majority of Chelonia are harmless, although surprisingly strong. Mediterranean species, the tortoise may be held with both hands, one on either side of the main part of the shell behind the front legs. To keep the tortoise still for examination, it may be placed onto a cylinder or stack of tins, raising its legs clear of the table as it balances on the centre of the underside of the shell (plastron).

For aggressive species (e.g. snapping turtle and the alligator snapping turtle), it is essential that you hold the shell on both sides behind and above the rear legs to avoid being bitten. Chemical restraint is necessary in order to examine the head region in these species.

For the soft-shelled and aquatic species, soft cloths and latex-free gloves should be used to prevent damaging the shell.

Crocodylia

The Crocodylia include fresh and saltwater crocodiles, alligators, fish-eating gharials, and caimans. Their dangers to the handler lie in their impressively arrayed jaws and often their sheer size – an adult bull Nile crocodile may weigh many hundreds of kilograms.

Small specimens may be restrained by grasping the base of the tail in one hand whilst the other is placed behind the head. For slightly bigger specimens, a rope halter or noose may be tied around the snout so securing it closed. All of the major muscles in the crocodylian jaws are involved in closing not opening them, hence relatively fine rope or tape can be used to keep the mouth closed. The rest of the animal is restrained by pinning it to the ground.

Always approach crocodylians from head on, as their binocular vision is poor (although the alligator family does have some). Care should be taken when close to the crocodylian for head and tail movements both are directed at the assailant at the same time!

Much larger crocodiles require teams of people, with nets and snout snares in order to quickly clamp the jaws closed and to restrain the dangerous thrashing tail. Chemical immobilisation via dart guns is another option to be seriously considered.

Principles of chemical restraint

Chemical restraint is necessary for many procedures in reptile medicine, ranging from minor procedures such as extracting the head of a leopard tortoise or box turtle from its shell, to enabling a jugular blood sample to be taken or to carrying out coeliotomy procedures because of egg binding. Before any anaesthetic or sedative is administered, an assessment of the reptile patient's health should be made. Considerations include

- Is sedation or anaesthesia necessary for the procedure required?
- Is the reptile suffering from respiratory disease or septicaemia?
- Is the reptile's health likely to be made worse by sedation or anaesthesia?

Before discussing the administration of chemical restraint it is important to understand the reptilian respiratory system.

Overview of reptilian respiratory anatomy and physiology

The reptilian patient has a number of variations on the basic mammalian respiratory system.

The reptile patient has a glottis similar to the avian patient, which lies at the base of the tongue. This is more rostral in snakes and lizards and more caudal in Chelonia. At rest, the glottis is permanently closed, opening briefly during inspiration and expiration. In crocodiles, the glottis is obscured by the basihyal valve which is a fold of the epiglottis. This fold has to be deflected before they can be intubated (Bennett, 1998).

The trachea varies between orders. In Chelonia and Crocodylia, complete cartilaginous rings similar to those of the avian patient are found, with chelonians having a very short trachea. In some species, this trachea bifurcates into two bronchi in the neck. Snakes and lizards have incomplete C-rings, with snakes having a very long trachea.

The lungs of snake and lizard species are simple and elastic in nature. The left lung of most snakes is absent, or vestigial in the case of members of the boiid family. The right lung of snakes frequently ends in an air sac. Chelonian species have a more complicated lung structure, and the paired lungs sit dorsally inside the carapace of the shell. Crocodylian lungs are similar to mammalian lungs and are paired.

No reptile has a diaphragm, although crocodylians have a pseudodiaphragm which changes position with the movements of the liver and gut so pushing air in and out of the lungs. Most reptiles use intercostal muscles to move the ribcage in and out in a manner similar to birds. The exception to this is members of the order Chelonia. These species need to move their limbs, neck and head into and out of the shell in order to bring air into and out of the lungs.

Some species can survive in oxygen-deprived atmospheres for prolonged periods – chelonian species may survive for 24 hours or more, and even green iguanas may survive for 4–5 hours. This makes induction of anaesthesia via inhalation of a gaseous anaesthetic agent almost impossible in these animals. The stimulus for respiration in reptiles is therefore predominantly driven by lowered $pO2$ rather than elevated $pCO2$ and many reptiles when breath-holding show right-to-left shunting of blood in the heart so by-passing the lungs.

Many snakes have both intrapulmonary chemoreceptors and stretch receptors whereas many chelonians have only stretch receptors, hence when there are high levels of carbon dioxide, snakes can override the volume related feedback and continue to breathe. Hypercapnia tends to increase the tidal volume by suppressing the stretch receptors. Hypoxia increases breathing frequency by reducing or eliminating the non-breathing periods and these effects are increased at higher environmental temperatures.

In snakes, the central control of respiration can also override the stretch receptors allowing them to control breathing even when constricting prey or swallowing large prey which may impinge on the lungs.

Pre-anaesthetic preparation

Weight measurement
This is important for accuracy as some species of reptile may be very small. Scales accurate to 1 g are therefore advised for smaller reptiles to ensure correct dosage.

Blood testing
It may be advisable to test biochemical and haematological parameters before administering chemical immobilising drugs. Blood samples can be taken from

- Jugular vein in Chelonia
- Dorsal tail vein in Chelonia
- Ventral tail vein in snakes, Crocodylia and lizards
- Palatine vein or cardiac puncture in snakes (although they frequently need to be sedated or anaesthetised to collect blood from these routes).

Fasting
Fasting is necessary in snakes to prevent regurgitation and pressure on the lungs or heart. It is advisable to ensure that no prey has been offered in the two days prior to anaesthesia. Other reptiles require less fasting, e.g. chelonians rarely if ever regurgitate. However, it is important not to feed live prey to insectivores such as leopard geckos 24 hours prior to an anaesthetic as the prey may still be alive when the reptile is anaesthetised.

Pre-anaesthetic medications
Premedications are used to provide cardiopulmonary and central nervous system stabilisation, a smooth anaesthetic induction, muscle relaxation, analgesia and a degree of sedation.

Antimuscarinic medications
Atropine (0.01–0.04 mg/kg IM) or glycopyrrolate (0.01 mg/kg IM) may be used to reduce oral secretion and to reduce bradycardia; however, these are not usually of concern in reptiles. Indeed, antimuscarinics may increase the thickness of mucus secretions, leading to more rapid blocking of the airways. In addition, in herbivores it can result in prolonged periods of ileus.

Tranquilisers
Acepromazine (0.1–0.5 mg/kg IM) may be given one hour before anaesthetic induction to reduce the levels of anaesthetic required, as can diazepam (0.22–0.62 mg/kg IM in alligators) and midazolam (2 mg/kg IM in turtles) (Bennett, 1998).

Alpha-2 adrenoceptor stimulants
Xylazine at 1 mg/kg can be used 30 minutes prior to ketamine in crocodylians to reduce the dose of ketamine needed. Medetomidine, used at doses of 100–150 mg/kg, markedly reduces the dose of ketamine required in chelonians, and has the advantage of being reversible with atipamezole at 500–750 mg/kg. They both create a drop in blood pressure and cardiac output and so should be used with caution in debilitated reptiles.

Opioids
Butorphanol (at 0.4 mg/kg IM) can be administered 20 minutes before anaesthesia; this provides analgesia and reduces the amount of anaesthetic required. This drug may be combined with midazolam at 2 mg/kg. It does not have any sedation or general anaesthetic properties but does seem to have anaesthetic sparing properties allowing reduced levels of gaseous anaesthetic to be used.

Fluids
Fluid therapy is very important, and correction of fluid deficits should be attempted prior to surgery. Maintenance levels in reptile patients have been quoted as 25–30 mL/kg/day (see chapter 22 for more information on fluid therapy in reptiles).

Induction of anaesthesia
It should be noted that reptiles should never be immobilised by chilling or cooling them down. This does not provide analgesia and has serious welfare implications.

Injectable agents
Table 19.1 describes the advantages and disadvantages of injectable anaesthetic agents.

PART III: REPTILES AND AMPHIBIANS

Table 19.1 Advantages and disadvantages of injectable anaesthetics.

Advantages	Disadvantages
Ease of administration	Recovery often dependent on organ metabolism
Prevention of breath-holding on induction	Difficult to reverse rapidly
Reduced costs	Often prolonged recovery times
Easy to administer	Muscle necrosis at site of injection
Low risk to anaesthetist	

Dissociative anaesthetics

Ketamine: Recommended levels range from 22 to 44 mg/kg IM for sedation to 55–88 mg/kg IM for surgical anaesthesia. Lower levels are needed if combined with a premedicant such as midazolam or medetomidine (Bennett, 1996). Doses in excess of 110 mg/kg will produce profound bradycardia and the death of the reptile.

Effects are seen in 10–30 minutes but may take anything up to 4 days to wear off, particularly at low environmental temperatures. Its main use is therefore at the lower dose range, to allow sedation, facilitate intubation and maintenance of gaseous anaesthesia in species such as chelonians that hold their breath during gaseous induction. Doses of 5–10 mg/kg have been used in Chelonia to allow extraction of the head from the shell.

It is, however, frequently painful on administration. Also, because ketamine is excreted by the kidneys, it is recommended that it is administered in the cranial half of the body. This is because blood from the caudal half of the body travels to the kidneys before returning to the heart and the anaesthetic may thus be excreted before it has a chance to work. In addition, as it is actively excreted by the kidneys, its use in reptiles with renal disease will result in prolonged recovery periods.

Ketamine (5 mg/kg) may be combined with medetomidine (100 ug/kg) to facilitate intubation of small reptiles (<2 kg) or at 7.5 mg/kg ketamine plus 75 ug/kg medetomidine for reptiles >2 kg.

Other injectable anaesthetics

Alfaxalone: This can be used to aid induction, allowing intubation within 3–5 minutes when administered intravenously. It may be administered intramuscularly but induction takes longer via this route (25–40 minutes). Doses of 9 mg/kg have been advised and it appears in many reptiles not to be capable of inducing full anaesthesia but rather permitting intubation and causing immobilisation (Sheelings *et al.*, 2010).

Propofol: Propofol produces rapid induction and recovery. Its advantages include a short elimination half-life and minimal organ metabolism, making it relatively safe to use in debilitated reptiles which often have some liver damage.

Its disadvantage is that it requires intravenous access, although use of the intraosseous route is useful in green iguanas at a dose of 10 mg/kg. Propofol also produces a transient period of apnoea and some cardiac depression. In this situation, intubation and positive pressure ventilation is necessary.

Doses of 10–15 mg/kg in chelonians given via the dorsal coccygeal (tail) vein have successfully induced anaesthesia in under 1 minute. This allows intubation and maintenance on a gaseous anaesthetic if required. Alternatively, propofol can be used alone providing a period of anaesthesia of 20–30 minutes. For giant species of Chelonia, lower doses of 1–2 mg/kg IV/IO have been used.

Depolarising muscle relaxants

Succinylcholine: This is a neuromuscular blocking agent and produces immobilisation without providing analgesia. Therefore, it should only be used to aid the administration of another form of anaesthetic or for transportation, and not as a sole source of anaesthesia. Recovery is dependent on liver metabolism and its use in animals with possible liver disease should be avoided.

It can be used in giant Chelonia at doses of 0.5–1 mg/kg IM and will allow intubation and conversion to gaseous anaesthesia. Crocodilians can be immobilised with 3–5 mg/kg IM, with immobilisation occurring within 4 minutes and recovery in 7–9 hours. Respiration usually continues without assistance at these doses, but is important to have assisted ventilation facilities to hand as paralysis of the muscles of respiration can easily occur.

Reversal of succinylcholine is not possible and the patient must be ventilated until the drug has been excreted.

Gallamine: This has been used in crocodiles (0.3–1.5 mg/kg) to achieve immobility in 15–30 minutes with a recovery time of 1.5–3 hours. Its advantage over succinylcholine is that it is reversible with neostigmine (0.25 mg/kg).

Table 19.2 Advantages and disadvantages of gaseous anaesthetic.

Advantages	Disadvantages
Ease of administration via face mask	Breath-holding (chelonia particularly)
Pain free	Environmental pollution
Minimal tissue trauma	Health risk to anaesthetist Risk with dangerous reptiles during handling

Gaseous agents

The gaseous anaesthetics used for induction will be discussed in the next section on maintenance of anaesthesia, however, a table listing their advantages and disadvantages is presented in Table 19.2.

Maintenance of anaesthesia
Injectable agents
Dissociative anaesthetics

Ketamine: Ketamine may be used on its own for anaesthesia at doses of 55–88 mg/kg IM. It is worthwhile noting though that as the dosages get higher the recovery time also increases, and in some cases it can be as long as several days. Also, doses above 110 mg/kg will cause respiratory arrest and bradycardia.

Ketamine may be combined with other injectable agents to provide surgical anaesthesia. Examples of these combinations include

- Midazolam at 2 mg/kg IM with 40 mg/kg ketamine in turtles (Bennett, 1996)
- Xylazine at 1 mg/kg IM, given 30 minutes prior to 20 mg/kg ketamine in large crocodiles (Lawton, 1992)
- Medetomidine at 100 mg/kg IM with 50 mg/kg ketamine in kingsnakes (Malley, 1997).

Other injectable anaesthetics

Propofol: Propofol may be used to give 20–30 minutes of anaesthesia after administration, allowing minor procedures such as wound repair, intraosseous or intravenous catheter placement, or oesophagostomy tube placement to be carried out.

It may be topped up at 1 mg/kg/min IV/IO, but apnoea is extremely common and intubation and ventilation with 100% oxygen is required.

Alphaxalone: This can be used for induction and also for short periods of anaesthesia (average 25 minutes) at 9 mg/kg IV/IO. Topping up of the anaesthetic allows

maintenance of light anaesthesia for longer procedures but caution should be observed as it may not produce enough anaesthesia to allow invasive procedures in all species. Kischinovsky and Bertelsen (2011) showed that 30 mg/kg was required in green iguanas to achieve surgical anaesthesia, but many became apnoeic. Recovery times are often 1–4 hours.

Gaseous agents
Isoflurane

Isoflurane is the gaseous maintenance anaesthetic of choice (see also Table 19.2). Isoflurane is minimally metabolised in the body (0.3%) and has a very low blood–gas partition coefficient (1.4 compared with 2.3 for halothane in human trials). This means that it has a very low solubility in blood, so as soon as administration is stopped the reptile starts to recover, excreting it from the lungs. In addition, it has low fat solubility and so is not stored. Isoflurane still has excellent muscle relaxing properties and is a good analgesic during anaesthesia. Apnoea precedes cardiac arrest, unlike the case with halothane anaesthesia.

It can be used to induce anaesthesia in those species not exhibiting breath- holding at levels of 4–5%, by induction chamber. It is also possible to adapt the cases of 20 mL and 60 mL syringes to form long, thin face masks to induce snakes. Isoflurane can then be used to maintain anaesthesia, preferably via endotracheal tube, at levels from 2–3% depending on the procedure.

Sevoflurane

As with isoflurane, this drug may be safely used. It is highly insoluble in the bloodstream though, and so ventilation rates may need to be increased above the usual 4–6 breaths per minute to maintain anaesthesia. In this author's experience, it cannot be used to maintain anaesthesia alone in certain species of reptiles (leopard geckos, bearded dragons and green tree pythons to name a few) and so care should be taken in selecting this gas particularly when using a different induction agent as once the induction agent wears off the patient may wake up!

Induction and maintenance levels of sevoflurane are higher than for isoflurane being typically 6–8% and 3–4% respectively.

Nitrous oxide

Nitrous oxide can be used in conjunction with isoflurane, reducing the percentage of gaseous anaesthetic required for induction and maintenance of anaesthesia. Its other advantages include good muscle relaxation and excellent analgesic properties, making it useful in orthopaedic procedures.

Disadvantages of nitrous include its tendency to accumulate in hollow organs. This may prove a problem for herbivorous reptiles as they often have capacious hind guts and nitrous oxide can accumulate there. Nitrous oxide also requires some organ metabolism for full excretion and so may be a problem in a seriously diseased patient. It also prolongs anaesthetic recovery times by up to 50%.

Aspects of gaseous anaesthesia maintenance for reptiles

Inhalant gaseous anaesthesia is becoming the main method of anaesthetising reptiles for prolonged procedures. The reptile patient should preferably be intubated to allow the inhalant anaesthetic to be delivered in a controlled manner.

Intubation

Intubation is straightforward in reptiles as they do not have an epiglottis and the glottis, which acts as the entrance to the trachea, is relatively cranial in the majority of species. It is useful to note that the glottis is kept closed at rest, so the operator must wait for inspiration to occur to allow intubation. Reptiles produce little or no saliva when at rest or not eating, so blockage of the tube is uncommon.

In snakes, the glottis sits rostrally on the floor of the mouth just caudal to the tongue sheath and is easily visible when the mouth is opened (Figure 19.3). Intubation may be performed in the conscious patient if necessary, as reptiles do not have a cough reflex. The mouth is opened with a wooden or plastic tongue depressor and the endotracheal tube inserted during inspiration. Alternatively, an induction agent may be given and then intubation attempted.

In Chelonia, the glottis sits slightly more caudally at the base of the tongue (Figure 19.4). The trachea is very short and the endotracheal tube should only be inserted a few centimetres, otherwise there is a risk that only one or the other of the bronchi will be intubated, leading to only one lung receiving the anaesthetic. An induction agent such as ketamine or propofol is advised for chelonians prior to intubation due to their ability to breath-hold and difficulty in extracting the head from the shell.

Lizards vary depending on the species, most having just a glottis guarding the entrance to the trachea (Figure 19.5). Some species possess vocal folds, notably

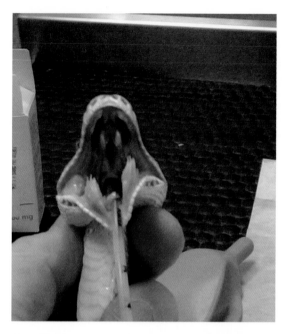

Figure 19.3 Intraoral views after intubation of a green tree python (*Morelia viridis*) showing glottal tube.

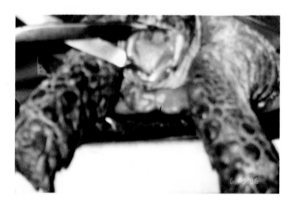

Figure 19.4 Intraoral view of a tortoise showing the fleshy tongue and the glottis at its base.

some species of gecko (Porter, 1972). Some may be intubated consciously, but most are better induced with an injectable preparation or by face mask using gas. Some species may be too small for intubation. The larger species may also require a mouth gag to avoid biting down on the tube (see Figure 19.6).

Crocodylia have a basihyal fold (Bennett, 1998) that acts as an epiglottis and needs to be depressed prior to intubation. Because they are potentially dangerous, these species require some form of injectable chemical sedation or induction prior to intubation.

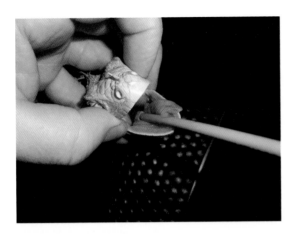

Figure 19.5 Intraoral views after intubation of a green iguana (*Iguana iguana*) showing fleshy tongue.

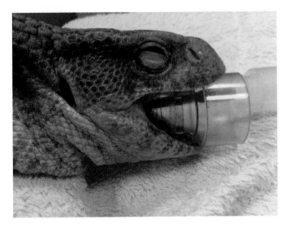

Figure 19.6 A mouth gag may be needed in larger species such as this Savannah monitor lizard (*Varanus exanthematicus*) to prevent them biting down on the tube.

Intermittent positive pressure ventilation

If intubation is performed on a conscious patient, anaesthesia may be induced, even in breath-holding species, by using positive pressure ventilation. This has some advantages as it leads to rapid post-operative recovery.

Tidal volume of reptiles varies between species (many boiids are around 12.5 mL/kg, many aquatic turtles are around 45 mL/kg). There is often right-to-left pulmonary shunting of blood which can be worsened by the presence of intracoelomic masses such as eggs, food or effusions. In addition, position of the reptile may also create a perfusion mismatch as many chelonians require to be placed in dorsal recumbency to expose the plastron for surgery, thus allowing the dorsally located lungs to be squashed by the liver and gastrointestinal tract. If intubation is performed

fully consciously, anaesthesia may be induced, even in breath-holding species, by using positive pressure ventilation, in a matter of 5–10 minutes. This does have some advantages as the avoidance of injectable induction agents leads to rapid post-operative recovery.

Many species therefore require positive pressure ventilation during the course of an anaesthetic. The aim of intermittent positive pressure ventilation (IPPV) is to inflate the lungs with an oxygen and anaesthetic mixture enough for an adequately oxygenated state to be maintained and for the animal to remain anaesthetised. To this end it is sufficient to ventilate most reptiles six times a minute and no more, at a pressure of 10–15 cm water. As with birds, a ventilator unit makes life much easier, but with experience, manual 'bagging' of the patient with enough pressure just to inflate the lungs and no more can be achieved (Figures 19.7 and 19.8a and 19.8b). A rough guide is to inflate the first two-fifths of the reptile's body at each cycle (Malley, 1997).

Anaesthetic circuits

For species weighing less than 5 kg, a non-rebreathing system with oxygen flow at twice the minute volume is suggested (Bennett, 1998). This approximates to 300–500 mL/kg/min for most species. Ayres T pieces, modified ('mini') Bain circuits and Mapleson C circuits may all be used.

NB: normal tidal volumes vary in reptiles widely (e.g., 12.5 mL/kg in boas to 45 mL/kg in freshwater turtles). They frequently have a ventilation–perfusion mismatch and right-to-left pulmonary shunts, all of which may be exacerbated by the presence of increased coelomic contents such as gravidity or recent large meals.

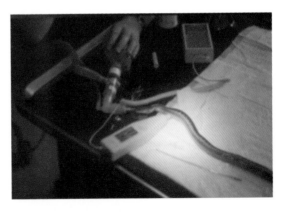

Figure 19.7 Manual bagging of a garter snake (*Thamnophis sirtalis*). Note Doppler probe to monitor heart sounds, and Mapleson C circuit for smaller species.

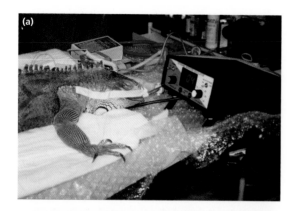

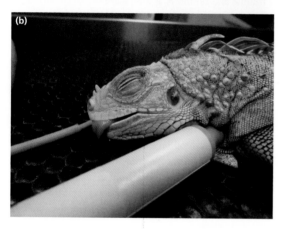

Figure 19.8 (a) and **(b)** Mechanical IPPV using a ventilator in the green iguana (*Iguana iguana*). Note again Doppler probe and cranial position of the heart in iguanids.

Additional supportive therapy

Recumbency

Many chelonians are placed in dorsal recumbency for intracoelomic surgery. Other groups of reptiles may also be placed in this position for similar techniques. The use of foam wedges, or positional polystyrene-filled vacuum bags, is essential to maintain stability.

Snakes may become extremely flaccid during surgery. In order to provide stability they may be strapped to a long board or wedged in place with foam wedges or vacuum bags. In any case, it is important to keep the body wall of non-chelonian species free of constraint and to use IPPV if necessary.

Maintenance of body temperature

Maintaining body temperature is important for successful recovery. Body temperature can be monitored using a cloacal probe attached to a digital thermometer.

Reptiles should be maintained as near to their preferred body temperature (PBT) as possible, which lies in the range 22–30°C for most species. This can be achieved by placing the reptile onto a circulating water or air heating pad during anaesthesia and room temperature should be kept up to reduce heat losses. Warmed subcutaneous or intracoelomic fluids can be given during and after surgery.

Hot water bottles or hot water-filled latex gloves may also be used, but must be wrapped in towelling to prevent direct contact with the reptile. Care should be taken when these cool down, as they may then draw heat away from the patient rather than provide it. The use of clear drapes will also help to keep heat in as will the utilisation of light sources for surgery, many of which radiate heat.

Fluid therapy

Fluid therapy is covered in more detail in chapter 22. However, it should be noted that, as with small mammals, post-operative fluid therapy will enhance the recovery rate and improve the patient's return to normal function. Recommended fluid volumes are 20–25 mL/kg every 24 hours across the species (Frye, 1991). They should not exceed 2–3% body weight in chelonians.

Monitoring anaesthesia

Box 19.1 shows the stages of anaesthesia seen in reptiles.

Monitoring the heart rate and rhythm can be difficult with a conventional stethoscope due to the rough scales of the reptile interfering with sound transmission and the three chambered heart of reptiles which reduces the clarity of the heart beat. Some of this can be overcome by placing a damp towel over the area to be auscultated so deadening the sound of the scales, but in many cases the best solution is to resort to using a Doppler probe which may be placed over the heart outlet at the base of the neck in lizards and Chelonia (Figure 19.9) and directly over the heart in snakes (Figure 19.10). Changes in rate and intensity of flow can then be monitored.

Pulse oximetry is not useful in reptiles due to the differences in haemoglobin structure, which makes interpretation impossible. General trends though may be monitored but this author finds them generally unreliable in reptiles.

Capnography is also debateable as to its usefulness due to cardiac shunting of blood in reptiles, which means that expired carbon dioxide levels do not reflect arterial levels.

ECG leads may be attached to the patient to give an electrical trace of heart activity. The alligator forceps on

Box 19.1 Stages of anaesthesia in reptiles

Stage 1

- Limb movements reduced
- Righting reflex present (reptile will flip back onto its feet after being inverted)
- Snake tongue withdrawn after being grasped
- Responds to noxious stimuli
- Muscles are tense
- Writhing movements occur
- Vent stimulation reflex present
- Palpebral reflex present

Stage 2

- Righting reflex ceases
- Tongue withdrawal reflex much reduced
- No response to noxious stimuli
- Muscles start to relax
- Writhing movements cease
- Vent reflex reduced
- Palpebral reflex diminished

Stage 3

- Righting reflex ceased
- No voluntary motion
- Tongue withdrawal reflex totally absent
- No response to noxious stimuli
- Muscles totally relaxed
- Snakes: Bauchstreich reflex (where stroking of the ventral scales produces movement in the body wall) much reduced
- Laryngeal reflexes lost in alligators
- Chelonia still have a corneal reflex
- Vent reflex much reduced – loss of this indicates anaesthesia is too deep

Stage 4

- Extreme depression and death (Chelonia lose corneal reflexes just before entering this phase).

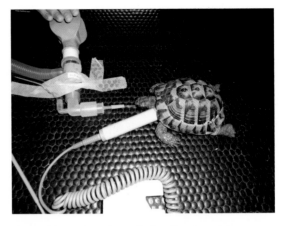

Figure 19.9 Doppler probe monitoring of heart sounds in an anaesthetised spur-thighed tortoise (*Testudo graeca*).

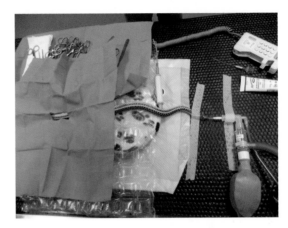

Figure 19.10 Doppler probe monitoring heart sounds in an anaesthetized garter snake (*Thamnophis sirtalis*). Note also the tape securing the ET tube and the snakes head to prevent dislodgement.

the leads may be attached to hypodermic needles which can then be attached to the patient to minimise the crushing effects of the forceps on small fragile patients. In snakes, these can still be used, even in the absence of limbs. The leads are placed two heart lengths cranial and caudal to the heart. In some lizards, such as iguanas, skinks, chameleons and water dragons, the heart is situated far cranially and hence the forelimb leads are better placed cervically. Heart rates may be measured and compared with the formula

$$HR = 33.4 \times [Body\ weight\ (kg)]^{-0.25}$$

Assuming the reptile is kept in its preferred optimum temperature, i.e. it is at its preferred body temperature.

Respiratory flow monitors are not so useful due to the need for IPPV in most reptile species.

Recovery and analgesia

Recovery

Reptiles often recover rapidly from isoflurane anaesthesia. But, if other injectable drugs were used, such as alphaxolone or ketamine, recovery may be prolonged. It is essential at this time to keep the reptile patient calm, stress free and at its optimum preferred body temperature. It is also necessary to keep the patient intubated and on IPPV with oxygen until the reptile is once again breathing for itself. The use of doxapram at dose of 5 mg/kg by intramuscular or intravenous injection is useful to help stimulate respiration. The stimulus for reptiles to breathe, however, is a falling blood partial pressure of oxygen, and not a rising partial pressure of carbon dioxide, so IPPV with 100% oxygen may actually inhibit respiration. Therefore, recovery using room air, or increasing the intervals between ventilations from one every 10 seconds to one every 20–30 seconds may be helpful in lowering pO2 and so aid in stimulating spontaneous breathing.

Fluid therapy during this period will also help to speed recovery, especially from agents such as ketamine which are cleared through the kidneys. Once recovery is complete, the reptile should be encouraged to eat, or, if anorectic, the patient should be assist fed, stomach tubed etc.

Many snakes will start to show sinuous movements from the tail end first as they recover. Chelonians will start to move hindlimbs and then forelimbs and lizards will start uncoordinated hindlimb movements followed by forelimb movements.

Analgesia for reptiles

Pain assessment in reptiles

Reptiles which have been provided with analgesia have been shown to have a quicker return to normality, eating, normal behaviour etc. than those who do not receive analgesia. However, assessing pain in reptiles is extremely difficult owing to the huge species variations. Mosley (2011) has derived an approach to pain assessment which tries to encompass behaviour (taking into account species variations, stage of ecdysis, hibernation status, socialisation, concurrent illness, and owner assessment of their pet), environmental considerations (enclosure and temperature range), locomotor activity (taking into account posture, gait) and miscellaneous attributes (including appetite, eyelid position, colour changes and abnormal respiratory movements). These are compared with the anticipation of pain levels based on our understanding in mammals and birds.

General but non-specific signs of pain in reptiles include immobility, anorexia, abnormal locomotion and posture, increased aggression and in those species which can control chromatophore expression in their skin, a dull or dark colouration (e.g. chameleons and bearded dragons). Many snakes with visceral pain will adopt an S-shaped position.

Analgesics used in reptiles

Buprenorphine

Buprenorphine at 0.01–0.02 mg/kg IM have been recommended but doses of 0.075–0.1 mg/kg were needed in red-eared terrapins in order to maintain therapeutic levels for 24 hours (Kummrow et al., 2008. Some difference was noted in concentrations needed, depending on where the drug was administered with significantly reduced levels being achieved, if injected in the hindlimbs versus the forelimb (thought to be hepatic removal) – also enterohepatic recycling has been noted.

Morphine

Morphine has been shown to be effective at high doses in bearded dragons (10 mg/kg) (Greenacre et al., 2008), but at 1.5–6.5 in turtles with a duration of activity which lasted 24 hours (Sladky et al., 2007). At high doses, morphine can act as a significant respiratory depressant in some species (Sladky et al., 2007; Sladky et al., 2008; Sladky et al., 2009) and that its onset of action can be prolonged (2–8 hours) due to unknown factors.

Butorphanol

The same studies suggested that butorphanol may not be an effective analgesic even at excessive dosages. However, it has been used at 0.4 mg/kg prior to anaesthesia and found to have anaesthetic sparing effects.

NSAIDs

All NSAIDs are potentially nephrotoxic and have gastrointestinal ulcerative side effects and hence fluid therapy and close monitoring should be performed. Carprofen at 2–4 mg/kg IM once, and then 1–2 mg/kg every 24–72 hours thereafter has been advised. Pharmacokinetic studies on meloxicam at 0.2 mg/kg orally every 24 hours have also been recommended (Hernandez-Divers et al., 2004). However, the same study showed that doses of 5 mg/kg meloxicam were administered orally for 12 days in green iguanas and produced no clinically apparent abnormalities of histopathological lesions associated with toxicity.

However, dosages of 0.3 mg/kg meloxicam in ball pythons (Python regius) showed no decrease in physiological stress after a surgical procedure suggesting it did not provide adequate analgesia (Olesen et al., 2008). This study did acknowledge that it was difficult to see any increase in physiological stress response, however, in the control animals after surgery!

Other analgesics

Tramadol has been used at 11 mg/kg in bearded dragons (Greenacre et al., 2008) and at 10–25 mg/kg in red-eared terrapins (Cummings et al., 2009) and found to increase the threshold to noxious stimuli and is thought to work via its weak opioid activity on mu receptors. Duration in the terrapins was between 6 and 96 hours when given orally (10–25 mg/kg) and 12–48 hours when given parenterally (10 mg/kg).

Ketamine appears to be well tolerated in reptiles and has been used as an adjunct to multimodal analgesia. The alpha-2 drugs may also be useful in analgesia but they do seem to produce similar undesirable effects as in mammals, i.e. bradycardia, hypotension and a reduction in arterial pO2 levels (Sleeman & Gaynor, 2000; Dennis & Heard, 2002).

Local anaesthesia

Local anaesthetics may be used as ring blocks around amputations to reduce the chances of post-operative self-mutilation. Doses should not exceed 4 mg/kg of lidocaine (known toxic doses in mammals are 10–22 mg/kg) and should be diluted to at least 1:10. Bupivicaine should not exceed 5 mg/kg.

Overview of amphibian anaesthesia

Techniques and equipment involved in restraining amphibian patients

Examination of the amphibian patient should be performed at that species' optimum preferred body temperature, as with reptile patients. A rough guide is between 21 and 24°C, which are lower than the more usual 22–32°C reptile housing conditions.

The examination table should be covered with paper towels (unbleached) that have been soaked in dechlorinated water – preferably purified water. More purified water should be on standby to be applied to the amphibian patient to prevent dehydration during the examination.

Initially, it is useful not to restrain the amphibian patient until the extent of any problem is assessed, as many have severe skin lesions that are extremely fragile. Once an initial assessment has been made, the patient may be restrained manually. First, it is advisable to put on a pair of latex-free gloves in order to minimise irritation to the amphibian's skin caused by either the handler's normal acidic skin environment or by the powder in many pre-packed latex gloves. The wearing of gloves is also essential in many species of anurans whose skin can produce irritant or even potentially deadly toxins which can be absorbed through unprotected human skin. It may also be necessary to wear goggles when handling some species of toad – the giant toad (*Bufo marinus)* can squirt a toxin from its parotid salivary glands over a distance of several feet.

When handling the amphibian patient, the method of restraint will obviously depend on the animal's body shape. The elongated form of salamanders and newts will require similar restraint to that of a lizard, with one hand grasping the pectoral girdle from the dorsal aspect, index finger and thumb encircling one forelimb, second and third fingers the other, with the opposite hand grasping the pelvic girdle, again from the dorsal aspect in a similar manner. Some salamanders will shed their tails if roughly handled, so care should be taken with these species.

Large anurans can be restrained by cupping one hand around the pectoral girdle immediately behind the front limbs with the other hand positioned beneath the hindlimbs. Care should be taken with some species which have poison glands in their skin, as mentioned above, and in the case of species such as the Argentinian horned frog, care should be taken as they bite. Aquatic urodeles should be examined only in water as removal causes skin damage. Some of the larger urodeles, such as the hellbender species (*Cryptobranchus* spp.) can also inflict unpleasant bite wounds on handlers, so firm restraint is required.

Smaller species and aquatic species may be best examined in small glass jars.

Aspects of chemical restraint in amphibians

There are three main routes of administration of anaesthetic and sedative agents to amphibians: Injections, inhalant gaseous anaesthetics and in-water methods.

In-water anaesthetic agents

There are two main anaesthetics – MS-222 and benzocaine.

MS-222

This is tricaine methanesulphonate, an anaesthetic used commonly in fish restraint. It is a water soluble white powder. A range of 1–2 g/L water is required to anaesthetise most frogs and urodeles, but a solution of 3 g/L is required for most toads (Wright, 1996). A much reduced level of 0.5 g/L can be used for tadpole anaesthesia. The same weight of sodium bicarbonate is often added to the water to counteract MS-222's tendency to acidify the solution.

It is best to use the amphibian's own water to minimise environmental changes, and to place this into a plastic bag, or plastic-lined box. This is useful as many amphibians go through an excitation stage during anaesthesia, and the slight give in the plastic bags reduces skin damage. It is also important to ensure any anurans and other non-gilled amphibians can raise their nostrils above the water, otherwise they will drown.

Anaesthesia induction will take 20 minutes or so, with reducing respiration rates. Respiration may even stop, although cardiac function persists. During the induction period, the ventrum of the amphibian will redden and anurans will become excited, making leaping movements.

Initial anaesthesia is manifested by the inability of the amphibian to right itself, and loss of the corneal reflex, but with pain reflexes still intact. A deep plane of anaesthesia is when all of these are abolished and only the heartbeat can be seen as a sign of movement. The level of anaesthesia can be maintained by trickling the anaesthetic solution over the amphibian's body once the amphibian is removed from the solution. Reversal is achieved by trickling fresh, distilled, oxygenated water over the amphibian's skin.

Benzocaine

This can be used to anaesthetise many adult amphibians at solutions of 0.2–0.3 mg/L water. It is more soluble in ethanol than in water and so is often dissolved in a small volume of this before it is added to the water. Recovery occurs some 60 minutes after rinsing the amphibian with benzocaine-free water.

It may be necessary to add a buffer solution to the water to correct acidification as with MS-222.

Injectable anaesthetic agents

Ketamine may be used, but is less preferable to MS-222. This is because relatively large volumes are required (75–100 mg/kg (Bennett, 1996)), and the anaesthetic takes a variable period to take effect, from 10 minutes to 1–2 hours. Injections may be made intramuscularly, intravenously into the midline ventral abdominal vein or subcutaneously.

Inhalant gaseous anaesthetic agents
Isoflurane

This may be used via induction chamber at dose of 2.5–3%, or, in the larger species of toads, by dripping it directly onto the toad's skin. Some of the larger species may also be intubated, but anaesthesia is often erratic, as alternative respiratory routes are available to amphibians (cutaneous or buccopharyngeal routes, i.e. the amphibian can breathe through its skin or oral membranes). Some of the more fragile species, such as the smaller urodeles or

caecilians may actually suffer severe skin damage during gas chamber induction due to the direct irritant effect of the anaesthetic on the skin.

Analgesia

There is limited research and knowledge into pain and its control in amphibians. Recognising pain in amphibians is also difficult, but studies by Pezalla (1983) showed that the wiping response (where the hindlimb wiped the affected limb) to increasing levels of acetic acid was a specific response to pain. These tests showed that opioids (e.g., morphine, butorphanol and buprenorphine) could raise the pain threshold in amphibians. Indications are that mu and kappa receptors exist in the spinal cord of amphibians.

In addition, other tests showed the analgesic efficacy of alpha-2 agonists such as xylazine (Terril-Robb *et al.*, 1996; Brenner *et al.*, 1994). NSAIDs produced weaker but still significant analgesic effects. Barbiturates, however, did not seem to provide analgesia in a similar study.

Suggested analgesics for frogs include butorphanol (25 mg/kg intracoelomically), buprenorphine (14 mg/kg intracoelomically), flunixin meglumine (25 mg/kg intracoelomically once) and xylazine (10 mg/kg intracoelomically q12—24 h) (Terril-Robb *et al.*, 1996; Stevens, 2011). This author has also used meloxicam at 0.2 mg/kg *per os* q24 h in Anurans and newts as post-operative analgesia.

References

Bennett, R.A. (1996) Anaesthesia. *Reptile Medicine and Surgery* (ed R. Mader), pp. 241–247. W.B. Saunders, London.

Bennett, R.A. (1998) Reptile anaesthesia. *Seminars in Avian and Exotic Pet Medicine*, **7**, 30–40.

Brenner, G.M., Klopp, A.J., Deason, L.L., *et al.* (1994) Analgesic potency of alpha adrenergic agents after systemic administration in amphibians. *Journal of Pharmacological Experimental Therapy*, **270**, 540–545.

Cummings, B.B., Sladky, K.K. and Johnson, S.M. (2009) Tramadol analgesic and respiratory effects in red-eared slider turtles (*Trachemys scripta*). *Proceedings of the Association of Reptilian and Amphibian Veterinarians*, Milwaukee, Wisconsin, p. 115.

Dennis, P.M. and Heard, D.J. (2002) Cardiopulmonary effects of a medetomidine–ketamine combination administered intravenously in gopher tortoises. *Journal of the American Veterinary Medical Association*, **220**, 1516–1519.

Frye, F. (1991). *Biomedical and Surgical Aspects of Captive Reptile Husbandry*. Krieger, Malabar, FL.

Greenacre, C.B., Massi, K., Schumacher, J.P., *et al.* (2008) Comparative antinociception of various opioids and non-steroidal anti-inflammatory medications versus saline in the bearded dragon (*Pogona vitticeps*) using electrostimulation. *Proceedings of the Association of Reptilian and Amphibian Veterinarians*, Los Angeles, California, p. 87.

Hernandez-Divers, S.J., McBride, A., Koch, T., *et al.* (2004) Single dose oral and intravenous pharmacokinetics of meloxicam in the green iguana (*Iguana iguana*). *Proceedings of the Association of Reptilian and Amphibian Veterinarians*, Naples, Florida, p. 106.

Kischinovsky, M. and Bertelsen, M.F. (2011) Alfaxalone anaesthesia in green iguanas and red-eared sliders. *Proceedings of the European Association of Zoo and Wildlife Vets, Lisbon*, Lisbon, Portugal, p. 113.

Kummrow, M.S., Tseng, F., Hesdse, L., *et al.* (2008) Pharmacokinetics of buprenorphine after single dose subcutaneous administration in red-eared sliders (*Trachemys scripta elegans*). *Journal of Zoo and Wildlife Medicine*, **39**, 590–595.

Lawton, M.P.C. (1992) Anaesthesia. *Manual of Reptiles*, 1st edn. BSAVA, Cheltenham, Glos.

Malley, D. (1997) Reptile anaesthesia and the practising veterinarian. *Practice*, **19**, 351–368.

Mosley, C. (2011) Pain and nociception in reptiles. *Veterinary Clinics of North America: Exotic Animal Practice*, **14**, 45–60.

Olesen, M.G., Bertelsen, M.F., Perry, S.F., *et al.* (2008) Effects of preoperative administration of butorphanol or meloxicam on physiologic responses to surgery in ball pythons. *Journal of the American Veterinary Medical Association*, **233**, 1883–1888.

Pezalla, P.D. (1983) Morphine-induced analgesia and explosive motor behaviour in an amphibian. *Brain Research*, **273**, 297–305.

Porter, K.R. (1972) *Herpetology*. W.B. Saunders, Philadelphia, PA.

Sheelings, T.F., Holz, P., Haynes, L., *et al.* (2010) A preliminary study of the chemical restraint of selected squamate reptiles with alfaxalone. *Proceedings of the Annual Conference of the Association of Reptilian and Amphibian Veterinarians*, South Padre Island, Texas, pp. 114–115.

Sladky, K.K., Kinney, M.E. and Johnson, S.M. (2008) Analgesic efficacy of butorphanol and morphine in bearded dragons and corn snakes. *Journal of the American Veterinary Medical Association*, **233**, 267–273.

Sladky, K.K., Kinney, M.E. and Johnson, S.M. (2009) Effects of opioid receptor activation on thermal antinociception in red-eared slider turtles (*Trachemys scripta elegans*). *American Journal of Veterinary Research*, **70**, 1072–1078.

Sladky, K.K., Miletic, V., Paul-Murphy, J.J., *et al.* (2007) Analgesic efficacy and respiratory effects of butorphanol and morphine in turtles. *Journal of the American Veterinary Medical Association*, **230**, 1356–1362.

Sleeman, J.M. and Gaynor, J. (2000) Sedative and cardiopulmonary effects of medetomidine and reversal with atipamezole in desert tortoises (*Gopherus agassizii*). *Journal of Zoo and Wildlife Medicine*, **31**, 28–35.

Stevens, C.W. (2011) Analgesia in amphibians: Preclinical studies and clinical applications. *Veterinary Clinics of North America: Exotic Animal Practice*, **14**, 33–44.

Terril-Robb, L., Suckow, M. and Grigdesby, C. (1996) Evaluation of the analgesic effects of butorphanol tartrate, xylazine hydrochloride and flunixin meglumine in leopard frogs (*Rana pipiens*). *Contemporary Topics in Laboratory Animal Science*, **35**, 54–56.

Wright, K.M. (1996) Amphibian husbandry and medicine. *Reptile Medicine and Surgery* (ed D. Mader), pp. 436–458. W.B. Saunders, Philadelphia, PA.

Chapter 20

Reptile and Amphibian Nutrition

Classification

Reptiles and amphibians may be classified in a number of different ways, one of which is according to their diet. Of the commonly seen species there are four main categories as defined by the diet. These are the following:

- Carnivores are predominantly the members of the snake family, which will eat whole avian, amphibian or mammalian prey. To do this they have powerful crushing jaws. Some have poison fangs while others, such as the boa and the python species, rely on suffocating their prey.
- Herbivores come from a variety of species, from the tortoise family (e.g. the Greek or spur-thighed tortoises), to the lizard family (e.g. the green iguana).
- Insectivores are predominantly from the lizard family (e.g. the leopard geckos, collared lizards, etc.), and from the amphibians (e.g. the frogs, salamanders, etc.)
- Omnivores are from a variety of reptile species, and the term may be used to refer to reptiles which change their eating habits during the course of their life. For example, the bearded dragon starts off as an insectivore, but becomes more and more dependent on fruit and vegetable matter as it gets older.

In all these cases, the individual species have become highly evolved to cope with certain types of food. We also know that many of these creatures in the wild have a changing food supply throughout the year, so what may form a staple diet in the summer does not necessarily apply come the winter.

General nutritional requirements

Water

As mentioned in the chapter on avian nutrition, the most important thing about the water provided is its quality. Reptiles may defaecate in their water bowls, and turtles and terrapins eat in their water. These habits cause pollution which leads to disease.

To prevent this, either the water must have a powerful filter system, or the terrapins/turtles be fed in a separate feeding tank which may be cleaned out after feeding.

Vitamin and mineral supplements administered in the water will allow rapid bacterial growth over 24 hours, so bowl hygiene must be rigorous.

The amount of water consumed by individual reptiles and amphibians will depend on the diets being offered as well as on the species. On dry, insect-based diets, water consumption will be much higher than for reptiles and amphibians, which consume large amounts of fruit and vegetables. Even so a leopard gecko may only consume 5 mL of water in a 24-hour period.

Tap water contains chlorine, which may irritate the skin of sensitive aquatic species such as amphibians or soft-shelled turtles. It is advised that tap water be allowed to stand for 24 hours to let the chlorine escape and to allow it to come up to room temperature.

Renal disease as a result of chronic dehydration is common in captive reptile species. Many of these animals, e.g. green iguanas and water dragons, come from parts of the world which have high relative humidity – anywhere from 60–100%. If these species are kept in vivaria at their correct temperatures (a high of 30°C to a low of 20°C), then the air can hold large amounts of water, consequently the relative humidity often drops at these temperatures. Combine this with the fact that many reptiles will not drink from water bowls, instead preferring to lick moisture from leaves or cage furniture, and we can see that chronic dehydration can occur. To prevent this, it is important not only to provide drinking bowls but also to mist the cage, the reptile and the cage furniture several times daily. This is of course less necessary for desert-dwelling species, such as leopard geckos, pancake tortoises, but even these species benefit from being misted every now and then.

Reptiles, like birds, are susceptible to renal disease because the waste product of protein metabolism is predominantly the insoluble uric acid. If the reptile is not kept adequately hydrated, it will reduce the excretion of uric acid through the kidneys. This leads to deposition of uric acid inside the body, a condition known as visceral

Veterinary Nursing of Exotic Pets, Second Edition. Edited by Simon J. Girling. © 2013 John Wiley & Sons, Ltd. Published 2013 by John Wiley & Sons, Ltd.

gout. Once deposited, the uric acid forms a tough miner-alised coating to the lining of blood vessels, the kidneys, the heart and many other organs, leading to hypertension and multiple organ failure.

Maintenance energy requirements

Every species has a level of energy consumption per day which is needed to satisfy the basic maintenance require-ments. This is the energy used purely to maintain current status under minimal activity and is the minimum en-ergy required to support the reptile's or amphibian's life. In reptiles, basic maintenance requirements vary widely depending on activity level and environmental tempera-ture, so calculations are made at that animal's optimum environmental temperature. Energy requirements will also vary according to the animal's stage of life. For ex-ample, the maintenance energy requirements (MER) will be more than doubled in active egg-laying females during disease or growth.

MER is dependent on the basal metabolic rate (BMR – the energy requirement when at complete rest) and meta-bolic body weight as follows:

The constant, k, varies with family groups, and has been estimated at 10 for reptiles in general.

If the foods offered are so low in kilojoules that the rep-tile or amphibian has to eat more of it than will fit into its digestive system in 24 hours, that animal will rapidly lose condition (Figures 20.1 and 20.2).

For example, vegetables such as lettuce and celery have an energy content of 12.6 kJ/g dry matter (or in real terms 0.75 kJ/g wet food), whereas meat-based foods such as rodent prey have a much higher energy density of 19–21 kJ/g dry matter (or in real terms 6–7.5 kJ/g wet

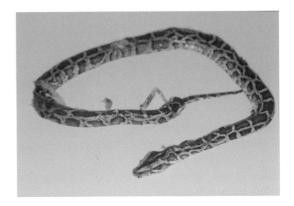

Figure 20.2 Malnutrition and blister disease in a Burmese python, *Python molurus bivittatus*.

food) (Donoghue, 1998). From this we can see that in 'as fed' terms, i.e. wet food, one would need to feed eight times as much weight of vegetable matter to give the same energy dose in animal prey. This volume may well exceed the gut capacity of the reptile or amphibian.

Conversely many pet reptiles and amphibians will con-tinue eating until their digestive tracts are full, and if all they are offered is high energy density food then they will rapidly achieve their MER, exceed it and become obese.

Protein and amino acid requirements

Proteins are assembled from groups of amino acids – indeed a protein can contain up to 22 amino acids. In general terms, for humans, and it seems for reptiles and amphibians, 10 amino acids are essential and need to be provided in the diet. The others may be manufactured from these 10. The essential amino acids are:

- leucine
- lysine
- methionine
- phenylalanine
- threonine
- tryptophan
- isoleucine
- valine
- arginine
- histidine

In addition, it is known that for diets low in the amino acids methionine or arginine, an extra supplement of the amino acid glycine is required.

Proteins are therefore assessed on their ability to pro-vide these essential amino acids, with poor proteins sup-plying only non-essential ones. This is quantified by the term biological value, a high-biological-value foodstuff containing more of the essential amino acids.

For herbivorous reptiles, levels of 25% protein content as metabolisable energy in the diet have been shown to be

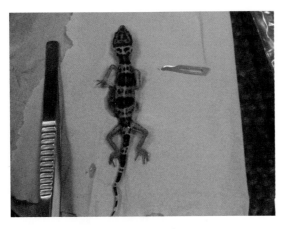

Figure 20.1 Malnutrition in a leopard gecko.

adequate (Donoghue, 1998). Most of this protein source in herbivores seems to come from leafy greens, but deficiencies are seen in herbivorous reptiles fed high cellulose, low-protein foods such as the ubiquitous lettuce, and fruits. Chronic protein deficiencies are often presented as gradual wasting conditions, with increased susceptibility to infections.

Deficiencies in amino acids in carnivorous reptiles and amphibians are extremely rare because they eat the whole prey. This gives them 30–60% protein content as metabolisable energy. Herbivorous deficiencies specific amino acids are possible, although not well documented.

In general, waste products of protein metabolism in land-based reptiles are converted into the relatively insoluble uric acid. Alligators may produce ammonia as the waste product, as may many amphibians, depending on their state of hydration, but adult frogs may excrete urea. Protein excesses, such as those produced by feeding cat- or dog foods to predominantly herbivorous species, can lead to an excess production of uric acid; visceral gout, renal failure and death may result.

Fats and essential fatty acids

Fats provide high concentrations of energy. They also supply the reptile or amphibian with essential fatty acids (EFAs), which are required for cellular integrity and as the building blocks for internal chemicals such as prostaglandins (which play a part in reproduction and inflammation). Fats also provide a carrier mechanism for the absorption of fat-soluble vitamins such as vitamins A, D, E and K.

The primary EFA for reptiles is linoleic acid, as it is for mammals, with the absolute dietary requirement of this fatty acid being 1% of the diet. If the diet becomes deficient in this EFA, a rapid decline in cellular integrity occurs. This is manifested clinically by the skin becoming flaky, inelastic, and prone to recurrent infections and also to fluid loss through the skin, which in turn leads to polydipsia (Wallach & Hoff, 1982).

In herbivores, less than 10% of the diet on a dry matter basis is composed of fats, the chief energy sources being carbohydrates and proteins. However, fermentation of fibre in the lower bowel produces short-chain fatty acids which can be used for energy. For carnivores, fat forms a major part of the energy source in the diet, as much as 40–70% of the calories, with protein chiefly making up the rest.

The problem of overconsumption of fats in pet reptiles which are not exercising regularly is well known, and high

fat foods such as dog- and cat food fed to herbivores, or extremely fat rodent prey fed to snakes, are prime culprits for this. Obesity can lead to a number of problems, high amongst which is fatty degenerative change in the liver (hepatic lipidosis), which can lead to liver failure. This is particularly common in tortoises.

Carbohydrates

Carbohydrates are primarily used for rapid energy production. This is particularly important in herbivores which consume plant matter only, and so gain the majority of their energy source from carbohydrates and proteins. Carnivorous reptiles do not utilise carbohydrates much at all.

Fibre

Dietary fibre is extremely important for herbivorous reptiles. Indeed, the presence of fibre acts both as a bulking agent, encouraging gut motility, and as a source for fermentation by the intestinal microflora, essential for fatty acid and B vitamin production. Snakes and other carnivores do not have a dietary fibre requirement, and indeed if provided fibre will not be utilised. Ultimately it will dilute the energy concentration of the diet, necessitating feeding more frequent and larger meals.

Vitamins

These compounds are grouped together although they are widely differing in nature, but all animals have a requirement for various numbers of these. They are categorised into fat-soluble (vitamin A, D, E and K) and water-soluble (the B vitamin complex and vitamin C).

Fat-soluble vitamins

Vitamin A: In herbivore reptiles, beta-carotene is the most important plant precursor in terms of how much vitamin A can be produced from it. Carnivorous reptiles and amphibians will gain the preformed vitamin A in their prey food.

Hypovitaminosis A is a frequently seen problem in chelonians, particularly in tortoises and young red-eared terrapins. If a deficiency in vitamin A occurs, then mucous membranes become thickened and oral and respiratory secretions dry up. This is due to blockage of salivary and mucous glands with cellular debris – a condition known as squamous metaplasia. This leads to poor functioning of the ciliary mechanisms which have a role in removing foreign particles from the airways. Swelling of the periorbital membranes – a condition known as xerophthalmia – is also seen.

Vitamin A's role in immune system function means that a deficiency makes respiratory and digestive tract infections more common. The most frequently seen example of this is the increased susceptibility to pneumonias seen in red-eared terrapins and manifested in the lopsided position they adopt when swimming. This is because of lung collapse or congestion which reduces buoyancy on the affected side.

Tortoises may suffer more frequently from upper respiratory tract infections when a deficiency is present. Evidence of sterile pustules and cornified plaques inside the mouth are commonly seen, with overgrowth of the beak due to hyperkeratosis.

Vitamin A also has a role in bone growth and structure, the normal function of secretory glands such as the adrenals and also in reproductive function. Finally renal damage may occur in hypovitaminosis A, with evidence of oedema in the inguinal and axillary regions secondary to failure of the renal tubular filtration system.

Because it is fat soluble, vitamin A can be stored in the body, primarily in the liver. Recommended minimum dietary levels are 200–300 IU/kg for reptiles (Wallach & Hoff, 1982).

Hypervitaminosis A rarely occurs naturally but may be induced by overdosing with vitamin A injections at 1000 times or more the daily recommended doses. If this occurs, acute toxicity develops with mucous membrane and skin sloughing and frequently death within 24–48 hours. Vitamin A supplements are therefore often given orally as, due to slower absorption, this reduces the risk of this condition developing.

Vitamin D: Vitamin D_3 is the most active form for calcium homeostasis, and plants are not effective as suppliers of this compound.

Cholecalciferol, the precursor of vitamin D_3, is manufactured in the reptile or amphibian's skin in a process enhanced by ultraviolet light. For this reason, indoor animals produce much less of this compound unless supplied with an effective artificial ultraviolet light source.

Hypovitaminosis D_3 causes problems with calcium metabolism, and leads to rickets. This is exacerbated by low calcium, high phosphorus-containing diets. A typical sufferer would be a young growing reptile, kept indoors with no ultraviolet light supplementation and fed on a low-calcium diet – e.g. lettuce/celery/cucumber for herbivores, or meat only a day old mice/chicks for carnivorous species. The condition so produced is referred to as 'metabolic bone disease'.

An animal so affected is frequently apparently 'well-muscled', due to poorly mineralised bones which increase their thickness to maintain their strength. There is often flaring of the epiphyseal plates at the ends of the long bones, with concomitant bowing of the limbs. Green iguanas and other herbivorous species such as terrestrial chelonians are particularly susceptible, with the lizards showing rachitic rosettes (Frye, 1991) due to flaring of the epiphysis in the ribs at the costochondral junction.

Chelonia develop 'lumpy shell', a deformity of the carapace in particular, where the edges roll upwards creating a 'Cornish pasty' effect, and the muscles which attach the limbs to the inside of the shell, pull the carapace downwards creating pits either side cranially and caudally (Figure 20.3). Recommended maximum levels are 50–100 IU/kg every other day.

Hypervitaminosis D_3 occurs due to over supplementation with D_3 and calcium and leads to calcification of soft tissues, such as the medial wall of the arteries, and the kidneys, creating hypertension and organ failure. This often occurs in herbivores such as tortoises fed on tinned cat and dog food.

Vitamin E: Hypovitaminosis E may occur due to a reduction in fat metabolism or absorption, such as can occur in small intestinal, pancreatic or biliary diseases, or due to a lack of dietary green plant material for herbivores. A relative deficiency will occur in species eating large amounts of polyunsaturated fats, e.g. marine fish such as tuna and mackerel. These use up the body's vitamin E reserves. A condition called steatitis, wherein body fat starts to necrose, has been seen in gharials (a fish-eating crocodilian) (Frye, 1991) and terrapins.

Hypervitaminosis E is extremely rare.

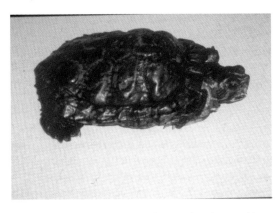

Figure 20.3 Red-eared terrapin, *Trachemys scripta elegans*, with hypovitaminosis D_3. (Reproduced with permission from Girling & Raiti, 2004, © BSAVA)

Vitamin K: Because of its production by gut bacteria, it is very difficult to get a true deficiency, although absorption will be reduced when fat digestion or absorption is reduced, as in biliary or pancreatic disease. The consumption of warfarin- and coumarin-derived compounds (as found in sweet clovers) can increase the demand for clotting factors, and this may also be seen in snakes consuming prey which has been killed by these rodenticides. Disease so caused is characterised by increased internal and external haemorrhage, but vitamin K also has some function in calcium/phosphorous metabolism in bone so this may also be affected. Frye (1991) has recorded disease in crocodiles exhibiting gingival bleeding without petechiation. Recommended minimum levels for reptiles are 1 ppm (Wallach & Hoff, 1982).

Water-soluble vitamins

Vitamin B_1 (thiamine): A source of thiaminases, enzymes which destroy thiamine, is raw saltwater fish which may be fed to some snakes, crocodilians and turtles, such as garter snakes, red-eared terrapins and gharials. There are thiamine antagonists as well in blackberries, beetroot, coffee, chocolate and tea when considering herbivores. When a relative deficiency occurs, neurological signs such as opisthotonus, weakness and head tremors may be seen. In garter and water snakes, a classical inability to right itself occurs, with the snake continually flipping onto its back. In addition, fungal infections are reported as more likely after a B_1 deficiency. The recommended minimum level for reptiles is 20–35 mg/kg food offered. In addition, if sea-fish such as smelt, which are high in thiaminases, are to be fed, cooking the fish for 5 minutes at 80°C deactivates the thiaminase. In a reptile with thiamine deficiency, doses of 50–100 mg/kg body weight should be given. Because of this problem it is often advised that garter and water snakes be fed on rodent prey rather than sea-fish. They may be encouraged to eat this by wiping the rodent prey with the fish to which it is accustomed to cover the scent.

Biotin: Deficiencies do occur commonly in Gila monsters, beaded lizards and monitor lizards, all of which enjoy raw eggs in the wild. In this state the majority of eggs are fertile, and contain little avidin (an antibiotin vitamin). However, unfertilised hen's eggs are high in avidin so a relative biotin deficiency may occur. Deficiencies produce muscular weakness, occasionally with skin lesions. It is therefore recommended that minimal levels of raw eggs are fed to such reptiles.

Folic acid: A deficiency of folic acid is rare but can lead to severely impaired cellular division. This can lead to a number of obvious problems, such as females' reproductive tracts not maturing, macrocytic anaemia due to failure of red blood cell maturation and immune system cellular dysfunction. A relative deficiency of folic acid may occur in some individuals fed a very high protein diet, as folic acid is needed to produce the waste products of protein metabolism in reptiles, uric acid. In addition, there are inhibitors of folic acid in some foods such as cabbage and other brassicas, oranges, beans and peas. The use of trimethoprim sulphonamide drugs also reduces gut bacterial folic acid production.

Vitamin B_{12}: Vitamin B_{12} is produced generally by intestinal bacteria and so deficiencies are uncommon but may occur after prolonged antibiotic medication. Deficiency produces slow growth, muscular dystrophy in the legs, poor hatching rates, high mortality rates and hatching deformities in young reptiles and amphibians.

Choline: Choline may be synthesised in the body, but not in enough quantities for the growing reptile. Because of interactions, the need for choline is dependent on levels of folic acid and vitamin B_{12}. Excess protein, therefore, as with folic acid, increases choline requirements, as does a diet high in fats. Deficiency causes retarded growth, disrupted fat metabolism and fatty liver damage.

Vitamin C: There is no direct need for this vitamin in reptiles and amphibians as vitamin C may be produced from glucose in the outermost portions of the kidneys. However, during disease processes, particularly those which affect liver function, it may be beneficial to the recovery process to provide a dietary source of vitamin C. It is required for the formation of elastic fibres and connective tissues and is an excellent anti-oxidant similar to vitamin E. Deficiency leads to 'scurvy' where there is poor wound healing, increased bleeding due to capillary wall fragility and bone alterations. Deficiency has been postulated as the cause of skin splitting in snakes fed rodent prey that had been starved for 24–48 hours before being fed (Frye, 1991). This allowed the emptying of their gastrointestinal tract, and hence reduced levels of vitamin C from the plant material therein. It has also been suggested that increasing vitamin C levels by supplementation at levels of 10–20 mg/kg intramuscularly or orally (Frye, 1991) may be useful in the treatment of chronic infections, such as 'mouth rot' in snakes.

Minerals

As with mammals there are two main groups of minerals, those classified as macro-minerals, i.e. those present in large amounts in the body, such as calcium and phosphorus, and micro-minerals, or trace elements, such as manganese, iron and cobalt, which are all necessary for normal bodily function.

Macro-minerals

Calcium: Calcium has a wide range of bodily functions, the two most obvious being its role in the formation of the skeleton and mineralisation of bone matrix, and its requirement for muscular contractions. The active form of calcium in the body is the ionic double charged molecule Ca^{2+}. Low levels of this form, even though the overall body reserves of calcium are normal, leads to hyperexcitability, fitting and death, conditions seen in gravid female egg-bound green iguanas.

The ratio of calcium to phosphorus is important – as one increases, the other decreases and vice versa. This is controlled by the hormones calcitonin, parathyroid hormone and the accessory hormone vitamin D_3. A ratio of 2:1 calcium to phosphorus is desirable in growing reptiles and 1.5:1 for adults. In high egg laying periods though, to keep pace with the output of calcium into the shells, a ratio of 10:1 may be needed.

Calcium deficiency causes nutritional osteodystrophy, or metabolic bone disease, and is often accompanied by deficiency in vitamin D_3. Normal levels of vitamin D_3, however, may exacerbate this disease as they encourage further calcium resorption. Deficiency may be seen in lizards such as green iguanas and water dragons, and chelonians fed on diets high in fruit, lettuce, celery, etc.. Diets with excessive levels of oxalates, compounds which bind up calcium and prevent it being absorbed, such as spinach and beetroot or rhubarb leaves, can also lead to a deficiency.

Calcium deficiency may also be seen in insectivorous species, such as geckos, and bearded dragons, fed on insects without supplementation (Figure 20.4). Insects have little or no calcium, their tough outer coat is made of a protein known as chitin. To provide adequate calcium therefore, the insect must be dusted with a calcium powder immediately before being fed (if not, by the time the reptile has caught the insect most of the powder has fallen off!). Alternatively, the insect is pre-fed on a calcium supplement. This is mixed in with the insect's food and fed for the 24–48 hours before feeding the reptile, so that the insect's gut is pre-loaded with calcium.

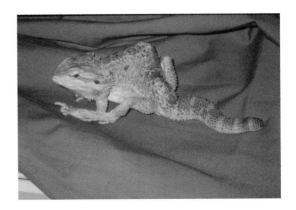

Figure 20.4 Bearded dragon, *Pogona vitticeps,* with metabolic bone disease and resultant spinal and limb deformity.

Extensive resorption of calcium occurs from the bones during dietary deficiencies, leaving only fibrous tissue. This is considerably weaker and so the 'bones' thicken to maintain their strength. Even so, the bones are weakened, and bowing of long bones and spontaneous fractures occur in lizards, collapsing of spinal vertebrae and deformities in most reptiles and deformed, lumpy shells in chelonians. Excessive calcium in the diet (>1%) though, reduces the use of proteins, fats, phosphorus, manganese, zinc, iron and iodine, and can lead to soft tissue mineralisation if in conjunction with adequate or excessive vitamin D_3 levels. Red-eared terrapins have been shown to have a requirement for 2% calcium on a dry matter basis (Kass *et al.,* 1982).

Phosphorus: Phosphorus is widespread in plant and animal tissues, but in the former it may be bound up in unavailable form as phytates. Levels of phosphorus are controlled in the body as for calcium, the two being in equal and opposite equilibrium with each other. Therefore, if dietary phosphorus levels exceed calcium levels appreciably, the parathyroid glands become stimulated to produce more parathyroid hormone and nutritional secondary hyperparathyroidism occurs. This leads to progressive bone demineralisation and renal damage due to high circulating levels of parathyroid hormone. High dietary phosphorus also reduces the amount of calcium which can be absorbed from the gut, as it complexes with the calcium present there. This can be a problem in reptiles fed pure meat with no calcium or bone supplement, and in herbivores which are predominantly fruit and lettuce consumers, as these are high phosphorus low calcium foods. Green vegetables or supplementation with calcium powders may therefore be necessary. In addition, low calcium/high phosphorus levels frequently allow bladder stones to form in those species (such as chelonians, green iguanas) that have a bladder.

Magnesium: Most magnesium is absorbed from the small intestine, and is affected by large amounts of calcium in the diet which reduce magnesium absorption. Deficiencies rarely occur, but muscular weakness can be the result.

Potassium: As with mammals, potassium is the major intracellular positive ion. Rarely is there a dietary deficiency, but severe stress can cause hypokalaemia through increased kidney excretion because of elevated plasma proteins. This can lead to cardiac dysrhythmias, muscle spasticity and neurological dysfunction.

Sodium: Sodium is the main extracellular positive ion and regulates the body's acid–base balance and osmotic potential. In conjunction with potassium, it is responsible for nerve signals and impulses. Rarely does a true dietary deficiency occur, but hyponatraemia may occur due to chronic diarrhoea or renal disease. Many reptiles have salt glands found outside the kidneys, responsible solely for the excretion of excess sodium whilst conserving water. The green iguana's salt glands, e.g. are present inside the nostrils, and white crystalline deposits of salt may be seen here and are frequently sneezed out. It may be necessary to supplement the diet of marine species with sodium chloride if kept in fresh water situations, or if fed freshwater plants or fish.

Chlorine: This is the major extracellular negative ion and is responsible for maintaining acid–base balances in conjunction with sodium and potassium. Deficiencies are rare.

Micro-minerals (trace elements)

These elements include zinc, copper, iron, manganese, cobalt and sulphur, all of which have an important part to play in cellular function. However, so far no actual deficiencies specifically related to these elements have been reported in reptiles or amphibians. The exception is iodine.

Iodine: Iodine's sole function is in thyroid hormone synthesis, which affects metabolic rate. Deficiency causes goitre and fluid retention (myxoedema). It has knock-on effects on growth, causing stunting and neurological problems and in amphibians may prevent metamorphosis from intermediate tadpole stages to the adult form. In reptiles it is most often encountered in giant terrestrial tortoises, which will exhibit goitre swelling of the neck. It can also occur due to overfeeding with iodine-binding plants, such as cabbage, cauliflower, broccoli, kale and Brussels sprouts. Excess iodine added to the water may cause species such as the amphibian axolotl (a neotenic salamander – i.e. its 'adult' form has the external gills more typical of a tadpole or intermediate life stage) to shed its external gills. Levels of 0.3 mg/kg body weight have been quoted (Donoghue & Langenburg, 1996).

Specific nutritional problems in reptiles

Below are some common presentations of nutritional problems in reptiles.

Post-hibernation anorexia

PHA (post-hibernation anorexia) occurs in the Mediterranean species of tortoise (Hermann's, Greek or spur-thighed, marginated and Horsfield's), which hibernate during the winter months. The commonest presentation is that of an inappetant tortoise after coming out of hibernation, often with signs of systemic or respiratory tract infections (such as the 'runny nose syndrome') and often with a low body weight in relation to length (a low Jackson's ratio). In addition the blood glucose levels are frequently below 3.2 mmol/L, which appears to be the minimum level required for appetite stimulation (Lawrence, 1987), with high levels of urea. More severe cases often have evidence of renal disease with elevated uric acid levels and potassium. Many have become ketoacidotic with the production of ketones such as beta hydroxybutyrate.

Dehydration is apparent in these cases, and treatment requires aggressive fluid therapy and nutritional support, using glucose-containing fluids and liquid food stomach tubing, as well as warming the tortoise to its optimum temperature (20–27°C) (Figure 20.5).

Causes of this condition could involve any one of the following:

- Disease during or prior to hibernation
- Poor nutrition leading to poor fat reserves prior to hibernation
- Owner failure to observe recovery from hibernation for several days, so no food offered at the critical time, or
- A period of cold weather immediately after recovery.

It is the rising plane of blood glucose post hibernation that acts as the stimulus for appetite in these chelonians, and failure of this rise, due to malnutrition or failure to eat whilst the levels are still high, may lead to unresponsive anorexia.

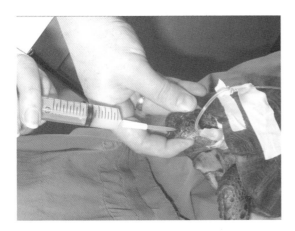

Figure 20.5 Spur-thighed tortoise, *Testudo graeca*, with post-hibernation anorexia being stomach tubed with Vetark's critical care formula. Note also the intravenous drip into the jugular vein.

To prevent PHA, therefore, it is important to attend disease prior to hibernation, and, if severely affected or underweight, the tortoise should not be hibernated, but kept indoors at its optimum temperature range and fed throughout the winter. The tortoise should also be checked regularly once in hibernation, around once or twice a week, to ensure if the tortoise does come out of hibernation early, it has food and water available immediately. Bathing the tortoise immediately after waking in warm water, cleaning the nose, eyes and mouth especially can also stimulate appetite, and no tortoise having recovered from hibernation should be allowed to re-hibernate that same winter. Finally, stomach tubing with fluids and soluble carbohydrates, such as the basic sugar and protein containing liquid food Critical Care Formula produced by Vetark Professional Ltd., or vegetable baby food porridges, early on in the course of the problem can be useful.

Visceral and articular gout
Gout is a condition caused by the unique way that many reptiles deal with the waste products of protein metabolism. Most reptiles are uricotelic, i.e. the main excretory product of protein metabolism is uric acid. This compound is relatively insoluble in water, which has its advantages as reptiles are therefore able to reduce the water lost in excreting it. Unfortunately, if the reptile becomes dehydrated, either acutely or chronically, or consumes diets with excessive protein levels, particularly a type of protein called purines, or suffers kidney damage, then uric acid levels build up in the bloodstream. If allowed to

do so, they will eventually exceed the precipitation point and form crystals inside the body.

Diet is important, as purine proteins, which are found mainly in animal protein, are converted readily to uric acid on degradation in the body. Therefore, if herbivorous species, such as green iguanas, which are not used to large volumes of purines, are fed a diet rich in animal protein, such as cat or dog food, they will produce excessive amounts of uric acid and develop gout.

There are two forms of gout, visceral and articular. Articular gout can easily be diagnosed ante-mortem, as it causes gross swelling and inflammation in the joints where the uric acid crystals form. Visceral gout is more difficult to diagnose ante-mortem, because it occurs where uric acid crystals are deposited in the soft tissues of the body, primary sites being the kidneys, the pericardial sac, the lungs, spleen and liver. Once deposited, it is almost impossible to move the crystals medically and permanent damage is often done.

Obesity
Obesity is a common problem in many reptiles and amphibians kept in captivity. Many species are overfed because of owners' ignorance of natural feeding intervals and of food types commonly eaten in the wild. Examples include feeding dog food to tortoises and green iguanas, both of which are totally herbivorous in the wild but both of which will eat meat if offered it. The resulting problems are as mentioned above, with excess protein causing gout, excess calcium and vitamin D_3 causing soft tissue mineralisation and excess animal fat causing fatty liver syndrome (hepatic lipidosis) wherein the liver cells are filled with fat deposits impeding their function. Snakes also suffer from these conditions when fed overly fatty laboratory rodents, or simply fed too often. A rough idea of feeding frequencies is given in Table 20.1.

The aim should be a reptile which does not appear emaciated, but lean.

Hypoglycaemia in crocodilians
It has been reported that crocodiles kept in high density conditions, or are otherwise stressed, are prone to hypoglycaemic fits (Scott, 1992). It is interesting to note that crocodiles' blood sugar levels vary throughout the year, being lowest in the winter and highest in the summer. A rising blood sugar level appears to be the stimulus to eat, as seems to be seen with Mediterranean tortoises after hibernation.

Table 20.1 Feeding frequencies and food types for various reptile species.

Species	Feeding frequencies and food types
Herbivores (e.g. iguanas, tortoises)	Daily grazing of food advised
Small insectivores (e.g. leopard geckos, collared lizards)	Fed 2–3 times weekly on live insect prey, supplemented with mineral/vitamins
Small carnivores (e.g. garter snakes, corn snakes)	Fed 2–3 times weekly on rat pups, fuzzies (furred baby mice) or pinkies (nude baby mice) up to adult mice according to size. Try not to feed anything more than 50% the maximum width of the snake
Medium carnivores (e.g. kingsnakes, rat snakes)	Fed 1–2 times weekly, adult mice or small rats according to size. Try not to feed anything more than 50% the maximum width of the snake
Large carnivores (e.g. boa constrictors, Burmese pythons)	Fed once weekly or fortnightly (the larger the snake the less often) on adult rats or small rabbits. Try not to feed anything more than 50% the maximum width of the snake

Environmental temperature and its effects on nutrition

Because reptiles and amphibians are ectothermic, i.e. they rely on their surroundings to maintain their body temperature, environmental temperature is important in all aspects of husbandry.

There is an optimum preferred temperature zone that will allow their enzymes and metabolic pathways to function at their optimum levels, so environmental temperature will influence the rate of digestion of the food offered. It may take 2–3 days for a rat consumed by a large boa constrictor to pass through its digestive system if kept within its preferred temperature zone of 25–30°C, but if kept 5–10°C cooler this will often slow down to 5–7 days, and if kept much lower than this, digestion may not occur before the prey item becomes rancid inside the snake. Similarly, if kept at too high a temperature, the reptile may not be stimulated to eat at all and dehydration and heat stress may set in.

A general guide to feeding reptiles

Fresh food should always be fed to reptiles. It should also be remembered that at the increased temperatures of most vivaria, the food offered will spoil very quickly and will need to be replaced frequently.

Snakes

It is important to note that it is illegal to feed live vertebrate prey to another animal in the United Kingdom. All rodent prey fed to snakes and lizards must therefore have been humanely killed first. In addition, live prey may damage the reptile if the latter is not hungry and does not kill the prey quickly.

To encourage anorectic snakes to eat, a number of tricks may be employed including:

- Warming the prey briefly before offering by heating it in a pot of hot water
- Breaking the prey item open to release the scent of blood
- Teasing the snake by moving the dead prey item around the cage with forceps, to mimic live prey
- Trying a variety of colours of prey – some snakes will only take dark-furred rodents
- To get a snake (such as a garter or water snake) used to eating rodent prey after only eating fish or amphibians (hog-nosed snakes), wipe the rodent to be offered with the previously taken food item to transfer scent
- Ensure that there are plenty of areas to hide; some boids and pythons like to consume their prey in a box or hide
- Leave the prey in overnight because some species prefer to hunt at night
- Choose the next smallest size of rodent, so if adult mice were previously offered try fuzzies; if juvenile rats, try adult mice, etc.

NB: The term 'pinkies' refers to nude neonatal rat and mice pups, 'fuzzies' refers to week-old rat and mice pups with a thin covering of fur, and 'furries' refers to juvenile rat and mice pups between 1 and 3 weeks of age which have a soft but longer covering of fur.

Refeeding syndrome

If anorexia in a snake or other reptile has persisted for some time it is essential to rehydrate the patient before attempting to feed. Indeed, initial feeding after this should be started off at very low levels. This is because excess calories and proteins cause a rapid uptake of glucose from the bloodstream into the cells, which takes potassium and phosphorous with it. After a prolonged period of anorexia, the whole body levels of potassium and phosphorus can be reduced and therefore this can lead to a life-threatening hypokalaemia and hypophosphataemia in the bloodstream which results in cardiac arrhythmias. The monitoring of blood phosphorus and potassium is therefore to be recommended when treating chronically anorectic reptiles, whether carnivores or herbivores.

Herbivores

If using a commercial pelleted food for iguanas or tortoises, then be sure to soak the pellets thoroughly before feeding, otherwise they swell up inside the reptile causing colic and bloat. Commercial pelleted diets are a useful adjunct to the diet of herbivorous reptiles and many companies now produce iguanid and chelonian diets which are well supplemented with minerals and vitamins and also contain moderate levels of fibre for gut motility enhancement. Any pelleted food should be thoroughly soaked in water before feeding; otherwise, they can dramatically swell inside the reptile. This also increases water intake which is important in many species.

The feeding of certain foods to herbivores should be prohibited. Animal proteins are one, as are certain fruit and vegetables. We have already discussed the problems of excessive volumes of largely water-containing vegetables such as lettuce, cucumber and celery, the goitrogenic properties of cabbage, kale, broccoli and cauliflower and the anti-calcium effect of oxalate-containing plants such as spinach, beetroot and rhubarb leaves. In addition, fruits such as banana can cause a sugar ferment in herbivorous reptiles causing colic, as well as adhering to the mouthparts and encouraging local infection. Avocados have an extremely high fat content and should not be fed to herbivorous reptiles due to potential secondary fatty degeneration of the liver.

Sample diet for green iguanas

Pelleted soaked commercial food may be fed at around 25% of daily intake. The rest can be based on the following: Up to half of the plant material offered can be made of calcium-rich vegetables such as kale, dandelions, chicory, watercress, cabbage, flat-leaved parsley, basil, and coriander. The other half may be made up of other vegetable matters such as peas, beans, carrots, sweet peppers, courgettes or marrows, cauliflower and florets and flowers of plants such as nasturtiums, dandelions and roses. To this mixture can be added small amounts of fruits such as apples, pears, tomatoes, plums, strawberries, raspberries, melon, passion fruit and papaya or fibrous foods such as bran cereals, brown bread and cooked brown rice.

This combination should be thoroughly mixed so as to prevent selective feeding, and to it should be added a supplement of calcium in the form of calcium lactate or gluconate, or a natural calcium source such as cuttlefish or oyster shells. In addition, the use of a vitamin D_3/calcium supplement once or twice a week, particularly for growing iguanas and egg-laying females, is advised.

Sample diet for Mediterranean tortoises

The majority of the diet is to be composed of vegetable matter of a leafy nature such as dandelions, kale, watercress, flat-leaved parsley, chicory and bok-choy. To this may be added peas, beans, hay or dried grass, fresh grass (not cut), grated carrot, grated pumpkin and sweet peppers.

To this may be added small volumes of fruit such as apples, pears, melon, papaya, passion fruit, strawberries and plums; flowers such as dandelions, nasturtiums and roses; and sprouted seeds such as mung beans, lentils and chick peas.

For more tropical species, such as the red and yellow footed tortoises (*Chelonoidis carbonaria* and *Chelonoidis denticulata*), the amount of fruit and flowers may be doubled.

For grassland species, such as leopard tortoises (*Stigmochelys pardalis*), African spurred tortoises (*Geochelone sulcata*) and Indian starred tortoises (*Geochelone elegans*), a good provision of fresh uncut grass or good quality hay is advised.

For more omnivorous species, such as box turtles (e.g. *Terrapene carolina* spp.), up to 50% of the above fruit and vegetable diet may be replaced with adult maintenance dry dog foods (soaked), mealworms, crickets, earthworms and even baby mice (pinkies). Juveniles of this species tend to be more carnivorous than the adults.

In all of these diets it is recommended that daily supplementation with calcium lactate or gluconate be included, with a calcium/vitamin D_3 supplement added once or twice weekly depending whether the tortoise is a juvenile (higher requirement) or an adult (lower requirement).

Diets for snakes and insectivorous species have been mentioned. The latter need calcium supplementation as discussed in the section considering calcium as a macromineral which may either be dusted onto the insects, or pre-fed to them to load their digestive contents with the calcium.

References

Donoghue, S. (1998) Nutrition of pet amphibians and reptiles. *Seminars in Avian and Exotic Pet Medicine*, 7, 3.

Donoghue, S. and Langenburg, J. (1996) Nutrition. *Reptile Medicine and Surgery* (ed. D. Mader), pp. 148–174. W.B. Saunders, Philadelphia, PA.

Frye, F. (1991) A practical guide for feeding captive reptiles. *Biomedical and Surgical Aspects of Captive Reptile Husbandry*, Vol 1. Krieger Publishing, Malabar, FL.

Kass, R.E., Ullrey, D.E. and Trapp, A.L. (1982) A study of calcium requirements of the Red-eared slider turtle (*Pseudemys scripta elegans*). *Journal of Zoo Animal Medicine*, **13**, 62.

Lawrence, K. (1987) Post hibernational anorexia in captive Mediterranean tortoises (*Testudo graeca* and *T. hermanii*). *Veterinary Record*, **120**, 87.

Scott, P.W. (1992) Nutritional diseases. *Manual of Reptiles* (eds P.H. Beynon, M.P.C. Lawton & J.E. Cooper), pp. 138–152. BSAVA, Cheltenham, UK.

Wallach, J.D. and Hoff, G.L. (1982) Metabolic and nutritional diseases of reptiles. *Non-infectious Diseases of Wildlife* (eds G.L. Hoff & J.W. Davis), pp. 155–168. Iowa State Press, Ames, IA.

Further reading

Barten, S.L. (1996) Lizards. *Reptile Medicine and Surgery* (ed. D. Mader), pp. 47–60. W.B. Saunders, Philadelphia, PA.

Boyer, J.H. (1996) Turtles, tortoises and terrapins. *Reptile Medicine and Surgery* (ed. D. Mader), pp. 61–77. W.B. Saunders, Philadelphia, PA.

Calvert, I. (2004) Nutrition. *Manual of Reptiles* (eds S. Girling & P. Raiti), 2nd edn, pp. 18–39. BSAVA, Quedgeley, UK.

Calvert, I. (2004) Nutritional problems. *Manual of Reptiles* (eds S. Girling & P. Raiti), 2nd edn, pp. 289–308. BSAVA, Quedgeley, UK.

Donoghue, S. (2006) Nutrition. *Reptile Medicine and Surgery* (ed. D. Mader), 2nd edn, pp. 251–298. Saunders Elsevier, St Louis, MO.

Girling, S. and Raiti (eds) (2004) *BSAVA Manual of Reptiles*, 2nd edn. Blackwell Publishing, Oxford.

McArthur, S. and Barrows, M. (2004) Nutrition. *Medicine and Surgery of Tortoises and Turtles* (eds A. McArthur, R. Wilkinson, J. Meyer, C. Innis & S. Hernandez-Divers), pp. 73–86. Blackwell Publishing, Oxford.

Zimmerman, E. (1995) *Reptiles and Amphibians: Care, Behaviour and Reproduction*. TFM Publishing, Neptune City, NJ.

Chapter 21　Common Reptile and Amphibian Diseases

Skin disease

Ecdysis

The process of ecdysis involves the forming of a new skin beneath the old one. Once this is complete, a series of proteolytic enzymes and lymphatic fluid is secreted between the new skin layer and the overlying old one. This lifts and separates the two, and makes the snake appear dull and lacklustre with the eyes noticeably bluing (Figure 21.1). This lasts for 5–7 days on average in the snake. Once complete, the fluid is reabsorbed, and the snake appears to return to its normal hue. After a further 5–7 days the skin is shed, in the case of the snake, in one whole go from the head end first. It is initiated in snakes by rubbing the face on an abrasive surface to loosen the first piece of skin (see Figure 21.2). The regularity at which the process of ecdysis occurs depends on a number of factors including:

1. Age of the reptile (younger animals shed more frequently as they are growing faster)
2. Nutritional status (high-protein and high-calorie diets increase the frequency of ecdysis)
3. Seasonal influences such as daylight length, humidity, temperature, etc. may all have an effect depending on the species involved.

When the separation fails to occur, whether in part or totally, the condition is known as dysecdysis.

Dysecdysis

Dysecdysis is when ecdysis fails. It occurs in snakes, and to a lesser extent, lizards.

The causes of dysecdysis are many and varied, but can include any condition which can cause dehydration so reducing lymphatic fluid available to separate the skin layers. If the reptile is malnourished, dysecdysis may occur due to a lack of proteolytic enzymes. Alternatively old scars, a lack of an abrasive surface in the vivarium upon which to start the process or severe ectoparasitism may also cause dysecdysis.

Scale rot

Scale rot is a colloquial term for a range of conditions affecting the reptile skin which result in severe infections.

Septicaemic cutaneous ulcerative disease

Septicaemic cutaneous ulcerative disease (SCUD) is seen in aquatic chelonians. *Citrobacter freundii* has been implicated which, once it has gained access to the bloodstream, produces ulcers in the skin and loosening of scales with debilitation and, in many cases, death. Other bacteria such as *Pseudomonas* and *Aeromonas* are also involved (Figure 21.3).

Blister disease

This is a form of scale rot seen in semi-aquatic species such as garter or water snakes. It can, however, occur in any species which is exposed to a persistently damp substrate. The outer layer of skin develops blisters of a clear fluid which become secondarily infected with environmental bacteria such as *Aeromonas* spp., *Serratia* spp., or *Pseudomonas* spp. These can progress to septicaemia. Occasionally these conditions may involve a fungus such as *Aspergillus* spp.

Abscesses

Reptile abscesses have recently been quoted as being more accurately termed fibriscesses (Huchzermeyer & Cooper, 2001). Instead of liquid pus, reptiles and birds form solid, caseous, dried pus surrounded by a thick shell of fibrous tissue. This is due to the lack of lysozymes and the secretion of huge amounts of fibrin into the abscess (Figure 21.4). These may form anywhere, but a common site in chelonians is the middle ear, causing a bulging of the ear drum (Figure 21.5). The pathogens involved are frequently Gram-negative species, although the presence of fungi has been well recorded.

Veterinary Nursing of Exotic Pets, Second Edition. Edited by Simon J. Girling. © 2013 John Wiley & Sons, Ltd. Published 2013 by John Wiley & Sons, Ltd.

PART III: REPTILES AND AMPHIBIANS

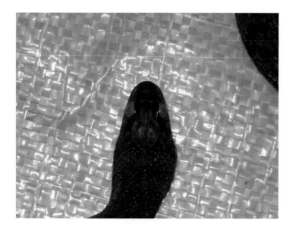

Figure 21.1 During the process of ecdysis in snakes, the eyes appear to go cloudy due to secretion of lymphatic fluid between the new and old spectacles.

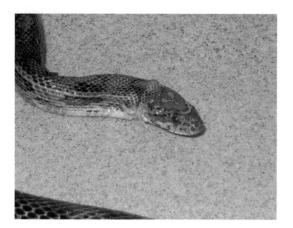

Figure 21.2 Ecdysis in a corn snake (*Pantherophis guttatus guttatus*).

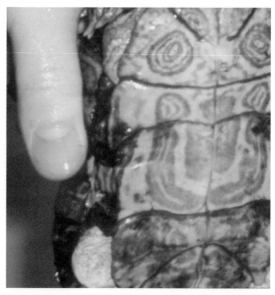

Figure 21.3 SCUD in a red-eared terrapin, *Trachemys scripta elegans*.

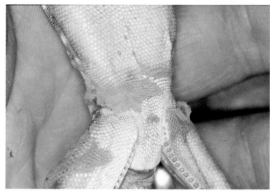

Figure 21.4 Dysecdysis in a green iguana (*Iguana iguana*).

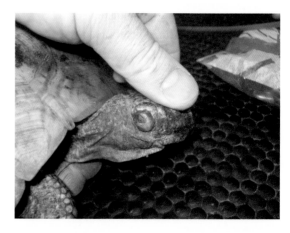

Figure 21.5 Aural abscess in a spur-thighed tortoise (*Testudo graeca*).

Erythema, petechiae and ecchymoses

These three conditions may all be present at the same time or may appear individually.

Erythema is the reddening of skin tissues due to vascular congestion beneath. It can be seen in reptiles as a pink hue to the areas between scutes in the case of chelonians (Figure 21.3) and crocodilians, or the more generalised reddening of the skin seen in snakes. Erythema is often suggestive of septicaemia.

Petechiae are pin-point subepithelial haemorrhages. They can be seen in the mouth, where they are often associated with oral infection such as 'mouth rot'. They may be seen over the body suggesting septicaemia. Other conditions producing petechiae include clotting deficiencies, for example, consumption of rodent prey which has itself consumed a warfarin-type poison.

Ecchymoses are larger areas of haemorrhage, and may be caused by severe local infection disseminated intravascular coagulation (DIC) or conditions mentioned above.

Overgrown beaks and claws

Overgrown beaks are common in chelonians, and are often due to a lack of abrasive foodstuffs or abrasive surfaces from which to eat them.

However, it should be noted that some species have perfectly normal apparently 'long' claws. An example is the male red-eared terrapin, which uses its claws as a display aid to attract and mate the female.

Pigment changes

An example of a physiologically normal colour change is seen in the Chamaeleonidae which will often darken in colour as they become stressed. Green iguanas often become yellow brown in colour as they become stressed or unwell, bearded dragons often become dark coloured and many of these species will exhibit darkening at the site of an injection. Areas of previous trauma may become whitened.

Ectoparasitic

Mites

The snake mite, *Ophionyssus natricis* appears as red to dark-coloured pin-head mites hiding under the overlapping edges of scales. They may be seen in water dishes in which the reptile has been bathing. They can cause severe irritation, pruritus and self-trauma, as well as causing anaemia and dysecdysis. In addition, they can transmit *Aeromonas* spp. bacteria, which may cause septicaemia and viruses, for example, inclusion body disease (IBD). Other mites include the cloacal mites of aquatic turtles of the family *Cloacarus* spp. In addition, there is of course the non-parasitic harvest mite or *Neotrombicula autumnalis*, which may be brought in on straw and hay bedding material. The adult itself is not an irritant but the six–legged larval stage is and may cause the reptile to traumatise itself.

Ticks

In the United Kingdom, *Ixodes ricinus* (the sheep or deer tick) and *Ixodes hexagonous* (the hedgehog tick) are seen. In tortoises, these are naturally the areas around the neck inlet and in front of the hind legs. They may cause local damage and can transmit pathogens. These include bacteria (*Staphylococcus aureus*, the cause of tick pyaemia and *Borrelia burgdorferi*, the cause of Lyme's disease) as well as haemoparasites and viruses. Some of the soft-bodied ticks (*Amblyomma marmoreum* and *A. sparsum*) have

been implicated in the transmission of *Cowdria ruminantium* the cause of heart water disease in mammals. These ticks are common on wild-caught imported reptiles.

Blowfly myiasis

Myiasis is a problem for any reptile kept in insanitary conditions or those with diarrhoea. Members of the blue bottle, black bottle and green bottle families are all capable of laying eggs on a tortoise. In peak conditions these can hatch into larvae or maggots within 1–2 hours. These then burrow away from the light, into the body of the tortoise causing severe trauma, infections, shock and ultimately death.

Leeches

Leeches tend not to be such a problem in the United Kingdom, but can affect aquatic species all over the world. The family Annelidae are the most dangerous, and cause large wounds which continue to bleed after the leech has detached. These may then become secondarily infected. They can also transmit haemoparasites, bacteria and viruses.

Traumatic and spontaneous damage

Traumatic damage can be due to attacks by predators or other reptiles, for example, males fighting over a female. In some species, for example, green iguanas, the male mounting the female during mating bites the shoulder area vigorously, causing open wounds. Dog attacks are common in tortoises (Figure 21.6). In the United Kingdom, it is unlawful to feed live vertebrate prey to any animal; but invertebrate live prey can be offered and these can still cause trauma to a sick or anorectic reptile. Unprotected heat sources frequently cause severe burns.

In some chelonians, scutes may be seen to lift off, often weeping clear fluid beneath them. This is frequently associated with underlying renal disease.

Iatrogenic causes of skin damage are also seen in some reptiles such as chelonians. This can occur after over-administration of vitamin A, which can cause sloughing of the epidermal layer on the head, neck and limbs, exposing the underlying dermis.

Tumours

Fibrosarcomas and squamous cell carcinomas of the head are seen in lizards and snakes. Melanomas are also seen in pigmented species such as the bearded dragon (*Pogona vitticeps*). Viral-induced fibropapillomas are frequently seen in green turtles (*Chelonia mydas*), where

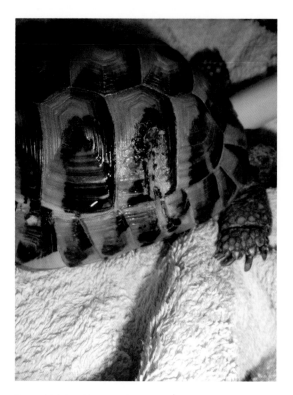

Figure 21.6 Dog bite wounds are common in juvenile tortoises.

herpesviruses have been implicated. Another herpesvirus is a common cause of 'grey-patch disease' in this species, where circumscribed papular grey lesions appear over the whole body. In addition, papillomata have been regularly reported in Lacertidae (sand, wall and emerald lizards), occurring over the dorsum of the individual lizard.

Bacteria associated with skin problems

Gram-negative bacteria can cause skin abscesses, septicaemia and areas of skin sloughing. Others such as *Mycobacteria* spp. may be seen associated with the appearance of classical tuberculous lesions. The mycobacteria found are more commonly environmental ones, for example, *Mycobacterium marinum* (Girling & Fraser, 2007) and *Mycobacterium chelonae*, rather than the human or cattle TB organisms.

Dermatophilus congolensis has been associated with skin disease in a number of lizards and snakes and *D. cheloniae* has been isolated from captive chelonians (Masters *et al.*, 1995).

Dermabacter spp. related bacteria have been associated with a proliferative cheilitis syndrome in Agamid lizards (Koplos *et al.*, 2000). This has also been seen to cause proliferative lesions around the cloaca and over the legs

(Pasmans *et al.*, 2010) and is now thought to be due to the bacterium *Devriesea agamarum*. Gram-negative bacterial infections of the hind feet of Savannah monitor lizards seems to be another common condition and is associated with an overly abrasive and damp substrate leading to foot abrasion and secondary infection (Stahl, 2003).

Fungal

The incidence of fungal infections in reptiles has been quoted between 0.4% (Austwick & Keymer, 1981) and 4% (Jacobson, 1980). These include: *Aspergillus* spp. (Austwick & Keymer, 1981; Tappe *et al.*, 1984; Girling, 2002; Girling & Fraser, 2009); *Mucor* spp. (Lappin & Dunstan, 1992; Heatley *et al.*, 2001); *Paecilomyces* spp. (Heard *et al.*, 1986; Schumacher, 2003; Diaz-Figueroa *et al.*, 2008); *Candida albicans* (Austwick & Keymer, 1981; Migaki *et al.*, 1984); *Fusarium* spp. and *Chrysosporium* spp. (Austwick & Keymer 1981; Schumacher 2003); *Sporothrix schenckii, Pestalotia pezizoides* and *Geotrichum candidum* (Cheatwood *et al.*, 2003); *Beauveria bassiana* (Gonzalez Cabo *et al.*, 1995); *Penicillium griseofulvum* (Oros *et al.*, 1996); *Alternaria* spp. (Rossi & Rossi, 2000); *Cryptococcus* spp. (Hough, 1998); *Scolecobasidium humicola* (Weitzman *et al.*, 1985) and the primary fungal pathogen the Chrysosporium anamorph of *Nannizziopsis vriesii* (CANV) in bearded dragons, brown tree snakes and chameleons (Pare *et al.*, 1997; Nichols *et al.*, 1999; Bowman *et al.*, 2007; Abarca *et al.*, 2009). CANV produces the so-called 'yellow skin disease' of bearded dragons and may be fatal to a wide range of reptiles (Figure 21.7).

Many of these fungal infections appear to enter the reptilian body via the skin (Austwick & Keymer, 1981). With increasing use of antibiotic therapy in pet reptiles and the discovery of new fungal species associated with disease (e.g., CANV), the incidence of fungal disease appears to be on the increase (Fraser & Girling, 2004).

Viral

There are more and more cases of viral associated disease being diagnosed in reptiles each day. Herpesviruses causing grey patch disease have been found in turtles, papilloma viruses in lizards, and pox viruses in caimans (a member of the family Crocodylia).

Hereditary

Many species exhibit scale and skin abnormalities. These vary from cleft palates, to failure of scales to develop at all. In addition, many colour variations have been specifically bred for.

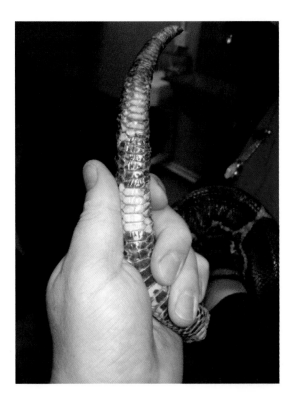

Figure 21.7 CANV fungal infection in a *Boa constrictor* is frequently fatal.

Hyperthyroidism

This has been diagnosed in green iguanas and corn snakes, although it is rare. It is associated with an increased turnover of skin and so an increase in ecdysis. It may also be associated with loss of dorsal spines in iguanas, tachycardia, increased aggression, polyphagia and weight loss overall (Hernandez-Divers *et al.*, 2001). Normal thyroid reference ranges are difficult to find, but 0.21–6.78 nmol/L have been reported for *Calotes* and *Sceloporus* lizards.

Hypothyroidism

This has been reported in giant chelonia (Frye, 1991). It may also be due to the presence of goitrogens in the diet such as brassicas. Myxoedema and heart failure are the most commonly seen clinical signs.

Thermal burns

Reptiles can sense pain but do not appear to respond to thermal pain in the way that birds and mammals do; that is, they do not remove themselves from the heat source even when it is resulting in severe burns. Unprotected heat lamps which allow reptiles close contact are dangerous, as

are so-called 'hot-rocks' when the thermostat breaks. Full skin thickness burns and even death of the reptile are not uncommon (Figure 21.8).

Hypovitaminosis A

This is mainly seen in aquatic chelonians and chameleons. The presenting signs include ocular oedema, xerophthalmia, middle ear abscessation, hyperkeratosis, lethargy and anorexia. It is preferable that vitamin A supplements should be given orally to minimise toxicity. Values of 200 IU/30 g bodyweight have been quoted dosed twice, 7 days apart (Harkewicz, 2001).

Hypervitaminosis A

This can occur if parenteral vitamin A is given in doses exceeding 10,000 IU/kg. Initially it presents as dry skin, but may progress to whole skin sloughing. Management is as for thermal burns.

Hypovitaminosis C

This has been reported by Frye (1991) as resulting in spontaneous splitting of the skin in anorexic/cachexic pythons and may be associated with a collagen defect. Injections of 10–20 mg/kg vitamin C per day are advised.

Hypovitaminosis E

This has been reported in caimans and other reptiles which eat marine fish. The presence of free radicals in oily frozen marine fish can result in a relative vitamin E deficiency which can lead to steatites, skin sloughing, and necrosis of fat and secondary infections. Dietary supplementation with vitamin E at 1 IU/kg until resolution of signs is recommended.

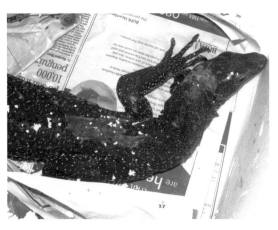

Figure 21.8 Full skin thickness burns can be seen where heat lamps are left unprotected as in this monitor lizard.

PART III: REPTILES AND AMPHIBIANS

Biotin deficiency

This may be seen in reptiles which consume large amounts of eggs, such as some snakes and monitor lizards. Unfertilised eggs contain avidin, an anti-vitamin to biotin which may lead to a relative deficiency. The main signs are neurological, but fracturing and splitting of keratin structures such as scales and claws and beaks along with abnormal sloughing may be seen. Removal of eggs from the diet results in a cure in most cases.

Hypocalcaemia/hypovitaminosis D

This can result in shell deformities in chelonians. See the section on musculoskeletal diseases for further information. In addition, calcinosis cutis and circumscripta have been reported in reptiles with multifocal crusting and thickened skin which can then ulcerate. These two conditions are often related to calcium imbalances – more often hypercalcaemia, but also to areas of skin damage.

Digestive disease

Oral (mouth rot)

'Mouth rot' is the colloquial term for stomatitis, commonly seen in many reptiles particularly in snakes and chelonians.

The causes are many and varied. It can be caused by secondary infections with Gram-negative bacteria. The initial cause of the damage can be rubbing of the snout on vivarium glass, particularly in snakes. The use of opaque tape stuck to the outside of the glass helps the snake to 'see it', preventing this injury.

Stomatitis may also be due to the overzealous force-feeding of anorectic reptiles, to other disease or stresses leading to reduced immune system function. Uric acid crystals deposited around the base of the teeth, due to visceral gout and renal failure can allow infections to occur. Herpesvirus and iridovirus infections in terrestrial tortoises are also a cause with oral ulceration and diphtherisis. Lytic agent X – a suspected virus – has also been associated with upper digestive tract lesions in chelonia. *Devriesea agamarum,* a bacterium, has been reported in agamid lizards as a cause of proliferative cheilitis, pericloacal disease and dermatitis.

Diagnosis is made on impression smears and bacterial swabs of samples. A polymerase chain reaction (PCR) for diagnosing chelonian herpesvirus has been produced at the RVC London, and reptile cell lines are available through the AHVLA Weybridge to attempt virus isolation.

Alternatively, electron microscopy of samples may aid the diagnosis.

Herpesvirus may also affect the central nervous system and organs such as the liver, kidneys and gonads. Depression and neurological signs are possible.

Periodontal disease

This is particularly common in Agamidae and Chameleonidae which possess acrodont teeth. These teeth are not replaced when lost during the course of the lizard's life. This is as opposed to pleurodont teeth (e.g., the Iguanidae) where the teeth are continually replaced. If inappropriate food is provided, such as soft fruit, which adheres readily to the teeth and rots, periodontal disease will develop. As the species with acrodont teeth cannot shed and replace the teeth, infection, often with osteomyelitis ensues.

Vomiting and regurgitation

In snakes, regurgitation may simply occur due to rough handling, particularly soon after the snake has eaten. Snakes will also regurgitate if fed, or force-fed and then kept at sub-optimal environmental temperatures. Lizards and chelonia rarely vomit.

Parasitic causes of vomiting and regurgitation

In snakes, one of the most important stomach diseases is cryptosporidiosis due to a single-celled parasite, *Cryptosporidia serpentes*, which invades the outer membrane of cells lining the stomach. With time, it causes a thickening of the stomach, narrowing the lumen and so reducing its elasticity and digestive powers and causing vomiting. In lizards, cryptosporidiosis mainly affects the intestines, making vomiting less likely. Cryptosporidiosis was implicated in an outbreak of vomiting in juvenile Hermann's tortoises (McArthur *et al.*, 2004). It is therefore currently thought that there is a lizard-, snake- and chelonian-specific form of *Cryptosporidia* spp.

Diagnosis is made on clinical signs and demonstrating oocysts shed in the faeces or recovered from a stomach wash, or biopsy of the stomach wall. In snakes, the course of the disease can vary from 4 days in severe cases to 2 years in chronic ones. Externally, the snake often shows signs of a mid-body swelling, due to the thickening of the stomach wall. The parasite is passed directly from one snake's faeces or regurgitated fluids to another. The condition is difficult to treat and frequently results in the death of the snake (Figure 21.9).

Other forms of parasitism may cause vomiting or regurgitation in snakes. For example, *Kalicephalus* spp. (the snake hookworm), which may cause extensive

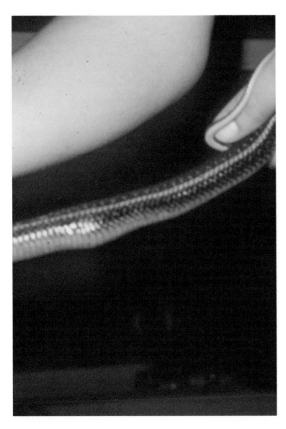

Figure 21.9 Cryptosporidiosis is a common cause of swellings in the stomach of snakes.

ulceration of the digestive system; ascarids; and in the python family, the tapeworm *Bothridium* spp., have been reported.

Bacterial and fungal causes of vomiting and regurgitation

Bacterial and fungal infections, granulomas and abscesses may also cause damage to the stomach, or pressure on it, and so lead to regurgitation or vomiting.

Viral causes of vomiting and regurgitation

Inclusion body disease, a retrovirus, has been associated with chronic regurgitation in boids although there are usually other clinical signs such as respiratory disease and neurological disease.

Tumours

Stomach tumours, for example, gastric adenomas and adenocarcinomas, have been reported and may cause swelling.

Intestinal disease
Parasitic causes of intestinal disease

Snakes: Species involved include the hookworm *Kalicephalus* spp.; ascarids; strongyles such as *Strongyloides* spp.; and tapeworms such as *Bothridium* spp. in pythons; and *Ophiotaenia* spp. in garter and water snakes.

Entamoebiasis caused by the single-celled parasite *Entamoeba invadens* can cause diarrhoea in snakes. Its life cycle is direct; that is, spread directly from one reptile to another. After incubating in the lining of the small intestine, each infective cyst produces eight uninucleate amoebae which invade cells lining the large intestine of the same snake. The amoebae may also penetrate into the blood stream and so end up in the liver, causing necrotising hepatitis. Diagnosis is by finding the small amoebae or cysts in the faeces ($\times$ 400 magnification is required).

Other single-celled parasites of snakes include the flagellate family, (e.g., *Trichomonas* spp.). Symptoms again include large bowel distension with fluid and gas, diarrhoea and increased thirst.

Chelonians: The ascarid family, for example, *Angusticaecum* spp. (10–20 cm in length!) is most significant. Oxyurid pinworms may be asymptomatic, but some may be large enough to debilitate a tortoise, particularly prior to and subsequent to hibernation. Roundworms are passed directly from chelonian to chelonian in the faeces in the infectious egg form, and may be diagnosed by the detection of these eggs in a faecal smear.

The most important group of intestinal parasites of Chelonia is the flagellate family. These include *Trichomonas* and *Hexamita* spp. The symptoms produced are rapid in onset and include anorexia, occasionally diarrhoea and frequently, the passage of undigested food in the faeces. There is often polydipsia, due partly to the inability of the damaged intestines to absorb water, and partly, in the case of *Hexamita parva*, due to kidney damage, as this organism migrates up the ureters from the cloaca into the kidneys. Diagnosis is made by viewing the very fast-moving organisms microscopically using $\times$ 400 magnification, although a fresh faecal specimen is required. Transmission is faecooral. The prognosis may be extremely poor for any chelonian severely parasitised by this organism, due to its ability to cause irreparable damage to the intestinal mucosa.

Another family of motile protozoa afflicting Chelonia are ciliates such as *Balantidium coli* and *Paramecium* spp. They may be seen normally in the stool of healthy animals, but they may be present in such large numbers as to cause weight loss and intestinal damage.

Entamoeba invadens has caused large intestinal and hepatic disease in herbivorous chelonians. However, this condition is less common than in snakes.

As mentioned, *Cryptosporidia* spp. can affect the small intestine and stomach of chelonia, and has been implicated in pancreatitis as well.

Lizards: Oxyurid nematodes are common. Due to the direct life cycle of these parasites, levels may become very high enough to produce intestinal damage and debilitation. Diagnosis is by finding the eggs in the faeces (Figure 21.10).

The coccidian family are also important parasites in lizards, particularly geckos and chameleons. Clinical signs include anorexia, weight loss, diarrhoea, dysentery and general debilitation. *Isospora amphiboluri* is a cause of stunting and runting in bearded dragon neonates. Diagnosis is by finding the typically isosporean oocysts in the faeces, and disease spread is direct.

Intestinal cryptosporidiosis is a problem in geckos. Symptoms include weight loss, diarrhoea and anorexia and typically affect young hatchlings that basically fail to thrive. The pathology has been described above.

Entamoeba invadens may also be seen in carnivorous lizards, producing colic and progressive weight loss with diarrhoea.

Bacterial causes of intestinal disease
In all species, but particularly snakes and chelonians, members of the zoonotic family Salmonellae are commonly recovered. Current advice is that providing they are not causing clinical disease, no antibiotics should be given. This is to prevent antibiotic resistance, and on a practical basis no one has satisfactorily proven that

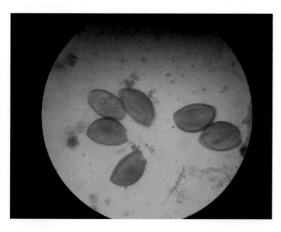

Figure 21.10 Oxyurid nematode infections are common in reptiles and may be diagnosed by finding these classical eggs in the faeces.

such treatment can clear a reptile permanently of the bacterium.

Salmonella spp. may be carried by perfectly healthy individuals, but during other disease processes, such as parasitism, or during periods of stress, they can become opportunistic pathogens. Other bacteria found in the normal digestive system of reptiles can act as opportunistic pathogens, including many members of the *E. coli* family, *Pseudomonas* spp., *Campylobacter* spp., *Clostridia* spp., and *Aeromonas* spp.

Fungal causes of intestinal disease
Published reports of gastrointestinal fungal disease are rare, but fungal overgrowth appears to be a relatively common finding. Documented cases of intestinal fungal overgrowth include *Penicillium*, *Basidiobolus ranarum* and *Paecilomyces*.

Physical causes of intestinal disease
Foreign bodies are not uncommon in chelonians and lizards, which may consume stones, sand, soil or any other substrate present. Surgery may be required to remove some foreign bodies, although many may be passed with the aid of oral liquid paraffin and fluid therapy.

Other physical obstructions include tumours within the intestines. These are not uncommon, particularly in snakes, and may present as a swelling, or produce symptoms such as vomiting, diarrhoea, constipation or anorexia.

Lead poisoning
This has been reported in chelonian such as common snapping turtles (*Chelydra serpentina*) and spur-thighed tortoises (*Testudo graeca*). Clinical signs included ileus, anaemia, lethargy and renal failure. Radiography will highlight larger lead particles.

Liver disease
Snakes
Possible causes of liver damage in snakes (*Entamoeba invadens*) have already been mentioned above.

Other parasitic causes include some forms of the coccidian family which gain access to the liver from the small intestine via the bile ducts.

A herpesvirus and an adenovirus have been isolated from damaged snake livers.

Chelonia
The protozoan *Hexamita parva* has been associated with intestinal, renal and hepatic disease in Chelonia.

Hepatic lipidosis is common in tortoises fed inappropriate high-fat diets. Fat becomes deposited within the liver cells themselves, enlarging the liver and, more importantly, severely affecting its function. This can lead to jaundice, anorexia and death.

Post-hibernation jaundice is often a temporary finding in tortoises however it may persist, indicating liver damage due to any one of the above or due to hepatitis from bacteria such as *Salmonella* spp. and *Aeromonas hydrophila*. In addition some forms of herpesviruses and iridoviruses have been isolated from damaged tortoise and other chelonian livers.

The liver may become calcified due to over-supplementation of the diet with calcium and vitamin D_3.

Lizards

Bacterial hepatitis due to *Salmonella* spp., *Aeromonas* spp. or *Pseudomonas* spp. has all been recorded. These may or may not be associated with heavy worm burdens, many of which may migrate through or to the liver, often carrying bacteria with them.

Viral hepatitis has been reported due to adenoviruses in bearded dragons (*Pogona* spp.). It is generally seen in young animals and often associated with coccidiosis resulting in poor thriving young. Serological tests are available for detection of this disease as is a PCR test. Herpesviruses have been associated with hepatitis as well as pneumonia in iguanids and agamids. Yellow-green urates may be seen in both snakes and lizards associated with hepatic dysfunction due to the presence of increased levels of biliverdin.

Hepatic lipidosis, or fatty liver syndrome, has been well documented in lizards, particularly monitors and bearded dragons. This is frequently seen when fed inappropriate high-fat diets. In bearded dragons, the feeding of excessive amounts of insects to adults (which are supposed to become more herbivorous once they reach maturity) has also been implicated (Figure 21.11). In lizards with pre-ovulatory stasis, lipidosis occurs due to the high levels of circulating yolk lipids. Lipidosis can lead to jaundice, anorexia and death. The liver may become calcified due to over-supplementation of the diet with calcium and vitamin D_3.

Pancreatic diseases

Pancreatitis

This may be associated with bacterial infections as well as herpesvirus disease and cryptosporidiosis in chelonia (McArthur *et al.*, 2004). Frye (1999) describes a spontaneous autoimmune pancreatitis and diabetes mellitus in a Western pond turtle.

Diabetes mellitus

This has been reported in chelonia and is thought to be due to a reduction in insulin secretion due to pancreatic

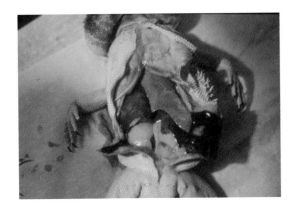

Figure 21.11 Hepatic lipidosis is common in species such as the bearded dragon (*Pogona* spp.). Note the tan coloured liver and fat deposits.

damage (McArthur *et al.*, 2004). Reptiles are insulin resistant; therefore, insulin therapy is rarely effective. Ketoacidosis and hepatic lipidosis are often also present.

Neoplasia of the digestive tract

Neoplasia of the pancreas has been mentioned. Neoplasia of the stomach and intestines are not uncommon, particularly in snakes. Hepatic neoplasia has been reported most frequently in chelonia. Onset tends to be gradual, and unless the neoplasm involves an intestinal obstruction, may pass unnoticed until advanced.

Respiratory disease

Signs of respiratory disease

Respiratory disease in reptiles is exacerbated by the lack of a cough reflex as reptiles have no true diaphragm (Figure 21.12). Secretions pool in the dependent parts of the lungs and so make the course of the disease more chronic and difficult to treat. Signs of respiratory disease are given in Table 21.1.

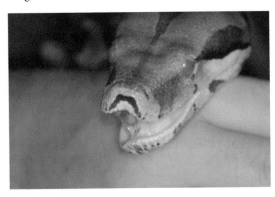

Figure 21.12 Mouth breathing and excess oral mucus are often seen in advanced cases of respiratory disease as in this boa constrictor.

Table 21.1 Signs of respiratory disease in reptiles.

Common signs of respiratory disease in reptiles	Less frequently seen signs of respiratory disease in reptiles
Mouth breathing (particularly snakes) Excess mucus at nares and mouth Lethargy Anorexia	Hypopyon (pus in the anterior chamber of the eye – particularly chelonia) Abscess beneath the eye spectacle

Causes of respiratory disease

Parasitic causes

Entamoeba invadens can cause respiratory disease in snakes. The commoner parasites though are nematodes. These are represented by:

- *Kalicephalus* spp.: This can migrate through the skin of the snake, or be eaten. The worm then migrates through body, often through the lungs as it develops, before finally ending up as the adult hookworm in the gut.
- The family Ascaridae: In carnivorous reptiles, ascarid infection is frequently acquired via amphibian or rodent prey, which acts as an intermediate/paratenic host. The worm larvae, once consumed, migrate through the liver and lungs of the reptile.
- *Rhabdias* spp. (lungworm of snakes): The snake ingests the infective eggs from the faeces of other snakes, or the infective larvae may penetrate the skin of the snake as with *Kalicephalus* spp. The larvae then migrate to the lungs, where they all develop into adult female worms. Eggs are therefore produced by parthenogenesis (female giving birth to female).
- *Entomelas* spp. (lungworm of lizards): The life-cycle is similar to the lungworm of snakes.

Other less common parasitic causes of respiratory disease in reptiles include:

- Flukes (e.g., *Dasymetra* spp.), which live in the oral cavity and respiratory tract of snakes. These parasites are rarely pathogenic. Diagnosis is made by finding the fluke eggs in the snake's faeces.
- Pentastomes, also known as 'tongue worms'. These are the adult stage of an arachnid organism related to spiders and ticks, rather than a true worm. It uses the lungs of snakes, crocodiles or lizards as the final host, shedding eggs which are coughed up and swallowed and passed in the faeces. These then are ingested by an intermediate host such as rodents, or even humans, making this a zoonotic disease. The larvae encyst in the intermediate host. If this is then consumed by the

reptile, the larvae are reactivated and migrate to the lungs where they can grow to several centimetres in length, causing severe damage. They are generally only found in wild-caught specimens, due to the lack of native prey to transmit the parasite in captivity.

- Intranuclear coccidiosis in the lungs has been reported in chelonia by biopsy, although a PCR test has been developed (Garner et al., 2006).

Bacterial causes

Examples of the bacteria seen in pneumonias include *Aeromonas* spp., *Pseudomonas* spp., *Klebsiella* spp., and *Pasteurella* spp.

Mycoplasmas are regularly recovered from chelonians with Herpesvirus infections, particularly *Mycoplasma agassizii*. One study suggested an incidence of 15.8% in UK tortoises (Soares *et al.*, 2003). This may result in oedema and swelling of the neck and tissues between neck and forelimbs in chelonian. *M. agassizii*-like mycoplasma has also been identified as a cause of a proliferative interstitial pneumonia and tracheitis in Burmese pythons (Penner *et al.*, 1997). PCRs and culture have been used to diagnose mycoplasmal infections.

Chlamydophila spp. infections have also been reported particularly in snakes resulting in pneumonia.

Bacterial sampling

There are two main techniques involved in sampling bacteria or parasites that cause pneumonias:

- Lung wash: A sterile catheter is passed into the trachea of the reptile and may be done in the conscious animal due to the lack of the cough reflex. Fractious animals may require sedation. Through this catheter, sterile saline may be infused, at doses equal to 0.5–1 mL per 100 g body weight, and immediately aspirated. This sample can then be cultured to identify the pathogen. Sample collection may be enhanced by holding the reptile upside down whilst aspirating.
- Direct sampling: This involves taking a swab directly from the site of the problem. This may be done via laparotomy or endoscopy. In the case of Chelonia, the reptile may be anaesthetised, the shell overlying the pneumonic lesion aseptically prepared and a small hole drilled through to enable the bacteriological swab to be passed.

Fungal causes

Fungal infections of the respiratory tract are more commonly seen in chelonians than in other species of reptile.

The infections are due to saprophytic opportunistic environmental fungi and so are often secondary to bacterial infections or traumatic injuries. Fungi associated with disease include *Aspergillus, Paecilomyces, Candida, Sporotrichum, Cladosporium* and *Penicillium* spp.

Viral causes

Paramyxovirus: This virus is highly infectious, being shed in respiratory secretions. It causes a haemorrhagic pneumonia and viraemia which affects other organs as well. Diagnosis is generally made at postmortem or by serological analysis of blood samples for the PMV-3 and PMV-7 strains (AHVLA Weybridge, United Kingdom). Seroconversion does take 6–8 weeks to occur post infection, so false-negative results early in the course of the disease are possible. Currently, two Ophidian and one Saurian paramyxovirus are known to exist, but probably many more await discovery.

A paramyxovirus related to parainfluenza 2 (PI2) virus was recovered from the lungs of two Ottoman vipers (*Vipera xanthena xanthena*) with interstitial pneumonia (Potgieter *et al.*, 1987).

Inclusion body virus: This retrovirus, which also causes digestive and CNS system diseases, has been associated with pneumonia in snakes – primarily pythons and boas. There is no treatment. It is thought to be spread by aerosol and by the snake mite *Ophionyssus natricis*. Diagnosis is made by biopsy of lung, liver, spleen or kidney tissue or occasionally it may be possible to see the characteristic eosinophilic virion 'inclusions' in pneumocytes dislodged during a lung wash, particularly in boids in this author's experience.

Herpes viruses: This has been recorded in tortoises with upper respiratory tract infections. Clinical signs include lethargy, rhinitis, conjunctivitis, stomatitis and anorexia. Diphtheritic plaques may form inside the oral cavity and oesophagus. *Testudo* spp. appear to be the most susceptible with one serological study reporting 42.5% of spur-thighed tortoises and 18.5% of Hermann's were positive (Frost & Schmidt, 1997). Routes of transmission are not fully understood but studies have shown success via oral, aerosol and intramuscular routes. Any infected tortoise should be considered as infected for life and so can spread herpesvirus particles even after resolution of clinical signs.

Diagnosis is by serology or PCR. A serum neutralisation test was the first to be developed, but a more effective and sensitive ELISA now exists. A PCR real-time assay also exists and is the most useful in an acute outbreak as serological conversion can take 6–8 weeks post infection to occur. Histopathology may also demonstrate classical eosinophilic intranuclear inclusion bodies.

Iridovirus: Iridoviral respiratory infections particularly *Ranavirus* infections produced a severe, extensive necrotizing ulcerative tracheitis, pneumonia, pharyngitis and oesophagitis in an adult male Gopher tortoise (*Gopherus polyphemus*). In other animals, such as *Testudo horsfieldii* and *Terrapene carolina* with iridovirus, no lesions were described. It seems that amphibians are the reservoir host as the *Ranavirus* isolated in cases of upper respiratory tract disease in chelonia is of amphibian origin. PCR and neutralization tests are available (Westhouse *et al.*, 1996).

Hypovitaminosis A

This has been reported in aquatic and semi-aquatic carnivorous chelonia. Typical lesions of squamous metaplasia, periocular oedema and xerophthalmia, and secondary bacterial infections of the gastrointestinal and respiratory tract are seen.

Trauma and respiratory tract disease in reptiles

Trauma to the carapace of chelonians is a frequent cause on non-infectious lung disease. It is often associated with dog attacks, car accidents or lawnmower injuries.

Cardiovascular disease
Congenital defects

These have been reported in a number of species and include atrial septal defects and valve dysplasias.

Cardiomyopathy

Dilated cardiomyopathy has been reported, particularly in snakes (Barten, 1980; Wagner, 1989). Causes appear to be similar to those described for birds and mammals. Management is as for congestive heart failure.

Infectious disease

Many pathogens which cause systemic illness and septicaemia are responsible for cardiac damage. Damage can be due to bacterial endocarditis causing micro-thrombi to seed off into the rest of the body. Many of the Gram-negative bacteria seen in reptiles, such as *Aeromonas* spp. *Salmonella* spp. and *Pseudomonas* spp., are associated with heart disease. Diagnosis requires ultrasonography and radiology to determine heart size and internal structure. Electrocardiograms may also be helpful. Final proof of the organism involved depends on blood culture.

Chlamydial myocarditis has been reported in Puff adders and mycoplasmosis has been reported in American alligators. Mycobacteriosis has also been reported as a cause of myocarditis.

Pneumonia often accompanies endocarditis and septicaemic situations in reptiles (Pees *et al.*, 2010).

Haemoparasites
Filarids
The adults often live subcutaneously and release microfilaria, microscopic young, which may be transmitted from reptile to reptile by mosquitoes and ticks. These parasites may cause thrombi to develop in any of the major blood vessels, causing ischaemic necrosis or cardiac damage.

Trematodes
Other parasites such as trematodes have been isolated in marine chelonia. The adult fluke is not normally the problem, but the eggs laid into the blood stream cause thrombi to form and so block capillary beds.

Plasmodium and haemoproteus
In chelonia, the haemoparasite family *Plasmodium* spp. has been shown to cause haemolytic anaemia and mortality. They are transmitted by mosquitoes predominantly and schizonts, gametocytes and trophozoites may be found in the peripheral blood. The gametocyte is the most obvious stage, as it is refractile with pigment granules in the cytoplasm of white and red blood cells and thrombocytes.

Haemoproteus spp. are found as gametocytes in the cytoplasm of erythrocytes and have refractile pigment granules. There is no known effective treatment for this condition but it is not common in reptiles.

Haemogregarines
These are probably the most commonly seen group of sporozoan haemoparasites in reptiles. They have an indirect life-cycle with intermediate hosts which vary from leeches and mosquitoes to mites and ticks. The three most commonly seen families include *Haemogregarina* (found in fresh water turtles, *Testudo* spp. tortoises, snakes and some lizards), *Hepatozoon* (found in snakes predominantly) and *Karyolysus* (Old World lizards). They difficult to differentiate between clinically. The gametocyte is found in the erythrocyte cytoplasm, often curling around the nucleus or displacing it.

Reptile haemogregarines rarely cause disease. Heavy infestations though have been associated with anaemia

Other haemoparasites
Trypanosomes, *Schellackia* spp., piroplasms (e.g., *Sauroplasma*) have all been reported in reptiles and are nearly always asymptomatic. Treatment is rarely needed.

Nutritional disease
Hypoiodinism in chelonians has been associated with cardiac disease and goitre. The feeding of mineral-poor foods such as cucumber and lettuce or goitrogenic foods such as brassicas (e.g., cabbage, Brussels sprouts), may lead to this.

Oversupplementation with vitamin D_3 and calcium may lead to calcification of the tunica media of the major arteries, causing a decrease in their elasticity and so increased blood pressure. This may lead to heart failure or aneurysm formation.

Dietary deficiencies in vitamin E and/or selenium can lead to a condition known as white muscle disease, and can cause a dilated cardiomyopathy to develop. It may occur due to a dietary deficiency, or to overfeeding with high-fat foods, such as snakes fed overweight rodents or fish, such as tuna and mackerel, which are high in polyunsaturates and increase the demand for vitamin E.

Atherosclerosis
This has been reported in green iguanas (Schuchman & Taylor, 1970) and bearded dragons (Schilliger *et al.*, 2010) and may be a precursor to mineralisation of major arteries.

Neoplastic disease
Leukaemias have been regularly reported in many reptiles, particularly in snakes. They are usually are tissue-bound lymphomas but these may become leukaemic over-spill cases with the presence of lymphoblast cells. There is some suggestion that as with birds, some lymphomas are virus associated.

In addition, other tumours have been reported including fibrosarcomas, mast cell tumours and chondrosarcomas in snakes (Schumacher *et al.*, 1998; Schmidt & Reavill, 2010). Fibrosarcomas seem to have a predilection for the right atrium.

Urinary tract disease
Renal disease and gout
Aetiology
Damage to kidney function in the average terrestrial reptile can lead to increasing blood levels of uric acid, the main excretory product of protein metabolism. Uric acid

is poorly water soluble, and so rapidly reaches its precipitation point whereby crystals form and come out of solution. This may occur in internal organs (visceral gout) and also the joints (articular gout).

Factors contributing to renal failure include:

1. Diets high in protein, fed to herbivores, automatically leading to excessive production of uric acid, the main waste product of protein metabolism

2. Diets with excessive levels of vitamin D_3 and calcium leading to calcification of soft tissue structures, such as the tunica media of the arterial walls, and the kidneys themselves.

3. Diets low in vitamin A resulting in squamous metaplasia of the proximal tubules

4. Glomerulonephritis occurred in approximately 27% of kidneys examined in one survey (Zwart, 2006).

5. Flagellates such as *Hexamita* spp., *Trichomonas* spp., and *Giardia* spp. have been reported in chelonia, snakes and lizards. *Hexamita* spp. are particularly damaging to the kidneys of chelonia.

6. *Entamoeba invadens* has also been reported in snakes where it often becomes systemic and so can cause extensive areas of renal necrosis.

7. Kidney flukes are found in Kingsnakes, and members of the Boidae. They may block renal tubules, and in high enough quantities, cause kidney failure.

8. Coccidial parasites (e.g., *Klossiella boae*) in boids which parasitizes the collecting ducts and ureters. Intranuclear stages of coccidia have also been found in chelonia causing tubular necrosis.

9. Myxosporidia of the genus *Myxidium* have been reported in the kidneys of chelonia but little is known about their pathogenicity.

10. Microsporidia have also been reported in bearded dragons associated with infection of renal epithelial cells.

11. Almost any bacteria found in the digestive system or environment of the reptile has the potential to cause renal disease if that reptile is stressed or debilitated in any way (e.g., *Salmonella* spp., *Aeromonas* spp., *Pseudomonas* spp. and E. coli). In some chelonia, the bacteria responsible for septicaemic cutaneous syndrome, *Citrobacter freundii* is also implicated. Mycobacteria have also been associated with renal disease in chelonia.

12. Inclusion body disease of snakes has been associated with inclusions and damage to the kidneys with glomerulonephritis. Herpesvirus has been seen in chelonia causing the same.

13. Any systemic mycosis or local extension from a fungal pneumonia may lead to infection of the kidneys. *Penicillium griseofulvin*, *Geotrichum nigra* and *Colletotrichium acutatum* have all been reported associated with renal disease in chelonia.

14. Iatrogenic causes – certain nephrotoxic drugs such as the aminoglycoside antibiotic family (e.g., gentamicin, amikacin etc.), and the diuretic furosemide.

15. If sufficient muscle bruising occurs, such as too firm a grasp of the patient when handling, then myoglobin is released. This causes damage to the kidney filtration membrane.

Diagnosis of renal disease

Clinical signs can include lethargy, polydipsia, polyuria, collapse, visceral and articular gout, obstipation due to renomegaly pressing on the cloaca/rectum and dystocia (remember, the kidneys are in the pelvis in lizards and chelonia) and fluid retention with oedema (Figure 21.13).

Haematological parameters may alter with a leukocytosis in acute infectious renal disease. Chronic renal failure may have a non-regenerative anaemia. Uric acid measurement will allow an assessment of the severity of renal damage with visceral gout starting when levels in the blood rise above 1500 µmol/L. Remember though, that uric acid measurement is not a sensitive indicator of early renal disease, as less than 25% of the renal mass has to be left functioning before the uric acid levels will rise significantly. Also any carnivore that has eaten a meal recently will have elevated uric acid levels. In aquatic chelonia, urea is a consistent fraction of nitrogen and therefore may be of use. In terrestrial species urea is not a useful indicator of renal disease.

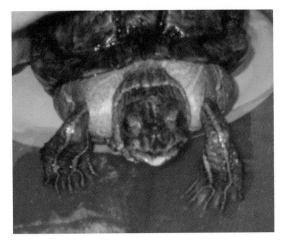

Figure 21.13 Chronic renal failure in a red-eared terrapin (*Trachemys scripta elegans*) with tissue oedema and fluid retention.

Calcium and phosphorus levels have been used as an early indicator of renal disease in reptiles. The product of calcium and phosphorus in mmol/L should be less than 9. If it exceeds this, and particularly if it exceeds 12, then metastatic mineralisation occurs and phosphate binders should be used. Gamma-glutamyl transferase is found in the brush border of the renal tubule and so is released when damaged. At this stage there is not enough evidence to determine what is significant.

Potassium levels may significantly elevate in chelonians with renal disease.

Urinalysis is less useful in reptiles than birds as there is usually post-renal modification of the urine in either the urinary bladder (where present) or the rectum, as urine is refluxed, and more water (and solutes) is absorbed. No urine sample will be sterile either. However, assessment for protein casts, haematuria and of course, for parasites is useful.

Radiography demonstrating renalomegaly can aid diagnosis. In lizards the kidneys should be within the pelvis. In renalomegaly the cranial pole often projects into the caudal coelomic cavity and can be seen. Radiopaque dye may be injected intravenously to perform a urogram (800–1000 mg/kg of aqueous iodine). Finally, loss of bone density may occur with secondary hyperparathyroidism, although there has to be a significant drop in bone density for conventional radiographs to detect it.

Ultrasound examination of kidney structure can also be helpful to indicate overall increases in echogenicity and size. It is particularly useful in chelonia where radiography is not useful in detecting changes in size. The probe is placed in front of the hindlimb and angled caudally onto the inside of the carapace to examine the kidneys.

Endoscopy and biopsy, as with birds, is perhaps the definitive technique to determine the cause and severity of renal disease in reptiles. Even then, they have their limitations; in lizards, the kidneys are in the pelvis and may be difficult to visualise due to the presence of the fat pads, and in chelonians, their position on the dorsum of the internal carapace means a rigid endoscope may find access difficult. Ultrasound-guided biopsy may also be attempted.

Bladder stones

These are common in reptiles – but obviously some reptiles do not have a urinary bladder. Chelonia and lizards such as the green iguana are the most commonly seen species. The stones are uric acid based and may form around a nidus of bacteria, a refluxed egg in females or a parasite. They may reach significant sizes, resulting in cystitis and cause considerable pain and discomfort.

Reproductive tract disease
Egg-binding or post-ovulatory stasis

Dystocia is common in many species of reptile. It is associated with hypocalcaemia, however other causes include malformed eggs, fractured pelvic bones, cystic calculi, lack of nesting material or malnutrition of the female.

Dystocias can be difficult to diagnose in snakes, as they tend to be relatively quiet creatures. This difficulty is exacerbated in those species (e.g., garter snakes) which are viviparous (that is give birth to live young rather than eggs) in that any abdominal swelling is much less pronounced. Any previous history of passing eggs, and then the presence of a persistent caudally-located mass is of course highly suggestive. In addition, any evidence of a prolapse of the cloaca or distal reproductive tract can indicate dystocia.

In lizards, the patient may be obviously distended with eggs, and become progressively more moribund and lethargic (Figure 21.14). Many snakes can survive prolonged periods of dystocia, but lizards are not so resilient and dystocia may prove fatal within days.

Chelonia may show signs of discomfort and straining or they may show no signs at all. Radiographs are often the only way to tell if a chelonian is gravid.

Pre-ovulatory stasis

A condition recorded in both lizards and Chelonia is pre-ovulatory stasis.

This is when the ovaries produce follicles, which enlarge but do not shed into the reproductive tract. This results in ovaries containing anywhere up to 30 or 40 yolks, displacing all other coelomic organs (Figure 21.15). Over time the affected reptile becomes anorectic and lethargic

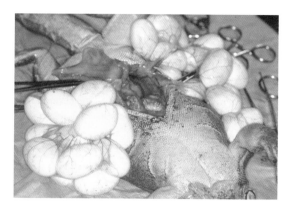

Figure 21.14 Post-ovulatory stasis/egg binding in a green iguana (*Iguana iguana*).

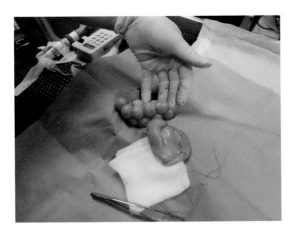

Figure 21.15 Pre-ovulatory stasis in a green iguana (*Iguana iguana*).

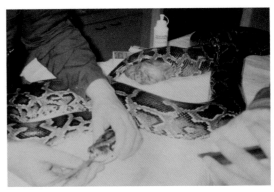

Figure 21.16 Oviduct prolapse in a Burmese python (*Python molurus bivittatus*).

and often succumbs to secondary diseases (e.g., egg yolk coelomitis) and malnourishment. The cause of the condition is not fully understood but is thought to be associated with a long-term absence of a male or a brief exposure to a male after prior isolation. Radiographs show spherical, rather than oval densities in the abdomen without the characteristic thin walled part-calcified shell.

Yolk coelomitis

This is often associated with pre-ovulatory stasis. Ultrasonography and radiography may help in identifying the cause. Clinical signs include lethargy, anorexia, coelomic distension and diarrhoea. There may be evidence of hyperproteinaemia, an increase in beta globulins, leucocytosis, hypercalcaemia and azotaemia.

Hemipenal and phallus prolapse

This is often seen in weakened cachectic reptiles, or those with gastrointestinal, urinary or cloacal disease which results in persistent straining. In addition, many reptiles prolapse their phallus due to sexual frustration or due to infection or due to the formation of dried secretions (so-called hemipenal plug) within the hemipene which are irritants.

Oviduct prolapse

This may be seen in female reptiles, as a result of conditions described for phallus prolapse in males, and as a consequence of dystocia/egg binding (Figure 21.16). Severe prolapses, which have been present for some time, may necessitate emergency surgery and replacement of the prolapse via a coeliotomy, with the possibility of a salpingectomy at the same time.

Musculoskeletal disease
Metabolic bone disease (MBD)
Aetiology

This is common in young growing lizards and chelonia on a calcium-deficient diet, often in conjunction with vitamin D3/ultraviolet light deficiency. This results in nutritional secondary hyperparathyroidism (NSHP).

Clinically in lizards, an individual is often weak and lethargic, and unable to support its body off the ground. The limbs are swollen due to fibrous thickening of the bones. Pathological fractures are common. Bowing of the lower jaw is also common in lizards due to tongue muscle contraction of softened bone. Hyperaesthesia may also be seen due to the hypocalcaemia manifested as twitching digits when standing at rest and this may extend to the gastrointestinal tract with ileus and cloacal prolapses made more likely.

In chelonia, the disease is seen as a softening and pyramiding of the shell. The plastron and carapace are weakened due to hypomineralisation, which allows the muscles to deform their structure. This is particularly obvious over the internal attachments of the fore- and hindlimb where depressions are seen. In some chelonia, for example, the softened shell allows the corners of the carapace to roll upwards.

Cholecalciferol source for most snakes and carnivorous chelonians is entirely from their food. For most diurnal insectivorous or herbivorous lizards and some chelonians UVB (280–315 nm wavelength) and UVA (315–400 nm wavelength) are necessary to activate the cholecalciferol pathway.

Diagnosis of MBD

Ionised calcium levels are a more accurate indicator of the bioavailable calcium than total. Values of 1.47 mmol/L have been calculated as mean ionised calcium in green iguanas (Dennis *et al.*, 2001). Hypocalcaemia, hyperphosphatemia and a Ca:PO ratio of less than 1:1 are all early indicators of MBD. Studies have also looked at calcitriol levels but these are currently difficult to measure outside of research institutes.

Radiography has been used as a primary, although not very sensitive, tool for diagnosing MBD. Poor bone mineralisation, widening of the bone diameter and deformity in the long axis of bones with kyphotic/scoliotic spines may be seen.

Prevention of MBD

Klaphake (2010) has described ultraviolet light provision for reptiles to prevent MBD as follows:

1. Desert diurnal lizards/chelonians – high UVB levels (10% or full unfiltered sun for 12 hours)
2. Diurnal arboreal lizards or semiaquatic basking chelonians – moderate UVB (5%, 12 hours)
3. Diurnal terrestrial lizards or chelonians from forests – low UVB (5%, 6 hours)
4. Nocturnal lizards – low levels UVB (2%, 6 hours)
5. Snakes – dietary calcium and vitamin D_3 is sufficient

Calcium supplementation should be provided for young growing lizards and chelonia, but unfortunately, little data exists to demonstrate in what form or how much is necessary. For insectivores, gut-loading their prey is preferred as this guarantees the reptile will get the nutritional supplement. Commercially available insects need supplementation as most have inverted Ca:PO ratios. Dietary deficiencies for herbivores in calcium can occur where large amounts of leaves containing oxalates (e.g., spinach and beetroot tops) that bind calcium in the gut and prevent absorption are present. Fruit should be kept to a minimum as it contains little or no calcium. Studies into shell pyramiding in chelonia (*Geochelone sulcata*) showed that pyramiding was more likely to occur in individuals kept under dry environmental conditions than those in more humid ones with small variations occurring due to higher levels of dietary protein. This study showed no significant impact on pyramiding of the dietary Ca:PO ratio just to add further confusion to the MBD debate! (Wiesner & Iben, 2003).

Fractures

These may be pathological, as is seen in cases of MBD, or truly they may be traumatic in origin. Repair of these fractures depends on their cause; see chapter 22.

Joint swelling

This can be due to tumours, sepsis and articular gout. Systemic or local mycobacteriosis due to *M. marinum* has also been reported (Girling & Fraser, 2007)

Autotomy (tail shedding)

Autotomy, or spontaneous shedding of the tail with subsequent regrowth, is seen in some Saurian species, for example, many geckos and iguanas. These lizards have 'fracture planes' in their tails which will allow a clean break, with minimal bleeding, to occur should a predator (or over-zealous restraint) attack. The tail will subsequently regrow, but when it does, the coccygeal vertebrae are replaced with a rod of cartilage, and the scale pattern is frequently much more haphazard (Figure 21.17).

When treating such lizards, it is important to avoid suturing the skin of the lizard over the stump of the tail left, as this may well prevent regrowth. Instead, the area should be treated as an open wound with topical antiseptics such as dilute povidone–iodine. In iguanids, once the individual matures, autonomy often ceases. This can occur over the age of 2.5–3 years in the green iguana, for example.

If the tail wound is very proximal, such as through the area where the inverted hemipenes are situated in the male species, or in species of lizard where autonomy does not occur (such as many species of Agamid lizards), routine closure of the skin over the stump under a general anaesthetic is required.

Neurological disease

Parasitic causes of neurological disease

Acanthamoebic meningoencephalitis is a condition seen primarily in snakes due to *Entamoeba invadens*. Fits and opisthotonic seizures are seen. Treatment is generally unsuccessful.

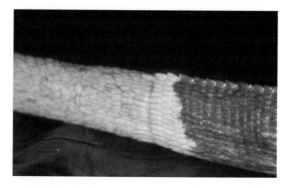

Figure 21.17 Autotomy in a green iguana (*Iguana iguana*). Note the haphazard arrangement of scales distal to the break and the lack of dorsal spines.

Toxoplasma and *Encephalitozoon* infections have also been reported as a cause of meningoencephalitis in reptiles.

Bacterial causes of neurological disease

Bacterial abscesses/granulomas of the spinal cord or the brain may result in neurological disease. These are usually as a result of septicaemia which is common in reptiles. Most are Gram negative in nature, but mycoplasma and chlamydophilal organisms have also been reported as have Mycobacterial infections.

Middle ear infections in aquatic chelonia are common and may result in peripheral vestibular disease. There is often an underlying vitamin A deficiency problem.

Fungal causes of neurological disease

Migration of fungal disease from other body organs such as the lungs can involve the spinal column or disseminate into the central nervous system and cause neurological disease.

Viral causes of neurological disease

Paramyxovirus

These have been reported in many species of snake. The virus causes haemorrhagic pneumonias but will also cause neurological signs such as the loss of righting reflexes. There is no current treatment.

Inclusion body disease

This has been seen in boas and pythons, elapids and colubrids. It is thought to be a retrovirus. In pythons, the disease is severe with infectious stomatitis, pneumonia and neurological signs such as loss of the righting reflex, disorientation and blindness often followed rapidly by death. In boas, the disease is fatal in young individuals. In older patients, the disease produces more chronic neurological signs with chronic anorexia, vomiting and pneumonias. Neurological signs are milder with a loss of ability to chew and swallow prey, and a loss of the striking reflex. Diagnosis is currently based on biopsy of affected organs, principally the liver, kidney, spleen and oesophageal tonsils which will show classical eosinophilic intracytoplasmic inclusion bodies. Early in the course of the disease there may be a leucocytosis (WBC > 30×10^9/L)

There is no treatment for this disease.

Other viruses

Chelonian herpesviruses have been associated with neurological disease. Adenoviruses have been associated with opisthotonus and death in chameleons (Jacobson & Gardiner, 1990).

Nutritional causes of neurological disease

Hypocalcaemic collapse

This is commonly seen in gravid lizards, such as green iguanas, when the blood calcium levels drop too low. The female becomes flaccidly paralysed, and unresponsive. Occasionally fine muscle tremors will be seen.

Hypovitaminosis B$_1$

It is seen in primarily fish-eating reptiles such as garter snakes. The thiaminases present in salt-water fish break down the vitamin B$_1$ present in the food leading to a functional deficit. The presenting signs include opisthotonus and a lack of a righting reflex.

Biotin deficiency

This is seen in species fed mainly on unfertilised hen's eggs that contain large amounts of the antibiotin vitamin, avidin. This produces a relative deficiency in biotin which leads to muscle tremor and general weakness. Monitor lizards are commonly affected.

Hypoglycaemia

This is a condition seen in crocodiles. It is unknown why it occurs, but muscle tremor and weakness are seen.

Environmental causes of neurological disease

This can occur due to freezing injuries. These are seen in chelonians overwintering outside in the United Kingdom. Frost damage causes blindness, vestibular disease and death. There is no treatment.

Toxic causes of neurological disease

Pyrethrin/organophosphate poisoning

These are most likely to be associated with mite treatments. Overdose will result in opisthotonus, head tilts, fits and death. Management with atropine in cases of organophosphate poisoning may be successful but is rarely so in pyrethrin cases. Supportive therapy in mildly affected animals may be sufficient to allow recovery.

Lead toxicosis

This has been reported in chelonians. It usually results in gut stasis and liver/kidney problems, but may present as neurological disease in reptiles. Treatment with 10–40 mg/kg sodium calcium EDTA q12 hours has been used. See the section in digestive tract disease for more details.

An overview of reptilian biochemistry

Blood for biochemical parameters is best collected in a heparinised container. This also applies for haematological parameter measurements as Ca-EDTA often causes lysis of reptilian red blood cells, particularly in chelonia.

Liver parameters

There are no liver specific enzymes in reptiles. Levels of AST in excess of 150–200 IU/L are suggestive of hepatocellular damage; but as there is much species variation and as AST is also found in the skeletal muscle, it is only a guide. Liver function may be assessed using bile acids. However, studies have shown that in reptiles the 3 alpha-hydroxyl bile acids isomer is important which is not the same as in mammals (McBride *et al.*, 2006). Creatinine kinase (CK) and lactate dehydrogenase (LDH) levels may be used to distinguish elevations of AST due to muscle (where both CK and LDH will be elevated) and liver (when only AST or AST and LDH will be elevated) damage. In addition, GLDH may be used to determine severe hepatic necrosis as may occur with herpesvirus/iridovirus infections in chelonia and in post hibernational anorexia (PHA).

Renal parameters

Uric acid is used for diagnosing kidney failure in uricotelic species. Levels over 450 µmol/L suggest renal problems, but in carnivores, recent meals will falsely elevate levels. With disease, uric acid levels will only be elevated if greater than 75% of the renal mass ceases to function and so it is not a sensitive test. Blood levels in excess of 1000 µmol/L should be given a guarded prognosis, and those over 2000 µmol/L are invariably fatal.

Potassium levels exceeding 7 mmol/L should be given a guarded prognosis and those exceeding 9 mmol/L usually die of cardiac failure.

Urea has been used in chelonia immediately after hibernation to assess pre-renal dehydration. Creatinine appears to be of no use in assessing renal function in reptiles.

Glucose

Levels below 3 mmol/L are seen in the hypoglycaemic syndrome of crocodiles. Fits, incoordination and weakness are a common sign in malnourished reptiles, which will also show low glucose levels. Diabetes mellitus has been recorded in some species.

Calcium and phosphorus

Total calcium levels vary between 2 and 5 mmol/L in most reptiles. Levels below 2 mmol/L can be seen in gravid female lizards with egg binding and young growing reptiles with MBD. Calcium levels will increase up to fourfold in females producing eggs. Phosphorus levels vary from 0.3 mmol/L to 1.8 mmol/L. Calcium to phosphorus ratios of less than 1:1 have been used to indicate early renal disease, and phosphorus levels are regularly elevated in cases of renal dysfunction. Ionised calcium levels have been shown to be a more accurate assessment of bioavailable calcium. Values of 1.47 mmol/L have been calculated as a mean ionised calcium in green iguanas in one study with no variation with sex or age (Dennis *et al.*, 2001).

Total proteins

These are used to indicate general nutritional status, and liver function. Dry chemistry techniques are not accurate for albumen and globulin levels. Values of total protein of 30–80 g/L have been quoted as normal. Plasma protein electrophoresis results in reptiles are proving promising in diagnosing early inflammatory disease, as has been documented in birds and mammals.

Other parameters

B-hydroxybutyrate (BHB) may be used in chelonia to assess the severity of ketosis during PHA, and these may be found in the urine, causing it to become acidic in nature (herbivorous reptile urine should be alkaline as with mammals). It is thought to be a good indicator of ketogenesis in reptiles and in desert tortoises (*Gopherus agassizii*), plasma levels varied from 0.4–0.75 mmol/L in times of significant rainfall (and food availability) but increased to 2.0 mmol/L after two months of drought (Christopher *et al.*, 1994). In contrast, ketogenesis did not appear to be important during hibernation.

Urinalysis

Urine pH may be measured to give an indication of catabolism in herbivores, as well as looking for BHB to diagnose ketosis in PHA chelonia cases. Urine specific gravity is likely to provide a sensitive indication of hydration status (Gibbons, 2000).

Specific gravity varies from 1.003–10.14 in most normal reptiles (Innis, 1997). Uric acid crystals and bacteria are normal findings, as urine is not sterile in reptiles owing to the mixing of urine and faeces in the cloaca. The presence of renal casts indicates renal disease, although leukocytes and low numbers of erythrocytes are not uncommonly seen in healthy reptiles.

Diseases of amphibians

Bacterial

Redleg

Redleg is caused by the bacteria *Aeromonas* spp. It produces ulcerating red wounds, which give it its name (Figure 21.18). The bacteria also cause a septicaemic syndrome with the amphibian becoming bloated and developing renal and hepatic failure. Poor environmental conditions are often blamed.

Mycobacteria

Mycobacterial infections due to environmental species such as *Mycobacterium marinum* cause classical tuberculous lesions mainly on the limbs or internal organs. The affected amphibian loses weight rapidly, becoming emaciated. There is no effective treatment.

Flavobacterium

These Gram-negative, yellow pigment–producing bacteria are widely present in aquatic environments and are a known cause of oedema disease in adult amphibians producing a syndrome which resembles some viral conditions and dermatosepticaemia. Diagnosis is based on detection of the bacteria either after culture or using PCR technology.

Chlamydiosis

The bacteria *Chlamydophila* spp. have been associated with disease in large Anurans including the European common frog. Clinical signs including petechiation, sloughing of the skin and abdominal swelling. Diagnosis is based on clinical signs, use of generic PCR tests on swabs of affected areas for chlamydophilal organisms and histopathology.

Fungal

Chytridiomycosis

This is the single most important fungal disease affecting amphibians in the world today and has resulted in a massive decline in amphibian numbers. The organism is *Batrachochytrium dendrobatidis* and may be diagnosed from a ventrum swab of the amphibian using a PCR test offered by the Institute of Zoology, Regent's Park, London. The fungus produces skin ulceration, and invades deeper tissues resulting in dehydration, secondary bacterial infections and death.

Saprolegniasis

This is a common environmental fungal disease seen in all aquatic species. It is seen classically as strands of white, cotton wool-like material adhering to the skin surface. The condition is worsened in warmer waters.

Phycomycosis

This is due to common moulds such as *Mucor* spp. These are often darkly pigmented. These moulds will often affect amphibian eggs.

Viral

Herpesvirus

A herpesvirus in the North American leopard frog induces a form of renal adenocarcinoma, known as Lucke's renal tumour. The tumour grows during the warmer months, with the virus being shed in the spring to infect other frogs. Renal failure occurs with chronic weight loss and death. There is no treatment for this condition.

Tadpole oedema virus

Again this is thought to be due to a Ranavirus in the family Iridoviridae. As its name suggests it produces oedema

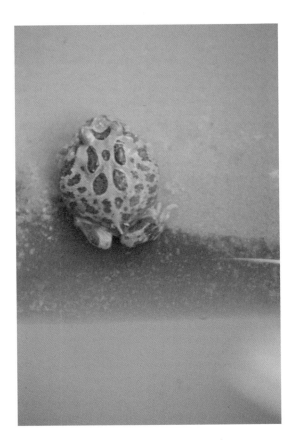

Figure 21.18 Redleg in an Argentinean horned toad (*Ceratophrys ornata*).

in affected tadpoles and internal haemorrhage. There is no treatment.

Spindly leg syndrome

This has been associated with a Ranavirus in the family Iridoviridae but other causes of this condition have also been suggested, such as poor diet – particularly vitamin B deficiencies. As its name suggests, it affects mainly young growing anurans by causing a failure in the development of the forelimbs. Once developed there is no treatment.

Parasitic
Nematodes

The commonest nematode seen in anurans is the lungworm *Rhabdias* spp. In large numbers, this parasite may cause pneumonia. The parasite has a direct life cycle.

Other nematodes of the Strongyloides family may parasitise the gut and coelomic cavity, with large burdens resulting in poor growth and intestinal blockages.

Protozoa

Entamoeba ranarum: Can cause damage to the large intestine of anurans, as well as the liver. These may lead to weight loss, diarrhoea with blood, anorexia and dehydration. It can also cause nephritis with ascites and oedema of the limbs.

Oodinium pillularis: Is a motile protozoan which affects many aquatic animals including amphibians. It damages the skin, and in tadpole stages damages the gills leading to anoxia. It is able to swim through the water from amphibian to amphibian and can therefore spread rapidly.

Metabolic bone disease

This is common, particularly in frogs and toads (anurans). There is often softening of the lower jaw which bulges laterally, weakness and paralysis of the limbs, with spontaneous fractures.

References

Abarca, M.L., Martorell, J., Castella, G., Ramis, A. and Cabanes, F.J. (2009) Dermatomycosis in a pet inland bearded dragon (*Pogona vitticeps*) caused by a Chrysosporium species related to *Nannizziopsis vriesii*. *Veterinary Dermatology*, **20**(4), 295–299.

Austwick, P. and Keymer, I. (1981) Fungi and Actinomycetes. *Diseases of the Reptilia* (eds J.E. Cooper & O.F. Jackson), pp. 93–231. Academic Press, San Diego, CA.

Barten, S. (1980) Cardiomyopathy in a kingsnake (*Lampropeltis calligaster rhombomaculata*). *Veterinary Medicine Small Animal Clinics*, **75**, 125–129.

Bowman, M.R., Pare, J.A., Sigler, L., *et al.* (2007) Deep fungal dermatitis in three inland bearded dragons (*Pogona vitticeps*) caused by the Chrysosporium anamorph of *Nannizziopsis vriesii*. *Medical Mycology*, **45**(4), 371–376.

Cheatwood, J.L., Jacobson, E.R., May, P.G., *et al.* (2003) An outbreak of fungal dermatitis and stomatitis in free-ranging population of pigmy rattlesnakes (*Sistrurus miliarius barbouri*) in Florida. *Journal of Wildlife Diseases*, **39**(2), 329–337.

Christopher, M.M., Brigmon, R. and Jacobsen, E. (1994) Seasonal alterations in plasma beta-hydroxybutyrate and related biochemical parameters in the desert tortoise *Gopherus agassizi*. *Compendium of Biochemical Physiology*, **108**, 303–310.

Dennis, P.M., Bennett, R.A., Harr, K.E., *et al.* (2001) Plasma concentration of ionized calcium in healthy iguanas. *Journal of American Veterinary Medical Association*, **219**(3), 326–328.

Diaz-Figueroa, O., Mitchell, M.A., Ramirez, S., Hananeh, W., Kim, D.Y. and Taylor, W. (2008) *Paecilomyces lilacinus* pneumonia in a free-ranging Gopher tortoise, *Gopherus polyphemus*. *Journal of Herpetological Medicine and Surgery*, **18**(2), 52–60.

Fraser, M.A. and Girling, S.J. (2004) Dermatology. *BSAVA Manual of Reptiles* (eds S.J. Girling & P. Raiti), 2nd edn, pp. 184–198. BSAVA, Quedgeley, UK.

Frost, J.W. and Schmidt, A. (1997) Serological evidence for susceptibility of various species of tortoises to infections by herpesvirus. *Verh Ber Erkrg Zootiere*, **38**, 25–28.

Frye, F. (1991) *Biomedical and Surgical Aspects of Captive Reptile Husbandry*, Volume 1. Krieger Publishing, Malabar, FL.

Frye, F.L. (1999) Spontaneous autoimmune pancreatitis and diabetes mellitus in a Western pond turtle *Clemmys m. marmorata*. *Proceedings of the Association of Reptilian and Amphibian Veterinarians,* Columbus, OH, pp. 103–106.

Garner, M.M., Gardiner, C.H., Wellehan, J.F.X., *et al.* (2006) Intranuclear coccidiosis in tortoises: nine cases. *Veterinary Pathology*, **43**, 311–320.

Gibbons, P.M. (2000) Urinalysis in Box Turtles. *Proc ARAV Reno*, Nevada, 2000, pp. 161–165.

Girling, S.J. (2002) A fungal granuloma in a corn snake (*Elaphe guttata guttata*) due to *Aspergillus fumigatus* associated with a previously treated abscess. *British Veterinary Zoological Society ZooMed Bulletin*, **2**(1), 27–35.

Girling, S.J. and Fraser, M.A. (2009) Treatment of *Aspergillus* species infection in reptiles with itraconazole at metabolically scaled dosages. *Veterinary Record*, **165**(2), 52–54.

Girling, S.J. and Fraser, M.A. (2007) Systemic mycobacteriosis in an Inland Bearded Dragon (*Pogona vitticeps*). *Veterinary Record*, **160**, 526–528.

Gonzalez Cabo, J.F., Espejo Serrano, J. and Barcena Asensio, M.C. (1995) Mycotic pulmonary disease by *Beauveria bassiana* in a captive tortoise. *Mycoses*, **38**(3–4), 167–169.

Harkewicz, K.A. (2001) Dermatology of reptiles: a clinical approach to diagnosis and treatment. *Veterinary Clinics of North America: Exotic Animal Practice*, **4**, 441–461.

Heard, D.J., Cantor, G.H., Jacobson, E.R., *et al.* (1986) Hyalophomycosis caused by *Paecilomyces lilacinus* in an Aldabran tortoise. *Journal of the American Veterinary Medical Association*, **189**, 1143–1145.

Heatley, J.J., Mitchell, M.A., Williams, J., Smith, J.A. and Tully, T.N. (2001) Fungal periodontal osteomyelitis in a chameleon *Furcifer pardalis*. *Journal of Herpetological Medicine and Surgery*, **11**(4), 7–12.

Hernandez-Divers, S.J., Knott, C.D. and MacDonald, J. (2001) Diagnosis and surgical treatment of thyroid adenoma-induced hyperthyroidism in a green iguana (*Iguana iguana*). *Journal of Zoo and Wildlife Medicine*, **32**, 465–475.

Hough, I. (1998) Cryptococcosis in an Eastern water skink. *Australian Veterinary Journal*, **76**(7), 471–472.

Huchzermeyer, F.W. and Cooper, J.E. (2001) Fibriscess, not abscess, resulting from localised inflammatory response to infection in reptiles and birds. *Veterinary Record*, **147**, 515–516.

Innis, C.J. (1997) Observations on urinalysis of clinically normal captive tortoises. *Proceedings of the Association of Reptilian and Amphibian Veterinarians*, Houston, TX, pp. 109–112.

Jacobson, E.R. (1980) Mycotic Diseases of Reptiles. *The Comparative Pathology of Zoo Animals* (eds R.J. Montali & G. Migaki), pp. 283–290. Smithsonian Institution Press, Washington, DC.

Jacobson, E.R. and Gardiner, C.H. (1990) Adeno-like virus in oesophageal and tracheal mucosa of a Jackson's chameleon (*Chameleo jacksonii*). *Veterinary Pathology*, **27**, 210–212.

Klaphake, E. (2010) A fresh look at metabolic bone diseases in reptiles and amphibians. *Veterinary Clinics of North America: Exotic Animal Practice*, **13**, 375–392.

Koplos, P., Garner, M., Besser, T., Nordhausen, R. and Monaco, R. (2000) Cheilitis in lizards of the Genus *Uromastyx* associated with filamentous Gram positive bacterium. *Proceedings of the Association of Reptile and Amphibian Veterinarians*, pp. 73–75.

Lappin, P.B. and Dunstan, R.W. (1992) Difficult dermatologic diagnosis. *Journal of the American Veterinary Medical Association*, **200**, 785–786.

Masters, A.M., Ellis, T.M., Carson, J.M., Sutherland, S.S. and Gregory, A.R. (1995) *Dermatophilus chelonae* sp. nov. isolated from chelonids in Australia. *International Journal of Systemic Bacteriology*, **45**, 50–56.

McArthur, S.D., McLellan, L. and Brown, S. (2004) Gastrointestinal system. *Manual of Reptiles* (eds S.J. Girling & P. Raiti), 2nd edn, pp. 210–229. BSAVA, Quedgeley, UK.

McBride, M., Hernandez-Divers, S.J., Koch, T., *et al.* (2006) Preliminary evaluation of pre and post-prandial 3a hydroxy bile acids in the Green Iguana (*Iguana iguana*). *Journal of Herpetological Medicine and Surgery*, **16**, 129–134.

Migaki, G., Jacobson, E.R. and Casey, H.W. (1984) Fungal diseases in reptiles. *Diseases of Amphibians and Reptiles* (eds G.L. Hoff & E.R. Jacobson), pp. 183–204. Plenum Press, New York.

Nichols, D.K., Weyant, R.S., Lamirande, E.W., Sigler, L. and Mason, R.T. (1999) Fatal mycotic dermatitis in captive brown tree snakes (*Boiga irregularis*). *Journal of Zoo and Wildlife Medicine*, **30**(1), 111–118.

Oros, J., Ramirez, A.S., Poveda, J.B., Rodriguez, J.L. and Fernandez, A. (1996) Systemic mycosis caused by *Penicillium griseofulvum* in a Seychelles giant tortoise (*Megachelys gigantean*). *Veterinary Record*, **139**(12), 295–296.

Pare, J.A., Sigler, L., Hunter, D.B., Summerbell, R.C., Smith, D.A. and Machin, L. (1997) Cutaneous mycoses in chameleons caused by the Chyrsosporium anamorph of *Nannizziopsis vriesii* (Apinis) *Currah. Journal of Zoo and Wildlife Medicine*, **28**(4), 443–453.

Pasmans, K., Hellebuyck, T., Haesebrouck, F. and Martel, A. (2010) Dermatitis and septicaemia caused by *Devriesea agamarum*: an overview including recent developments in disease management. *Proceedings of the 1st International Conference on Reptile and Amphibian Medicine*, Munich, Germany, pp. 105–106.

Pees, M., Schroff, S., Kiefer, I. and Krautwald-Junghanns, M.E. (2010) Ultrasonopgraphic examination of the heart and the great vessels in boid snakes and demonstration of a case of valvular insufficiency in a Burmese python (*Python molorus bivittatus*). *Proceedings of the 1st International Conference on Reptile and Amphibian Medicine*, Munich, pp. 211–212.

Penner, J.D., Jacobson, E.R. and Brown, D.R. (1997). A novel *Mycoplasma* sp. associated with proliferative tracheitis and pneumonia in a Burmese python (*Python molurus bivittatus*). *Journal of Comparative Pathology*, **117**, 283–288.

Potgieter, L.N., Sigler, R.E., and Russell R.G. (1987). Pneumonia in Ottoman vipers (*Vipera xanthena xanthena*) associated with a parainfluenza 2-like virus. *Journal of Wildlife Diseases*, **23**, 355–360.

Redrobe, S.P. & Frye, F.L. (2001) Hepatic thrombosis and other pathology associated with severe periodontal disease in the Bearded dragon, *Pogona vitticeps*. *Proceedings ARAV*, Orlando, FL, pp. 217–219.

Rossi, J. and Rossi, R. (2000) Fungal dermatitis in a large collection of Brazos water snakes, Nerodia harteri harteri housed in an outdoor enclosure, and a possible association with slugs. *Proceedings of the Association of Reptilian and Amphibian Veterinarians* (eds M.M. Willette & L.C. Boyer), pp. 81–83 Reno, Nevada.

Schilliger, L., Lemberger, K., Bourgeois, A. and Charpentier, M. (2010) First case of atherosclerosis associated with pericardial effusion in a Bearded dragon (*Pogona vitticeps* AHL 1926). *Proceedings of the Annual Conference of the Association of Reptilian and Amphibian Veterinarians*, pp. 70–74.

Schmidt, R.E. and Reavill, D.R. (2010) Metastatic chondrosarcoma in a corn snake (*Elaphe guttata*). *Proceedings of the 1st International Conference on Reptile Amphibian Medicine*, Munich, Germany, p. 147.

Schuchman, S.M. and Taylor, D.O. (1970). Arteriosclerosis in an iguana (*Iguana iguana*). *Journal of the American Veterinary Medical Association*, **157**, 614–616.

Schumacher, J. (2003) Fungal diseases of reptiles. *Veterinary Clinics of North America: Exotic Animal Practice*, **6**(2), 327–355.

Schumacher, J.R., Bennett, A., Fox, L.E., *et al.* (1998) Mast cell tumor in an eastern kingsnake (*Lampropeltis getulus getulus*). *Journal of Veterinary Diagnostic Investigation*, **10**, 101–104.

Soares, J.F., Chalker, V.J., Erles, K., Holtby, S., Waters, M. and McArthur, S. (2003) Prevalence of *Mycoplasma agassizii* and chelonian Herpesvirus in captive tortoise (*Testudo* spp.) in the United Kingdom. *Proceedings of the Association of Reptilian and Amphibian Veterinarians*, p. 91.

Stahl, S.J. (2003) Pet lizard conditions and syndromes. *Seminars in Avian and Exotic Pet Medicine*, **12**(3), 162–182.

Tappe, J.P, Chandler, F.W., Lui, S.K. and Dolensk, E.P. (1984) Aspergillosis in two San Esteban Chuckwallas. *Journal of the American Veterinary Medical Association*, **185**(11), 1425–1428.

Wagner, J. (1989) Clinical challenge case number one. *Journal of Zoo and Wildlife Medicine*, **20**, 238–239.

Weitzman, I., Rosenthal, S.A. and Shupack, J.L. (1985) A comparison between *Dactylaria gallopava* and *Scolecobasidium humicola*: first report of an infection in a tortoise caused by *S. humicola. Sabouraudia*, **23**(4), 287–293.

Westhouse, R.A., Jacobson, E.R., Harris, R.K., *et al.* (1996). Respiratory and pharyngoesophageal iridovirus infection in a gopher tortoise (Gopherus polyphemus). *Journal of Wildlife Diseases*, **32**, 682–686.

Wiesner, C.S. and Iben, C. (2003) Influence of environmental humidity and dietary protein on pyramidal growth of carapaces in African spurred tortoises (*Geochelone sulcata*). *Journal of Animal Physiology and Animal Nutrition*, **87**, 66–74.

Zwart, P. (2006) Renal pathology in reptiles. *Veterinary Clinics of North America: Exotic Animal Practice*, **9**, 129–159.

Chapter 22

An Overview of Reptile and Amphibian Therapeutics

FLUID THERAPY
Maintenance requirements

Every reptile or amphibian has a fluid maintenance requirement. These losses, as for cats and dogs, occur in several ways; for example, urine output, insensible losses through respiration, panting (i.e., gular fluttering) and salivation.

In most reptiles very little water is lost through the skin; reptiles have little to no true sweat glands. Amphibians, however, will lose fluid readily across their semi-permeable skin membranes, and so need to remain close to a water source for nearly all of their lives.

Some reptiles will lose water through gular fluttering; for example, members of the Crocodylia as well as many desert-dwelling lizards.

Reptiles are extremely good at conserving water. Most species are uricotelic, excreting uric acid instead of urea as their main form of urinary protein waste product. Uric acid requires very little water to be excreted with it, unlike urea in mammals, and so maintenance requirements are very much lower for these reptiles than mammals. Many aquatic and semi-aquatic species of reptile excrete ammonia and urea. In the case of totally aquatic amphibian species such as caecilians, ammonia is excreted, whereas the more terrestrial amphibian species such as toads excrete urea and one or two may produce uric acid.

Maintenance requirements can vary widely. A desert-dwelling, uricotelic species may be able to cope with some water deprivation, while an ammonotelic species, such as an aquatic turtle or amphibian, is used to large, regular fluid intakes and outputs and therefore has a higher maintenance requirement.

However, if a uricotelic reptile is deprived of water for prolonged periods of time, uric acid waste will not be excreted. This leads to a buildup of uric acid in the bloodstream. Once levels exceed 1200–1500 μmol/L of uric acid, precipitation of uric acid crystals occurs inside the body, a condition known as 'visceral gout'. Once uric acid crystals are deposited in and around vital organs, such as the kidneys and heart, they cannot be removed and permanent damage has been done.

The volume of water consumed daily varies from species to species as do the sources of water. Herbivorous reptiles such as Mediterranean tortoises get the majority of their daily fluid requirement from their diet. However, other herbivorous species, such as the green iguana, are used to living in tropical rainforest conditions where the relative humidity is 100%. Place this reptile into an arid vivarium and it will, with time, lose fluid through its skin if it is not also provided with daily misting of its tank. Many reptiles will not drink from water bowls, only taking water from droplets on leaves in the wild; for example, many chameleons as well as the green iguana.

To add to this, whenever ectothermic species such as reptiles are kept, it is important to take into account the environmental temperature requirements of that species. If the reptile is not kept within its preferred optimum temperature zone (POTZ), then it cannot achieve its preferred body temperature (PBT) and its internal physiological processes will not operate at their optimal rates, leading to inefficient water usage and consumption. A list of optimum temperature requirements can be found on page in Table 22.1.

The effect of disease on fluid requirements

Fluid loss may be rapid, due to water loss alone, for example, with acute diarrhoea, thermal burns or vomiting. In this case, the remaining extracellular fluid (ECF) becomes reduced, but is still of the same composition (isotonic). Alternatively, fluid loss may be due to long-term anorexia, producing a reduction in electrolytes and creating a hypotonic ECF. Finally, water deprivation or oral trauma preventing drinking will lead to increases in the tonicity of the ECF, and create a hypertonic dehydration.

With any disease, the need for fluids increases, even if no obvious fluid loss has occurred. This is due to

Veterinary Nursing of Exotic Pets, Second Edition. Edited by Simon J. Girling. © 2013 John Wiley & Sons, Ltd. Published 2013 by John Wiley & Sons, Ltd.

Table 22.1 Examples of normal packed cell volumes (PCV) and total blood proteins in selected species of reptiles.

Species	PCV L/L	Total protein (g/L)
Green iguana (*Iguana iguana*)	0.25–0.38	28–69
Tortoise (*Testudo* spp.)	0.19–0.4	32–50
Rat snake (*Elaphe* spp.)	0.2–0.3	30–60
Boa constrictor (*Boa constrictor constrictor*)	0.2–0.32	46–60

a number of reasons. It may involve renal changes, such as increases in the glomerular filtration rate or reduction in water reabsorption by the collecting ducts so causing increased urine output. Or there may be reduced absorption of water from the small or large intestine.

Respiratory disease is common in reptiles, with increased respiratory secretions being the result. Fluid loss via this route can be appreciable.

Another less obvious route is fluid and electrolyte loss through skin disease. Reptiles often suffer from serious burns from unprotected basking lamps and faulty heaters. Not only will there be serious fluid and electrolyte loss via full-thickness skin burns but these reptiles will succumb to secondary skin infections from environmental bacteria such as *Pseudomonas* spp. These produce lesions which resemble chemical or thermal burns, and leave large areas of weeping exudative skin for further fluid loss.

Finally, we have to consider the need for fluid therapy during other forms of medical therapy, such as antibiotic treatment. Many bacterial infections in reptiles are caused by Gram-negative bacteria; therefore, the aminoglycoside family of antibiotics (gentamicin, tobramycin, amikacin etc.) has been widely used for treatment. This family of antibiotics has several serious side effects. The most serious of these is renal damage. This can happen if there is reduced renal perfusion because of dehydration. The renal damage so caused can be strong enough to kill even a healthy reptile.

Post-surgical fluid requirements

Causes of fluid loss include the possibility of intrasurgical haemorrhaging. This will call for vascular support with an aqueous electrolyte solution or, in more serious blood losses (greater than 10% blood volume), colloidal fluids or even blood transfusions.

Even if surgery is relatively bloodless, there are inevitable losses via the respiratory route. This is due to the drying nature of gases used in anaesthesia. As many of these species are small in size, they have a large lung surface area in relation to volume and hence a greater loss of fluid per unit time/per breath than larger animals. To exacerbate the situation, many patients are not able to drink immediately after surgery, and so the period without water or food intake may stretch to several hours. Finally, some forms of surgery will lead to inappetence for a period, for example, oral surgery.

Electrolyte replacement

Other diseases, such as diarrhoea, will cause fluid loss and metabolic acidosis due to the prolonged loss of bicarbonate. This is often due to parasitism, such as amoebiasis, in snakes. There may also be chronic losses of potassium, in cases of chronic diarrhoea, due to the reduced absorption of this electrolyte by the large intestine.

Snakes will vomit after a meal if stressed, and may suffer from diseases of the stomach such as cryptosporidiosis, causing loss of fluid and hydrogen ions, and a resultant metabolic alkalosis. Other reptiles such as tortoises will rarely vomit, so the likelihood of fluid loss via this route is less common.

Fluids used in reptilian practice

Lactated Ringer's/Hartmann's

As with cats and dogs, lactated Ringer's solution is useful as a general purpose rehydration and maintenance fluid. It is particularly useful for reptiles and amphibians suffering from metabolic acidosis, such as those described above with chronic gastrointestinal problems, but can also be used for fluid therapy after routine surgical procedures.

Glucose/saline combinations

Glucose/saline combinations are useful for reptiles and amphibians, as they may have been through periods of anorexia prior to treatment, and therefore may well be borderline hypoglycaemic.

There is some evidence that in reptiles, and probably amphibians, the isotonicity of the ECFs is lower than that of mammals. Studies on non-marine reptiles suggest that isotonicity for the majority is 0.8% rather than the 0.9% saline assumed for mammals. Because of this, a number of fluid combinations utilising the above two types of crystalloid support have been derived as follows:

- One-third each of 5% glucose with 0.9% saline, lactated Ringer's solution and sterile water and
- Nine parts 5% glucose with 0.9% saline to one part sterile water.

Many texts still advise that straightforward, undiluted lactated Ringer's solution or 4% glucose with 0.18% saline may be used, and glucose/saline solutions are particularly useful for amphibia, where the use of potassium-containing fluids should be avoided initially.

It is important that whatever fluid is administered, it be warmed to the reptile or amphibian's PBT (approximately 30–35°C) before being given.

Hypertonic saline

This may be used in reptiles with acute hypovolaemia. It works by rapidly drawing fluid from the cellular and pericellular space into the circulation to support central venous pressure. See Chapter 24 on reptile emergency and critical care medicine for further details of its use. It must be administered intravenously or intraosseously.

Protein amino acid/B vitamin supplements

Protein and vitamin supplements are useful for nutritional support. Products such as Duphalyte® (Fort Dodge) may be used at the rate of 1 mL/kg/day. They are used to replace nutrients in cases where the patient is malnourished or has been suffering from protein-losing enteropathy, such as may occur with heavy parasitism, or a protein-losing nephropathy, as in renal failure. It is also a useful supplement for patients with hepatic disease or severe exudative skin diseases, such as heater burns, in which blood proteins will be reduced.

Colloidal fluids

Colloidal fluids have been used in reptilian practice when intravenous administration has been possible. This limits their usefulness, as some reptiles are just too small to gain full vascular access, although there is some evidence that they may be used via the intraosseous route. They are used when a serious loss of blood occurs, in order to support central blood pressure. This may be a temporary measure whilst a blood donor is selected, or, if none is available, the only means of attempting to support such a patient. Use of Hetastarch® which has a larger colloid particle size and so stays in the circulation for up to 24 hours is preferred where this is available. See Chapter 24 for shock fluid therapy.

Blood transfusions

Blood transfusions are indicated when the packed cell volume (PCV) has dropped below 0.05–0.1 L/L, and they may be given via intravenous or intraosseous routes. Cross-matching of blood groups does not appear to be necessary for one-off transfusions, but the same species should be used each time; that is, green iguana to green iguana, boa constrictor to boa constrictor. Up to 2% body weight as blood may be taken from healthy species (Klingenberg, 1996), preferably into a pre-heparinised or citrate–phosphate anticoagulant-coated syringe before immediately transfusing into the recipient.

Oral fluids and electrolytes

Oral fluid administration may also be used in reptile and amphibian practice for those patients experiencing mild dehydration, and for home administration. Many products are available for cats and dogs, and may be used for reptiles. However, as with the crystalloid fluids, it is advisable to dilute these oral electrolytes by approximately 10%, otherwise their concentration will be greater than the reptile's ECF and so water will move from the body into the gastrointestinal tract rather than the other way around. The inclusion of a probiotic/prebiotic with the electrolytes may aid recovery by normalising gut flora and digestion.

Calculation of fluid requirements

Fluid requirements may be calculated as for cats and dogs. It is worth noting that a lot of the fluid intake is normally consumed in food, for example, in the form of fresh vegetation for herbivorous species. This is difficult to take into consideration, and therefore it is safer to assume that the debilitated reptile will not be eating significant enough amounts for this to matter in the calculation. In any case, levels of fluid replacement rates have received relatively little research.

Frye (1991) recommends that levels of 20–25 mL/kg/day be used for hydration purposes in both reptiles and amphibians, and current literature suggests that rates across several species vary from 10–50 mL/kg/day.

The factor that limits the volume of fluids that can be administered is that, although intravenous and intraosseous routes may also be used, most fluids are given intracoelomically to the debilitated reptile. Reptiles and amphibians do not possess true diaphragms; therefore the thorax and abdomen are all interconnected in a coelom. When fluids are placed in this cavity, it is equivalent to giving intraperitoneal fluids to a mammal, but as there is no diaphragm, these fluids can cause pressure to build up on the lungs. Excessive fluids may severely compromise respiration.

Excessive fluids given intravenously or intraosseously may also overload the circulation and cause pulmonary oedema. It can result in cardiac and renal overperfusion and solute wash-out, with potassium in particular being excreted with the increased diuresis causing a hypokalaemic crisis to develop. This may manifest itself initially as an anorectic reptile, but will progress to cardiac arrhythmias, coma and death.

One can assume that 1% dehydration equates with a need to supply 10 mL/kg fluid replacement in addition to the maintenance requirements. It is also possible to make some qualitative assessment of the level of dehydration from the elasticity of the skin. Although reptile skin is not as elastic as mammalian, it should be freely mobile and recoil, albeit slowly, after tenting particularly over the epaxial muscles in snakes, the thigh of lizards and antebrachium of chelonia. Other factors to assess are the brightness of the corneas in species with mobile eyelids. In those without mobile eyelids (e.g., snakes) the collapse of the spectacle (the clear fused eyelids) is suggestive of dehydration. Other assessments of thirst and urate output can be made over 24 hours.

It is possible to estimate the degree of dehydration of a reptile patient as follows:

- 3% dehydrated – increased thirst, slight lethargy, decreased urates
- 7% dehydrated – increased thirst, anorexia, dullness, tenting of the skin with slow return to normal, dull corneas, loss of turgor of spectacles in snakes
- 10% dehydrated – dull to comatose, skin remains tented after pinching, desiccating mucous membranes, sunken eyeballs, no urate/urine output.

The alternative is to compare PCVs and total protein levels to assess dehydration (Table 22.1), again with 1% increase in PCV suggesting 10 mL/kg fluid replacements are needed (this assumes no anaemia in the patient).

It is important not to exceed 25–30 mL/kg/day as a maximum for reasons mentioned above, whatever the level of dehydration of the patient. So rehydration of severely debilitated reptiles may take days to weeks. As with avian patients, therefore, making good the fluid deficit may need to be split over several days.

Equipment for fluid administration

Catheters

Butterfly catheters are very useful for the small and fragile vessels in these patients, as they have a short length of tubing attached to the needle. If the syringe or drip set is connected to this piece of flexible tubing, rather than directly to the catheter, there is less chance of the catheter becoming dislodged if the reptile moves. Also, the piece of clear tubing on the catheter allows you to see when venous access has been achieved, as blood will flow back into this area without the need to draw back thus collapsing the fragile veins.

To make effective use of a butterfly catheter, it is advisable to flush it with heparinised saline prior to use to prevent clotting. 25–27 gauge sizes are recommended. They may also be used to give intracoelomic fluids to reptiles, as the conscious patient may continue to move (particularly a problem in snakes), without dislodging the needle.

For larger patients, such as adult iguanas, monitor lizards and Crocodylia, 21–25 gauge over-the-needle Teflon®-coated catheters can be used.

Hypodermic or spinal needles

Hypodermic needles are useful for the administration of intraosseous, intracoelomic or subcutaneous fluids.

Intraosseous fluids may be the only method of central venous support in very small patients or patients in which vascular collapse is occurring. The proximal femur, tibia or humerus may be used. Entry can be gained using spinal needles. These have a central stylet to prevent clogging of the lumen of the needle with bone fragments after insertion. 23–25 gauge spinal needles are usually sufficient.

Straightforward hypodermic needles may also be used for the same purpose, although the risks of blockage are higher. Hypodermic needles may also be used, of course, for the administration of intracoelomic and subcutaneous fluids. Generally 23–25 gauge hypodermic needles are sufficient for the task.

Pharyngostomy or oesophageal tubes

Pharyngostomy tubes are often used in reptiles in order to provide nutritional support in as stress-free manner as is possible. They are also useful as a route for some fluid administration, as only liquid formulas will pass through these narrow (3.5–6.5 French) tubes. It should be noted though that in severely dehydrated individuals there is a real possibility that gut pathology may exist, so this route may need to be supplemented by others. This route therefore has limited use in facilitating fluid replacement, and is used mainly for nutritional support and rehydrating and replenishing the gut microflora.

Syringe drivers

For continuous fluid administration, as is required for intravenous and intraosseous fluid administration, syringe drivers are advisable. Their advantage is that small volumes, such as a fraction of a millilitre may be administered accurately per hour. An error of 1–2 mL in some of the smaller species dealt with over an hour could be equivalent to over-perfusion of 50–100%! In addition, it is almost impossible to keep gravity-fed drip sets running at these low rates without blockage every few minutes.

Intravenous drip tubing

Particular fine drip tubing is available for attachment to syringes and syringe-driver units. It is useful if these are luer locking as this enhances safety and prevents disconnection when the patient moves.

Routes of fluid administration in reptile

As with cats and dogs, the same medical principles broadly apply with five main routes of administration available as follows:

- Oral
- Subcutaneous
- Intracoelomic
- Intravenous
- Intraosseous.

Table 22.2 gives the advantages and disadvantages of each of the five routes.

Table 22.2 Advantages and disadvantages of various fluid therapies for reptiles and amphibians.

Route of fluid administration	Advantages	Disadvantages
Oral	Minimal stress with experienced handler Physiological route for fluid intake Less risk of tissue trauma Home therapy possible Rapid administration	Stressful with inexperienced handler No use in cases of digestive tract disease May damage stomach if the stomach tube is inserted too roughly Rehydration rates are slow Risk of aspiration pneumonia Limited volumes may be administered at any one time
Subcutaneous	Large volumes may be given at one time Rapid administration possible, minimizing stress Uptake may be better than oral in cases of digestive tract disease Minimal risk of internal organ damage during administration	May be uncomfortable for the patient Risk of muscle and subcutaneous tissue trauma Rates of rehydration poor if severely dehydrated and peripheral vessels are collapsed Only isotonic or hypotonic fluids may be administered Darkening of the skin at the injection site particularly in lizards such as iguanas and chameleons
Intracoelomic	Large volumes may be administered at one time increasing dosing intervals Uptake is faster than subcutaneous Minimally painful route of administration	Large volumes may cause pressure on the lungs (no diaphragm) Rehydration rates may still be slow in severe cases of dehydration Only isotonic or hypotonic fluids may be administered Increased risk of organ damage
Intravenous	Rapid rehydration in even severely dehydrated patients is possible Colloidal and hypertonic fluids and blood transfusions possible Use of intravenous catheters and syringe drivers makes for accurate delivery	Size of reptile may prevent venous access Species of reptile (e.g., snakes) may make venous access difficult without minor surgery Veins are more fragile than mammalian vessels Increased skill levels and equipment required
Intraosseous	Rapid rehydration possible even with collapsed peripheral vasculature Colloidal and hypertonic fluids and blood transfusions possible Use of intraosseous catheters and syringe drivers makes for accurate delivery Useful in smaller species or species where venous access is difficult	Not useful in the presence of infection (osteomyelitis) or metabolic bone disease Sedation, local or general anaesthesia is required for catheter insertion Tolerance may be poor in some species

Oral

Snakes

The oral route is not useful for seriously debilitated animals, but is for those with pharyngostomy feeding tubes in place, or if the owner or handler is experienced in stomach tubing. Mild cases of dehydration, where owners wish to home treat their pet, are ideal. A stomach tube is passed by restraining the snake's head gently but firmly, and then inserting a plastic or wooden tongue depressor to open the mouth. A lubricated feeding tube is then passed through the labial notch (the area at the most rostral aspect of the mouth without teeth) and to a depth of one third of the snake's length.

Lizards

Gavage (stomach) tubes or avian straight crop tubes or straightforward feeding tubes can be used to administer fluids directly into the oesophagus or stomach. The reptile needs to be firmly restrained to keep the head and oesophagus in a straight line. The mouth is opened with a plastic or wooden tongue depressor and the tube inserted to a depth of one third to one half the torso length of the reptile. This method is often stressful for the reptile. The alternative is to syringe fluids into the mouth, but this risks inhalation in a debilitated reptile. A pharyngostomy tube may be placed for nutritional support, and so may be used for fluid therapy.

Chelonians

An oesophagostomy tube may be implanted as described below, and levels of 10 mL/kg at any one time can be administered. Alternatively, a stomach tube may be inserted each time it is needed. The feeding tube is first measured from the tip of the extended nose to the line where the pectoral and abdominal ventral scutes connect. It can then be lubricated and passed after extending the head and gently prising the mouth open with a wooden or plastic speculum (Figure 22.1).

Placement of oesophagostomy tubes: Oesophagostomy tubes may be placed in any species of reptile, but are particularly useful in chelonians which can retract its head deep inside its shell, making repeated stomach tubing impossible. It also significantly reduces the stress and trauma of repeatedly passing a stomach tube in long-term anorectic reptile patients.

The steps for placement are as follows:

1. Sedation or anaesthesia is required and good analgesia post implantation.

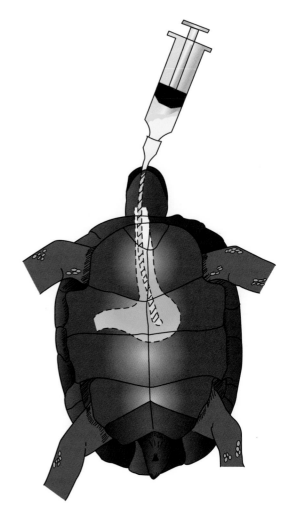

Figure 22.1 Placement and depth of insertion of a stomach tube in a chelonian.

2. Surgically prepare the site with 0.25–0.5% povidone-iodine, being particularly scrupulous as reptile skin is notoriously dirty. In chelonians, the implantation site is the ventral aspect of the lateral neck, 3–4 cm caudal to the angle of the jaw. In snakes and lizards it is the ventrolateral aspect of the throat region, 5–10 cm caudal to the angle of the jaw.

3. A pair of curved haemostats is placed in through the mouth and pushed laterally and ventrally, tenting the skin above them.

4. A sharp incision is made with a scalpel blade, over the point of the haemostats, through the skin and the underlying muscle.

5. The tubing, preferably as large a diameter as will comfortably fit down the oesophagus (Foley catheters are

useful in tortoises), is grasped with the haemostats as they protrude out through the incision, and then pulled into the pharynx and pushed down into the oesophagus.

NB: The tube should be measured prior to implantation so the depth of insertion is known. It is measured in tortoises from the site of the tube incision to the midportion of the plastron, halfway through the abdominal scutes. A further length should then be allowed, in order to attach the end of the feeding tube to the dorsal aspect of the carapace.

6. Once in place, two pieces of zinc oxide tape may be attached to the tube close to the skin surface. Through this, sutures may be placed, attaching this to the skin itself. The tube may then be attached to the midline cranial carapace in tortoises, or taped to the side of the neck for snakes and reptiles, and a bung inserted (Figures 22.2a and 22.2b). Care of the tube is as for nasogastric tubes in cats and dogs, that is, plain water should be flushed through the tube prior to administering food to ensure correct placement. This should also be done after feeding to flush food debris out of the tube.

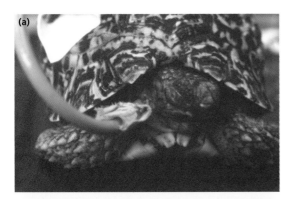

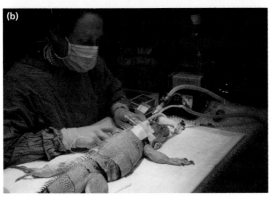

Figure 22.2 (a) An oesophagostomy tube in place in an anorectic leopard tortoise (*Stigmochelys pardalis*). **(b)** An oesophagostomy tube in place in an anorectic green iguana (*Iguana iguana*).

Subcutaneous
Snakes

The lateral aspect of the dorsum of the snake, in the caudal third of its body, is the ideal site for subcutaneous fluid administration. This is a good technique for use for routine post-operative administration of fluids to patients undergoing minor surgical procedures such as skin mass removals. If positioned correctly, there is a lymph sinus running lateral to the epaxial muscles on either side, just subcutaneously, which can be used for moderately large volumes. It may, however, still be necessary to use several sites.

Lizards

The lateral thoracic area is easily used for smaller volumes of fluids at any one site. There is a risk of the reptile developing a darkened, pigmented area over the injection site, particularly in chameleons.

Chelonians

The subcutaneous route is easily used for post-operative fluids and mild dehydration in this species. Fluids may be given in the area just cranial to the hind limbs, or in the skin folds just lateral to the neck. Relatively large volumes may be given via this route.

Intracoelomic
Snakes

The intracoelomic route is useful for more seriously dehydrated reptiles, as there is a greater vasculature at this site for absorption. The needle or butterfly catheter is inserted two rows of lateral scales dorsal to the ventral scutes in the caudal third of the snake, but cranial to the vent. The needle is inserted so that it just penetrates the body wall, the plunger of the syringe is pulled back to ensure no organ puncture has occurred and the fluids administered. If correctly inserted, there will be no resistance to the injection.

Lizards

Because of the positioning necessary for administration, the intracoelomic route may be a stressful method of fluid administration. As for small mammals, the lizard should be placed in dorsal recumbency with its head downwards to encourage the gut contents to fall cranially and away from the injection site. The needle, preferably 25 gauge or smaller, is advanced slowly to just pop through the abdominal wall in the lower right ventral quadrant. The syringe plunger should be pulled back to ensure that no organ has been penetrated, and the fluids can be administered without any resistance.

Chelonians

The intracoelomic route can be used in tortoises up to a maximum of 20–25 mL/kg/day only; otherwise, due to the confines of the rigid shell, the fluids will place too much pressure on the lung fields. The area cranial to the hind limbs is used, that is, the same site as for subcutaneous routes, but the chief difference is depth. The concern with this route is that the bladder lies in this area, and if full may be punctured. The other route is the cranial access site. This is located lateral to the neck and medial to the front limb and is more epicoelomic than truly intracoelomic. The needle is kept close and parallel to the plastron and a 3/4-inch needle may be inserted to the level of the hub.

Intravenous

Snakes

There are no major vessels for intravenous use in snakes which are easily accessible. If an intravenous route is to be used, one of the following is required.

Ventral tail vein: This is more of a plexus of veins, and may be accessed from the ventrum. The needle is inserted midline, one-third of the tail length from the vent, and advanced until it touches the coccygeal vertebrae at a 90-degree angle. The needle is then retracted slightly whilst drawing back on the syringe until blood flows into the hub. Fluids may then be given slowly.

Palatine vein: This is present on the roof of the mouth, as its name suggests, and is paired. Cannulation may be performed with a 25–27 gauge butterfly catheter although the snake has to be sedated or anaesthetised to gain access.

Jugular vein: These can only be accessed in an anesthetised or sedated snake. A full-thickness skin cut-down procedure is performed 5–7.5 cm caudal to the angle of the jaw, two rows of scales dorsal to the ventral scutes. The jugular vein can then be seen medial to the ribs. An over-the-needle catheter is best for this, and should then be sutured in place.

Intracardiac: This site can be used in emergencies. The heart may be catheterised under sedation or anaesthesia only. On turning the snake onto its back, the heart may be seen to beat against the ventral scale, approximately one quarter of its length from the snout. A 25–27 gauge over-the-needle catheter may be inserted between the scales, ventrally, in a caudocranial manner at 30 degrees to the body wall into the single ventricle. A bolus may be administered, or it may be taped, glued or sutured in place for 24–48 hours.

Lizards

The intravenous route can be difficult in small lizards, and frequently requires sedation or anaesthesia. Several veins may be tried.

Cephalic vein: This is approached in the anaesthetised lizard by performing a cut-down procedure on the cranial aspect of the middle of the antebrachium, perpendicular to the long axis of the radius and ulna. The vessel may then be catheterised using an over-the-needle catheter, which is then sutured in place. This technique is really only useful for lizards over 0.25 kg in weight.

Jugular vein: This vessel may be accessed via a cut-down technique in the anaesthetised or sedated lizard. An incision is made in a craniocaudal direction 2.5 cm caudal to the angle of the jaw. An over-the-needle catheter may then be sutured in place.

Ventral tail vein: This is more of a plexus of veins. It is accessed from the ventral aspect of the tail and can be performed in the conscious lizard. It is frequently only suitable for one-off bolus injections, and special care should be taken with species which exhibit autotomy (spontaneous tail shedding). The needle is inserted at 90 degrees to the angle of the tail and advanced until it touches the coccygeal vertebrae. It is then withdrawn slightly while drawing back on the syringe. When blood flows into the syringe, the infusion may begin (Figure 22.3).

Chelonians

There are two main intravenous routes: the dorsal tail vein and the jugular veins.

Jugular vein: These may be accessed for catheter placement in the sedated or anaesthetised tortoise. The neck is extended and the head tilted away from the operator to push the neck towards him or her. The jugular vein runs from the dorsal aspect of the eardrum along the more dorsal aspect of the neck (Figure 22.4). An over-the-needle catheter may be placed directly, or, in thicker-skinned animals, a cut-down technique employed.

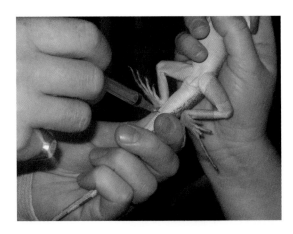

Figure 22.3 Basilisk restrained for ventral tail vein fluid administration or blood sampling.

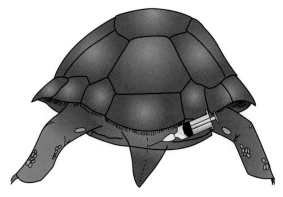

Figure 22.5 Access to dorsal tail vein in chelonian for fluid administration or blood sampling.

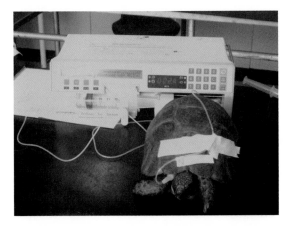

Figure 22.4 Placement of a jugular catheter in a chelonian. Note the taping of the drip tubing to the dorsal carapace midline and the attachment to the syringe driver.

Dorsal tail vein: This is more of a plexus of veins. Therefore it is often not possible to give large volumes of fluids, and certainly not possible to place a catheter. Access is midline, on the dorsal aspect of the tail. The needle is inserted at a 90-degree angle until it hits the coccygeal vertebrae. The needle is then pulled back, drawing back on the syringe at the same time, until blood flows into the hub (Figure 22.5).

Intraosseous

Snakes

The intraosseous route is not possible in the snake.

Lizards

The intraosseous is a good route for smaller species of lizards, where venous access is restricted or difficult. There are a few access points to choose from. Hypodermic or spinal needles of 23–25 gauge sizes may be used.

Proximal femur: This may be accessed from the fossa created between the greater trochanter and the hip joint. This route may be difficult due to the 90-degree angle the femur often forms with the pelvis.

Distal femur: This is relatively easy to access from above the stifle joint. It does restrict the movement of the stifle, but it is easier to bandage the catheter into this site and access to the medullary cavity of the femur is certainly easier via this route. Sedation or anaesthesia is required. See below for the placement technique.

Proximal tibia: This again is possible in the larger species. Anaesthesia and sedation is needed, and the spinal needle or hypodermic needle may be screwed into the tibial crest region in a proximodistal manner.

Placement of distal femoral intraosseous catheters in lizards (Figure 22.6): The technique for placement of a distal femoral intraosseous catheter in a lizard is explained in detail below.

1. Sedation or anaesthesia (local or general) is needed, and in all cases it is advised that good analgesia is administered.
2. Surgically scrub the area overlying the craniolateral aspect of the stifle joint using dilute povidone-iodine. It is important that placement of the catheter or needle is performed as aseptically as possible.
3. Take a 20–23 gauge spinal or hypodermic needle and insert it through the ridge just proximal to the stifle joint, screwing it into the bone in the direction of the long axis of the femur proximally.

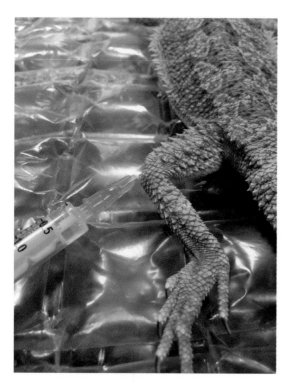

Figure 22.6 Distal femoral intraosseous fluid administration in an inland bearded dragon (*Pogona vitticeps*).

4. Flush the needle with heparinised saline (the advantage of a spinal needle is that it has a central stylet which helps prevent it from becoming plugged with bone fragments).

5. Tape the needle securely in place and apply an antibiotic cream around the site. It may be worthwhile radiographing the area to ensure correct intramedullary placement of the needle.

6. Once the needle or catheter has been correctly placed, attach the intravenous tubing and bandage it securely in place by wrapping bandage material around the leg of the patient.

7. It may be necessary to immobilise the limb by bandaging it to a splint to prevent dislodgement of the catheter, which should now be attached to a syringe driver.

Chelonians

Two main intraosseous sites can be used.

Plastrocarapacial junction/pillar: This is the pillar of shell which connects the plastron to the carapace. It is approached from the caudal aspect, just cranial to one of the hind limbs. The spinal or hypodermic needle (21–23 gauge) is screwed into the shell attempting to keep the

angle of insertion parallel with the outer wall of the shell, so entering the shell bone marrow cavity (Figure 22.7). In larger, older species, the shell may be too tough to allow penetration.

Proximal tibia: This may be approached as for lizards. The area is thoroughly scrubbed with 0.25–0.5% povidone-iodine and the hypodermic or spinal needle is screwed into the tibial crest in the direction of the long axis of the tibia distally.

Routes of fluid administration in amphibians

Cutaneous

The cutaneous route is unique to amphibians and makes use of their semi-permeable skin. It can be used only with mildly dehydrated amphibians, and should only involve the use of dechlorinated, plain water. It should be warmed to the amphibian's PBT and be well oxygenated before immersing the patient. Absorption will occur across the skin membranes.

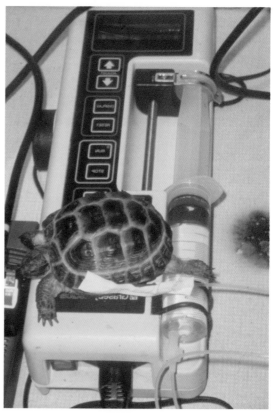

Figure 22.7 Intraosseous fluid administration via the plastrocarapacial pillars. Note the syringe driver in background.

Oral

This route can be used for hypotonic fluid therapy via a small feeding tube inserted orally. The danger is that trauma can easily occur during restraint and opening of the amphibian's mouth during this procedure. In addition, the process is moderately stressful.

Intracoelomic

This is accessed in the right lower ventral quadrant of the 'abdomen'. The amphibian should be placed in dorsal recumbency and with its head down to allow coelom contents to fall away from the injection site.

Intravenous

In the larger anurans and some salamanders, the midline ventral abdominal vein may be used for bolus fluids or blood transfusions. The vessel lies midline, just below the skin surface and runs from the pubis of the pelvis to the xiphoid of the sternum. A 25–27 gauge insulin needle may be used to gain access, although the vessel is very fragile and care should be taken not to rupture it.

Treatment of reptilian diseases

As this text is aimed at the veterinary nurse or technician, it is not intended to give exhaustive lists of treatments or drug dosages, rather to give an idea of the treatments possible and the techniques useful to aid recovery. For drug dosages, the reader is referred to one of the many excellent texts listed in the additional reading list at the end of this chapter.

Metabolic scaling of drug dosages

Many drugs have not been evaluated in reptiles and amphibians; however, drug doses may (with care) be extrapolated from known doses in other species. However, to do this, the differences in basal metabolic rate (BMR) or metabolism should be taken into consideration (see Chapter 20). Reptiles have a much lower metabolic rate than mammals, and this is reflected by the fact that they excrete drugs at slower rates. The environmental temperature at which the reptile or amphibian is kept, due to their ectothermic nature, will also greatly affect its metabolic rate and hence excretion of any drug administered. Therefore, dosages and dose rates are often much lower in reptiles than in mammals.

A formula has been derived though to 'metabolically scale' the dosage of a drug in a tested species, such as a dog, to an untried one, such as a snake. This is derived from the formula used to calculate the BMR which is:

$$BMR = K(W_{kg}^{0.75})$$

where K is a constant dependent upon the order of animal being considered (K is 70 for placental mammals, 78 for non-passerine birds and 10 for reptiles).

From this, it is possible to calculate an animal's specific minimum energy cost (SMEC) as:

$$SMEC = K(W_{kg}^{0.75}/W_{kg}) = K(W_{kg}^{-0.25})$$

This then allows you to calculate a SMEC *dose* for any drug by dividing its known dose rate in mg/kg in a species (say a human) by that species' SMEC. For example, if the dose rate of ceftazidime in a human being is 20 mg/kg, and that humans' SMEC is 24.2, then the SMEC dose is 0.8. Therefore, by simply balancing equations, if you then know the weight of your reptile (say a 2 kg iguana), you can calculate its SMEC as:

$$Iguana\ SMEC = K(10) \times (2^{-0.25}) = 8.4$$

And therefore, the dose rate of drug required by multiplying the iguana's SMEC by the SMEC dose as:

$$8.4 \times 0.8 = 6.72\ mg/kg$$

The next stage is to calculate the dose frequency. Again by extrapolation from a known dose frequency in humans for the drug of three times per 24 hours, the SMEC *frequency* may be calculated as:

$$SMEC\ frequency = treatment\ frequency/SMEC$$
$$= 3/24.2 = 0.1$$

Therefore to calculate the treatment frequency for the iguana you simply multiply the iguana's SMEC by the SMEC frequency for the drug:

$$Dose\ frequency\ iguana = 8.4 \times 0.1$$
$$= 0.84\ times\ in\ 24\ hrs$$

which is equivalent to 1 dose (of 6.72 mg/kg) every 28.6 hours.

The technique is crude, but does allow some attempt to derive a dose more suited to the lower metabolic rate of reptiles in comparison with mammals, when extrapolating drug doses.

Reptile dermatological disease therapy

Table 22.3 highlights some of the treatments and therapies commonly used for the management of reptilian dermatological diseases.

Table 22.3 Treatment of skin diseases.

Diagnosis	Treatment
Ectoparasites	
Mites	Ivermectin 0.2 mg/kg injection on 2–3 occasions at 10–14 d intervals Can spray environmental mixture of 0.5 mL ivermectin + 1 L water with 1–2 mL propylene glycol to aid mixing to remove remaining mites Fipronil has also been used topically, sprayed onto a cloth and wiped over the reptile
Ticks	Manual removal, ivermectin or fipronil on a cloth. Treat for secondary bacterial infection
Blowfly miasis	Manual removal, often under sedation, antibiosis and treatment of initiating cause
Leeches	Manual removal after applying lignocaine to leech
Dysecdysis	1. Rehydrate patient 2. Treat underlying cause 3. Lukewarm water shallow bathing; allow access to abrasive surfaces for snakes, e.g., wet towels 4. Retained spectacles in snakes may be removed carefully with viscous tear drops and moistened cotton buds
Scale rot	1. Isolate bacteria/fungi involved and obtain sensitivity 2. Blisters treated topically dilute povidone-iodine, silver sulfadiazine/enilconazole washes 3. Parenteral antibiosis 4. Prevention geared to reducing substrate moisture and increasing hygiene
Abscesses and bacterial infections	Surgical therapy for most abscesses due to their fibrous nature. Requires debridement and topical antiseptic with systemic antibiosis based on culture and sensitivity – many are Gram-negative infections; therefore fluoroquinolones and third-generation cephalosporins are useful. *Devriesea agamarum* require debridement and application of topical doxycycline mixed in with a gel such as Orabase. Alternative treatment with ceftiofur at 5 mg/kg q24h has been effective (Pasmans et al., 2010)
Erythema, ecchymoses and petechiae	Finding the cause of the condition which has lead to septicaemia If anticoagulant poisoning is suspected, then injections of vitamin K 0.25–0.5 mg/kg
Fungal skin infections	Superficial infections may respond to enilconazole washes Most are deeper and require systemic medication with itraconazole at metabolically scaled doses (Girling & Fraser, 2009) Voriconazole has been shown to be effective against CANV in bearded dragons
Viral skin infections	Some herpes virus infections may be treated with acyclovir topically or orally once daily at 80 mg/kg (Stein, 1996) Some have suggested three times daily treatment to be more effective (McArthur et al., 2004)
Hyperthyroidism	Case of the green iguana: a thyroid adenoma was surgically removed (Hernandez-Divers et al., 2001) Case of the corn snake: methimazole was used at 1–1.25 mg/kg q24h for 30 d (Frye, 1991)
Thermal burns	Management of large skin deficits using skin grafts or porcine xerograft patches (veterinary Biosist® Cook) or suturing granulation pads, e.g., Granuflex® over the wounds once infection has been contained. Antibiotics suitable for Gram-negative infections should be used systemically and topically (e.g., silver sulfadiazine). Repair of large skin deficits may take up to 6 mo

Reptile digestive tract disease therapy

Table 22.4 highlights some of the treatments and therapies commonly used for the management of reptilian digestive tract diseases.

Reptile respiratory and cardiovascular disease therapy

Table 22.5 highlights some of the treatments and therapies commonly used for the management of reptilian respiratory and cardiovascular diseases.

Table 22.4 Treatment of digestive system diseases.

Diagnosis	Treatment
Oral diseases	
Mouth rot	Antibiosis based on culture and sensitivity
	Necrotic tissue debrided under sedation/anaesthesia
	Topical compounds containing silver sulfadiazine and framycetin are useful
	Intralesion injections of antibiotic and vitamin C advised (Frye, 1991)
	Chelonian herpesvirus, use topical iodine washes and acyclovir ointment/systemic acyclovir 80 mg/kg s.i.d-t.i.d
Periodontal disease	Ultrasonic scaling of debris and calculus is advised. The use of antibiotics effective against Gram-negative bacteria is advised. The diet should also be corrected
Stomach diseases	
Neoplasia	Surgical excision
Granulomas (bacterial/ fungal)	Surgical excision for large granulomas, culture and sensitivity testing and antimicrobials for small
Nematodes	Ivermectin 0.2 mg/kg once; repeat after 2 wk – NEVER USE IVERMECTIN IN CHELONIA AS IT IS LETHAL. Or fenbendazole 50–100 mg/kg once and repeat after 2 wk
Cryptosporidiosis	Metronidazole orally at a dose of 260 mg/kg given twice 2 wk apart has been reported successful. Extreme care should be taken due to toxic reactions to this high dosage (Bone, 1992). In indigo snakes (Drymarchon corais spp.) and kingsnakes (Lampropeltis spp.), it is probably better to avoid using metronidazole as they are especially sensitive to its toxic side effects which include neurological signs and liver damage
	Paromomycin at 100 mg/kg daily for 7 d and then twice weekly for 3 mo was also successful in Gila monsters (Pare, 1997)
	Increasing the environmental temperature to >80°F, whilst ensuring prevention of dehydration and provision of easily digestible liquid foods has increased the success rates by reducing environmental survival of the organism and speeding up the life cycle. Hospital enclosures should be disinfected between cases. Few disinfectants can be guaranteed, only ammonia (5%) and formol-saline (10%) were considered effective at low temperatures by Cranfield and Graczyk (1996). Most effective method of disrupting the parasite life cycle includes steam cleaning, freezing and desiccation
Intestinal diseases	
Nematodes	See stomach diseases. NEVER USE IVERMECTIN IN CHELONIA AS IT IS LETHAL
Entamoebiasis	Metronidazole 160 mg/kg orally once daily for 3 d. In indigo and kingsnakes reduced dose of 25 mg/kg q96h metronidazole plus iodoquinol at 25–50 mg/kg q24h can be used to minimise metronidazole toxicity
Cryptosporidiosis	See section under 'Stomach diseases'
Coccidiosis	Sulfadimidine, orally, 50 mg/kg once daily for 3 days. Clazuril at 2–3 mg/kg q48h on three occasions has also been used
	Toltrazuril diluted down to poultry concentrations for drinking water and dosed for 2 d has also been used
Flagellates	Flagellates may be treated using metronidazole as a single dose of 100–275 mg/kg orally (Cranfield & Graczyk, 1996) – beware toxicity in indigo and kingsnakes
Liver diseases	
Entamoebiasis	See 'Intestinal diseases' above
Hepatic lipidosis	Hepatic lipidosis may be treated with supportive fluid and nutritional therapy. In addition, use of anabolic steroids at doses of 0.5–1 mg/kg orally every 7 days and the use of levothyroxine at 20 µg/ kg orally every 2 days may be helpful. In chelonians during this period the diet needs to be a high fibre vegetarian one. It may be necessary to prevent hibernation if the problem occurs in the autumn, and the placement of a pharyngostomy tube for ease of food administration is advisable. The use of milk thistle extract, inositol and L-carnitine in cases of liver disease also appear beneficial

Table 22.5 Treatment of respiratory and cardiovascular system diseases.

Diagnosis	Treatment
Respiratory disease	
Nematodes	Ivermectin may be used at 0.2 mg/kg EXCEPT IN CHELONIA. Alternatively, fenbendazole and oxfendazole may be used (see intestinal disease treatment, Table 14.4)
Pentastomes	Manual removal. Levamisole has been used at 5 mg/kg
Bacterial respiratory disease	Based on culture and sensitivity results. Lung washes may be used to collect samples and to flush out infection. Gram-negative bacterial infections predominate; therefore fluoroquinolones, aminoglycosides and third generation cephalosporins may be useful
Fungal respiratory disease	Itraconazole or voriconazole preferred as ketoconazole is ineffective against *Aspergillus* spp. which are commonly found
Cardiovascular disease	
Heart failure	With little information regarding suitable therapeutics, the following provides a guide only: 1. Maintain at lowest extent of POTZ 2. Enrich local environment with oxygen 3. Minimise stress with minimal handling 4. Withhold food (for the short term) 5. Short-term diuresis when signs of congestive failure are present – frusemide 2–5 mg/kg IV or IM 2–3× daily, (may also use hydrochlorothiazide 1 mg/kg every 24–72 h) 6. Broad spectrum antimicrobial 7. Parasiticides (if suspect haemoparasites/microfilaria, or blood-sucking ectoparasites/endoparasites) 8. Fluids (15–30 mL/kg/d) 9. Digoxin has been used at empirical cat and dog dosages for a case of diagnosed dilated cardiomyopathy in a python, but extreme care should be taken with all of these drugs as no proper studies have been performed to ascertain safe dosages
Filariasis	Nematode filariasis treatment attempted with ivermectin 0.2 mg/kg intramuscularly. Alternatives include raising the environmental temperature to 35–37°C for 24–48 h causing death of the adult worms. Watch for signs of heat stress and dehydration at these temperatures.
Other haemoparasites	Chloroquine 125 mg/kg, PO, every 48 h on three occasions for haemoparasites, e.g., *Plasmodium* spp. (Girling & Raiti, 2004) Quinacrine 20–100 mg/kg PO, every 48 h for 2 wk for haemogregarines in snakes (Raiti, 2002)
Goitre	Iodine supplement at 2–4 mg/kg orally once weekly (Stein, 1996)
Leukaemia	Vincristine (0.025 mg/kg intravenously once weekly), and prednisolone (0.5–1 mg/kg once daily). Resistance can occur with this regime and more success has been achieved by adding in cyclophosphamide (10 mg/kg) and chlorambucil (0.1–0.2 mg/kg *per os* once daily) (Willette *et al.*, 2001). Doxorubicin has been used at 1 mg/kg intravenously once weekly for two treatments, then once every 2 wk for two treatments and then once every 3 wk for two treatments (Rosenthal, 1994)

Reptile urinary tract disease therapy

Table 22.6 highlights some of the treatments and therapies commonly used for the management of reptilian urinary tract diseases.

Treatment of renal disease

Fluid therapy is an essential part of this (see above and Chapter 24). In severely dehydrated reptiles, an initial fluid rate of 5 mL/kg/hour may be attempted for the first

Table 22.6 Treatment for urinary tract diseases.

Diagnosis	Treatment
Renal disease	See text
Urinary bladder stones	Treatment by surgical removal, or if small enough via endoscope via the cloaca. Antibiotic therapy often required due to concurrent cystitis

Table 22.7 Treatment for reproductive system diseases.

Diagnosis	Treatment
Dystocia (post-ovulatory stasis)	See text
Pre-ovulatory stasis	Surgical ovariectomy
Egg yolk coelomitis	Similar to the condition in birds; however, reptiles will often be more tolerant of advanced disease Surgical option is an ovariectomy to prevent recurrence – also allows debridement and flushing of the coelomic cavity. Covering antibiotics with fluid therapy and assist feeding also required
Hemipenal/phallus prolapse	If hemipene/phallus is non-reducible then amputation is advised
Oviductal prolapses	Severe prolapses, which have been present for some time may necessitate emergency surgery, and replacement of the prolapse via a coeliotomy, +/– salpingectomy at the same time

1–3 hours. Beware of reptiles with hyperkalaemia that potassium-containing fluids are avoided.

If anuria is present, then diuretics such as furosemide (2–5 mg/kg intravenously or intramuscularly q24h) or mannitol (20% as 2 mL/kg intravenously q24h) can be given.

Allopurinol can be given to reduce blood uric acid levels (20 mg/kg orally q24h).

Bladder lavage, involving the cloacal insertion of a Foley catheter into the bladder and lavage of its contents, offers possibilities for the stabilisation of hyperuricaemic, hyperkalaemic patients (Dantzler & Schmidt-Nielson, 1966). Bearing in mind the function of the lower urinary tract, it should be possible to remove excess potassium and uric acid, and to administer fluids (and possibly even medications such as allopurinol) by this route.

Hypocalcaemia is a common finding with renal failure and can cause seizures and tetany. Calcium gluconate therapy with 100 mg/kg q6h along with aluminium hydroxide (15–45 mg/kg orally q24h) to reduce phosphate absorption is advised.

In chronic renal failure, anabolic steroids and vitamin B injections may also be given to enhance appetite and stop catabolism and reverse anaemia.

Reptile reproductive tract disease therapy
Table 22.7 highlights some of the treatments and therapies commonly used for the management of reptilian reproductive tract diseases.

Treatment of dystocia (post-ovulatory stasis) (Figures 22.8 and 21.15)
Medical treatment revolves around the administration of oxytocin at 5–30 IU/kg intramuscularly or intracoelomically (Stein, 1996). Prior to this, calcium gluconate at 100 mg/kg, particularly in lizards and chelonia where hypocalcaemia is a problem, is administered. In addition, the use of sterile lubricants injected into the reproductive tract via the cloaca may be helpful. The provision of nesting material such as damp sand or bark chippings for the female to dig into is also useful and maybe all that is needed in uncomplicated cases, particularly in chelonia.

Atenolol at 7 mg/kg orally with calcium gluconate has been used in chelonians followed by 1–3 IU/kg of oxytocin intramuscularly the following morning. This protocol is continued daily, assuming eggs are produced, until all eggs are out.

As with birds, the application of prostaglandin E gel to the oviduct sphincter per cloaca may help dilation if this is the cause of dystocia.

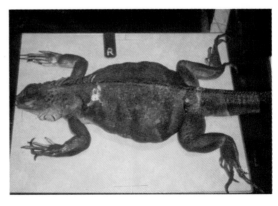

Figure 22.8 Heavily pregnant female green iguana with post-ovulatory stasis. See Figure 21.15 for the intra-operative view of this reptile.

Surgical methods include percutaneous aspiration of the egg contents by bringing the egg to the abdominal wall, surgically scrubbing the skin surface and passing a 21 gauge needle through the body wall into the egg. The needle should be attached to a syringe which should be used to aspirate the yolk and albumen contents. Once collapsed, the egg shells will often be passed of their own accord.

Other methods include salpingotomy. In the case of snakes, this means making very long incisions to ensure removal of all of the eggs. In the case of chelonians, this means entering into the shell via the plastron by creating a trap door.

Reptile musculoskeletal system disease therapy

Table 22.8 highlights some of the treatments and therapies commonly used for the management of reptilian musculoskeletal system diseases.

Treatment of metabolic bone disease

This is by correction of the dietary deficiency in calcium and by ensuring that susceptible species are provided with ultraviolet artificial lighting on the inside of the vivarium. Injectable calcium should not be used for routine metabolic bone disease (MBD) cases as it is both painful and if given intravenously, may cause fatal arrhythmias. Injectable calcium should only be used if there is evidence of hypocalcaemic tetany or collapse. Treatment should focus on dietary correction of calcium imbalance in combination with vitamin D_3 provision (UV light or dietary). Salmon calcitonin has been used once blood calcium levels have been corrected to encourage deposition of calcium in the bones. Doses of 50 IU per green iguana once weekly for 2 weeks have been quoted (Mader, 2006). A typical protocol for a green iguana with MBD is to administer 400 IU/kg vitamin D_3 intramuscularly plus

Table 22.8 Treatment of musculoskeletal diseases.

Diagnosis	Treatment
Metabolic bone disease	See text
Fractures	In cases of metabolic bone disease, it is better to correct diet and splint fractures than repair surgically
Lizards	For one forelimb fracture, bandage limb to body wall (see Figure 22.9). For bilateral humeral fractures, use a coaptation splint. For one hindlimb fracture, bandage limb to tail base. For digital fractures ball bandage as for avian patients
Chelonians	Possible to bandage limb into shell. This is useful in cases of metabolic bone disease. Spinal fractures should be splinted as neural control may be regained. All species may require external coaptation or internal surgical fixation to mend fractures
Tail loss	Young iguanids and geckos treat stump as an open wound and dress with topical silver sulfadiazine cream or iodine antiseptic (dilute) For agamids or species not showing autonomy and older iguanids which lose this ability, suture the stump surgically

23 mg/kg calcium gubionate orally twice daily plus supportive therapy. The first week after, repeat the vitamin D_3 injection, and assuming normalised blood calcium, give the first salmon calcitonin injection and continue with the oral calcium. The second week, just the calcitonin injection, is repeated plus the oral calcium (Mader, 2006).

Unfortunately, some of the shell deformities seen in chelonia are not correctable. Fractures are best repaired by splinting and dietary corrections.

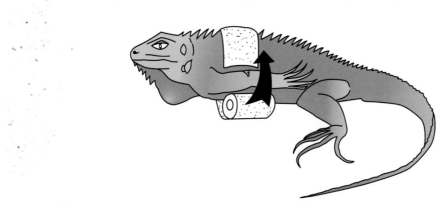

Figure 22.9 Bandaging a forelimb to the body wall as a conservative method of treating a humeral fracture in a lizard.

Internal fixation is not advised due to the fragility of the bones.

Prevention of metabolic bone disease

Klaphake (2010) has described ultraviolet light provision for reptiles to prevent MBD as follows:

1. Desert diurnal lizards/chelonians – high ultraviolet B-wave (UVB) levels (10% or full unfiltered sun for 12 hours)
2. Diurnal arboreal lizards or semiaquatic basking chelonians – moderate UVB (5%, 12 hours)
3. Diurnal terrestrial lizards or chelonians from forests – low UVB (5%, 6 hours)
4. Nocturnal lizards – low levels UVB (2%, 6 hours)
5. Snakes – dietary calcium and vitamin D_3 is sufficient

Calcium supplementation should be provided for young growing lizards and chelonia in particular, but unfortunately little data exists to demonstrate in what form or how much is necessary. For insectivores, gut-loading their prey is preferred as this guarantees the reptile will get the nutritional supplement. Commercially available insects need supplementation as most have inverted calcium:phosphorus ratios. Dietary deficiencies for herbivores in calcium can occur where large amounts of leaves containing oxalates (e.g., spinach and beetroot tops) that bind calcium in the gut and prevent absorption. The feeding of fruit should be kept in check as most fruit contains little or no calcium.

Reptile neurological system disease therapy

Table 22.9 highlights some of the treatments and therapies commonly used for the management of reptilian neurological system diseases.

Treatment of amphibian diseases

Table 22.10 highlights some of the treatments and therapies commonly used for the management of amphibian diseases.

Table 22.9 Treatment of nervous system diseases.

Diagnosis	Treatment
Hypocalcaemic tetany	Over short term use calcium gluconate 100 mg/kg intramuscularly. Over long term, administer dietary calcium, vitamin D_3 and UV-light supplementation
Hypovitaminosis B_1	Over short term, thiamine injections 25 mg/kg once daily. Over the long term change to a non–thiaminase-containing diet, or supplement with thiamine at 35 mg/kg of food given. Biotin deficiency: over short term give a vitamin B complex by injection. Over long term supplement the diet with vitamin B complex powder or stop feeding unfertilised hen's eggs
Hypoglycaemia	Oral administration of 3 g/kg glucose solution
Lead poisoning	10–40 mg/kg sodium calcium edentate every 12 h
Meningoencephalitis	There are many causes: entamoebiasis – see section on treatment of intestinal diseases; viral causes, e.g., inclusion body disease are not treatable; bacterial causes may be treated early on with antimicrobials

Table 22.10 Treatment of diseases of amphibia.

Diagnosis	Treatment
Redleg	Enrofloxacin at 5 mg/kg orally daily. Tetracyclines, e.g., oxytetracycline, at 50 mg/kg
Saprolegnia	Dilute topical malachite green
Phycomycosis	Phycomycosis: dilute topical malachite green (not always successful)
Parasitic nematodes	Fenbendazole orally 50 mg/kg once, or ivermectin 0.2 mg/kg orally once
Protozoal diseases	*Entamoeba ranarum* in anurans treated with metronidazole at 100 mg/kg orally once. Note: may be toxic. *Oodinium pilularis* treated with mild salt solutions of 0.4–0.6% for 2–3 d or a 0.15% formalin dip every 48 h are useful
Metabolic bone disease	Dietary supplementation with calcium and vitamin disease D_3. Flaked fish foods also contain these two nutrients

References

Bone, R.D. (1992) Gastrointestinal system. *Manual of Reptiles* (eds P.H. Beynon, M.P.C. Lawton & J.E. Cooper), pp. 101–116. BSAVA, Cheltenham, UK.

Cranfield, M.R. and Graczyk, T.K. (1996) Cryptosporidiosis. *Reptile Medicine and Surgery* (ed. D.R. Mader), pp. 359–363. WB Saunders, Philadelphia, PA.

Dantzler, W.H. and Schmidt-Nielson, B. (1966) Excretion in the fresh-water turtle (*Pseudemys scripta*) and desert tortoise (*Gopherus agassizii*). *American Journal of Physiology*, **210**, 198–210.

Frye, F.L. (1991) Infectious diseases. *Biomedical and Surgical Aspects of Captive Reptile Husbandry*, 2nd edn, Vol 1. Krieger Publishing, Malabar, FL.

Girling, S.J. and Fraser, M.A. (2009) Treatment of *Aspergillus* species infection in reptiles with itraconazole at metabolically scaled dosages. *Veterinary Record*, **165**(2), 52–54.

Girling, S.J. and Raiti, P. (2004) Appendix 2 A formulary of drugs for use in reptiles. *BSAVA Manual of Reptiles* (eds S.J. Girling & P. Raiti), 2nd edn, pp. 352–356. BSAVA, Quedgeley, UK.

Hernandez-Divers, S.J., Knott, C.D. and MacDonald, J. (2001) Diagnosis and surgical treatment of thyroid adenoma-induced hyperthyroidism in a green iguana (*Iguana iguana*). *Journal of Zoo and Wildlife Medicine*, **32**, 465–475.

Klaphake, E. (2010) A fresh look at metabolic bone diseases in reptiles and amphibians. *Veterinary Clinics of North America: Exotic Animal Practice*, **13**, 375–392.

Klingenberg, R.J. (1996) Therapeutics. *Reptile Medicine and Surgery* (ed. D.R. Mader). WB Saunders, Philadelphia, PA.

Mader, D. (2006) Metabolic bone disorders. *Reptile Medicine and Surgery* (ed. D. Mader), 2nd edn, pp. 841–851. Saunders, Elsevier, Philadelphia, PA.

McArthur, S., McLellan, L. and Brown, S. (2004) Gastrointestinal disease. *Manual of Reptiles* (eds S.J. Girling & P. Raiti), 2nd edn, pp. 210–229. BSAVA, Quedgeley, UK.

Pare, J. (1997) Treatment of cryptosporidiosis in gila monsters (*Heloderma suspectum*) with paromomycin. *Proceedings of the Association of Reptilian and Amphibian Veterinarians*, Houston, TX, pp. 23–24.

Pasmans, K., Hellebuyck, T., Haesebrouck, F. and Martel, A. (2010) Dermatitis and septicaemia caused by *Devriesea agamarum*: an overview including recent developments in disease management. *Proceedings of the 1st International Conference on Reptile and Amphibian Medicine*, pp. 105–106.

Raiti, P (2002) Snakes. *Manual of Exotic Pets* (eds A. Meredith & S. Redrobe), 4th edn, pp. 241–256. BSAVA, Quedgeley, UK.

Rosenthal, K. (1994) Chemotherapeutic treatment of a sarcoma in a corn snake. *Proceedings of the American Association of Zoo Veterinarians/Association of Reptilian and Amphibian Veterinarians*, p. 46.

Stein, G. (1996) Reptile and amphibian formulary. *Reptile Medicine and Surgery* (ed. D.R. Mader), pp. 465–472. WB Saunders, Philadelphia, PA.

Willette, M.M., Garner, M.M. and Drew, M. (2001) Chemotherapeutic treatment of lymphoma in a king cobra (*Ophiophagus hannah*). *Proceedings of the American Association of Zoo Veterinarians/Association of Reptilian and Amphibian Veterinarians*, pp. 20–24.

RADIOGRAPHY

Introduction

The rationale behind diagnostic imaging of reptiles and avian patients is much the same as that behind any species commonly seen in general practice. The main aims are to ensure the rapid detection of internal foreign bodies, the presence of growths, whether they be tumours, granulomas or abscesses, as well as the enlargement/reduction of internal organs due to diseases. In addition, the detection of gravidity and the confirmation of fractures are common reasons for radiographing a patient.

There are many considerations which need to be made prior to attempting to radiograph a reptile or avian patient. These include

- Is the patient an aggressive or even venomous species and therefore will require anaesthesia or chemical sedation to safely radiograph?
- Is the patient in respiratory distress, and therefore the stress of manual restraint or chemical restraint may be too high to allow safe radiography?
- What is the area that is to be viewed? In the case of reptiles in particular, the absence of a diaphragm makes viewing the lung fields (which are situated generally in the dorsal coelom) almost impossible on normal lateral views, and horizontal x-ray beam radiography with a standing patient is required in lizards and chelonians (see Figure 23.1). Snakes due to the presence of fascia which holds the coelomic organs in place can be radiographed in a conventional vertical beam for both lateral and dorsoventral views.
- What is the size of the patient to be radiographed?

Physical restraint

Many of the more docile reptiles will remain motionless for long enough to take dorsoventral radiographs without the need for chemical restraint. The use of perspex or even cardboard boxes to constrain the reptile, particularly if they are some of the smaller lizards such as anoles and day geckos, is very useful, although minor reduction in the quality of the radiographs will occur.

Chelonians may be easily positioned for horizontal beam radiography in the conscious state by balancing the mid part of the plastron on a block or small pile of upturned feeding bowls so as to lift all four feet off the ground!!

Snakes may be constrained manually or encouraged to crawl into a perspex or plastic tube, such as can be made from syringe cases taped together. This has two advantages. One is that the snake is adequately restrained enough to allow the handler to leave the snake whilst the radiograph is being taken. The second is that it ensures the snake is stretched out and avoids the confusion of interpretation which occurs in the coiled individual.

Lizards such as the green iguana (*Iguana iguana*) may present more difficulty to restrain physically. However, many will quieten down when placed into a dimmed environment. Alternatively, the use of a heavy towel to restrain the iguana initially, long enough to gently close the eyelids and apply firm but careful pressure to the eyeballs through the eyelids, can be employed. This may be maintained manually, or replaced by a ball of cotton wool over each eyelid and the whole wrapped in an elasticated bandage to keep the pressure on. This process is known as the vagovagal reflex as the pressure on the eyeballs stimulates the vagus nerve and consequently leads to the reduction in respiration rate and heart rate, so creating a semi-sedated condition. This is sufficient to allow the iguana to be placed in lateral recumbency for limb radiographs, etc., without the need for chemical restraint. However, as soon as a loud noise or other form of stimulation occurs, the effect is abolished and the iguana becomes alert again.

Chemical restraint

This may be necessary for very aggressive species or poisonous ones. There are many combinations of sedatives and anaesthetic regimes available to practitioners, and it

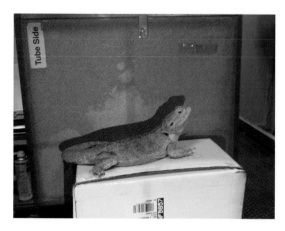

Figure 23.1 Horizontal beam radiography is necessary in lizards and chelonians to obtain anatomically correct views of the coelomic cavity due to the absence of a true diaphragm.

is impossible to go into them all at this time. However, some of the more commonly used methods in this author's practice are as follows.

- Propofol – given intravenously or intraosseously at 5–10 mg/kg will produce a short plane of near surgical anaesthesia, allowing radiography and minor surgical procedures to be performed. It is advised that the reptile is intubated and oxygenated during this time (and this may require manual oxygenation) to prevent hypoxia. Duration of sedation is from 20 to 40 minutes. Recovery times are 30–40 minutes on average.
- Ketamine – used at doses ranging from 22 to 44 mg/kg, preferably the lower end of the range if radiography is the most invasive technique intended. Duration of deep sedation is from 2 to 20 minutes. Recovery may take 1–4 days, particularly at the higher doses and in debilitated patients.

Positioning

As with small mammals, the need is to obtain a three-dimensional view of the area under investigation. To obtain this the traditional two views at right angles to each other are required.

However, although a dorsoventral view is performed as for a small mammal patient, a lateral view is often better performed in the standing patient as mentioned above. This is due to the anatomy of the average reptile patient, which does not possess a diaphragm separating the lung fields from the gastrointestinal system, so creating a common cavity or coelom. Thus, if placed in lateral recumbency, the gut contents will fall dorsally and obliterate the

lung field, making radiographic evaluation impossible. Instead, if the x-ray machine (and local safety protocols) will allow, the head of the machine should be moved to fire x-rays horizontally, so allowing the reptile to be imaged standing upright. This is also extremely useful in cases of coelomic fluid effusion where fluid lines become readily apparent.

In chelonia, an additional third view is recommended. This is the craniocaudal view, again utilising the horizontal beam x-ray. This view allows comparison of the right and left lung fields, which are situated in the dorsal aspect of the shell, and is useful for diagnosing one-sided lesions such as granulomas or focal pneumonias (Figure 23.2).

In snakes, it is advised that the snake be extended in form before radiography is performed, as the traditional coiled-up view of a snake makes for poor interpretation of internal organs and the position of lesions (Figure 23.3).

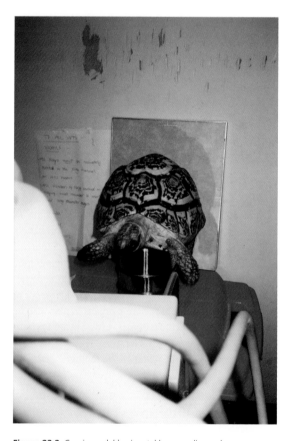

Figure 23.2 Craniocaudal horizontal beam radiographs are an additional useful view to compare the right and left lung fields in chelonians. Note that the tortoise is restrained by placing it on a pedestal so its feet are clear off the ground.

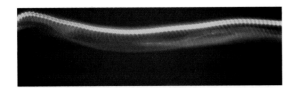

Figure 23.3 Right lateral view of a boa constrictor. Snakes do not have to undergo horizontal beam radiography due to the fascia which holds body organs in place no matter what the snake's orientation. Note the paired ribs along the whole body, the prominent lung and air sacs surrounding the heart shadow to the left of the radiograph. As the lung moves caudally the radio-dense stomach and liver can be seen ventral to it.

Positive contrast techniques

Barium

The use of barium sulphate is useful for positive contrast radiography of the gastrointestinal tract in all reptiles.

Chelonia

The use of 5–7 mL of a 25–30% solution of barium, administered by stomach tube, is useful for most Mediterranean tortoise species. Stomach emptying time may take up to a day, and the gut transit time from mouth to cloaca may take nearly a month! Barium studies are especially useful in chelonians due to the lack of detail encountered on plain radiographs.

Lizards

As for chelonia. Transit times are faster, particularly in insectivorous species such as geckos, and may take 24–36 hours if kept at optimal temperatures. Useful for highlighting foreign intestinal bodies in iguanas.

Snakes

As for chelonia, with doses of barium at 5 mL/kg, although transit times are much faster with gastric emptying occurring in 2–3 hours and full transit time taking 4–7 days. Air may be injected into the stomach immediately after barium to create a positive contrast technique – useful when examining thickening of the stomach wall as is found with some tumours, cryptosporidiosis and abscesses.

Iodine-based contrast

Useful where minimal irritation is required, such as when gut/intestinal surgery may be planned shortly after using positive contrast techniques.

Chelonia

Transit times are faster with stomach emptying occurring in 1.5–4 hours and full gut transit time taking 3–8 hours at 21°C. A positive contrast urocystogram may be seen some 8–10 hours after oral administration as the aqueous iodine is absorbed and excreted through the kidneys.

Lizards

Intravenous techniques have been used to determine blood flow through the kidneys and may be used to assess the cardiovascular system. Doses of 0.5–1 mL/kg intravenously have been used.

Snakes

As for chelonia, although gut transit times are even faster, with stomach emptying occurring within 30–45 minutes.

Normal and abnormal radiographic findings

Chelonia

It is difficult to view many of chelonians' internal organs due to the density of their shell. However, the heart and liver may be seen on lateral views using horizontal beam radiography, and the liver shadow may be enhanced by the use of positive contrast studies and lies in a dumb-bell shape across midline in the caudal part of the cranial half of the chelonian.

Metabolic bone disease (MBD) will cause deformities of the carapace and lucencies in the pelvis and pectoral girdle. Over-supplementation with vitamin D_3 and calcium may lead to renal and cardiovascular mineralisation. Bladder stones and gravidity are most easily seen in dorsoventral radiographs.

Lung fields are best assessed on the lateral horizontal beam radiograph and the craniocaudal horizontal beam radiographs. Eggs are easily seen in gravid chelonians, and the most useful view is the dorsoventral (see Figures 23.4–23.6).

Radiography may, of course, also be used to assess whether intraosseous catheters are correctly sited (Figure 23.7).

Lizards

Internal organs of most lizards are best viewed on the lateral horizontal beam radiographs. These allow good visualisation of the dorsal lung fields and the liver shadow (Figure 23.8). The dorsoventral view, due to the absence of a diaphragm, results in superimposition of the lung fields over the liver and digestive tract, making interpretation difficult (Figure 23.9).

The caudal coelom is occupied by the gut, which may be extensive in herbivorous species such as the green

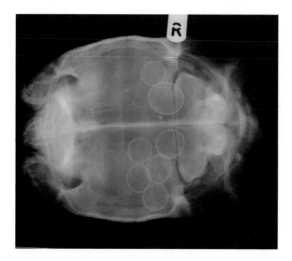

Figure 23.4 Dorsoventral view of a female gravid spur-thighed tortoise (*Testudo graeca*) showing the outlines of seven eggs. Note the radiolucent line across the plastron which is the plastral 'hinge' typical of this species which facilitates oviposition.

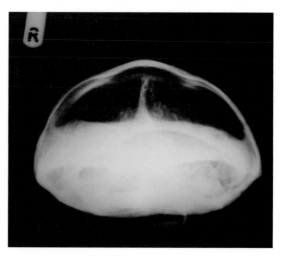

Figure 23.6 Horizontal beam craniocaudal view of the tortoise in Figure 23.4. This view is useful for comparing the left and right lung fields to pinpoint a lesion.

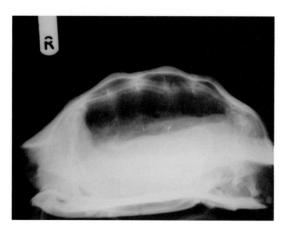

Figure 23.5 Horizontal beam lateral view of the tortoise in Figure 23.4. Note the dorsally situated lungs. The eggs are more difficult to see in this view as they are masked by the intestinal mass.

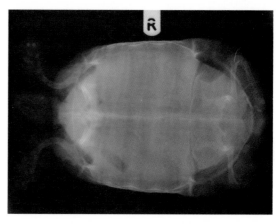

Figure 23.7 Dorsoventral view of a spur-thighed tortoise (*Testudo graeca*) showing the correct placement of an intraosseous catheter in the distal right femur.

iguana, and may contain gas. In insectivorous and more omnivorous species such as geckos and monitors, the gut may be smaller. Large fat bodies fill the ventral and caudal abdomen in many lizards and may make outlining the gut more difficult in obese individuals. The horizontal beam radiograph may also be used to view the renal shadow, which if enlarged projects cranially from the pelvis on the dorsal surface of the coelomic cavity.

The heart in lizards may be placed so far cranially that it is hidden within the sternal plate (e.g., green iguanas and bearded dragons) and so is not visible on either horizontal beam radiographs or dorsoventral views. In other species (e.g., monitor lizards) the heart is more caudally placed and so better seen. The stomach of many lizards such as the green iguana is actually quite far caudal (Figures 23.10 and 23.11). Loss of coelomic detail can be associated with coelomitis such as will occur due to a perforated bowel (Figures 23.12 and 23.13).

There are members of the order Geckonidae (*Uroplatus* and *Phelsuma* spp), which store calcium in specialised structures called endolymphatic sacs. These organs lie in the cervical area and are readily visible (Figure 23.14).

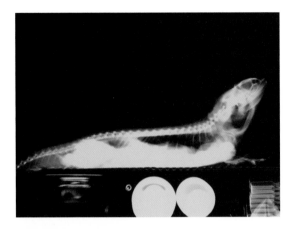

Figure 23.8 Horizontal beam lateral view of an inland bearded dragon (*Pogona vitticeps*) showing the lung fields.

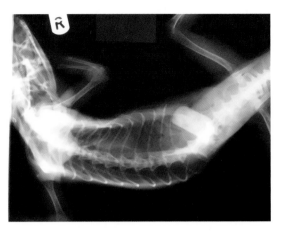

Figure 23.11 Dorsoventral view of the green iguana in Figure 23.10 showing again the foreign body located in the caudally situated stomach.

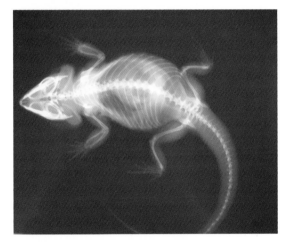

Figure 23.9 Dorsoventral view of the bearded dragon in Figure 23.8 showing the now obscured lung fields due to superimposition of the digestive tract.

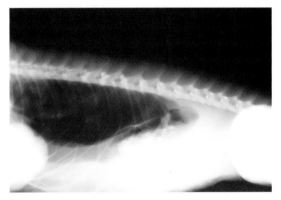

Figure 23.12 Horizontal beam lateral view of a green iguana (*Iguana iguana*) showing loss of caudal coelomic detail due to coelomitis from a perforated bowel. Note the small stones in the stomach which have been pushed dorsally to the mid coelom by the fluid in the coelomic cavity.

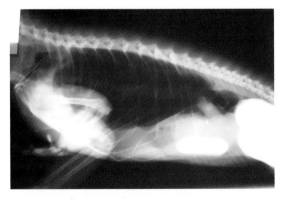

Figure 23.10 Horizontal beam lateral view of a green iguana (*Iguana iguana*) showing the extensive lung fields and the presence of a foreign body (an eraser) located in its caudally situated stomach lying on the ventral coelomic floor.

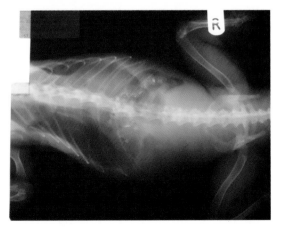

Figure 23.13 Dorsoventral view of the green iguana in Figure 23.12.

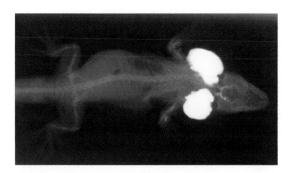

Figure 23.14 Dorsoventral view of a Standing's day gecko (*Phelsuma standingi*) demonstrating the calcium storage glands in the neck. This is a normal radiographic finding in this species.

MBD can be confirmed by radiography, with the dorsoventral radiographs being the most useful, and by comparing soft-tissue density with bone density (Figure 23.15). Long bone deformities are common in this condition, as are swellings and flaring of the epiphyseal plates in cases of rickets due to vitamin D3 deficiencies (most commonly seen on the costochondral junctions of green iguanas). The exoskeleton often has a moth-eaten appearance with MBD causing the ribs to appear more prominent. In lizards, demineralisation is followed by fibrous tissue proliferation around the shafts of the long bones. Folding fractures are common, particularly in chronic cases of MBD. Fractures in adult reptiles are most commonly due to trauma.

Infectious diseases of bones (osteomyelitis) are characterised by lysis and soft-tissue swelling. With septic arthritis, there is destruction of the epiphyses of the bones which form the joint. Articular gout may be another

skeletal abnormality easily detected on radiography as radiopaque uric acid crystals form in the joint spaces.

In addition dorsoventral views allow the confirmation of pre- and post-ovulatory stasis, two common reproductive diseases of lizards, particularly the green iguana. Preovulatory stasis is shown by up to 70 spherical soft-tissue densities in the cranial-mid coelom, and post-ovulatory stasis is shown by more ovoidal soft-tissue densities with very thin calcium cortices as reptile shells are poorly mineralised in comparison to their avian counterparts (Figure 23.15). This radiographic view also allows visualisation of bladder stones in species possessing a urinary bladder, such as the green iguana.

Some monitor lizards (*Varanus indicus*, *V. prasinus*, *V. gouldii*) can be sexed radiographically because there is calcification of the hemibacula of the hemipenises.

Snakes

The most useful view for snakes is the lateral radiograph as the dorsoventral view is obscured by the ribs and spinal column. However, both views are recommended to obtain a three-dimensional image.

In the lateral beam radiograph, the lung fields are clearly seen occupying the caudal half of the first third of the snake, with the heart shadow clearly outlined (Figure 23.3). Pneumonia and fluid lines are occasionally seen (Figure 23.16). Caudal to the heart shadow lie the liver shadow and stomach followed by the gall bladder and small intestine. Blockages of the bowel may be seen on plain radiographs if food material is held back, but determining their severity often requires positive contrast techniques as described above (Figure 23.17).

In the cranial half of the caudal third of the snake lie the kidneys and reproductive organs along the dorsal surface of the coelom. Radiolucent areas may represent follicular activity, and regular ovoidal soft-tissue densities along the caudal third of the snake may indicate gravidity. For livebearers, such as garter snakes and boa constrictors, it is

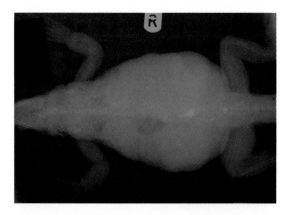

Figure 23.15 Dorsoventral view of a female gravid green iguana (*Iguana iguana*) with metabolic bone disease. Note the faint outlines of the eggs giving a scalloped appearance to the body wall, the poorly mineralised bones and the presence of fractures in the long bones (recent left femur and part healing left humerus).

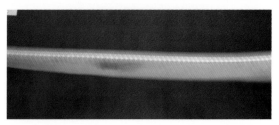

Figure 23.16 Lateral view of a Burmese python (*Python molurus bivittatus*) with pneumonia. Note the increased radiodensity of the lung field in comparison with the snake in Figure 23.3.

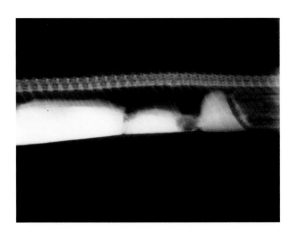

Figure 23.17 Lateral iodine contrast view of a reticulated python (*Python reticulatus*) with an intestinal obstruction. Note the partial blockage to the passage of the contrast to the right of the picture.

possible to see the skeletons of the foetuses in this region when gravid. The large intestine and rectum occupy the ventral surface.

ULTRASONOGRAPHY
Physical restraint

This is the preferred method for ultrasound examination as it allows easy positioning and the observation of gut movements, which may not be possible in a sedated or anaesthetised reptile.

Equipment

The use of a hard work top area with a section cut out to allow the ultrasound probe to be applied to the dependent side of the patient is preferred.

As far as the ultrasound equipment is concerned, the preferred size of probe is a 7.5 MHz transducer, as most reptile patients are relatively small. Indeed it may still be necessary to use a 'standoff' (an acoustic coupling device) in patients under 50 g in weight and the narrower snakes. A standoff may be cheaply made from a latex glove finger filled with coupling gel, or more expensive purpose-built ones may be bought. In patients over 1.5 kg, it may be necessary to use a 5 MHz transducer to see internal organs such as the liver.

In chelonia, the heart and thyroid gland may be examined via the thoracic inlet and the abdomen, particularly the liver, reproductive tract and urinary bladder, may be examined via the inlet cranial to a hindlimb. The rest of the shell obviously limits the amount of internal organs examinable.

Lizards are easy to examine by ultrasound, although the high placement of the heart behind the sternal shield in species such as the green iguana may make these organs more difficult to visualise.

Snakes are again easy to examine by ultrasound, but only from the ventral aspect as the presence of ribs along their length prevents lateral or dorsal examination.

Normal and abnormal ultrasound findings
Chelonia
Thoracic inlet

The thoracic inlet allows the heart to be visualised. As with other reptiles (except the Crocodylia), there are two atria and only one ventricle. This may be seen midline, on the floor of the plastron, and just cranial to this area is the oval thyroid gland (Figure 23.18). Enlargement is seen in the thyroid in cases of goitre such as overfeeding of brassicas. The atrioventricular valves appear hyperechoic. It may be possible to examine some of the liver behind the heart structure, allowing the assessment of focal lesions such as abscesses, as well as general increased density as will occur in mineralisation, gout and hepatic lipidosis. The anechoic gall bladder is easily visible in the right lobe.

Inguinal inlet

The inguinal inlets will allow the urinary bladder to be examined, which can be an extensive bilobed structure. Bladder stones are not uncommon.

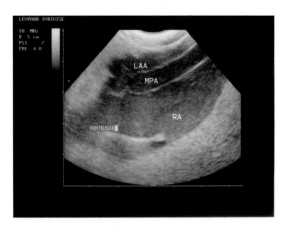

Figure 23.18 Two-dimensional echocardiogram sagittal view from the right side of the neck in a leopard tortoise (*Stigmochelys pardalis*). LAA, left aortic arch; MPA, main pulmonary artery; RA, right atrium; V, ventricle. (Reproduced with permission from Girling & Raiti, 2004, © BSAVA)

The kidneys appear homogenous in outline with a very narrow hypoechoic medulla. They are attached to the dorsal aspect of the caudal shell. Again, gout, abscesses and enlargement may be visualised by changes in density and outline.

The female reproductive tract can be visualised easily when gravid. There are two ovaries, suspended from the underside of the carapace, caudal to the lung field and cranial to the kidneys. Pre-ovulatory stasis will present as the 'cluster of grapes' effect with more than 10–15 follicles in each ovary. From each ovary, a uterine body extends down to the cloaca, and it is here that shelled eggs and post-ovulatory stasis or gravidity may be determined. Shelled eggs are readily apparent, with the lightly mineralised shell, surrounding the hypoechoic albumen, around the denser yolk.

Lizards

The heart again is a three-chambered organ, and may be found anywhere from the thoracic inlet in the case of the green iguana, to the midsection of the body in the case of many monitor lizards.

The liver sits on the ventral body wall just caudal to the ribcage, and is a bilobed structure with the gall bladder and caudal vena cava appearing as hypoechoic structures in the right lobe. Abscesses, gross enlargement and tumours as well as gout may be visualised.

The kidneys may be located in the pelvic region in species such as the green iguana, or on the caudal coelomic wall dorsally in species such as bearded dragons and chameleons. As the kidneys enlarge due to inflammation or growths, they will protrude out from the pelvis region and be easier to examine. Gout crystals indicative of advancing renal failure appear as scintillating hyperechoic areas.

The bilateral fat pads extend cranially from the pelvis. In cachectic animals they are reduced in size and may even be absent. Adipose tissue is hyperechoic compared to other coelomic organs and is divided into lobes by hyperechoic septae. In obese animals the fat bodies extend to the liver and heart and can significantly interfere with imaging of the coelomic cavity.

The female reproductive tract may be easily visualised. There are two ovaries, suspended from the dorsal body wall caudal to the rib cage, follicles appearing as echogenic densities, increasing in density as they mature. Eggs have a hyperechoic rim. In viviparous lizards (e.g., blue-tongue skinks – *Teliqua scincoides*), foetuses are identified by their hyperechoic signals surrounded by anechoic fluid and membranes. In the later stages of gestation, the

skeletons and beating hearts become visible. Pre- and post-ovulatory stasis may be determined as described for chelonia.

In sexually monomorphic lizards such as Gila monsters (*Heloderma suspectum*) and prehensile-tailed skinks (*Corucia zebrata*), the hemipenises can be identified in the ventral tail base. They appear as elongated heterogeneous structures compared to the surrounding homogenous muscle tissue.

Snakes

The heart is situated in the caudal section of the first third of the length of the snake. Under sedation and in relaxed snakes the heart apex beat may be seen moving the ventral scutes. Again the heart is a three-chambered structure (see Figures 23.19 and 23.20).

The liver is a short distance caudal to the heart and is an elongated structure of homogeneous echogenicity. Abscesses, tumours and gout crystals may all disturb this homogeneity. The gall bladder is a separate, hypoechoic spherical organ situated immediately caudal to the liver, adjacent to the splenopancreas.

The kidneys are elongated flattened structures extending the proximal half of the caudal third of the snake.

The female reproductive system is again suspended from the dorsal body wall, with the paired ovaries located cranial to the kidneys and caudal to the stomach. Pre-ovulatory stasis is uncommon, but ultrasonography is useful to determine gravidity as the thin-shelled eggs

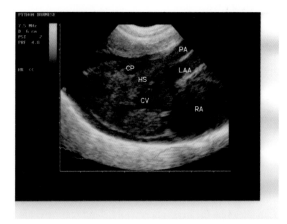

Figure 23.19 Two-dimensional echocardiogram (midline long axis or sagittal view) of a normal Burmese python (*Python molurus bivittatus*). CP, cavum pulmonale; CV, cavum venosum; HS, horizontal septum; LAA, left aortic arch; PA, pulmonary artery; RA, right atrium. (Reproduced with permission from Girling & Raiti, 2004, © BSAVA)

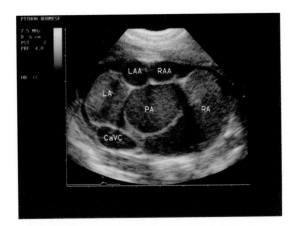

Figure 23.20 Two-dimensional echocardiogram short axis view demonstrating the normal echocardiographic anatomy of a Burmese python in Figure 23.19. CaVC, caudal vena cava approaching the sinus venosus; LA, left atrium; LAA, left aortic arch; PA, pulmonary artery; RA, right atrium; RAA, right aortic arch. (Reproduced with permission from Girling & Raiti, 2004, © BSAVA)

are easily visualised. Hyperechoic reflections may be seen in viviparous species such as the garter snake and boa constrictor due to reflections from the ribs/skeleton of the foetus.

The hemipenises may be seen as hyperechoic areas caudal to the vent and either side of midline. The female has no similar structure, and this method may be used to sex snakes.

MRI AND CT SCANNING

Both of these techniques are useful, particularly CT scanning in chelonia due to its ability to penetrate the bony shell without distortion, allowing examination of the internal organs. Normal chelonian lungs appear as radiolucent air-filled cavities with CT images, separated by septae consisting of pulmonary vasculature and smooth muscle. Soft tissues do not emit high-contrast signals; however, pre-ovulatory follicles and dystrophic calcification may be easily defined with CT images.

MRI scanning is useful as in other species for determination of soft-tissue growths within organs and may be applied to reptiles in a similar manner.

Both techniques require that the reptile is completely immobilised, and therefore chemical restraint is necessary.

RIGID ENDOSCOPY

This is a useful technique in lizards and particularly chelonia. Similar equipment to that used in avian patients is used; however, due to the absence of air sacs, it is more difficult to perform laparoscopic procedures in reptiles. For this, the use of a positive pressure system to pump either carbon dioxide or room air into the coelomic cavity and so separate the internal organs to aid visualisation is helpful. Snakes, due to their elongated nature and multiple internal connective tissue compartments, are not so suited to this modality.

Further reading

Frye, F. (1991) *Biomedical and Surgical Aspects of Captive Reptile Husbandry*. Krieger Publishing, Malabar, FL.

Girling, S and Raiti, P. (eds) (2004) *BSAVA Manual of Reptiles*, 2nd edn. Blackwell Publishing, Oxford.

Mader, D. (2006) *Reptile Medicine and Surgery*, 2nd edn. WB Saunders, St Louis, MO.

McArthur, S., Wilkinson, R. and Meyer, J. (2004) *Medicine and Surgery of Tortoises and Turtles*, 2nd edn. Blackwell Publishing, Oxford.

Raiti, P. (2004) Non-invasive imaging. *Manual of Reptiles* (eds S.J. Girling & P. Raiti), 2nd edn, pp. 87–102. BSAVA, Quedgeley, UK.

Triage

Any reptile presented unconscious, fitting, with evidence of head trauma or respiratory distress should be attended to immediately. Reptiles which are off colour and dull should be moved into a quiet, warm (32–38°C) vivarium with supplemental oxygen if there is any evidence of tachy/hyperpnoea and should be examined as soon as possible.

Emergency protocol 'ABC'

A for airway and B for breathing

It should be noted that the impetus for respiration in the reptile is not the detection of raised $PaCO_2$ levels as with mammals, but detection of a lowered PaO_2. This means that if 100% oxygen is administered to a reptile, it will in effect not want to breathe of its own accord!

Intubation of reptiles is straightforward and should be attempted where there is any doubt over whether the reptile is breathing or not (Figure 24.1). The glottis is situated at the base of the tongue and is easily visualised, particularly in snakes. The only problems encountered are that the glottis is held closed at rest-only opening for inspiration so an introducer may need to be used to allow intubation. Positive-pressure ventilation is necessary and should aim to allow a 30% increase in body diameter with snakes and lizards, equivalent to 10–12 cmH$_2$O pressure on a mechanical ventilator. Doxapram does work in reptiles and may be dosed as for birds and mammals.

C for cardiovascular

The prognosis for respiratory arrest without cardiac arrest in reptiles is good. With intermittent positive-pressure ventilation (IPPV) and 100% oxygen, reversal of any anaesthesia and administration of doxapram, recovery is likely.

However, cardiac arrest in reptiles carries a worse prognosis than for mammals. This is partly due to the robustness of the heart in most reptiles, meaning that should arrest occur, there is usually significant myocardial

hypoxaemic damage. Most reptiles become bradycardic immediately before arrest, and if this is recognised, rapid administration of atropine at 0.02 mg/kg can be effective. Epinephrine may be given intravenously, intraosseously or often more effectively intratracheally.

D for drugs

See Table 24.1 for a list of commonly used 'emergency' drugs in reptiles. It should be noted that most sick reptiles are borderline or fully septicaemic. They tend to be attacked by their own gut bacteria, which are generally Gram negative in nature, and often contain the Salmonella and Pseudomonad bacterial family. Therefore, a bacteriocidal antibiotic with good action against Gram-negative bacteria should be used. These include the fluoroquinolones and third-generation cephalosporins. However, other injuries may be sustained such as dog attacks, and so anaerobic bacteria may also be implanted into wounds (Figure 24.2).

Garter and water snakes, who are fed salt-water fish which has been previously frozen, may suffer from a relative deficiency of vitamin B_1 (thiamine), which can lead to a neurological condition (similar to cerebrocortical necrosis in grain-gorged cattle) manifesting as an inability to right itself and continual star gazing. Injections of vitamin B_1 at 25–35 mg/kg may be effective if administered quickly, and sedation with midazolam/diazepam or anaesthesia may be necessary to prevent seizuring (Figure 24.3).

Cardiovascular and respiratory diseases are relatively common, and pneumonia or lung oedema may result. Use of diuretics such as furosemide and hydrochlorothiazide may be helpful. Oxygen therapy can be used, but care should be taken as the impetus for breathing in reptiles is a lowered PaO_2 rather than an elevated $PaCO_2$ as in mammals, therefore providing 100% oxygen for even short periods of time can stop breathing altogether. As reptiles do not have a cough reflex (no diaphragm) and are relatively easy to intubate, conscious intubation of collapsed

Table 24.1 Commonly used emergency and recovery medications for reptiles.

Drug	Dosage	Notes
Adrenaline	0.05–0.5 mL depending on size of reptile	Use intratracheally after intubation and IPPV with 100% oxygen
Allopurinol	10–50 mg/kg PO SID	Reduces uric acid production to aid management of gout
Calcium gluconate	100 mg/kg IM/SC/intracoelomically	Hypocalcaemic tetany especially in female egg-bound green iguanas
Ceftazidime (Fortum® Pfizer)	20 mg/kg SC/IM/IV q72h	Broad-spectrum bacteriocidal third-generation cephalosporin; particularly effective against Gram-negative bacteria
Diazepam	0.2–0.5 mg/kg IM/IV	Muscle necrosis if given IM
Doxapram	0.5 mg/kg PO/IV	Intubate and use IPPV
Enrofloxacin	5–10 mg/kg SID	Licensed antibiotic for reptiles. Useful against Gram-negative bacteria but not against anaerobes. Can cause muscle necrosis
Furosemide	1–5 mg/kg	Diuretic but action not known
Hydrochlorothiazide	1 mg/kg	Diuretic
Midazolam	0.2–0.5 mg/kg IM/IV	Less likely to cause muscle necrosis than diazepam
Meloxicam	0.2–0.3 mg/kg IM/PO SID	Beware use if already has renal damage
Oxytocin	Chelonians 10 IU/kg IM Lizards 5–20 IU/kg IM Snakes 20–40 IU/kg IM	Uterine muscle stimulant. May be repeated on max of four occasions. Useful to administer calcium gluconate first
Silver sulfadiazine cream (Flamazine® Smith & Nephew)	Topical on burns/wounds	Effective cream against Gram-negative bacteria and some fungi
Vitamin B$_1$	25–35 mg/kg IM/PO/SC	Thiamine deficiency (fish-eating snakes)

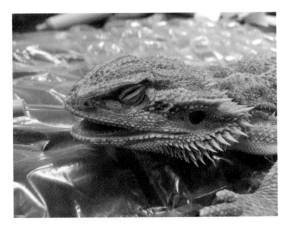

Figure 24.1 Intubation to secure an airway is important in any reptile where there is doubt over respiration.

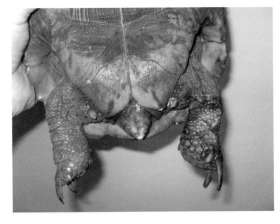

Figure 24.2 Dog-attack wounds in terrestrial chelonians are common and may result in serious trauma and infections.

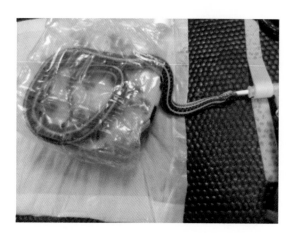

Figure 24.3 Hypovitaminosis B₁ is common in garter snakes fed previously frozen salt-water fish and may require sedation with midazolam/diazepam or anaesthesia in addition to vitamin B1 injections to control seizuring and star-gazing neurological signs.

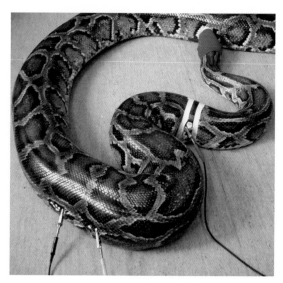

Figure 24.4 Placement of ECG leads in a snake. (Reproduced with permission from Girling & Raiti, 2004, © BSAVA)

reptiles can be performed and IPPV administered for a short period.

If cardiac arrest occurs, intubation and intratracheal administration of epinephrine should be attempted. Reptiles can cope with a degree of hypoxia beyond that tolerated by mammals. IPPV after intubation is essential, although chest massage in the case of lizards and moving limbs into and out of the shell in chelonians may also be successful, aiding the pumping of air into and out of the lungs.

Many nutritional and husbandry diseases are common in reptiles, including metabolic bone disease and hypocalcaemic tetany in egg-bound mature lizards such as the green iguana. Calcium gluconate at 100 mg/kg may be administered in an emergency. Some of these lizards may fit, and diazepam or midazolam may be administered (see Table 24.1).

E for ECG

ECG deflections are generally small and rates, of course, slow. The rate is dependent on the external temperature the reptile is kept at.

In snakes, lizards and chelonians, metal crocodile clips with filed teeth may be used. Coupling gel or surgical spirit is required to optimise contact, and prolonged contact time is necessary to allow the gel to penetrate the keratin skin layer.

- Snakes: a base-apex reading is taken with electrodes placed two heart lengths cranial and caudal to the heart on the lateral aspect (Figure 24.4).

- Lizards: cranial leads are placed on the skin of the axilla, forelimb or neck, caudal leads on the crural or popliteal fold.
- Chelonians: cranial leads are placed on the cervical or axillary skin folds and caudal leads on the skin fold caudal to the hind limb.

Reptile ECGs demonstrate a P wave, QRS complex and T wave pattern familiar to cardiologists. An additional SV waveform preceding the P wave representing depolarisation of the sinus venosus has been described but is a rarely seen.

Normal ECG findings include pleomorphism of the P wave, which may be single, peaked or biphasic. The QRS complex is often represented as a single R wave. Long repolarisation phases (longer QT and ST intervals) are present.

Allometric scaling may be used for the prediction of heart rate (HR = $33.4 \times [\mathrm{Wt}_{kg} - 0.25]$, Sedgwick, 1991), assuming the reptile is maintained at its optimal body temperature.

Other useful drugs and techniques

Initial assessment of the collapsed reptile

An initial assessment should be made of the reptile patient before it is removed from its carry cage/box. This should focus on the following points:

1. Is it potentially hazardous/dangerous to the handler? (e.g., male green iguanas, snapping turtles, aggressive snakes and unlikely but possibly venomous)

2. Is it mouth breathing and therefore in possible respiratory distress?

3. Is it a fragile species? (many geckos will shed their tails very easily, as will many iguanas)

4. Is it suffering from metabolic bone disease making it a risk to handle? (deformed limbs, shell, spine, etc., and inability to support its own weight in a lizard or chelonian may suggest this condition is present)

5. How large is the animal? (many larger species of tortoise are surprisingly heavy and strong, and snakes longer than 3–4 feet require more than one handler to avoid damaging the patient and putting the handlers at risk).

Whilst examining the patient from a distance to ascertain if it is safe to handle, it is a good idea to question the owner about the husbandry of the reptile at home, i.e.,:

1. What do they feed it?

2. Do they feed vitamin/mineral supplements?

3. Is there a UV lamp? (may not be necessary for most snakes but is necessary for most lizards and chelonians)

4. What temperature range do they keep the vivarium at?

5. What hides/cage furniture is present in the tank?

6. What humidity do they keep the vivarium at?

7. Do they have any other reptiles/pets?

8. If a snake – when did it last shed its skin, and was it a complete shed?

Detailed examination of the collapsed reptile
Manual restraint

This is covered in the section on anaesthesia and analgesia.

Detailed examination

1. An intra-oral examination using a mouth gag or a pen/pencil to encourage the reptile to open its mouth (be careful with chelonians as they have powerful jaws). This should allow a close examination of the tongue, the roof of the mouth/nasal passages (there is no hard palate in reptiles other than Crocodylia). The glottis may also be visualised at the base of the tongue. Abnormalities such as a discharge from the nasal passages, petechiae or haemorrhages in the mouth, an abnormal or foul odour, and evidence of white or yellow plaques on the mucosa should all be noted and if possible sampled with a swab dampened with sterile water. Note that many lizards have a two-coloured tongue, e.g., the green iguana has a bright red tongue tip and a pale pink body to the fleshy tongue.

2. A detailed examination of the nares and the eyes. This will allow an assessment of any upper respiratory tract disease. Clinical signs of this include: abnormal shaped nare(s), sinking of the globe of the eye, swelling below the globe of the eye (the region of the infraorbital sinus), discharge from the eye itself, swelling of the conjunctiva, corneal blemishes and in the case of snakes evidence of a retained spectacle.

3. A detailed examination of the skin/shell. This may allow you to see areas of retained slough (snakes should shed in one complete go, lizards in small patches and chelonians only in small patches from the limbs and head/neck/tail). It will also allow any petechiae or ecchymoses to be observed which may indicate septicaemia. Abscesses appear as firm, inspissated subcutaneous masses.

4. A detailed auscultation of the lungs and air sacs. The lungs are best auscultated from the dorsum in chelonians and lizards. To improve sound conductivity, a damp towel/cloth may be placed over the reptile and the diaphragm of the stethoscope applied to this. Snakes are difficult to auscultate owing to their long thin lungs.

5. The heart is very difficult to auscultate, and it is often preferable to use a Doppler probe to assess blood flow throughout the heart to determine heart rate. Note that heart rate and sounds for reptiles are significantly different from mammals owing to the three-chambered heart (one ventricle and two atria) and its different construction. In addition, environmental temperatures will significantly alter heart rates.

6. A detailed examination of the limbs may be made. Palpate the long bones as metabolic bone disease is common producing fibrous dystrophy where the poorly ossified bone swells due to cartilage deposition making the limb look fat and muscular. Palpation reveals, however, that it is merely bone mass and not muscle. Shells of chelonians may be deformed and soft to touch. Mandibles of lizards may be bowed and malleable with this condition as well.

7. A detailed examination of the vent and caudal coelom should also be made. Many lizards have kidneys tucked into the pelvic area, and so these should not be palpable in front of the iliac wings in a normal animal. Snakes may be palpated by running a finger along the ventrum to feel for masses or obstructions. Chelonians are obviously difficult to palpate, although gentle ballottement of eggs or masses by placing a finger cranial to a hind limb and rolling the animal onto its side and away again is possible.

Monitoring and vital sign assessment

Pulse assessment

This is best performed using a Doppler ultrasound probe. It should be attached to the skin with a generous amount of coupling gel. The main site of attachment is around the outflow of the heart. This is located immediately caudal to the neck inlet in chelonians, around the mid-point of the first third of a snake (measured from the snout), or just in front of the point of the shoulder in most lizards.

Cardiac and respiratory auscultation

It is difficult to auscultate reptiles owing to their scaly skin. To aid the passage of sound, wrapping the reptile in a damp cloth first and applying the diaphragm of the stethoscope to the outside of the towel can improve sound transference. Alternatively, a Doppler probe applied over the heart (base of the neck in most lizards and chelonians and 20–30% of the snout-vent length in snakes) can provide an assessment of blood flow which can give an indication of the intensity of flow and turbulence.

The lungs of snakes are particularly challenging to auscultate due to their long drawn out nature. Chelonian lungs are situated in the dorsal aspect of the carapace, and lizard lungs are encased in the ribcage.

The heart is not possible to auscultate in the same way a bird's or mammal's heart can due to the slow rate at which it beats and the fact that the heart is three-chambered (there is only one ventricle). Therefore, Doppler probes should be used to gain an idea of cardiac output, strength and any variations in flow.

Neurological assessment

This can be very difficult in reptiles, particularly if they are not within their preferred optimum temperature zone as they will be sluggish and lethargic if too cold. All critically ill reptiles should be gradually warmed to their preferred body temperature to assess them fully and to support their normal physiological functions (Figure 24.5).

One of the commonest neurological problems is loss of the righting reflex in snakes, i.e., they continually flip onto their backs. This may be associated with the following conditions:

1. Vitamin B_1 deficiency (garter/water snakes who are fed defrosted frozen fish as this contains large amounts of thiaminases)
2. Permethrin/organophosphate toxicity (overzealous owners treating their snakes for mites)

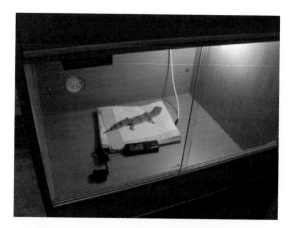

Figure 24.5 Warming all reptiles to their preferred body temperature is an essential part of their critical care.

3. Meningoencephalitis (usually associated with Acanthamoeba invadens or Gram-negative bacteria)
4. Inclusion body disease (a retrovirus, particularly prevalent in pythons and boas).

Blindness and head tilts may be seen in tortoises associated with frost damage.

Hypocalcaemic tremors are common in female iguanas on low-calcium diets or where no ultraviolet light has been provided.

Panniculus reflexes can be tested as for cats and dogs in snakes and lizards, although of course with less success in chelonians!

Pulse oximetry

This is not so useful in reptiles as reptile haemoglobin is significantly different to a mammalian. However, trends of readings are of some help as with birds. The clips/probes may be applied to the vent, tongue (if anaesthetised) or in thin-skinned smaller reptiles, the extremities.

Blood biochemistry

It should be noted that, as with birds, uric acid is the only useful indicator of renal function, although usually less than one quarter of the kidneys need to be left functioning before uric acid levels become elevated. Urea and creatinine levels do not provide information on renal function in reptiles.

As with birds, no one parameter is specific for liver damage, although AST is more useful than ALT.

A very rough guide to average plasma biochemistry values is provided in Table 24.2.

Table 24.2 Broad range plasma biochemistry values for reptiles.

Parameter	Value	Notes
Total protein (g/L)	44–65	
Albumin (g/L)	13–30	
AST (IU/L)	20–80	Not liver specific, also found in muscle
CK (IU/L)	400–600	Only found in muscle
LDH (IU/L)	200–350	Not liver specific, also found in muscle including cardiac
Calcium (mmol/L)	2–3	May be elevated in female reptiles around egg production
Phosphorus (mmol/L)	1–1.85	
Glucose (mmol/L)	8–18	Budgerigars may be seen with glucagon-associated diabetes mellitus; birds of prey may be seen with hypoglycaemia associated with exercise when malnourished – glucose levels usually <2 mmol/L
Uric acid (μmol/L)	150–350	Gout (precipitation of uric acid) occurs when levels exceed 1500 May be transiently elevated in snakes immediately after a meal

Haematology

All blood samples in reptiles should be collected in heparin as potassium EDTA lyses the red cells of many reptiles.

As with biochemistry, values vary between species. Some indication of PCV across reptile species has been given in Chapter 17. In general white cell counts are in the range of $2–8 \times 10^9$/L. During an infection, there is often no change in the overall white cell count and, therefore, creating a blood smear is a vitally important diagnostic technique.

The reptile equivalent of the neutrophil, as in birds, is the heterophil.

Erythrocytes and platelets in reptiles are nucleated. The erythrocytes are rugby ball shaped with a similar shaped nucleus. The platelets are oval and smaller. Other cells are similar to those seen in mammals except occasionally you may see a circulating plasma cell (type of lymphocyte which produces antibodies), particularly in the face of a chronic infection. Also in snakes, large numbers of so-called 'azurophils' (darkly basophilic staining monocytic cells) may indicate chronic infection.

Urinalysis

This is less useful than for mammals owing to the faecal contamination which occurs with reptile urine. However, it is important to look at the urates (white portion of the dropping) to see if there is any blood, or if the urates have turned mustard yellow or lime green. If the latter has occurred, this is evidence of biliverdinuria, which in reptiles as in birds is an indicator of liver inflammation/damage. Biliverdin is the main excretory product of the liver as opposed to bilirubin in mammals.

Volumes of water/true urine should be small in a healthy reptile's dropping. If they are very watery, as opposed to diarrhoea, then this may indicate polyuria. Specific gravity of reptile urine is around 1.005–1.010.

Monitoring and treatment of acute hypovolaemia

Central venous and arterial pressure monitoring in reptiles is technically difficult to measure. Non-invasive blood pressure monitoring is also poorly understood in reptiles, and some evidence suggests discrepancies between invasive and non-invasive methods. Part of the problem is that reptiles are ectothermic, and this means the environmental temperature has significant effects on systemic blood pressure. A study in green iguanas indicates that systolic mean blood pressure is 43 mm Hg and diastolic mean blood pressure is 29 mm Hg (Mosley et al., 2004). In snakes there appears to be a relationship between the size of the snake and its blood pressure: the larger the snake, the higher the blood pressure (Mosley, 2005).

Non-invasive methods can be applied as follows: in chelonians and lizards, a cuff may be placed at the most proximal point on the forelimb and the Doppler probe applied above the carpus on the ventral aspect to cover the brachial artery. The cuff is inflated as with mammals to occlude blood flow and then deflated until flow occurs which is the maximum systolic pressure. In snakes the cuff is applied just caudal to the cloaca, and the probe is applied to the ventral tail artery distal to this.

Various studies have suggested that indirect systolic pressure varies from 30 to 63 mm Hg (Martinez-Jimenez & Hernandez-Divers, 2007).

Reptiles can survive significant haemorrhage because of the rapid shift of interstitial fluids into the circulation. However, this does not remove the need to replace fluid or blood losses to stabilise blood pressure. The amounts required can be assessed using blood pressure and heart rate. Expected heart rates can be calculated as mentioned in the section on ECGs above. However, it is important that reptiles are maintained at their preferred body temperature to accurately assess this due to their ectothermic nature. Bolus administration of fluids should be attempted intravenously or intraosseously until correction of blood pressure. Crystalloids are administered at a rate of 10 mL/kg and colloids, such as Hetastarch or Oxyglobin®, can be administered at 5 mL/kg – usually one or two boluses are required. In larger species 5 mL/kg of 7.5% hypertonic saline may be used once or twice to increase systolic blood pressure.

Calculation of fluid requirements for reptiles
Please see Chapter 22 for fluid therapy in reptiles.

Supportive therapy
Ongoing medication
Some antibiotics effective against Gram-negative bacteria include the third-generation cephalosporins, third-generation penicillins, aminoglycosides and fluoroquinolones. It is important to note that many reptiles will need to be on antibiotics for considerable periods of time (months rather than weeks) due to their often advanced state of infection – once finally seen – and due to their slower metabolism.

Ongoing fluid therapy is also very important whether it be regular warm water baths in the mildly dehydrated individuals, or intravenous/intraosseous fluids in the severely dehydrated ones as kidney failure is common.

Analgesia is also vitally important where there are serious injuries (Figure 24.6).

Critical care nutrition including calculation of energy requirements
Calculation of energy requirements can be made using the formula:

$$BMR = k \times (\text{weight [kg]})^{0.75}$$

where k the constant is 10 for all reptiles.

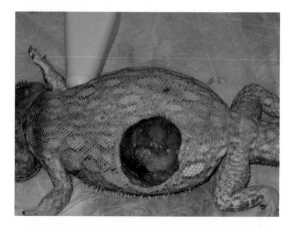

Figure 24.6 Analgesia in addition to antibiotics and fluid therapy is essential to aid the recovery of serious injuries such as this full-thickness skin and muscle thermal burn in a bearded dragon (*Pogona vitticeps*) due to a broken thermostat in a heated artificial rock.

Remember that MER (metabolic energy requirement) is generally 1.5–2× the BMR (basal metabolic requirement), and if disease is present then this further amplifies the required calories (sepsis and burns for example may increase MER by 2–3×).

Nebulisation
Achieving therapeutic levels of any antibiotic in infected reptile lungs is difficult. The blood–air barrier is thicker in reptiles than in mammals, plus reptiles have a poorly developed or absent cough reflex. Add to this the fact that caseous, impenetrable purulent discharges are common, and many of the most effective antibiotics such as aminoglycosides are potentially toxic if given in effective doses systemically, it can be seen that a topical respiratory method such as nebulisation of a drug is attractive. Although the possibility exists that a significant proportion of the drug could be absorbed across an inflamed respiratory epithelium, signs of e.g., aminoglycoside-related nephrotoxicity are not seen following aerosolised administration of these drugs. Other drugs suitable for nebulisation include antiseptic-disinfectants (F10®; Health & Hygiene Ltd.), soluble steroids in inflammatory conditions, bronchodilators and agents aimed at reducing the viscosity of respiratory secretions.

Assisted feeding techniques and foods
For information on oesophagostomy tubes placement – please see Chapter 22. For initial emergency nutrition,

as with birds, the use of products such as Vetark Professional Ltd's Critical Care Formula® is useful to give simple sugars and amino acids. For further nutrition, the carnivorous species may be administered products such as Hills a/d or Virbac's Reanimyl®, and the herbivores/omnivores may be given vegetable-based baby foods such as Milupa® or Cow and Gate® (avoid lactose-containing products).

To encourage anorectic snakes to eat, a number of tricks may be employed including:

1. Warming the prey before offering by heating it in a pot of hot water.
2. Breaking the prey item open to release the scent of blood.
3. Teasing the snake by moving the dead prey item around the cage with forceps, to mimic live prey.
4. Try a variety of colours of prey, some snakes will only take dark furred rodents.
5. To get a snake used to eating rodent prey after only eating fish (such as garter and water snakes) or amphibians (Hog-nosed snakes), wipe the rodent to be offered with the previously taken food item to transfer scent.
6. Ensure that there are plenty of areas to hide; some boids and pythons like to consume their prey in a box/hide.
7. Leave the prey in overnight, some species prefer to hunt at night.
8. Going to the next smallest size of rodent, so if adult mice were previously offered try fuzzies, if juvenile rats, try adult mice, etc.

The term 'pinkies' refers to nude neonatal rat and mice pups, 'fuzzies' refers to week-old rat and mice pups with a thin covering of fur and 'furries' refers to juvenile rat and mice pups of a few weeks of age (1–3) which have a soft but longer covering of fur.

If the reptile will not eat, then most species of snakes and chelonians may be stomach tubed relatively easily if they do not want to feed of their own accord.

In snakes, a dog urinary catheter is used and inserted to approximately the caudal end of the first third of the snake (roughly where the stomach lies). The volume given depends on the size of the snake with a 100 g garter snake getting a maximum of 4–5 mL and a 30 kg Burmese python getting up to 100–200 mL.

It is very important to ensure that in snakes in particular, the patient is rehydrated before feeding high-protein meals. This is because of the refeeding syndrome which briefly is as follows: if anorexia in a snake or other reptile has persisted for some time, it is essential to rehydrate the patient before attempting to feed. Initial feeding after this should be started off at very low levels: 50% of the requirement for the current weight of the reptile. Otherwise, excess calories and proteins cause a rapid uptake of glucose from the bloodstream into the cells, which takes potassium and phosphorous with it. This can lead to a life-threatening hypokalaemia/hypophosphataemia. The monitoring of blood phosphorus and potassium is therefore to be recommended when treating chronically anorectic reptiles whether carnivorous or herbivorous.

Tortoises can be stomach tubed by measuring from the extended tip of the head to the caudal edge of the large abdominal scutes on the plastron. Most tortoises of 2–3 kg may be stomach tubed with 10–15 mL of feed at one time.

Lizards may be gavaged liquid feed as for mammals, or again tubed. It is important to use a mouth gag when tubing reptiles to prevent the tube being bitten in half.

In all cases, feeding by stomach tube should be the last thing you do to a reptile before putting it back into its vivarium, otherwise the reptile will become distressed and regurgitate its feed.

Nursing of wounds

Open wounds are generally of two main types in reptiles: thermal burns and infections. It is important therefore to ensure correct antibiotic coverage for these wounds. As most reptile infections are due to Gram-negative bacteria, it makes sense to use fluoroquinolones and third-generation cephalosporins.

Povidone-iodine diluted to 1:30 with water may be used to clean infected wounds. Topical medications such as silver sulfadiazine creams have good efficacy against Gram-negative bacteria as does the use of topical eye drops containing gentamicin. Where an infected wound is present, daily changing of any dressings is advised.

Dressings which may be sutured to the skin around large wound deficits include Granuflex®, Melolin® and Veterinary BioSISt®. The former should be used where the infection is under control and is excellent for encouraging granulation tissue to form. In many cases this primary dressing is all that is required, particularly when sutured to the patient as reptiles rarely remove dressings, the problem being, especially in snakes, that dressings are difficult to attach in the first place unless sutured.

Gels such as Intrasite® or Nugel® may be used to cover the surface of wounds and promote further healing.

References

Martinez-Jimenez, D. and Hernandez-Divers, S.J. (2007) Emergency care of reptiles. *Veterinary Clinics of North America: Exotic Animal Practice*, **10**(2), 557–586.

Mosley, C. (2005) Anaesthesia and analgesia in reptiles. *Seminars in Avian and Exotic Pet Medicine*, **14**, 243–262.

Mosley, C., Dyson, D. and Smith, D. (2004) The cardiovascular dose-responsive effects of isoflurane alone and combined with butorphanol in the green iguana (*Iguana iguana*). *Veterinary Anaesthesia and Analgesia*, **31**, 64–72.

Sedgwick, C.J. (1991) Allometrically scaling the database for vital sign assessment used in general anesthesia of zoological species. *Proceedings: American Association of Zoo Veterinarians*, USA, pp. 360–369.

Further reading

Girling, S. and Raiti, P. (eds) (2004) *BSAVA Manual of Reptiles*, 2nd edn. Blackwell Publishing, Oxford.

Appendix 1 Legislation Affecting Exotic Pet Species in the United Kingdom

Convention on International Trade in Endangered Species (CITES)

Broadly this is the list of endangered species around the world, categorised into

- Appendix 1 contains those species highly endangered in which international trade is banned.
- Appendix 2 contains those species considered seriously threatened in which trade is again banned or at least heavily controlled.
- Appendix 3 contains those species which are at risk, and in which international trade is restricted.

In the United Kingdom, these lists are enforced by European Union Control of Trade in Endangered Species laws or COTES regulations (Council Regulation 339/97 and Commission Regulation 939/97) wherein the species are divided into four groups:

- Annex A includes species such as the Mediterranean tortoises, for example, the Greek or spur-thighed tortoise (*Testudo graeca*). It also includes many endangered species of native bird, such as the red kite.
- Annex B includes all species under CITES Appendix 2 and some other species.
- Annex C includes all species barring one or two under CITES Appendix 3.
- Annex D includes non-CITES species which are considered as needing protection by the European Union.

It is important to note that any person selling a species listed in Annex A must have a licence, as well as having some form of permanent identification of that individual to prove its identity.

In the case of the Mediterranean tortoise species, the vendor must have a licence to prove that the mother of the hatchling is captive bred, or was obtained before the regulations came into force. The hatchling must be sold currently with a licence from the government and with an electronic identification chip that is to be implanted in a standard site. The British Veterinary Zoological Society currently recommends subcutaneously in the left thigh region. The chip is to be implanted as soon as the plastral length of the tortoise exceeds 100 mm. New so-called 'mini' microchips are now available making implantation of smaller individuals possible.

Health and Safety at Work Act 1974

It is important to remember that many wildlife cases carry zoonotic diseases, such as Salmonella spp., rabies-related viruses in some wild bat populations, Yersinia pseudotuberculosis in many rodents and lagomorphs, chlamydiosis in many wild birds and psittacine species, etc. Many species of exotic pet may be aggressive when stressed or ill, and will readily turn on the handler. Unpleasant bites, scratches or worse can result.

The veterinary nurse (and other members of staff) has an obligation to avoid hazards and prevent accidents and accidental cross infection in the workplace. In addition, the employer has an obligation to ensure that facilities and training of staff are sufficient to minimise the risks of handling and treating these animals.

Welfare of Animals Act 2006/ Welfare of Animals (Scotland) Act 2006

This is now the primary UK legislation regarding the welfare of animals in captivity. As such, it covers all of the species we deal with in this text but also deals with wildlife cases during the time they are held in captivity for treatment or rehabilitation. It not only makes it an offence to have treated any such captive animal cruelly, but also makes it an offence to omit or do something which will lead to suffering at some point in the future.

Protection of Animals Act 1911–1964

Under this legislation, it is an offence to treat a captive animal cruelly or to cause it unnecessary suffering. This

Veterinary Nursing of Exotic Pets, Second Edition. Edited by Simon J. Girling. © 2013 John Wiley & Sons, Ltd. Published 2013 by John Wiley & Sons, Ltd.

ensures that all cases receive proper care and attention, and that their accommodation is of the correct dimensions and provides suitable shelter from other animals as well as excessive noxious stimuli. Most of its points of legislation have been reinforced or amended by the Animal Welfare act 2006.

Abandonment of Animals Act 1960

Under this legislation, it is an offence to release any wild animal that is not in a fit state to survive in the wild. Examples include release of birds of prey with foot injuries or beak injuries, release of mammals with fractures etc. Most of its points of legislation have been reinforced or amended by the Animal Welfare act 2006.

Wildlife and Countryside Act 1981

With regard to exotic pets, this legislation prohibits the release of non-native species into the wild in the United Kingdom (as listed in Schedule 9 of the Act). With regard to UK wildlife, it also prohibits the release of so-called non-native species such as the grey squirrel, the sika deer and the Canada goose amongst others. This makes treatment of such animals only sensible if they are to then be kept in captivity for the rest of their lives.

Dangerous wild Animals Act 1976 as amended

This applies to the private keeping of species, other than those in pet shops, zoos, circuses or areas designated under the Animals (Scientific Procedures) Act 1986 considered dangerous to public health and welfare and listed in the legislation. This includes all venomous species of reptile as well as Crocodylia and some of the ratite family of birds. It does not affect the veterinary profession's ability to treat these animals but does licence and restrict private ownership and care to people deemed fit to do so.

Appendix 2 Useful Addresses

British Veterinary Zoological Society
(This society welcomes veterinary surgeons, students, and veterinary nurses alike)
Mr. D.G. Lyon BVSc, MRCVS, Administrative Director
Website: www.bvzs.org

British Chelonia Group
Website: www.britishcheloniagroup.org.uk

Tortoise Trust
Website: www.tortoisetrust.org
Forum: www.tortoisetrustforum.org

Rabbit Welfare Association & Fund
(Incorporating the British House Rabbit Association)
Website: www.rabbitwelfare.co.uk

Association of Avian Veterinarians
(This association welcomes veterinary nurses/technicians and produces a quarterly peer-reviewed journal as well as an annual conference)
Website: www.aav.org

Association of Reptilian and Amphibian Veterinarians
(This association welcomes veterinary nurses/technicians and produces a quarterly peer-reviewed journal as well as an annual conference)
Website: www.arav.org

Index